SOCIAL & BEHAVIORAL ASPECTS OF PHARMACY PRACTICE

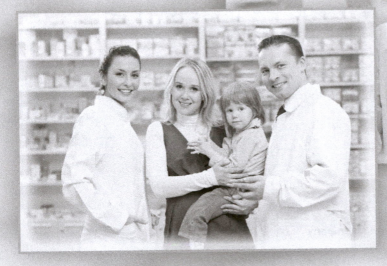

NATHANIEL M. RICKLES
PharmD, PhD, BCPP
University of Connecticut
School of Pharmacy

ALBERT I. WERTHEIMER
Professor, Dept. of Sociobehavioral
and Administrative Pharmacy,
College of Pharmacy,
Nova Southeastern University

JON C. SCHOMMER
PhD, Professor
University of Minnesota
College of Pharmacy

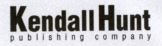

Kendall Hunt
publishing company

Book Team

Chairman and Chief Executive Officer	Mark C. Falb
President and Chief Operating Officer	Chad M. Chandlee
Vice President, Higher Education	David L. Tart
Director of Publishing Partnerships	Paul B. Carty
Senior Developmental Editor	Lynnette M. Rogers
Vice President, Operations	Timothy J. Beitzel
Production Editor	Elizabeth S. Cray
Senior Permissions Coordinator	Brianna M. Kirschbaum
Cover Designer	Faith Walker

Cover images © Shutterstock, Inc.

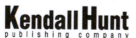
publishing company

www.kendallhunt.com
Send all inquiries to:
4050 Westmark Drive
Dubuque, IA 52004-1840

DEDICATION

I would like to dedicate this book to my wife Jenny Rickles for all her unconditional support in allowing me the time and energy to dedicate to projects like this book. Without such support, I am certain my contributions to the textbook would not have been possible.

I also dedicate this book to my children, Evan and Susanna Rickles, whose curiosity and fun spirits enabled me to engage all my projects with a child's eye of being open to new ways of doing things and smiling and laughing as often as possible to ward off the anguish and stress of many deadlines and daily needs to multitask.

Nathaniel M. Rickles

I am grateful to my wife Joaquima for permitting me to divert so many hours to this endeavor from other family activities.

Albert I. Wertheimer

To Lisa

Jon C. Schommer

CONTENTS

PART II APPROACHES TO RESOLVE HEALTH PROBLEMS 89

PART III   TARGETING CARE OF SPECIFIC PATIENTS   375

FOREWORD

Lucinda Maine, PhD, AACP,
Alexandria, VA

The fascinating evolution in the roles of medications and pharmacists in our health care system over the past century can be traced in phrases contained in three iterations of the Code of Ethics for the profession. From 1922 to 1969 the Code maintained that: *Pharmacists should never discuss the therapeutic effect of a physician's prescription with a patron or disclose details of composition which the physician has withheld.* The power in the physician/pharmacist/patient relationship was clearly and completely in the medical doctor's hands.

The Code of Ethics adopted in 1969 represents a significant change in the expectations of pharmacists and the use of their knowledge, skills and abilities: *A pharmacist should always strive to perfect and enlarge his knowledge. He should utilize and make available this knowledge as may be required in accordance with his best judgment.* In the decade that followed, *Pharmacists for the Future* was published and provided a roadmap for the evolution of pharmacy practice aimed at insuring that the growing armamentarium of medications becoming available could be used in the prevention and treatment of illness in the most safe and effective manner.

The current code of ethics, adopted in 1994, moves conceptually to a completely new expectation of the relationship between pharmacists and the consumer of medicines: *Considering the patient-pharmacist relationship as a covenant means that a pharmacist has moral obligations in response to the gift of trust received from society. In return for this gift, a pharmacist promises to help individuals achieve optimum benefit from their medications, to be committed to their welfare, and to maintain their trust.*

Each edition of *Social and Behavioral Aspects of Pharmacy Practice* has similarly evolved, reflecting our expanding appreciation of the relationships between individuals and their health, between pharmacists and patients, and between pharmacists and other health professionals. Each is complex and warrants examination and understanding, without which achievement of optimal health outcomes is not possible.

There have been dramatic changes in health care in the past 15 to 20 years. The Institute of Medicine (now the National Academy of Medicine) stimulated significant change in our systems as first To Err is Human (1999) and then Crossing the Quality Chasm (2001) gave voice to the failings in the US health care organization, delivery and financing models. These reports as well as other analyses highlight the fact that medication misuse is a leading cause of error, resulting in avoidable harm including loss of life. Our profession finally achieved agreement that 21st century pharmacists would need doctoral level education to establish themselves as the medication use specialists in contemporary health systems.

In the early 1990's pharmacists began to appreciate that they could play a significant role in improving access to public health services, specifically by increasing the rate of adult immunization for flu and other infectious disease prevention. While only 14 states empowered pharmacists to immunize in that era, today over 280,000 pharmacists have been certified and are allowed to administer a widening array of vaccines in every state and US territory. Additional public health services available from pharmacists include smoking cessation programs, drug abuse interventions, and health screenings for early detection of diabetes, heart disease and other conditions.

It has only been in the last ten years that pharmaceutical coverage has been part of the Medicare program which provides the primary insurance coverage for elderly and disabled Americans. Omitted initially from the program because drug costs were such an insignificant percentage of overall health care costs, the inability of significant numbers of Medicare beneficiaries to pay for needed medications tipped the balance and markedly changed federal pharmaceutical and health policy. Subsequently it has been documented that the addition of Medicare Part D drug coverage has had a modest but positive impact on the spending trend for both Parts A and B (hospital and outpatient health coverage) in the Medicare program.

The fact that medication use is central to safe, quality health care has not been lost on a variety of stakeholders in the health system. Attention to quality and safety has driven the field of performance measurement. A striking number of quality measures for hospitals, physicians, group practice organizations and others either directly assess the appropriate utilization of medications or are impacted by effective medication management. And evidence grows that when pharmacists are integrated into these care models with the empowerment to fully utilize their knowledge and skills, patient outcomes improve, costs are reduced, and patients and providers report greater satisfaction.

The pace of change in the next 10 to 20 years is expected to be even more dramatic. This will be driven in large measure by data, dollars and diversity. "Big data" is the term in use reflecting the profound amount of data that is generated, collected and analyzed related to virtually every aspect of our lives. Computational power offers insights into our genetics, cellular and subcellular aspects of health and disease, our behavior, our communities and our world.

Dollars reflects the growing belief that our spending on health care simply cannot be sustained. Despite the fact that we have just exceeded $10,000 per person per year on health services in the US, we have close to third world outcomes in many morbidity and mortality statistics. This will drive changes in both public policy and private sector approaches to achieve more rational cost control and better outcomes.

As our society becomes increasingly diverse, changes in how individuals engage as decision-makers with regard to their health care will also have an impact on pharmacists and other providers. Literacy levels, access to and the ability to interpret and apply health information, behavioral health status and many other factors will need to be understood by clinicians in the delivery of services to individuals and populations.

The magnitude of change confounds attempts to effectively answer important questions and anticipate how pharmacists' roles will continue to change. That said, there are things that we do know. Medications will continue to play a central role in health and wellness and pharmacists will become even more effectively integrated into patient care teams. Whether "precision medicine" or personalized dosage forms tailored to the unique genomic profile of an individual comprises a significant component of care delivery or only plays a selective role in patient management (e.g., oncology) is yet to be seen. Pharmacists will remain the clinician with the deepest and broadest knowledge of pharmacotherapy and will also parlay our accessibility into more prevention and wellness services. Pharmacists have the opportunity to play important roles as well in this period of enhanced health informatics, especially in the context of population health and decision-making.

This edition of *Social and Behavioral Aspects of Pharmacy Practice* is timely and essential to the education of today's pharmacist. The authors of each chapter have analyzed all of the forces of change noted above and they tease out the most salient issues pharmacists must know and do to fully engage in the covenantal relationship with individuals that our current Code of Ethics requires.

PREFACE

The present textbook, *Social and Behavioral Aspects of Pharmacy Practice Third Edition*, has been on the market under different titles since 1974. The first title was called *Pharmacy Practice: Social and Behavioral Aspects* published by University Park Press. The authors changed to Williams and Wilkins for the second edition and Haworth Press for the third edition. In 1996, the textbook changed titles to *Social and Behavioral Aspects of Pharmaceutical Care* reflecting the new buzz word that began the 1990s that defined the pharmacist's clear and significant role and responsibility for the patient's drug therapy outcomes. Interestingly, we are now 42 years later and have returned to a rearrangement of the original title. In many ways, the core concept has not changed so the return to original words of the first title makes a lot of sense. The first title placed the initial emphasis on pharmacy practice and a secondary and separate focus on the social and behavioral aspects as denoted symbolically by the colon. Our current title reverses the foci a little with the initial emphasis on the social and behavioral aspects and a secondary but melded (no colon) focus on pharmacy practice. The need for the current title change should become apparent over the next paragraphs.

This newly revised and updated edition brings to both the student and practitioner a host of different but related topics related to the social and behavioral aspects of medication use and pharmacy services. The reader will find some chapters have concepts that overlap with one another but for which the primary focus is unique. One key objective of the book is to bring together social and behavioral theories and principles together and integrate them into how pharmacists provide collaborative medication therapy management services to diverse patient populations. A second key objective is to provide an update of key topics discussed in prior editions. Several chapters are similar to the first edition of this textbook because they represent basic applications of social and psychological theory to pharmacy practice. Long ago, it was established that patients are people, not objects, and that their opinions, biases, cultures, and trust influence their collaborations with pharmacists and other health professionals. However, the passage of seven years since the last edition has brought about much new literature that continues to strengthen our understanding of the psychosocial world linking pharmacists to healthcare teams involving patients, caregivers, other health professionals, and the many others working within the healthcare industry that we hope will contribute to daily impacts on patient-centered and safe medication use.

A third important objective of this new edition is to tailor the book with emerging topics such as social networks and the removal of topics that were not as focused on the US healthcare experience. The addition of the social network chapter (Chapter 22) allows us to explore the science of understanding connections or relationships between individuals and how such connections contribute to human experiences and outcomes. We removed a previous chapter on international healthcare disparities since it pulled the book into a broader focus that prior readers felt distracting from a clear focus of the book on the U.S. and North American healthcare experience. There are other textbooks available that more specifically connect pharmacy to the international experience. There are still references to the literature and experiences from our international colleagues but intermixed in chapters rather than a sole chapter focus. The other change to note is that there are several new authors who add very different perspectives to past and new topics.

This edition, as with the last one, structures the book into four parts with the genesis starting from the initial interpretation of the health problem and need for treatment (Part 1), approaches to resolve health problems (Part II), targeting care of specific patients (Part III), and a final part exploring public policy perspectives on medication use (Part IV). The intent of this structure is to provide the reader flow from the individual, to the interpersonal/group perspectives, and end with the larger macro societal perspectives. Despite this overall structure, authors do infuse the individual, interpersonal, and macro perspectives even within chapters. We do anticipate educators and students may not use all chapters and select specific ones as they relate to their courses. The book's four-part structure provides overall thematic connection between chapters and sections but still allows readers to identify specific chapters to read without feeling lost having not selected other chapters.

The first part of the textbook includes several chapters that focus on describing how health and illness behaviors intersect across individual and societal perspectives given the known empirical and theoretical literatures on health behavior. The second and largest part of the textbook explores more specifically the different alternatives and experiences that individuals and social systems use when engaging in treatment options. This part of the book takes the reader through patient access to a variety of healthcare services that complement medication use. Chapters in this part consider how pharmacy practice has evolved and factors affecting the provision of various pharmacy services.

The third part builds on the prior parts' foundations on general considerations affecting pharmacy practice and explores the challenges of providing optimal pharmacist's care to specific patient populations. The last part of the textbook examines the complex macro issues of ethical issues faced by today's pharmacists and how patients, pharmacists, and others in healthcare services develop and interact in networks that can affect outcomes. A future edition may expand this section to include a chapter on how technology has changed patient and provider behaviors.

There is a great deal of material presented across the 22 chapters. The editors do hope that some of the concepts presented will assist readers in their journey toward reaching a stronger understanding of the complex and dynamic interactions between patients, pharmacists, medications, healthcare teams, organizations, and larger social systems. As we noted in the previous 2009 edition, we desire that the chapters challenge readers to continually ask questions, to find answers, and explore new ways to change the pharmacy profession so it can best meet the ever changing needs of patients and contribute to greater efficiencies in the healthcare system that optimize quality at the lowest cost. If there are aspects of this textbook that make the reader uncomfortable, perhaps that is okay since it is through such discomfort that we are often empowered to think critically and make improvements.

We always welcome feedback regarding the book and how we can make it stronger for a future edition. We do hope the chapters enable you to celebrate pharmacy's rich history, provocatively engage the reader in the psychosocial challenges of pharmacist care and patient medication use, and leave the reader thinking critically and creatively about how pharmacy can emerge with even greater impact in population health over the next decade.

Nathaniel M. Rickles

Albert I. Wertheimer

Jon C. Schommer

September 2016

ACKNOWLEDGMENTS

The completion of this textbook would not have been possible without the dedication and hard work of several individuals. The editors would like to first thank Paul Carty, the Director of Publishing Partnerships, who was our first point of contact with Kendall Hunt and continued with warm and enthusiastic support throughout the development and production process. The editors would also like to thank Elizabeth Cray, our production editor, for her positive energy and engagement to ensure we were staying on track and navigate through various challenges. She was always upbeat and generous about facilitating different deliverables. We would also like to thank others at Kendall Hunt such as Brianna Kirschbaum for her many tireless effort to assist in verification of copyrights and Ashley Hatteberg for her marketing guidance. There is simply not enough paper to thank the many others at Kendall Hunt who were involved in the book development process. To all our colleagues at Kendall Hunt, we appreciate your flexibility and all you did to ensure the best textbook of our discipline was delivered.

We also want to extend much appreciation to Anh Ho, a pharmacy student at Northeastern University School of Pharmacy, who assisted the editors in collecting needed documents and information from authors. She was persistent with several authors who needed reminders to send in materials, etc. Without her tireless support, we might still be collecting documents.

The editors also acknowledge this third edition may not have existed without the initial work of Dr. Mickey Smith, a professor emeritus of pharmacy from the University of Mississippi. Drs. Smith and Wertheimer were the first editors of the textbook in 1974 and their visionary effort with that edition and subsequent editions allows countless numbers of students and professionals across the country and overseas to have a rich resource for which they can use to learn, practice, and research the psychosocial aspects of medication use.

ABOUT THE EDITORS

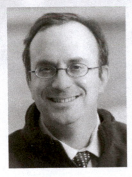

Nathaniel M. Rickles, PharmD, PhD, BCPP is an associate professor in pharmacy practice at the University of Connecticut. He received a BS degree from Dickinson College in chemistry and psychology, PharmD from the Philadelphia College of Pharmacy and Science in Pharmacy, and his MS and PhD in the social and administrative sciences from the School of Pharmacy at the University of Wisconsin-Madison. He also completed a psychiatric pharmacy practice residency at the University of Texas Health Science Center in San Antonio and board certified in psychiatric pharmacy practice. His primary research interests are to develop, implement, and evaluate intervention programs that improve pharmacist collaboration with patients and other professionals, patient medication adherence, and patient safety. Dr. Rickles also explores educational methods to improve the teaching of communication skills and patient safety.

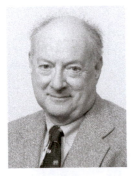

Albert I Wertheimer, B.S., M.B.A., Ph.D. is a professor at Nova Southeastern University in Fort Lauderdale, Florida. He is one of the founders of the discipline of social and behavioral pharmacy, having participated in the very first edition in 1974. He has guided nearly 100 Ph.D. students and has written over 100 journal articles and written or edited 36 books in this and closely related areas.

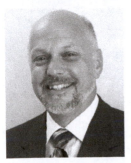

Jon C. Schommer, R.Ph., PhD, is a professor at the University of Minnesota. He received his BS, MS, and PhD degrees from the University of Wisconsin-Madison. His research is related to provision, use, and evaluation of drug products and pharmacist services. The work is grounded in health behavior theories, behavioral economics, behavioral psychology, and marketing models of organizational and consumer behavior.

CONTRIBUTING AUTHORS

Ilene Abranson, PhD
Adult Education/Anthropology
Lecturer
Wayne State University

H. John Baldwin, PhD*
Associate Dean
Nova Southeastern University
College of Pharmacy, Health Professions Division

Judith Barr, ScD, MEd
Professor Emeritus, School of Pharmacy
Director, National Education and Research Center for Outcomes Assessment
Northeastern University

Susan J. Blalock, PhD, MPH
Professor and Vice Chair
Pharmaceutical Outcomes and Policy
UNC Eshelman School of Pharmacy

Nicole J. Brandt, PharmD, MBA, CGP, BCPP , FASCP
Professor, Geriatric Pharmacotherapy, Pharmacy Practice and Science UMB School
of Pharmacy
Director, Clinical and Educational Programs of Peter Lamy Center Drug Therapy
and Aging

Patricia J Bush, PhD
Professor Emeritus Georgetown University School of Medicine

Angeline Carlson, PhD
Professor
College of Pharmacy, University of Minnesota

Karishma Desai, PhD, M.S., B.Pharm
Post-Doctoral Research Fellow,
Surgical Health Services Research Unit,
Department of Surgery,
Stanford School of Medicine.
Stanford University,

Marcus Droege, PhD, MBA
Sr. Director, Global Knowledge & Strategic Intelligence
Corporate Medical Affairs
Celgene Corporation

Kevin C. Farmer, PhD
Professor and Vice-Chair, Pharmacy: Clinical and Administrative Sciences-
OKC & Tulsa
Department of Pharmacy: Clinical and Administrative Sciences – Tulsa

Elizabeth A. Flynn, PhD
Affiliate Clinical Associate Professor
University of Florida

Sally-Anne Francis, PhD
Honorary Senior Lecturer
UCL School of Pharmacy, Department of Practice and Policy

John-Michael Gamble, BScPharm, PhD
Assistant Professor
School of Pharmacy
Memorial University of Newfoundland
Health Sciences Centre
St. John's, Newfoundland and Labrador

Emma Sheldon Gentry
Master's Candidate
Doctoral Program in Gerontology
University of Maryland, Baltimore
Department of Epidemiology and Public Health

Michael R. Gionfriddo, PhD, PharmD
Assistant Professor
Center for Pharmacy Innovation and Outcomes
Geisinger Precision Health Center

Kent E. M. Groves, PhD
Vice President, Strategy
Merkle Inc.

Amy Haddad, PhD
Director, Center for Health Policy and Ethics and the Dr. C.C. and Mabel L. Criss
Endowed Chair in the Health Sciences
Creighton University

Katri Hämeen-Anttila, Adjunct Professor, PhD (pharm.)
Finnish Medicines Agency Fimea

Chamika Hawkins-Taylor, MHA PhD
Assistant Professor
Chamika Hawkins-Taylor, MHA PhD
Assistant Professor
South Dakota State University

Carol J. Hermansen-Kobulnicky, PhD, RPh
Associate Professor, School of Pharmacy
Director of Interprofessional Education, College of Health Sciences
University of Wyoming

Gregory J. Higby, PhD
Adjunct Professor
Executive Director of the American Institute of the History ofPharmacy
University of Wisconsin-Madison

Xiaoban Hu, M.D., MPH.
Ph.D. Student
School of Public Health
University of Southern California

Rasheeda Joihnson, PhD
Health Insurance Specialist
Centers for Medicare and Medicare Services

Jan Kavookjian, MBA, PhD
Associate Professor of Health Outcomes Research & Policy
Harrison School of Pharmacy

Andrea Kjos, PharmD, PhD
Associate Professor of Social and Administrative Sciences
Department of Pharmaceutical, Biomedical, and Administrative Sciences
Drake University
College of Pharmacy and Health Sciences

Sean T. Leonard, PhD
Assistant Dean for Assessment
ST. JOHN FISHER COLLEGE| Wegmans School of Pharmacy

John M. Lonie, RPh, EdD
Associate Professor
Long Island University
College of Pharmacy

Amanda M. Loya, PharmD, BCPS
Clinical Associate Professor
The University of Texas at El Paso – Pharmacy

Neil J. MacKinnon, PhD
Dean and Professor
James L Winkle College of Pharmacy
University of Cincinnati

Linda Gore Martin, PharmD, MBA, BCPS
Dean and Professor, Social and Administrative Pharmacy
University of Wyoming School of Pharmacy

Anthony W. Olson, PharmD, MEd
PhD Student
University of Minnesota, College of Pharmacy

Denise Orwig, PhD
Associate Professor
Director of the Doctoral Program in Gerontology
Department of Epidemiology and Public Health
University of Maryland School of Medicine

Lourdes G. Planas, RPh, PhD
Assistant Professor
University of Oklahoma
College of Pharmacy

Daniel G. Ricci, PharmD
Graduate Fellow
Department of Social and Administrative Sciences
School of Pharmacy
University of Wisconsin-Madison

Jenny O. Rickles, MPH, CPHQ Consultant

Nathaniel Rickles, PharmD, PhD, BCPP
University of Connecticut
School of Pharmacy

Kraig L. Schell
Professor of Psychology
Angelo State University

Jon C. Schommer, PhD
Professor
University of Minnesota
College of Pharmacy

Jeri J. Sias, PharmD, MPH
Clinical Professor / PGY1 Community Pharmacy Residency Program Director
Provost's Faculty Fellow-in-Residence, UTEP Center for Civic Engagement
The University of Texas at El Paso/University of Texas at Austin Cooperative
Pharmacy Program

Piia Siitonen, MSc (Pharm.), PhD (Cand.)
University of Eastern Finland

Ingrid Sketris, PharmD, MPA(HSA)
Professor and Associate Director, Research
Dalhousie University

Felicity Smith, PhD
Professor of Pharmacy Practice
Department of Practice and Policy
UCL School of Pharmacy

Abigail E. Strate, PharmD
Clinical Pharmacist

Benjamin S. Teeter PhD
Assistant Professor
Department of Pharmacy Practice,
University of Arkansas for Medical Sciences

Gina Paola Torres Rubiano, MD
Universidad Militar Nueva Granada

Andrew P. Traynor, PharmD, BCPS
Chair and Associate Professor, Department of Pharmacy Practice
Director, PGY1 Pharmacy Residency Program
Concordia University Wisconsin School of Pharmacy

Cherie Tsingos-Lucas, PhD
B.Pharm, Graduate Certificate in Educational Studies (Higher Ed) PhD,
University of Sydney, Sydney, Australia

Albert I. Wertheimer
Professor, Dept. of Sociobehavioral and Administrative Pharmacy,
College of Pharmacy,
Nova Southeastern University

Salisa C. Westrick PhD
Associate Professor
Health Outcomes Research and Policy
Department Harrison School of Pharmacy, Auburn University

Amy F. Wilson, PharmD
Assistant Dean for Academic Affairs
Office of Academic and Student Affairs
Creighton University School of Pharmacy and Health Professions

PART I INTERPRETATION OF THE HEALTH
PROBLEM AND NEED FOR TREATMENT

SECTION A

CONCEPTS OF HEALTH AND ILLNESS

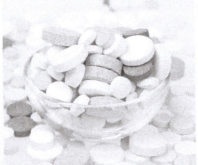
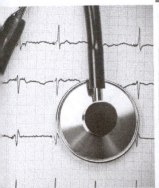
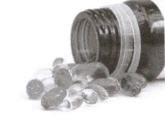
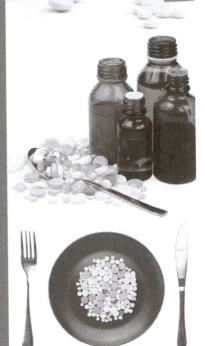
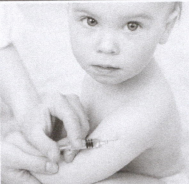
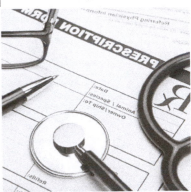

CHAPTER 1

DEFINITIONS AND MEANING OF HEALTH AND ILLNESS

Marcus Droege, PhD, MBA, Sean T. Leonard, PhD, and H. John Baldwin, PhD

LEARNING OBJECTIVES:

1. Define health and illness.
2. Evaluate the social dimension affecting health and illness.
3. Describe how people behave during illness.
4. Analyze the sick role concept and its ramifications for health care.
5. Identify cultural and contextual factors affecting health and illness.

KEY TERMS:

Acute illness

Addiction

Chronic disease

Disease

Fundamental Attribution Error (FAE)

Illness

Lifestyle drugs

Sick role

Signs

Sociology

Symptoms

THE GENESIS OF SOCIAL PHARMACY

Perhaps no other health profession in recent history has been challenged with changes as profound and momentous as the profession of pharmacy. A significant transformation involving a professional shift in focus from the product to the patient has occurred, pharmacists have assumed new roles as patient care providers, and pharmacy education has faced formidable challenges subsequent to this transition, particularly the transition to the Doctor of Pharmacy as the first professional degree. A basic understanding of historical events that have shaped contemporary pharmacy education reveals edifying insights into the pharmacist's role in society today.

Pharmacy educators formed the Millis Study Commission in an attempt to (re-)align pharmacy education with contemporary drug-related needs of patients. The commission set out to revise pharmacy curricula that were historically oriented to basic sciences and devise a road map to the profession's future. The Millis Commission, convened by the American Association of Colleges of Pharmacy (AACP), had a most significant impact on contemporary pharmacy education, and many believe that pharmacy education today has been shaped by the numerous recommendations of the commission. The commission was charged with addressing the perceived lack of "insight and foresight" in pharmacy education pertaining to the role of the pharmacist as integral members of the health care team. In addition to the many recommendations related to the need for an outcomes based pharmacy curriculum, student recruitment, and a six-year first professional doctor of pharmacy degree, the commission recommendations were for "curricula with less knowledge of science and more knowledge of patients and well people."[1] Deemphasizing the basic science focus of pharmacy curricula while focusing more on knowledge about how people make decisions about their health was deemed to be an important early step toward the differentiation of pharmacists while they are still students. Successful behavioral interventions have been shown to result in far greater improvements in patient health outcomes than increased access to health care. The care patients received from their pharmacist was no exception and pharmacy education at the time was perceived to be all about drugs and very little about people, an outcome in stark contrast with the need for a qualified practitioner possessing the skills and knowledge necessary to identify, resolve, and prevent patients' medication therapy problems.

This view, therefore, required pharmacy curricula to include topics such as social and behavioral aspects of health care delivery and communication skills. Discussion on curricular change and the Millis Commission report coincided with the creation of graduate programs and a disciplinary focus area in the social and administrative sciences as they pertain to pharmacy. These social pharmacy programs address in their full scope the problems of pharmacy and medicines in society.

DEFINITIONS OF HEALTH AND ILLNESS

Health and Illness are central themes of human existence, with various definitions and interpretations spanning all cultures. Addressing concerns arising from ill health receives much attention in virtually every society around the world and substantive resources are devoted to health professions education. The raison d'être for any health care professional to practice in his or her respective fields can be found in the very existence of health and illness along a continuum of definitions. In fact, the conceptualization of health and illness delineates the wide-ranging spectrum of practitioner activities across disciplines. Underlying decisions about someone's healthcare needs, irrespective of who made this determination, drive interventions. In the case of pharmacy, practitioner responsibilities can be found in the identification, resolution, and prevention of drug therapy problems, which should logically coincide with the focus of pharmacy education.

Given the universality, prevalence, and frequency of illness and disease for both an individual and society, it perhaps seems strange that they are considered to be abnormal conditions. One could argue, as René Dubois has, that disease and sickness are normal; it is health that is the abnormal condition. However, it is socially necessary that each individual within a society contribute to that society for the society to flourish. Thus, each person has one or more roles that define who that person is, what he or she does, and what is expected of him or her, e.g., student, spouse, wage earner, parent. These roles have two characteristics of relevance to this discussion, namely, societal expectations of one occupying a particular role, and the reciprocal nature of any role.

A review of the literature reveals that definitions of health and illness vary largely on the basis of cultural background. Disease is a medical term, meaning there is a pathologic change in the structure or function of the body or mind. The World Health Organization's (WHO) definition of health, "A state of complete physical, mental, and social well being, not merely the absence of disease or infirmity" reflects this mechanistic view of the body where ill health is treated as the mechanical failure of some part of one or more of these systems of the body and the medical task is to repair the damage.[2] Yet at the same time, the definition expands the role of healthcare providers beyond the traditional role of treating disease.

Illness is the response of the person to a disease; it is an abnormal process in which the person's level of functioning is changed. Talcott Parsons' 1972 definition of health, "The state of optimum capacity of an individual for the effective performance of the roles and tasks for which he (sic) has been socialized" expands earlier definitions to address social needs of individuals, i.e., normal role functioning. This shift from an individualistic toward a more collectivistic view of the effects of health and illness had far reaching consequences for health care practitioners as they were no longer limited to treating disease, but could engage in preventive measures.

THE SOCIAL DIMENSION OF PHARMACY

Just as individual actions collectively form and affect the society in which individuals live, society also affects the actions of individuals. Sociology is the social science that examines the organization and mores of a society and sociologists study a variety of issues with which pharmacy is concerned and occasionally obsessed.

Among the many areas of study, sociologists have focused on a number of areas which merit pharmacy's attention, for example, professions and role theory.

Sociology is a social science focused on theory whereas pharmacy can be viewed as a "field of application," taking concepts and facts from other fields and applying them to practice. As stated earlier, pharmacy education has tended to focus on chemical and biological sciences, with little input from the social sciences. It was not until the mid-1960s when the first seminal papers on social pharmacy topics were published in the pharmacy literature.

Harding and Taylor discussed the social dimensions of pharmacy and pointed out that our actions as health care professionals are embedded in a social context. Societal change and increased risk averseness have prompted providers of healthcare to re-think their professional roles and define their activities as an "examplar of social action."[3] The process by which human conditions come to be considered medical conditions is known as "medicalization," in which medical authorities effectively function as agents of social control. It is through that influence that a human condition becomes the subject of medical research, meets the criteria of a medical diagnosis, or becomes eligible for treatment.[4] A major theme in sociology has therefore been the process of becoming a patient. It has been suggested that the sick role be the focus of medical sociology. Certainly the patient may be considered as a central concept in any discussion of health care, pharmacists' role, or medication use.

Perhaps the best known and cited characterization of the concept of "patient" is that of Talcott Parsons (1951), a sociologist interested in social systems and the development of societies. To oversimplify, all societies consist of "actors" with multiple roles, each with a complementary role, adhering to a common or normative set of characteristics, and with reciprocal expectations. Each role has associated rights and obligations. The rights of a particular role are the responsibilities of its complementary role. There is some degree of tolerance for deviance from the norm. However, every society must have some means of enforcement of what Parsons calls the "societal normative order." As stated earlier, it is socially necessary that each individual within a society contribute to that society for the society to flourish and illness or sickness is a deviation from what is considered normal. Consequently, the sick role is a method of social control over illness as a deviant behavior. There are two rights and two obligations or responsibilities inherent in the sick role: the right to not be responsible or blamed for the condition and the right to be excused from normal role responsibilities; the obligations are to seek competent help and the responsibility to "want to get well."

Another sociologist, Edward A. Suchman, formulated illness behavior as consisting of five stages: the symptom experience, assumption of the sick role, medical care contact, dependent patient, and recovery or rehabilitation.[5] Each stage necessitates a decision by the "could-be patient," and illustrates the importance of the "lay referral" system, made up of family and friends, and which constitutes the complementary role to the sick role.

Symptom experience	Assumption of the sick role	Medical care contact	Dependent patient	Recovery or rehabilitation

FIGURE 1-1 SUCHMAN'S MODEL OF STAGES OF ILLNESS EXPERIENCE

SYMPTOM EXPERIENCE
AND ILLNESS BEHAVIOR

At the Symptom Experience Stage, the initial stage of illness behavior, the decision is made that something is wrong, or not normal. There are three aspects to this stage: physical experience, cognitive aspects, and emotional response. The most common physical experience indicating that something is wrong is pain. Cognitively, the experience is interpreted based on what the physical manifestations are, their severity, and the course they take, as well as previous personal experience or knowledge about the signs. Symptoms are recognized and defined in terms of their interference with normal role functioning. The emotional response includes fear, concern, or anxiety. When symptoms are extremely severe, felt to be serious, and perceived to interfere with other role responsibilities, the most common first inclination is to seek medical care, with a smaller number considering self-medication. However, even then there is a tendency to delay seeking treatment and engage in self-denial, at least until one has discussed the symptoms with a lay person, typically a relative, and most frequently a spouse.

Health care practitioners distinguish between signs and symptoms of disease. Signs are measurable changes of physiologic functioning and are detectable using diagnostic procedures, often involving medical instruments and diagnostic methods, e.g., stethoscope, glucometer. Many times, signs have little to no meaning to patients and may not even be noticed by them. Symptoms, however, are inherently subjective and not easily quantifiable. In most cases, patients will notice symptoms, (such as pain, fatigue, nausea, etc.) as an expression of ill health; a practitioner will then seek to derive a sense of the symptoms by asking the patient, for example, to rate pain during an examination. Healthcare professionals rely on patients reporting symptoms during an examination as they will use both signs and symptoms in formulating a hypothesis of a likely diagnosis.

An acute illness has a rapid onset of symptoms and lasts only a comparatively short time whereas characteristics of chronic disease often include permanent change(s) to the body's functioning. Chronic disease causes, or is caused by, irreversible alterations in normal anatomy and physiology. Although a cure is possible in most cases of acute illness, chronic diseases tend to require special patient education for rehabilitation as well as long periods of care or support.

Symptom experience varies widely from individual to individual and so do descriptions of symptoms along the continuum of acute versus chronic conditions. A determining factor in this regard for most people is the "return to normal" and their ability to assume normal role functioning without permanent change. In most cases, chronic symptoms result in sustained changes in one's life. In addition, patients will likely be able to communicate the underlying cause (disease) of which the symptoms are a consequence. This is in contrast to an acute illness where patients are often unaware of the underlying cause of their symptoms and will in most cases rely on expert practitioners to combine signs and symptoms as evidence for disease.

The Assumption of the Sick Role Stage is where the individual makes the decision that he or she is sick. As the individual seeks information and advice and relief of symptoms, the individual's lay referral system is paramount because few individuals are sufficiently confident to decide on their own that they are sick. Also, consistent with Parsons' formulation, sickness excuses them from their normal role obligations and imposes concurrent obligations on these significant others. Thus, the sick individual seeks permission (technically, "provisional validation" or "provisional legitimization") from these individuals to be sick and excused from his or her normal responsibilities. In most cases, the sick individual follows the advice given by his or her discussant.

At the Medical Care Contact Stage, the sick individual contacts a professional within the health care system seeking advice and permission to be sick from a "scientific" rather than a lay source, i.e., an authoritative definition or diagnosis of his condition, a proposed treatment, and official sanctioning or "legitimization" to be sick. If legitimization is denied, he is expected to return to his or her normal role activities. This stage may continue if the sick individual is not satisfied with the initial clinician's diagnosis or recommended treatment; that is, the individual may begin to "doctor shop." Interestingly, a significant minority of treated individuals indicate that they never received a diagnosis, or prognosis from their health care practitioner. The most common treatment is medication with the physician writing one or more prescriptions for the diseased or ill person.

At the Dependent Patient Stage, a decision is made to transfer control to the clinician and accept and follow the prescribed treatment. The most important aspects of this stage are that (1) only at this stage does the sick individual become a patient; (2) most patients believe, or claim, that they adhere to the prescribed treatment, and (3) the family and "lay referral system" continue to play an important role. Most patients do not accept the patient role easily as they are reluctant to give up their normal roles, but may see the only way to health and a return to these roles is to surrender his or her autonomy to the professional and lay caregivers. Also significant are the variety of barriers—social, administrative, logistical, psychological—that may easily affect the treatment process.

Of course, it is not always desirable to be assigned to the role of patient, or one who suffers from an illness. For example, until relatively recently individuals in the United States who were not heterosexual could be diagnosed with a mental illness. It was not until 1973 that the American Psychiatric Association voted to change the diagnostic system to allow homosexuality to be considered "normal."[6] Before that time a diagnosed homosexual could be assigned to the sick role and consequently lose social rights and privileges. He or she could be committed to psychiatric institutions, arrested and detained as a "sexual deviant" for engaging in homosexual behavior, etc.[7]

It is important for the student in pharmacy to recognize that the nature of sexuality did not somehow change in the early 1970s—it was the social context and values surrounding sexual orientation that are what changed. Homosexual orientation had been medicalized as an illness by Western clinicians for nearly a century, and some historians have argued that this reflects a pervasive bias within Western medicine against non-conventional sexual expression.[8] This bias may have its origins in moral or religious values about what is "right" and proper, yet the values are expressed in the form of a clinical diagnosis. In this way, diagnoses can be used as a social tool to regulate behavior. Personal values of the clinician may intersect or even conflict with standards of clinical practice, as may be observed in the assertion by some pharmacists that their moral and/or religious values prohibit them from dispensing certain kinds of contraceptive medications.

The final stage of illness, Recovery or Rehabilitation, requires a decision to relinquish the patient role. Because of the patient's desire (and responsibility) to return to health, this decision is generally easy in comparison to the necessary decisions at other stages. Also at this point either, or both, the health care professional and the lay person caregivers, withdraw their legitimization of the right to be excused from normal role responsibilities and the patient is expected to resume their old roles or, in chronic conditions or disability, accept a long period of convalescence or rehabilitation or a new role as an invalid.

Both Suchman's and Parsons' formulations have withstood the test of time for the last several decades. It must be noted however that Suchman validated his formulation based on a well-defined sample of people who had experienced a specific episode of illness and passed through all five stages. There is no requirement that all five stages be involved, nor are specific time frames associated with each phase, which may be very brief or very lengthy. Suchman pointed out that, for the ill person, social concerns seem to predominate over medical or health concerns and that responses to minor illness would seem to be even more likely to be governed by social rather than medical concerns. Additionally, Suchman dealt with people with an acute condition, or an acute episode of a chronic condition. However, Suchman also points out that individuals have a natural tendency to under-estimate (dismiss/ignore/disregard/deny) symptoms that are neither severe nor incapacitating. Because many chronic diseases are characterized by a lack of, or seemingly minor, virtually-unrecognizable symptoms at the onset of an illness, they are more easily denied and people are therefore unlikely to seek medical care early.

Indeed, this same characteristic would appear to be an explanation for some types of non-compliance, together with the natural responsibility to want to return to a healthy status and normal role functioning. The classic example is high blood pressure and patient non-adherence to blood pressure medications, which serve as a constant reminder that one is sick, despite the lack of overt symptoms.

The recovery/rehabilitation stage also holds special significance for those with chronic conditions. Since the ill person is expected to do everything possible to return to health, and yet chronic conditions by definition mean that there is no cure, special strain is put upon both the ill person and the lay person care giver. Frequently this seems to be resolved by a redefinition of what is "normal" for the afflicted individual. The classic example may be individuals with diabetes, who most frequently are able to control the disease with medication, and despite the continued reminders (regular medication, blood glucose readings) and relatively minor life style changes (diet, exercise), generally are able to resume their previous social roles with only minor, if any, restrictions.

The sick role, as formulated by Parsons, carries within it an inherent potential conflict. The ill person has the right to be excused from normal role responsibilities while at the same time has the responsibility to seek competent help and do everything possible to return to health and resume normal role responsibilities. For some people, the care and attention they receive when sick, coupled with being excused from doing things they would normally be expected to do (for example, in the case of children, going to school when they are unprepared for an upcoming test or haven't done the expected homework), is an attractive proposition. For these people, they accept the rights of illness, but seek to avoid the responsibility. Thus, these people adopt the "negative sick role."

Relinquishing the sick role appears to provide most people with less difficulty than assuming it. Convalescence, while not enjoyable, proceeds smoothly in most cases and ends with the patient's return to his former well status. Although there may be some concern about picking up where one had left off, this is not a problem for most people.[9]

Succinctly stated, health and Illness exist along a continuum; they are inherently constrained by interference with social action, and are much less objective than most people recognize.

CULTURAL AND CONTEXTUAL FACTORS IN HEALTH AND ILLNESS

There is much to be learned about health and illness in the process of becoming a health care professional. Even in training programs that last for years, there may be relatively little time devoted towards recognizing that definitions of health and illness are subjective in many ways. It may be tempting for students to assume that the diagnoses they learn in training are objective, free from bias, and durable over time. The most common philosophical approach to these issues reflected in medical schools and textbooks has been described as naïve normalism, where illness connotes abnormal functioning and health is suggestive of "normal" functioning.[10] However, the actual definition of "normal" is hardly clear, and in fact may be largely subjective and influenced by prevailing cultural factors.

For example, what constitutes a disease or illness in one culture may be considered normal and healthy in another. In Germany, low blood pressure is often interpreted as an illness while in the United States, it typically is not. An individual in Germany with this condition may be permitted to assume the sick role: He or she may be excused from some social responsibilities and receive treatment from health care professionals. Yet if the same individual was part of a different culture, he or she may not be afforded the sick role. Similarly, interpretations of a disease state may vary as well.[11] Students may be surprised to learn that a fairly large proportion of adults (as many as 50%) are colonized by Helicobacter pylori (H. pylori) yet relatively few of these individuals develop duodenal and peptic ulceration. Therefore, the mere presence of H. pylori in a patient does not necessarily mean that she or he is "sick."

Clinicians are afforded social status and power by virtue of their training and expertise, which means that their personal values are often given greater weight—even when those values and opinions are not informed by their professional training or scientific findings. We can expect that when there are significant, widespread changes in social values within a culture, then definitions and standards for health and illness will also be in some way affected.

This may be a humbling point for health care professionals to accept: The nature of our role and work is not strictly objective, and our current understandings of health and illness will likely change over time. It is sound advice to new students that one ought to avoid the temptation of being overly confident in their knowledge and work. A tragic example from history is the fact that the genocide perpetrated by the Nazis during World War II was in no small way facilitated by health care professionals.[12] Physicians and other health care professionals were recruited by the Nazi party to medicalize the process of killing socially undesirable people: The sick and feeble were "euthanized" in hospitals; sterilization was forced upon certain social and cultural groups; and physicians routinely evaluated new arrivals to concentration camps to determine their fitness for work (where the alternative to work was execution). By giving the genocide process a medical façade, the Nazi social and political agendas were more easily disguised and adopted on a large scale. Of course, this was only possible because some health care professionals adopted the Nazi value system (and extreme biases) as their own. History warns health care professionals that we are not immune to having our expert knowledge swayed and distorted by larger social forces.

This lesson may be especially relevant to today's pharmacists. There is considerable controversy surrounding the marketing of medications to laypersons, and how direct-to-consumer advertisements about medications contribute to the social context in which pharmacists practice. Connections have been drawn between direct-to-consumer advertising and the creation or exaggeration of the prevalence of diseases and symptoms. This is in contrast to the stated goals of such advertisements to better inform patients about available treatments options. The controversy has largely focused upon psychiatric conditions, such as adult variants of attention deficit disorder, but also has extended to diagnoses such as "low" testosterone, male hair loss and baldness, and the medical treatment of menopause. The argument is that marketing efforts by pharmaceutical companies have perpetuated the wide-spread belief that "there is a pill for everything" and therefore there has been a proliferation of new disease states and symptoms that merit medication treatment.

It can be observed that there are some common conditions that do not have medication treatments available (e.g., celiac disease), yet these are not as well-known within the lay public as diagnoses that carry with them known medication treatments. Also, it is not unusual to group collectively non-medication treatments as "alternative therapies," even when those treatments (such as psychotherapy, occupational therapy, behavioral modification, etc.) demonstrate equal or better responses. It is also interesting to note that symptoms of an illness are portrayed in many advertisements as being as "serious" as the illness itself (such as "fatigue"), or that associations between symptoms and diseases are overstated—such as that a vaccine for the human papilloma virus is essentially a vaccine for cervical cancer or asserting that depression is a medical condition. Although the diagnosis of major depressive disorder has been substantiated as a disease, the lay use of the term depression tends to be situational and usually refers to less severe emotional experiences, for example, distressing news etc. that generally do not satisfy the diagnostic criteria.

The controversy about pharmaceutical marketing is ongoing and we certainly cannot offer the reader any firm conclusions about it, yet we can point out that this demonstrates that definitions of health and illness do not exist in a vacuum. Even business and economic forces influence our interpretations of what is healthy and what is pathological.

It is interesting that people may define health and illness in ways that are different than clinicians. For example, it has been found that older adults who have multiple health problems may still describe themselves as "healthy." On the other hand, some people define themselves as suffering from a medical condition where the nature of the "illness" is poorly defined or subjectively understood. This is best observed in the ubiquity of the word "addiction" in Western society, where addiction implies a biological and/or medical condition. When one is "addicted" to something, he or she may be afforded the sick role and thereby partially or fully excused from responsibility for their actions due to uncontrollable biological forces. Addiction has been applied to alcohol and other substances, but more recently has also been used to explain behaviors that do not involve a known substance—such as addictions to shopping, television, the Internet, sexual behaviors and pornography, gambling, etc. Such definitions of addictions are controversial among clinicians and researchers, yet it is not at all unusual to encounter laypersons who use these terms to explain their own or someone else's behavior.

Body image is another area where the medicalization of common problems and concerns may be observed. Standards of beauty change over time and it is interesting to note that several centuries ago, women who were large in physique ("Rubenesque") were considered more attractive than slender, slim women. In modern Western civilization that standard for beauty has essentially reversed, and perhaps it is no coincidence that drugs and medical procedures that alter physical appearance have become increasingly popular. Elective surgery (such as liposuction) and other cosmetic procedures are rendered largely within a medical context. Procedures are performed by professional clinicians, recipients of elective cosmetic procedures may undergo surgery, receive prescription medications, and even be identified by clinicians as "patients"—yet they typically are not defined as "ill," "sick," or being "in need of treatment." It is worth stating that an abundance of research finds that most people are in some way disappointed with their physical appearance (it is "normal" to be dissatisfied with some feature of one's own appearance), but whether or not this constitutes a "medical" problem has yet to be substantiated.

Nonetheless, modern pharmacists will recognize that concerns about body image pervade Western culture, and increasingly people are turning to either medical or pseudo-medical solutions. A new term in the pharmacy lexicon is "lifestyle" drugs, which are not indisputably medically necessary yet may be prescribed for other (e.g., cosmetic) reasons. Lifestyle drugs may include those that decrease wrinkles in skin, promote hair growth, etc. Examples of pseudo-medical solutions include advertisements for "nutritional supplements" that look surprisingly like advertisements for prescription medications, and offer guarantees of weight loss, increased sexual performance, and even increases in penis or breast size.

Beyond medications and supplements, perceptions about pregnancy and child-birth may be changing. Over the past century or so, pregnancy and delivery had become medicalized in most Western cultures. The social benefits of medicalizing pregnancy have been clear: Infant and mother mortality rates have been significantly reduced, for example. Yet the drawbacks to the medicalization of pregnancy and childbirth are subtle and still important: The models offered by Parsons, or Suchman, do not always "fit" the desires of expectant parents very well. A growing number of pregnant women (and their partners) are unwilling to conform to the expectations of the patient role, such as handing over decision-making power to their obstetrician, on the basis that most pregnancies and deliveries are uncomplicated and do not necessitate medical involvement. The extent to which that perception is valid is beyond the scope of our discussion: What matters is that a significant minority of people perceive the role of the physician in pregnancy and delivery as intrusive, or "unnatural," and most physicians believe themselves to be "essential." This may be why some hospitals are now adopting marketing techniques to soften the role of medicine in pregnancy and delivery, by using terms such as "birthing center," "delivery suites," and so on. So it can be seen that individuals interact with health care professionals for diverse reasons, and the nature of those interactions is shaped by numerous external forces (such as culture, society, morality, economics, etc.). Further, definitions of health and illness are not limited to clinical interactions: One can define him or herself as "sick" without any formal clinical diagnosis, or one can define her or himself as "healthy" even in the presence of a formal diagnosis. Suffice it to say that objectively understanding health and illness is remarkably complicated—even though clinicians routinely interact with patients as though there is little or no subjectivity involved in the process.

We have been building up to a point that by now should make intuitive sense: As a pharmacist, it is both prudent and necessary to consider clinical interactions of all kinds as a type of social experience. Social experiences are not strictly objective, and consequently even the most skilled and competent pharmacist is susceptible to making errors during clinical interactions. Being mindful of the social context in the practice of pharmacy can help one reduce the risk of errors, and thereby enhance the quality of treatment.

In this sense of the word, "errors" is not limited to medical errors. Rather it refers to the universal problem that human perception is not reliably objective: Nobody is perfect. Sociologists, social psychologists, and other social scientists can tell us much about the ways in which we are prone to perceiving social experiences inaccurately. While the list of perceptual errors and distortions that all of us are susceptible to is quite long, we can benefit from focusing upon a few.

The fundamental attribution error is sometimes abbreviated as FAE, and is also known as either personality overattribution or correspondence bias. It has been defined in different ways but essentially, the FAE is the tendency to overlook situational factors in favor of more durable personality traits in explaining human behaviors. In short, the FAE is the tendency to believe that someone's observed behavior is entirely representative or descriptive of who they are as a whole person. The problem with such sweeping conclusions is that behavior changes significantly according to its context, and in reality, most people are very complex and their behaviors are multiply-determined.

For example, imagine that you are working in a community pharmacy and that you are confronted with a frustrated patient. The patient complains about the costs of his pain medications, and also about having to wait for the prescription to be filled. The FAE may lead you to conclude, "This is the kind of person who complains about everything—he's just an irritable person and nothing will satisfy him." Those would be attributions about the patient's personality, which are more durable and unlikely to change. The reality may be that this patient is actually very reasonable and likeable in most other contexts—it's just that right now, he is in pain and distress. These are situational factors. You might not fully appreciate the FAE until a time when you are in pain and distress while waiting for treatment, at which point you become frustrated and demanding towards your caregivers. The FAE might lead you to believe that you are normally a patient, calm individual except that now, you are in a frustrating situation.

Practically everyone is susceptible to the FAE, and it has a clear implication for clinicians. As a pharmacist, you will be interacting with patients when they are sick, and being sick commonly induces distress. That is, being sick is a situational factor that may influence behavior, yet the behavior you observe among your patients may not be at all descriptive of their entire personalities. The individual who presents to you as irritable and demanding at the pharmacy counter may, under most other contexts, be quite calm and patient.

Similar to the FAE is confirmatory bias, where one's attention is focused upon supporting initial impressions about someone else—even to the exclusion of disconfirming evidence. There was the case where a patient attempted to fill a prescription that the pharmacy did not have on hand; when informed of the problem, the patient complained and demanded to speak to the pharmacy manager. The pharmacy manager first met with her staff who advised her that "this patient is slurring his words and is probably drunk." Upon meeting with the disgruntled patient the pharmacy manager fell victim to the confirmatory bias: She operated from the first impression that this patient was intoxicated, and disregarded the patient's assertions to the contrary. It turned out that the patient was dysarthic due to a cerebral vascular accident and he was not intoxicated at all. This part of the patient's medical history might have been revealed had the pharmacy manager assessed him more objectively. Another way of expressing the thinking behind the confirmatory bias is "Don't confuse me with the facts—my mind is made up." The lesson here is to be wary of operating too strongly from first impressions.

Other sources of bias frequently come into play as clinicians interact with patients, and so it is not surprising to learn that clinicians are often more confident in their assessments of patients than they are accurate in those assessments.

SUMMARY

Both Parsons' Sick Role and Suchman's Illness Behavior have stood the test of time. But times have changed, and patient pharmacist interactions are more than ever influenced by social forces. As future roles are expected to expand and direct patient care is predicted to increase, an understanding of the patient as well as social and behavioral aspects of pharmaceutical care are highly pertinent to today's practicing pharmacist. It is important to acknowledge the inherently subjective nature of health care and health care delivery despite the presumed objectivity that is implied in today's science driven approach. Pharmacists are relatively new to direct patient care, and as such there is an increased responsibility on the profession to recognize the dynamic social context of health care practices. Culture has changed and has become more complex and some norms have changed over time. Major changes include (1) recognition of the patient's right to make decisions about his or her treatment; (2) an emphasis on preventive medicine and wellness; (3) recognition of non-adherence; (4) acknowledgment that the traditional Western medicine is only one choice for the ill person, and that rather than true choices people tend to use both conventional medicine and alternative therapies concurrently or complementarily; (5) increase in the use of health insurance, including federal and state programs; (6) the emphasis on cost containment by third parties, including HMOs and managed care; (7) the change from a preponderance of acute conditions to chronic conditions; (8) emphasis on self care; (9) direct-to-consumer advertising; (10) life style drugs; (11) proliferation of "allied health" professionals and paraprofessionals; and (12) demographic changes, incl. aging of America.

Each of these changes is associated with a social dimension relative to pharmacy practice and will be addressed in subsequent chapters of this text.

REFERENCES

1. D. B. Worthen, ed., *The Millis Study Commission on Pharmacy: A Road Map to A Profession's Future* (Binghamton, NY: Pharmaceutical Products Press).

2. L. Doyal, *What Makes Women Sick: Gender and the Political Economy of Health* (New Brunswick, NJ: Rutgers University Press, 1995).

3. G. Harding and K. Taylor, "Social Dimensions of Pharmacy (1) The Social Context of Pharmacy," *The Pharmaceutical Journal* 269 (2002): 395–97.

4. I. Illich, "The Medicalization of Life," *Journal of Medical Ethics*; 1 (2) (1975): 73–77.

5. E. A. Suchman, "Stages of Illness and Medical Care," *Journal of Health and Human Behavior* 6 (1965): 114–128.

6. American Psychiatric Association,"Position Statement on Homosexuality and Civil Rights," *American Journal of Psychiatry* 131 (1973): 497.

7. J. Pratt, "The Rise and Fall of Homophobia and Sexual Psychopath Legislation in Postwar Society," *Psychology, Public Policy, and Law* 4 (1998): 25–49.

8. V. L. Bullough, *Science in the Bedroom: A History of Sex Research* (New York: Harper Collins, 1994).

9. H. J. Baldwin, L.E. Cosler, and R.M. Schulz, "Opinion Leadership in Medication Information," *Communication Quarterly* 35 (1987): 84–102.

10. K. Sadegh-Zadeh, "Fuzzy Health, Illness, and Disease," *Journal of Medicine and Philosophy* 25 (2000): 605–638.

11. M.J. Cherry, "Polymorphic Medical Ontologies: Fashioning Concepts of Disease," *Journal of Medicine and Philosophy* 25 (2000): 519–538.

12. R.J. Lifton, *The Nazi Doctors: Medical Killing and The Psychology of Genocide* (New York: Harper Collins, 1986).

CHAPTER 2

SOCIAL EPIDEMIOLOGY

Angeline Carlison, PhD University of Minnesota College of Pharmacy;
and Chamika Hawkins-Taylor, PhD, South Dakota State University College of Pharmacy

LEARNING OBJECTIVES:

1. Describe the discipline of social epidemiology and its influences on health.
2. List the key historical developments for the field of social epidemiology.
3. Evaluate the influences of social determinants on the health care system, the delivery of health care and disparities in health care.
4. Analyze the societal, economic, cultural and environmental conditions that influence health.
5. Apply concepts of social epidemiology and social determinants of health to pharmacy practice.

KEY TERMS

Health disparities

Health equity

Health-In-All policies

Secondary data analysis

Social determinants of health

Social epidemiology

This chapter provides an orientation to social epidemiology and its influences on health, the healthcare system, and the delivery of health care. Throughout the chapter there will be a broad emphasis on social structures because every aspect of the social world in which we live, work and play has the potential to affect our health. The intent is to apply the concepts introduced in this chapter to the practice of pharmacy.

We will begin with a definition of social epidemiology. Social epidemiology is a branch of epidemiology that studies the distribution and determinants of health and disease in populations while considering the social context in which they occur (Succer, 1973; Krieger, 2001). Social epidemiologists focus on the underlying patterns of health and disease and the root causes for differences in experiences among groups of people (Galea, 2013).

HISTORICAL CONTEXT

Even though social epidemiology was not widely recognized as a discipline until the 1980s, thinking about disease causation within a social context has a long history (Syme, 2005). In 1662, for example, John Graunt, the demographer for London, used "Bills of Mortality" to develop the first lifetable of probabilities of death. He also quantified disease patterns and investigated their association with age, sex, and other factors (Graunt, 1665). In 1840, Louis Rene Villerme, a French physician, published a study of the working conditions of French cotton, wool and silk workers and their elevated levels of illness. His report was the first to stress the importance of the work environment (Coleman, 1982). As a last example, the location of disease outbreaks was investigated by John Snow in London leading to his publication of the Germ Theory of disease in 1849. Snow predicted the mortality impact of cholera in Britain and in 1854 correctly identified the source of a cholera outbreak in London to contaminated water at a street pump. His work led to public action to limit the spread of communicable disease, establishing one of the first priorities of public health (Hempel, 2007).

As a pure definition, the occurrence of disease is biological—disease is an alteration of the anatomy or physiology of the human body (Diez-Roux, 1998; Galea and Link, 2013) and, therefore, 'good health' is simply the absence of disease or illness (Grad, 2002). This bio-medical model of health postulated that a disease or illness was the result of a single, causal factor and the removal of the causal factor would return an individual to a healthy state (Porter, 1997; Wade and Halligan, 2004). Studying disease from the individual perspective led to important understandings of the role of working conditions on disease and mortality.

There have also been important relationships identified for the role that an individual's lifestyle plays in not only the occurrence of the disease but the disease experience (i.e., the manifestation of the disease, the decision to seek health care, the decision to accept treatment recommendations, and the outcomes resulting from these decisions). Today we place great importance on aspects of our lives that contribute to disease. A good example is cardiovascular disease, where lifestyle decisions including diet, exercise, and other risk behaviors such as smoking are recognized as strong contributors to disease risk and ultimately diagnosis.

Beginning in the years following World War II, a new paradigm of health emerged, the 'social model of health' (WHO, 2002). The World Health Organization first described this less biologically dependent idea of health in its constitution signed in 1946. Health was not merely the absence of disease; health was a "complete state of physical, mental and social well-being." This represented a world-wide recognition that disease and illness are, in part, the result of psycho-social factors and not necessarily obvious medical causes. The introduction of the social model of health forced epidemiologists to again consider the dimensions of populations or societies that had been part of the early pioneering efforts to establish epidemiology.

The blending of the two health models (the biologic model and the social model) helps inform our current view of health. The two models are complementary—neither one alone can fully explain the differences in the impact that disease has on the health and well-being of individuals and communities. Both have contributed to a mounting array of evidence arguing for the need to understand and consider the social determinants of health and their role in the public response to community health needs.

SOCIAL DETERMINANTS OF HEALTH AND HEALTH DISPARITIES

Understanding health problems and the etiology of disease requires a critical study of the social determinants of health. A population's health care needs exist within an ever-changing social and environmental backdrop (Kaplan and Lynch, 1997). There are longstanding features of society--poverty, social class, gender, race, and culture—that have been associated with differences in the incidence, prevalence and the treatment of disease and illness that are always present. Other features—environmental, political and economic—carry differing weights of influence over time. These features of society, identified collectively as social determinants, impact the health of populations to differing degrees and work in tandem to impact an individual's or a population's vulnerability to disease and illness (Diez-Roux, 1998).

Numerous models have been developed to explain the interactions among social determinants and prevalence of disease, since the first model was introduced by WHO. They all identify dominant social contributors impacting population health including individual factors; social and community influences; and economic, cultural and environmental conditions at the societal level (Table 2-1). It is important to remember that no one factor works on its own—there are always multiple factors at work. There are strong correlations, for example, between social networks and the experience of disease. Race and ethnicity are factors that are influenced by social norms, and impacted by multiple economic, cultural and environmental conditions that exist at the societal level. Even so, while poor health outcomes may be related to race and ethnicity, they do not explain all instances of poor health, in which case other social determinants are more likely at play (McCartney et al, 2013).

TABLE 2-1: LAYERS OF SOCIAL DETERMINANTS AFFECTING HEALTH

SOCIETAL ECONOMIC, CULTURAL AND ENVIRONMENTAL CONDITIONS						
Agricultural and food production	Education	Environmental Conditions	Employment opportunities	Water and sanitation	Health care services	Housing
SOCIAL AND COMMUNITY INFLUENCES						
Electronic Media	Social Media	Friend and Family Relationships	Community Affiliations	Social Norms	Religious/Spiritual Organizations	Socioeconomic Factors
INDIVIDUAL FACTORS						
Age	Sex	Gender and sexual orientation	Race and Ethnicity	Socioeconomic Status	Educational Attainment	Religious Affiliation

It is also important to note that there are numerous competing needs that must be addressed within a society to achieve what is determined to be an acceptable standard of living. In communities with high unemployment rates, there may be a willingness to give up air quality for the establishment of an industry bringing jobs. More jobs may lead to increases in income for residents. Unfortunately, there will also be an increase in respiratory health concerns. Another example is in the raising of animals for meat. Government regulators may allow the use of antibiotics to address problems introduced with large scale production but in doing so may expose consumers to harm from these drugs.

SOCIOECONOMIC STATUS

Social epidemiology assumes that the distribution of health and disease in a society reflects the distribution of wealth and resources in that society (Honjo, 2004). In general wealthy individuals enjoy good health and the means to satisfy all of their health care needs. In that regard, the United States should be considered the healthiest of nations given its status as one of the world's wealthiest countries. This is not the case, however, because of the many levels of disparities that exist within this nation's borders. Therefore, social epidemiology seeks to understand and explain the impact of socioeconomic status on health.

Despite America's wealth, millions of American families are food insecure with family incomes below poverty level. This same population is more likely to bear the consequences of obesity and poor diet, develop chronic diseases at a faster rate and be treated at later stages of disease (Abegunde et al, 2007). Foods most readily available to low-income persons are those high in fat, calories, sodium and sugar, and may not provide adequate nutrition.

On a daily basis, persons of low economic status face difficult decisions—buy food or buy medications; pay for heat or go hungry—decisions not faced by higher SES individuals. According to the USDA the cost of food at home for a family of four with a low cost food plan was $722 per month or $8,664 per year (USDA, 2015). For a family of 4 earning the 2014 median US income of $53,600 (DeNavis-Walt and Proctor,

2015), this expense represents 16% of their income. For a family of 4 at 133% of the federal poverty level of $32,252 (the ACA expanded coverage level) this expense represents 27% of their income—more than one-fourth of the income needed to provide for all of the needs of a family.

Socioeconomic status (SES) also encompasses educational attainment, employment, and other social benefits that are directly related to factors like social standing, and the ability to satisfy basic life needs like housing (Phelan et al, 2010). For example, a person with a high SES can afford to live in a neighborhood populated by persons of similar SES status. Collectively they are able to exert social and political influence to ensure that crime, noise, violence, pollution, traffic and unsanitary conditions are minimized. Their shared collective influence also ensures high quality social activities, recreational opportunities (parks, playgrounds), community resources like grocery stores and service companies and health-care facilities in close proximity, all of which are associated with better health (Phelan et al, 2010). Thus, a person with high SES receives health benefits in less obvious ways that lower SES persons cannot.

Research has established relationships between SES and health that help to explain differences in the etiology of diseases or illnesses, the personal and community experience of diseases and illnesses, the access to health care services to treat diseases and illnesses, and ultimately the causes of death (Susser and Susser, 1996; Diez-Roux, 1998; Honjo, 2004; Phelan et al, 2010). Since the earliest studies of SES and health, health status improves as economic means increase (Adler and Ostrove, 2006). Widespread manifestations of disease, some urinary and bladder afflictions (Ansari and Gupta, 2003), for instance are linked to lack of wealth and diet deficiencies. Social environment and economic conditions have also gained greater attention as important causal factors in the pathway from chronic kidney disease risk to the development and complications of the disease (Nicholas et al, 2015).

Individuals are born into social classes where they may live in environments overwhelmed with air pollution and chemical contaminants affecting their food and water, leading to differential exposure to pathogens and carcinogens. They also will live in poor housing where contaminants like lead and carbon monoxide are more evident. Persons may also have the unfortunate reality of residing in communities where crime is rampant, educational opportunities are few and household stress is virtually unmanageable (Hilfiker, 2000). These environmental concerns, largely outside of the individual's control, have large impacts on health.

As a result of their social standing, individuals may practice certain health behaviors that have a damaging effect on their health. Smoking, unhealthy eating, physical inactivity, alcohol and drug use are regular culprits of poor health and all have an effect on a person's mortality. The *Health and Retirement Study*, a longitudinal, biennial survey of a national sample of adults born between 1931 and 1941, investigated the extent to which these factors supported the association between SES and all-cause mortality. Researchers found that after ten years, the most economically disadvantaged had a higher risk ratio, most of which was due to their poor health practices (Nandi et al, 2014). A retrospective analysis of data from the Whitehall II study showed similar results among British subjects, where approximately one-half to three-quarters of the association between SES and mortality were mediated by poor health behaviors (Nandi et al, 2014).

Social programs have attempted to address health-related SES disparities. Government programs in the U.S., like Medicare and Medicaid, were originally created in an attempt to mitigate income and resource challenges experienced by elders and low-income families with children. Medicare, established by the Johnson Administration in 1965, has provided universal access to health care services primarily for the age group sixty-five and older. Medicaid, also established in 1965, is a shared state and federal program providing coverage to nearly 60 million Americans, including children, pregnant women, parents, seniors and individuals with disabilities.

The Affordable Care Act (ACA) is the latest U.S. national policy attempt to bring forward changes to the nation's health care system. It aims to decrease the number of uninsured, improve quality of care, diversify the workforce and incentivize providers to better serve underserved urban and rural areas. For lower income individuals the ACA subsidizes private based insurance premiums, allowing them greater access to health insurance policies that meet acceptable standards of coverage (HHS, 2015). The ACA, for instance, authorizes the federal government to offer resources to states so that they may expand their Medicaid programs. However, even with government support, a number of states have rejected the notion of expansion citing its potential high cost. Proponents of expansion suggest that the likely cost reductions in prevention of mortality, particularly with the use of prescription drug therapies in underserved or vulnerable populations, far outweigh the costs required to expand the program (Kesselheim et al, 2015).

Even with local, national and international efforts, SES continues to have a measurable impact on health. This idea is demonstrated in Medicare patients with recurring myocardial infarction (MI) where access to care services was not a challenge; still patients with lower educational levels had both higher reoccurrence of MI and higher mortality rates (Coady et al, 2014). The same is true for chronic conditions like diabetes where, despite the availability of health insurance through Medicaid and Medicare and in spite of increased funding for research and prevention initiatives, approximately 14 million people suffer from the disease—6% of whom are Native American and Alaskan Native (CDC, 2014). The Department of Health and Human Services, Indian Health Service Division, offers low cost or no cost disease prevention and management programs, but still the American Native population suffers from diabetes prevalence and complications at alarming rates (Chow et al, 2012). Socioeconomic inequalities in health are very large, very robust, and have remained remarkably unchanged over time. Society's poor and less privileged members live in worse health and die earlier than more privileged members (Phelan et al, 2010).

RACE AND ETHNICITY

There is a large body of evidence demonstrating the influence of race and ethnicity on health; the incidence and prevalence of disease; the individual, family and community experience of disease and illness; access to health care services; the quality of health care services received; and the level of patient participation in shared decision-making and self-management of disease. Various indicators of race and ethnicity have been used in these studies including native language; cultural norms; religious and spiritual traditions and values; geographic origin; ancestral and family patterns;

relationship formation and the quality of relationships; attitudes toward illness and disease; and attitudes toward treatment (Williams, 2005). Other indicators related to race and ethnicity, such as life stress and psychological, social and emotional stress related to the experience of discrimination, have also been included in these studies.

Race and ethnicity also play a role in the choice of treatment, the effectiveness of treatment and treatment outcomes of chronic diseases. The Institute of Medicine's 2002 report, *Unequal Treatment: Confronting Racial and Ethnic Disparities in Health Care*, highlighted studies assessing health disparities from each stage of the care process. Effectiveness of treatment was poor in many minority patients for a wide variety of reasons including low health literacy, mistrust in the provider, a history of unpleasant experiences with the health care system, poor knowledge on how to navigate the health care system, and poor provider-patient communication (IOM, 2002). Many non-white individuals delayed seeking necessary care, did not comply with treatment regimens, or sought care when a positive outcome was not likely (IOM, 2002).

Many studies find that the process of selecting the appropriate treatment for a patient is often a difficult one. Providers compare the risks and benefits for each treatment option while considering the individual patient's characteristics. Unfortunately, in many cases, this practice is tainted by clinical uncertainty, provider bias and perpetual stereotypes (Balsa and McGuire, 2003). Health professionals' interactions with patients and caregivers are influenced by their own views of race, ethnicity, gender, sexuality, socioeconomic status, and spirituality. These concepts--what social psychologists call "group characterizations"—can have a negative impact on the entire health care experience (Balsa and McGuire, 2003). It is a two way street, however. Minority patients' responses to healthcare providers can also be a source of disparities. Minority patients can convey mistrust of the health care system in general and individual providers. That mistrust can result in the refusal of treatment or affect medication taking behaviors, which in turn can lead to provider disengagement and less willingness to pursue vigorous treatment options (IOM, 2002).

In a study assessing breast cancer treatment choices by race, for example, patients who were African American, Mexican, and Puerto Rican were 20% to 50% more likely to receive or elect a treatment not meeting the national standard of care (Li et al, 2003). Mortality rates among these groups were also higher than white patients, although it has often been reported that non-white patients tend to seek medical treatment at later stages of disease and often only in emergent situations (Li et al, 2003).

Heart failure is another of many examples (Hawkins-Taylor and Carlson, 2013). Heart failure is suggested to manifest differently in black patients than in other races. The disease tends to occur due to the interplay of co-morbidities such as high blood pressure, high cholesterol, diabetes and poor management of those conditions. There are even instances of response differences to drug therapy for heart failure based on racial group. For instance, a retrospective analysis of Veterans Heart Failure Trial data in the 1990s, suggested that a fixed-dose combination of isosorbide dinitrate and hydralazine (later branded BiDil®) produced significantly better treatment outcomes when added to an established heart failure treatment protocol. These findings were later confirmed in the African American Heart Failure Trial in early 2004 and led to a modification of heart failure guidelines to include this drug therapy as part of the treatment plan. These same studies identified diuretics as a more effective first-line therapy for black patients than the established ACE Inhibitor drug class (Hawkins, 2010; Hawkins-Taylor and Carlson, 2013).

Race and ethnicity indicators may also determine or explain perpetual disadvantages and barriers. Considering race disparities, African Americans live shorter lives than whites and this rate is even greater at younger ages. The death rate for Blacks between ages one to four and twenty-five to fifty-four is more than two times that of white individuals. While historical accounts suggest that the health disparities due to race may be attributed to underlying biological characteristics (Kriegar, 1987), the census data has shown that socioeconomic factors--housing, home ownership, education, employment status and poverty—all facilitate health gaps that persist among minority racial and ethnic groups.

The literature on racial disparities details the problems that constantly plague minority care seekers. Research not only brings to bear problems of access, inadequate treatment, and cultural biases, it also tells a frightening tale of unequal and unethical treatment. There are historical, documented instances of physicians, often motivated by social or political agendas, performing immoral and unethical acts without regard for the human beings who were subject to their experiments. In *The Immortal Life of Henrietta Lacks*, Rebecca Skloot identified experimentation on vulnerable, often minority patients, calling them "illegal, immoral, deplorable." Skloot was referring to the long history of so-called clinical trials where the mistreatment of patients led to worsening disease states or death. She told the story of Henrietta Lacks and the unethical cultivating and use of her cells for research long after her death in 1951 (Skloot, 2010). Henrietta's cells, known in the science community as "HeLa Cells," are an immortal cell line whose scientific study has resulted in remarkable advances such as a vaccine for Polio, the development of chemotherapy as a course of cancer treatment, gene mapping among countless others (Skloot, 2010).

Among the abusive clinical trials, the most infamous of cruel and unethical schemes was the Tuskegee Syphilis Experiment where black men from Tuskegee, Alabama, infected with syphilis, were kept in hospital research settings and observed for symptoms, but were denied treatment long after a cure was discovered. Beginning in 1932, this experiment would continue for forty years without the affected being offered the curative penicillin. Discovery of this experiment was the turning point for the development of rules and standards for the responsible and ethical conduct of research and implementation of an institutional review board to approve studies regarding human subjects (Howard-Jones, 1982). This particular study is blamed for the reluctance of many African Americans to participate in clinical trials even today.

Henrietta Lacks and the Tuskegee trials are part of an unfortunate legacy of unethical treatment for research purposes in the United States. In the early 1900s to around the 1940s researchers were known to infect captives with infectious diseases such as cholera and bubonic plague. There was also a practice of starving prisoners of war to cause vitamin B-1 deficiency, ultimately resulting in the cardiac-affecting disease beriberi. These scandals of the past, generations of discriminatory behavior towards minority groups, and a lack of transparency about medical research have led to a lack of trust between patients and their health care providers and far worse, a failure to seek care until conditions are exacerbated if care is sought at all.

The overall goal in addressing health disparities associated with race and ethnicity differences has always been to achieve fair and equitable treatment for all. The basic premise of the literature is that vulnerable groups receive lower quality health care often due to lack of health insurance, inadequate access to affordable care and numerous other complicating issues like language barriers, poor health literacy, stereotyping and bias that contribute to poor patient-provider communication.

AGE

Age is generally considered a demographic variable but as a social determinant it is a powerful driver of health and health care needs. Age is associated with cultural roles, social position and wealth, all of which impact access to important resources. Age is, therefore, a vital factor in determining a population's burden of disease.

Specific risk factors and determinants of health vary across the life span. An inability to reduce the burden of illness for a number of diseases and illnesses can be due to the influence of age in combination with other individual and social determinants of health that can accumulate over time. Social epidemiologists are challenged to identify specific points of intervention in the life course, a Life Span approach, and interventions that will reduce risk factors and promote health (Healthy People 2020). An example is the increasing prevalence of Type II diabetes, identified as a public health epidemic in the United States and world-wide. Interventions earlier in the lifespan to reduce childhood obesity and increase physical activity coupled with education about nutritional choices, improved access to nutritional resources, and preventive health care to monitor for known risk factors are all considered important strategies in efforts to address this epidemic.

At the same time there is a need to balance the competing needs of all age segments. As people age they require an increasingly larger share of health care funds, resources, and attention to address the age-related burden of chronic diseases. The political influence of older citizens is strong, and there are researchers who believe that, because of this political clout, health care programs will focus on elderly health care issues at the expense of the needs, primarily preventive, of younger generations. For proponents of health care rationing this larger share is problematic and they propose that Medicare refrain from paying for life-extending medical care in the late stages of life. These individuals argue that the economy is already taxed to capacity in its attempt to support life-extending therapeutics and technologies for the elderly and should only cover routine or palliative care (Callahan, 1996). Many have found this idea unethical. Before the implementation of the Affordable Care Act in 2013, health care rationing largely forced the unhealthy to pay higher costs for health services— the smoker, the obese, and the chronically ill, for instance paid more. Coincidentally, many in this unhealthy group were older individuals.

Rationing of healthcare was considered a concept of the 1990s, but there is actually a long history of health care policy decisions resulting in rationing, and the concept has been reborn in the dialog regarding health care reform. Supporters of health care rationing suggest giving greater support to the young who mostly require preventive care and can be more productive in society, in their opinion (Bowling, 1997). The challenge for public policy is the need to provide adequate opportunities to ensure the social well-being of all citizens (Knickman and Snell, 2002).

SEX, GENDER, AND SEXUAL ORIENTATION

Sex categories, male and female, are biologically and physiologically determined definitions of men and women while gender categories, masculine and feminine, are socially constructed self-characterizations of an individual (WHO, 2015). As social determinants, sex and gender classifications impact income earnings, social power and influence. They also impact access to health promoting resources, health prevention and care access, most often negatively impacting those identifying as feminine or woman. Numerous medical study and treatment practices are based on research done on males. Even the dynamics of social relationships are different among genders, considered more emotionally supportive among and more stressful among women (Umberson et al, 2014).

How sex and gender characterizations play out in society may have significant implications for health. The patterns of health and disease are different among men and women and therefore, must be understood and treated uniquely in the case of many chronic diseases. Considering women, it was not until the year 2000 with the launch of *The Heart Truth* campaign by the National Institutes of Health that heart disease, the leading cause of death among women, made this a priority for and about women (Long et al, 2008). Even today the campaign continues to increase awareness among women that heart disease is a primary death threat for them. It also encourages women to know their risk, speak to their physicians and take action. Before *The Heart Truth* campaign, heart disease was thought of as a man's disease and gave little attention to women as a priority group (Long et al, 2008).

In recent years, understanding of sex and gender differences has called for greater priority to be given to reframing health service delivery toward more gender sensitive care. There is a need to have practitioners care for patients with an eye toward biological characteristics, sexual orientation (heterosexual, homosexual, and transgender persons) and gender roles (Doyal, 2003). In the Lesbian, Gay, Bisexual and Transgender (LGBT) community efforts to improve care have focused on changing attitudes among practitioners and minimizing stereotypes and biases (Lim et al, 2014).

EDUCATION

Education or academic achievement is a social determinant that strongly influences other social elements impacting health. Some have called education the most important social determinant of health because of its robust connection to and impact on health behaviors—diets, daily physical activity, attention to mind and body.

Level of education determines how well an individual will take care of basic health needs and take personal responsibility for their own health. From 2007–2010 higher levels of education for the head of household resulted in lower rates of obesity among boys and girls 2–19 years of age. In 2010, 31 percent of adults 25–64 years of age with a high school diploma or less education were current smokers, compared with 24 percent of adults with some college and 9 percent of adults with a bachelor's degree or higher.

Conversely, health may impact potential for academic achievement. Thus, the relationship between health and education goes in two directions (Ickovics et al, 2014). People with higher levels of education and higher income have lower rates of many chronic diseases according to a 2011 report of the CDC's National Center for Health Statistics. Reports suggest that students with disabilities or chronic diseases have poor academic achievement, and those who do not do well in school tend to have more comorbid conditions as adults and premature mortality (Fiscella and Kitzman, 2009). Even from an early age health and education are influenced by conditions such as school readiness, family structure and poverty level almost shaping an individual's destiny from the very start of life (Ickovics et al, 2014).

Besides school readiness and socioeconomic factors, indicators of education have included kindergarten to high school attendance and academic performance, high school graduation rates, college or post-secondary education and completion. The most used academic achievement indicator, however, is self-reported grades (often as grade point average), although recent studies have suggested that standardized test scores should be used instead (Ickovics et al, 2014). Regardless of how they are defined, academic influences are determinants of where employment status is attained, in what communities one lives, the social circle and social relationships that are formed and ultimately the socioeconomic status and planning for posterity. College graduates live at least five years longer than high school dropouts (RWJF, 2013). Similar studies suggest that higher achieving individuals are more likely to avoid common acute and chronic disease diagnoses such as heart disease and diabetes. This group is also less likely to struggle with weight issues and is more likely to lead healthy lifestyles (Burgard and Hawkins, 2014).

Given that academic achievement is associated with lifestyle, it would appear that health prevention methods during the formative academic years would have a positive impact on academic achievement. Indeed, healthy eating and regular physical exercise were associated with high cognitive functioning and academic success (Edwards et al, 2011). To the contrary, obesity and low activity level were associated with low cognitive functioning and lower overall achievement (Edwards et al, 2011). In a randomized, controlled trial, students participated in a short term exercise program. After just thirteen weeks, students showed increased brain functioning, execution function and mathematic achievement (Davis et al, 2011).

Recognition of the strong connection between education and health has recently led to a push for policy development promoting positive health practices as a means to improve academic proficiency in United States schools. First Lady Michelle

Obama's *Let's Move* campaign, launched in 2010 to address the growing epidemic of childhood obesity, targeted schools in efforts to promote healthier school foods and increased physical activity before, during and after school. Now five years since its inception schools nationwide have committed to making nutrition and fitness a priority to improve the health of all children (www.let'smove.gov). The Institute of Medicine 2012 report, *Accelerating Progress in Obesity Prevention*, evaluated obesity prevention strategies and concluded that we must "strengthen schools as the heart of health" (IOM, 2012).

SOCIAL GAPS IN THE DELIVERY OF HEALTH CARE

Health inequalities have been remarkably resistant to change or to geography, being demonstrated worldwide (McCartney et al, 2013). Acknowledgement of the theory of social determinants of health has challenged the field of epidemiology to more comprehensively assess the underlying reasons for the experience of disease and poor health. Individual characteristics and responsibility for health must be considered within a larger context of social, political and economic conditions. Populations are made up of individuals making personal choices about diet, exercise and smoking that are associated with chronic diseases like diabetes and hypertension. These individual decisions are made within a larger social context—as a member of a social group that may have a cultural propensity for rich, high-fat diets or, because they are living in a community with poor economic development characterized as a food desert, are limited in their access to nutritious foods. They may also be persons of racial or ethnic groups working in low-income jobs that do not provide adequate financial resources to afford more nutritious, but generally more expensive, foods.

The inequities in how society is organized means that the freedom to lead a flourishing life and to enjoy good health is unequally distributed between and within societies. The inequities are seen early—in access to prenatal care, in birth outcomes, and in the conditions of early childhood and schooling. They continue throughout the lifespan—in the nature of employment and working conditions, access to housing, and the quality of the natural environment in which people reside. Depending on the nature of these environments, different groups will have varied experiences of material conditions, psychosocial support, and behavioral options, which make them more or less vulnerable to poor health (WHO, 2008).

Since 1979, the federal *Healthy People* initiative has guided the United States' approach to improving population health. A new version of Healthy People is issued each decade and features updated goals and identifies topic areas and quantifiable objectives for health improvement for the succeeding ten years (Green and Fielding, 2011). The current version, *Healthy People 2020*, has been informed by the body of work on the role of disadvantage and health—how social and economic conditions affect our health and survival (Koh et al, 2011;Fielding et al, 2013). *Healthy People 2020* has been organized using a "Health Determinants and Health Outcomes by Life Stages" conceptual framework (Healthy People 2020). There are 12 Leading Health Indicator (LHI) topics that help draw attention to both individual and societal determinants that affect the public's health and contribute to health disparities from infancy through old age (Healthy People 2020). These LHI topics include indicators addressing access to health services, environmental quality, injury and violence, nutrition/physical activity/obesity and educational attainment (Healthy People 2020).

ACHIEVING HEALTH EQUITY

Traditionally, society has looked to the health sector to deal with its concerns about health and disease. The focus of public policy has been directed at the delivery of health care and the dominant view of modern health care facilities as repair shops for bodies gone wrong. Policies directly aimed at a health concern will not be adequate to address the influences that the social determinants of health present. Even if the incidence and prevalence of disease were equally distributed among all social levels, the experience of the disease would be unequal due to the imbalance of the influences of the social determinants of health. Barriers that make it impossible for some persons to make healthy choices must be addressed (IOM, 2014).

Attention is now being focused on addressing the greater influences of the social determinants of health. To achieve health equity, action must involve the whole of government, civil society and local communities, business, and international agencies. Policies and programs must embrace all the key sectors of society—health and non-health sectors alike. The unequal distribution of health-damaging experiences is the result of a combination of poor social policies and programs, unfair economic arrangements, and politics (WHO, 2008). Agencies focused on transportation, the environment, consumer protection, and agriculture have an equal share in the responsibility for the health of society on a global basis (WHO, 2008; International Fund for Agriculture Development, 2011). To recognize this multi-layered, multi-factorial need, recent public health and social writing has introduced the concept of "Health in All Policies" (APHA, 2013).

Health in All Policies (HiAP) is often identified as multi-sectored and multi-layered because it is an approach to improve population health that should develop seamlessly from other initiatives and across government policy issues. A number of definitions of HiAP exist, but all have in common the considerations of health implications across policy sectors. Fully operationalizing HiAP requires new frameworks, leadership structures, processes and measurement. It requires a shared understanding of health determinants in non-health sectors such as transportation, environment, and agriculture. This movement requires the removal of the typical silo culture among government areas.

At its origins is a spirit of multi-sectored collaboration—alignment of interests and focus on health inequities (Storm et al, 2011). European countries, who are leaders in their commitment to a HiAP government approach, consider a broad vision of health and the influence of health in all governmental areas (Storm et al, 2011). HiAP is large scale action to improve health through attention to the full range of health determinants. It should develop seamlessly out of other initiatives that are not primarily health focused (Greaves and Bialystok, 2011). According to the leading models, foundations of HiAP should include a strong cross-governmental focus; central government mandate and central coordination; flexible and adaptable methods of inquiry; mutual gain and collaboration; dedicated resources; and joint decision-making and accountability.

Fully operationalizing HiAP requires new organizational frameworks, leadership structures, processes and measures. It requires horizontal (cross-governmental) approaches and vertical (hierarchical) commitment. Addressing health through public policy makes health an all-encompassing goal for policymakers. All policies contribute to health in some way. Some, like the 2013 Affordable Care Act (ACA) in the United States, have a direct connection. The ACA has attempted to temper socioeconomic health determinants by improving access to health insurance and health services for economically disadvantaged families.

A primary goal of HiAP is to equip decision-makers with information about how choices made within *non-health policy* sectors also influence health and health equity (WHO, 2008; APHA, 2013). Policies that address minimum wage, safe work environments, housing for homeless and low-income persons, parenting leaves of absence, educational financing, environmental protection and even the regulation of lending practices have implications for health improvements because of their mediating effects on social determinants. Health disparities that lead to reduced productivity and premature death represent a substantial loss of talent that impacts all of society. Socioeconomic inequalities are also costly—more than $1 trillion dollars per year to the US economy by some estimates (IOM, 2014).

DATA AND MEASUREMENT IN SOCIAL EPIDEMIOLOGY

Social epidemiologists and other researchers have had great difficulty investigating the role of the social determinants of health and other aspects of health care utilization and expenditures due to a lack of complete, timely, and large population-based surveillance data (Placzek and Madoff, 2014). Social structures continually change and so do health care systems, health care delivery and how health care is financed in response to demographic trends, political pressures and other forces.

The evolution of health information technology has changed the way social epidemiologists study the health of populations and the social factors that impact health care use (Barrowman, 2014). Social epidemiologists are not presented with opportunities to manipulate large-scale social influences or political factors to study outcomes (Galea and Link, 2013), so using what is now referred to as big data, researchers can study health outcomes and health care utilization on large groups of people by age, sex, geographic location, health insurance status and benefits, and other demographic characteristics over time. Large databases suitable for epidemiologic research are available from a number of sources. In the United States, population-based health surveys like the *Behavioral Risk Factor Surveillance System* (BRFSS), the *National Health Interview Survey* and the *National Health and Nutrition Examination Survey*, are available from the Centers for Disease Control and Prevention. Technology also allows social epidemiologists to combine information from large databases with information recorded in national surveys and demographic information obtained from census reports and other sources of vital statistics.

Large databases offer social epidemiologists and other health service researchers a number of advantages. The data is more easily obtainable than collecting primary data for a single study and, therefore, the overall cost of conducting the research is less expensive. The number of patients that will meet study inclusion criteria is large and events that would otherwise go unnoticed may become visible. Large databases may offer, for instance, a chance to examine the health care utilization of persons with relatively uncommon health conditions and to obtain a better understanding of the health care services provided to them. Small populations that engage in unique health behaviors may emerge through modelling efforts with large databases and small clusters of illness and/or rare adverse events to medical treatments may also become noticeable.

In using large databases, however, it is important to remember that the data has usually been collected for purposes other than social epidemiology studies. Health insurance claims databases contain information about health service use for the purpose of providing payment to providers. Electronic medical record databases contain archival information about health encounters from the health provider perspective only; an EMR is both a patient care record and a detailed document to substantiate requests for payment. Census data is collected to provide an enumeration of a large population group and underlying demographic characteristics of that group. Large national health surveys have underlying purposes for the data gathering exercise defined by a government agency or a legislative need. Combining data from multiple sources that was collected for widely differing purposes can be problematic and raises questions about data ownership for the original and the enhanced data sets.

Conducting research on data collected for other purposes can also introduce problems with the interpretation of findings. Epidemiology studies are generally observational and, therefore, cannot demonstrate causality. While this is true for any observational study, the number of observations contained in large databases can lead to false assumptions about the truth of the findings; researchers who work with large databases must guard against interpretation of findings that go beyond the data, no matter how large it may be (Barrowman, 2014). With very large samples, relationships between variables can easily be statistically significant so that relying on p-values can lead to conclusion with no practical usefulness (Lin et al, 2013). Patterns that are identified in large databases may also be difficult to apply in clinical practice where the population of interest is much smaller. This area of social epidemiology efforts, called translational science, is still in its infancy.

Working with large databases also requires large capacity computing resources and the technical skills needed to manipulate the data. Computer technology has advanced significantly, increasing the ability to collect, download, analyze and report on extremely large numbers of health care occurrences. The application of privacy and security rules under the Health Insurance Portability and Accountability Act (HIPAA) must be carefully considered given the advances that have occurred. A balance between data security and data availability is delicate. The highly personal nature of the underlying patient-professional exchanges that lead to the data used to study health care means that concerns about patient privacy and data security must be thoughtfully addressed (Neff, 2013).

Despite these concerns large databases provide an opportunity to identify underlying care delivery differences that exist between disparate social groups, geographic areas, health insurance status and other aspects of social structures. These differences, that in the past were hypothesized or shown to exist in smaller isolated population studies, are now readily visible in large databases and, as the results become more widely disseminated, will help inform our collective response to the unequal impact of the social determinants of health and the wide variation and quality of health care practices that are present today.

SUMMARY

This chapter presented a review of social epidemiology's focus on the root causes for differences in the experience of disease and illness by groups of people. Longstanding features of society—poverty, social class, gender, race, and culture—have been associated with differences in the incidence, prevalence, and the treatment of disease and illness. Other features—environmental, political and economic—carry differing weights of influence over time. These features of society, identified collectively as social determinants, impact the health of populations to differing degrees, however, the discipline of social epidemiology is founded on the assumption that all health outcomes are inextricably tied to social context. A full understanding of health problems and the etiology of disease requires a critical study of these social determinants of health, because a population's health care needs exist within an ever-changing social and environmental backdrop.

REFERENCES

1. Adler, N.E. & Ostrove, J.M. (2006). Socioeconomic status and health: What we know and what we don't. *The Annals of the New York Academy of Sciences.* 896(1): 3–15.

2. American Public Health Association. (October 1, 2013). New guide helps state and local governments incorporate health in all policies. Available at: http://www.apha.org/NR/rdonlyres/7D35E8A9-9429-4072-993B-0211214E1CDF/0/HiAPGuide_4pager_FINAL.pdf

3. Ansari, M.S. & Gupta, N.P. (2003). Impact of socioeconomic status in etiology and management of urinary stone disease. *Urology International,* 70(4): 255–261.

4. Balsa, A.L. & McGuire, T.G. (2003). Prejudice, clinical uncertainty and stereotyping as sources of health disparities. *Journal of Health Economics* 22: 89–116.

5. Bambra, C., Gibson, M., Sowden, A., et al. (2010). Tackling the wider social determinants of health and health inequalities: Evidence from systematic reviews. *J Epidemiol Community Health* 64: 284–291.

6. Barrowman, N. (2014). Correlation, causation, and confusion. *The New Atlantis* (No. 43): 23–44.

7. Braveman, P., Egerter, S., & Williams, D.R. (2011). The social determinants of health: coming of age. *Annu Rev Public Health* 32: 381–398.

8. Burgard, S. & Hawkins, J.M. (2014). Race/ethnicity, educational attainment, and foregone health care in the United States in the 2007–2009 Recession. *American Journal of Public Health*. 104: e134–e140.

9. CDC. (2014). *Estimates of diabetes and its burden in the United States.* Available at: http://www.cdc.gov/diabetes/pubs/statsreport14/national-diabetes-report-web.pdf

10. Chow, E.A., Foster, H., Gonzalez, V., & McIver, L. (2012). The disparate impact of diabetes on racial/ethnic minorities. *Clinical Diabetes* 30: 130–133.

11. Coady, S.A., Johnson, N.J., Hakes, J.K., & Sorlie, P.D. (2014). Individual education, area income, and mortality and recurrence of myocardial infarction in a Medicare cohort: The National Longitudinal Mortality Study. BMC Public Health, 14: 705–716.

12. Coleman, W. (1982). *Death is a social disease: Public health and political economy in early industrial France.* Madison, Wis.: University of Wisconsin Press.

13. Covey, L.S., Botello-Harbaum, M., Glassman, A.H., et al. (2008). Smokers' response to combination bupropion, nicotine patch, and counseling treatment by race/ethnicity. *Ethnicity and Disease* 18(1): 59–64.

14. Davis, C.L., Tomporowski, P.D., McDowell, J.E., et al. (2011). Exercise improves executive function and achievement and alters brain activation in overweight children: a randomized controlled trial. *Journal of Health Psychology*, 30(1): 91–98.

15. deFortuny, E.J., Martens, D.E., & Provost, F. Predictive modeling with big data: Is bigger really better? *Big Data* 1 (4): 215–226.

16. Department of Health and Human Services. Indian Health Service. (2015). Division of Diabetes Treatment and Prevention. http://www.ihs.gov/medicalprograms/diabetes.

17. Doyal, L. (2003). Sex and gender: The challenges for epidemiologists. *International Journal of Health Services*, 33(3): 569–579.

18. Edwards, J.U., Mauch, L., & Winkelman, M.R. (2011). Relationship of nutrition and physical activity behaviors and fitness measures to academic performance for sixth graders in a Midwest city school district. *Journal of School Health*, 8(2): 65–73.

19. Fielding, J.E., Kumanyika, S., & Manderscheid, R.W. (2013). A perspective on the development of the Healthy People 2020 framework for improving U.S. population health. *Public Health Reviews* 35 (1): 1-24.

20. Fiscella, K. & Kitzman, H. (2009). Disparities in academic achievement and health: the intersection of child education and health policy. *Pediatrics*, 123(3): 1073–1080.

21. Galea, S. & Link, B.G. (2013). Six paths for the future of social epidemiology. *American Journal of Epidemiology* 178 (6): 843–849

22. Graunt, J. (1665). *Natural and political observations mentioned in a following index, and made upon the bills of mortality: With reference to the government, religion, trade, growth, air, diseases, and the several changes of the said city* (4th. impression. ed.). Oxford: [publisher not identified].

23. Greaves, L.J. & Bialystok, L.R. (2011). Health in all policies—All talk little action? *Canadian Journal of Public Health*, 102(6): 407–9.

24. Green, L.W. & Fielding, J. (2011). The U.S. Healthy People initiative; its genesis and its sustainability. *Annual Review of Public Health* 32: 451–70.

25. Hawkins, C. (2010). *Targeted drugs and market failure: The case of BiDil (RTM)*. University of Minnesota, ProQuest, UMI Dissertations Publishing.

26. Hawkins-Taylor, C. & Carlson, A. (2013). Communication strategies must be tailored to a medication's targeted population: lessons from the case of BiDil. *American Health & Drug Benefits* 6 (7): 401–412.

27. *Healthy People 2020.* Available at: https://www.healthypeople.gov/http://www.hhs.gov/healthcare/rights. (2015). About the law. Accessed: March 24, 2015.

28. Hempel, S. (2007). *The strange case of the Broad Street pump: John Snow and the mystery of cholera.* Berkeley: University of California Press.

29. Hilfiker, D. (2000). *Poverty in Urban America: Its causes its cures.* The Potter's House Book Service. Washington, D.C.

30. Ickovics, J.R., Carroll-Scott, A., & Peters, S.M., et al. (2014). Health and academic achievement: Cumulative effects of health assets on standardized test scores among urban youth in the United States. *Journal of School Health*, 84: 40–48.

31. Institute of Medicine. (2002). *Unequal treatment: Confronting racial and ethnic disparities in health care.* Washington, DC: The National Academies Press.

32. Institute of Medicine. (2012). *Accelerating progress in obesity prevention: Solving the weight of the nation.* Washington, DC: The National Academies Press.

33. Institute of Medicine. (2014). *Applying a health lens to decision making in non-health sectors: Workshop summary.* Washington, DC: The National Academies Press.

34. International Fund for Agricultural Development. *Rural poverty report*. Rome, Italy, (2011). Available at: http://www.ifad.org/rpr2011/report/e/rpr(2011).pdf.

35. Kesselheim, A.S., Huybrechts, K.F., Choudry, N.K. et al. (2015). Prescription drug coverage and patient health outcomes: A systematic review. *American Journal of Public Health* 105: e17–e30.

36. Kingston, R.S. & Smith, J.P. (1997). Socioeconomic status and racial and ethnic differences in functional status associated with chronic diseases. *American Journal of Public Health* 87 (5): 805–810.

37. Knickman, J.R. & Snell, E.K. (2002). The 2030 problem: caring for aging baby boomers. *Health Services Research* 37 (4): 849–884.

38. Koh, H.K., Kumanyika, S., & Fielding, J.E. (2011). Healthy People: a 2020 vision for the social determinants approach. *Health Education & Behavior* 38 (6): 551–557.

39. Kriegar, N. (1987). Shades of difference: Theoretical underpinnings of the medical controversy on black/white differences in the United States, 1830–1870. *International Journal of Health Services*, 17, 259–278.

40. Krieger, N. (2001). Theories for social epidemiology in the 21st century: An ecosocial perspective. *International Journal of Epidemiology* 30: 668–671.

41. LaViest, T.A., Gaskin, D.J., & Richard, P. (2009). *The economic burden of health inequalities in the United States*. Joint Center for Political and Economic Studies. Available at: http://hsrc.himmelfarb.gwu.edu/sphhs_policy_facpubs/225/

42. Le-Scherban, F., Diez-Roux, A.V., Y Li, Y., & Morgenstern, H. (2014). Does academic achievement during childhood and adolescence benefit later health? *Annals of Epidemiology* 24(5): 344–355.

43. Li, C.I., Malonem, K.E., & Daling, J.R. (2003). Differences in breast cancer stage, treatment and survival by race and ethnicity. *Archives of Internal Medicine* 163 (1): 49–56.

44. Lim, F.A., Brown, D.V., & Kim, S.M.J. (2014). Addressing health care disparities in the lesbian, gay, bisexual and transgender population: A review of best practices. *American Journal of Nursing*, 114(6): 24–34.

45. Lin, M., Lucas, H.C., & Shmueli, G. (2013). Too big to fail: Large samples and the p-value problem. *Information Systems Research*. Available at: http://dx.doi.org/10.1287/isre.(2013).0480

46. Long, T., Taubenheim, A., Wayman, J., Temple, S., & Ruoff, B. (2008). "The Heart Truth:" Using the power of branding and social marketing to increase awareness of heart disease in women. *Social Marketing Quarterly*. 14(3): 3–29.

47. McCartney, G., Collins, C., & Mackenzie, M. (2013). What (or who) causes health inequalities: Theories, evidence and implications. *Health Policy* 113: 221–227.

48. Michael, F.H. (2012). Using social determinants in a public health program to reduce infant mortality. *N C Med J.* 73(5): 390–391.

49. Nandi, A., Glymour, M.M., & Subramanian. S.V. (2014). Association among socioeconomic status, health behaviors, and all-cause mortality in the United States. *Epidemiology*, 25(2):170–177.

50. National Institutes of Health. The Heart Truth®. Available at: http://www. nhlbi.nih.gov/health/educational/hearttruth/

51. Neff, G. (2013). Why big data won't cure us. Big Data 1(3): 117-122. DOI: 10.1089/big.2013.0029.

52. Nicholas, S.B., Kalantar-Zadeh, K., & Norris, K.C. (2015). Socioeconomic disparities in chronic kidney disease. *Advances in Chronic Kidney Disease*, 22(1): 6–15

53. Pampel, F.C., Krueger, P.M., & Denney, J.T. (2010). Socioeconomic status and health behaviors. *The Annual Review of Sociology*. 36: 349–370

54. Pan, C.X. & Leo-To, W.F. (2014). Cross-cultural health care for older adults: strategies for pharmacists. *The Consultant Pharmacist* 29 (10): 645–657.

55. Phelan, J.C., Link, B.G., & Tehranifar, P. (2010). Social conditions as fundamental causes of health inequalities: theory, evidence, and policy implications. *Journal of Health and Social Behavior* 51 (S): S28–S40.

56. Placzek, H. & Madoff, L. (2014). Effect of race/ethnicity and socioeconomic status on pandemic H1N1-Related Outcomes in Massachusetts. *American Journal of Public Health*, 104(1): e31–e38.

57. Skloot, R. (2010). *The immortal life of Henrietta Lacks*. New York: Crown Publishers.

58. Storm, I., Aarts, M., Harting, J., & Schuit, A.J. (2011). Opportunities to reduce health inequalities by 'Health in All Policies' in the Netherlands: An explorative study on the national level. *Health Policy*, 103: 130–140.

59. Succer, M. (1973). *Causal thinking in the health sciences: concepts and strategies in epidemiology*. New York: Oxford Press.

60. Umberson, D., Williams, K., Thomas, P.A., Liu, H., & Thomeer, M.B. (2014). Race, gender, and chains of disadvantage: Childhood adversity, social relationships, and health. *Journal of Health and Social Behavior* 55(1): 20–38.

61. Williams, D.R. (2005). The health of US racial and ethnic populations. *Journals of Gerontology*, 60B (Special Issue II): 53–62.

62. World Health Organization. *Working for health: An introduction to the World Health Organization*. Available at http://www.who.int/about/brochure_en.pdf?ua=1

63. World Health Organization. (2008). *Closing the gap in a generation: Health equity through action on the social determinants of health. Final report of the commission on social determinants of health*. Geneva, Switzerland: World Health Organization.

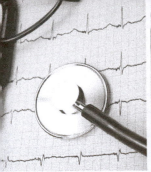
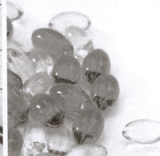
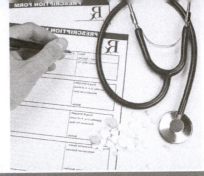
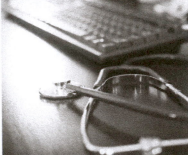
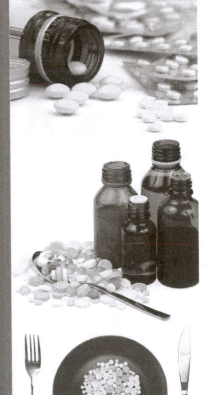
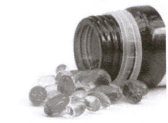

MODELS AND FRAMEWORKS FOR HEALTH AND ILLNESS BEHAVIORS

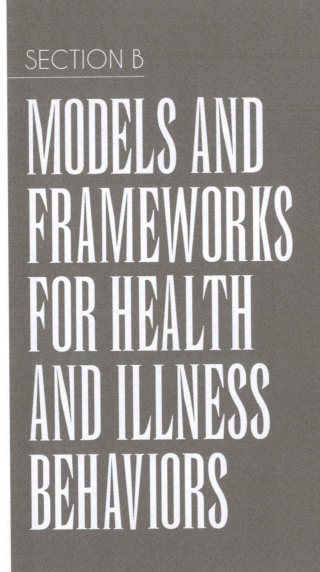
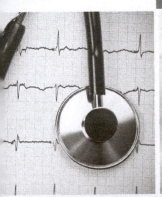
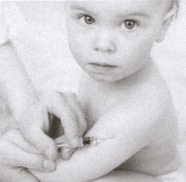
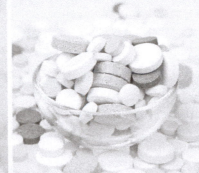
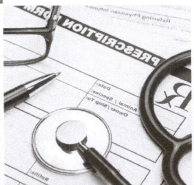

CHAPTER 3

INDIVIDUAL/INTERPERSONAL MODELS OF HEALTH AND ILLNESS BEHAVIOR

Nathaniel M. Rickles, PharmD, PhD, and Susan J. Blalock, PhD

LEARNING OBJECTIVES:

1. Describe the characteristics of an ideal theory.
2. Distinguish between value-expectancy and stage theories.
3. Identify the key features of: Rotter's Social Learning Theory, Social Cognitive Theory, Theory of Reasoned Action, Theory of Planned Behavior, Health Belief Model, Transtheoretical Model of Change, and Precaution Adoption Process Model.
4. Compare and contrast the strengths and limitations of different theories presented in the chapter.
5. Apply the individual/interpersonal theories presented in the chapter to the provision of care in a pharmacy practice setting.

KEY TERMS

Action

Attitudes toward the behavior

Behavior

Behavior potential

Behavioral belief

Behavioral capability

Behavioral intention

Contemplation

Control beliefs

Cues to action

Emotional coping responses

Expectancy

Health belief model

Health locus of control

Learned helplessness

Learned resourcefulness

Maintenance

Medication adherence

Motivation to comply

Normative beliefs

Outcome evaluation

Outcome expectations/expectancies

Perceived barriers

Perceived behavioral control

Perceived benefits

Perceived health threat

Perceived power

Perceived severity

Perceived susceptibility

Pessimistic explanatory style

Precaution adoption process model

Precontemplation

Preparation

Reciprocal determinism

Reinforcement

Reinforcement value

Self-efficacy

Social cognitive theory

Social learning theory

Stage theory

Subjective norm

Theory of planned behavior

Theory of reasoned action

Transtheoretical model of change

Value expectancy theory

In this chapter, we will focus on individual and interpersonal theories of health and illness behavior. Theories identify distinct sets of interrelated concepts, define these concepts using precise terminology, specify how the concepts are related to one another, and identify the conditions under which these relationships apply.[1,2] Theories are abstract and can be applied to a wide variety of behavioral phenomena, helping us understand why people behave in certain ways under specified conditions and how they are likely to respond when those conditions change. Theories, frameworks, and models can range from explaining very simple behaviors to very complex interactions changing over time. Ultimately, theories are ideal when they are based on clear assumptions, specify predictive relationships between variables based on evidence and experience, can be tested, and are relatively simple.

Theories can be useful to help clinicians and researchers better understand what contributes and maintains negative health behaviors and, therefore, guide interventions to address the negative health behaviors.[3] Specifically, theories might guide best ways to design interventions to reduce negative health behaviors and measure outcomes.[3]

By providing a systematic way to examine health behaviors, as well as guidance on developing interventions and assessing their effects, health behavior theories save practitioners from having to reinvent the wheel every time a new problem is faced.

This chapter will review several contemporary individual-interpersonal theories that are useful in understanding and predicting human health behavior. We start with value-expectancy theories since they are often a basis for other health behavior theories. Value-expectancy theories are based on the very simple notion that individuals are more likely to engage in a behavior if they believe that performing the behavior is likely to lead to desirable outcomes. When faced with a choice between two or more behavioral options, value-expectancy models posit that individuals will tend to adopt the behavior that maximizes the likelihood of obtaining desired outcomes and avoiding undesired ones.[4] We then introduce two stage models of health and illness behavior. Stage theories view behavior change as a process and posit that, in the process of moving from inaction to action, people pass through a series of stages—sometimes moving forward toward change, sometimes moving backward away from change, and sometimes remaining in the same stage indefinitely. A central premise that underlies stage theories is that the factors that influence behavior change depend on one's current stage in the behavior change process. Towards the end of the chapter, we examine models that are not value-expectancy models and incorporate emotion and/or temporal changes in outcomes and expectations. Finally, we provide a critique of the theories reviewed, emphasizing issues that they do not consider such as how organizations, networks or community-level factors and policies affect individual health behavior.

VALUE-EXPECTANCY THEORIES

ROTTER'S SOCIAL LEARNING THEORY

A central assumption underlying Rotter's social learning theory is that, through the course of their life experiences, people develop expectations concerning the types of outcomes that are most likely to occur if they perform a particular behavior in a particular situation. Consequently, when given an option, people usually choose to perform those behaviors that maximize the perceived likelihood of obtaining desired outcomes, and minimize the perceived likelihood of obtaining undesired ones. As described previously, this is the core tenet underlying all value-expectancy theories.

Rotter summarized this notion in the formula shown below where: BP=*Behavior Potential*, E=*Expectancy*, and RV=*Reinforcement Value*.

$$BP = f (E, RV)$$

The formula hypothesizes that the likelihood that a person will perform a particular behavior in a particular situation is a function of the person's judgment of how likely the behavior will lead to a specific outcome and the reinforcement value attached to that outcome.

When using value-expectancy theories, it is important to remember that *expectancies* and *reinforcement values* are subjective. Thus, different people will vary in their assessments of the likelihood that a particular behavior will result in a particular outcome. They may also differ in terms of the reinforcement value attached to different outcomes. Even for a single individual, *expectancies* and the *reinforcement value* attached to different outcomes will vary across situations, depending on the person's subjective interpretation of the environment. Moreover, expectancies and values may change as individuals gain life experience, including experience with an illness and the medications used to treat it. Thus, behavior is best viewed as a learned response to environmental contingencies.

Most research on health behavior that has used Rotter's social learning theory as a theoretical framework has focused largely on one key concept derived from the theory, *health locus of control*. *Health locus of control* is a generalized expectancy concerning the factors that a person believes influence his/her health. As originally conceptualized by Rotter, these generalized expectancies were viewed as existing on a continuum.[4] At one end of the continuum, individuals believed that health outcomes were totally within one's personal control. At the other end of the continuum, individuals believed that health outcomes were totally under the control of factors external to oneself (e.g., powerful others, chance, fate). Thus, this conceptualization did not allow for the possibility that one could strongly believe that health outcomes are influenced by both internal and external factors.

In the 1970s, this unidimensional conceptualization of *health locus of control* was replaced by a multidimensional one that recognized that individuals could believe that both internal and external factors influence health outcomes. The Multidimensional Health Locus of Control Scales (MHLC) have been widely used to assess this concept.[5] The MHLC assesses perceptions of three different sources of control: internal (e.g., If I get sick, it is my own behavior that determines how soon I get well again), powerful others (e.g., Health professionals keep me healthy), and chance (e.g. When I am sick, I just have to let nature run its course). Studies have examined the relationship between health locus of control and medication adherence in the context of a wide variety of chronic health problems, including: cardiovascular illness[6,7], asthma[8], renal disease[9,10], cancer[11–13], mental health conditions[14,15], and HIV/AIDS[16,17]. Typically, it has been hypothesized that adherence would be positively associated with beliefs in internal control over health outcomes and negatively associated with beliefs in powerful other or chance control. However, only mixed support has been found for these hypotheses. As noted by others, it seems likely that any effect locus of control may have on medication adherence will depend on other factors, such as whether individuals believe that they have the ability and resources needed to adhere.[18, 19] Thus, research is needed to better understand how locus of control beliefs may interact with other individual beliefs as well as environmental factors to influence medication adherence.

An early theory that brings the social interaction piece forward is the Theory of Reasoned Action (TRA). TRA was introduced in the 1970s and extended the value-expectancy notion considerably.[20] As shown in Figure 3-1, this theory posits that the best predictor of behavior is *behavioral intention*, which is a person's self-rated likelihood of performing the specified behavior. As we move backward in the model, from right to left, we gain insight into the factors that influence behavior through their effects on *behavioral intentions*. According to the model, *behavioral intentions* are influenced by two factors: *attitude toward the behavior* and *subjective norms*. *Attitude toward the behavior* is an overall judgment of the extent to which a person believes that his performance of the behavior is a good or bad idea. *Attitude toward the behavior* is influenced by a set of salient *behavioral beliefs*, reflecting how likely individuals believe specific outcomes are to occur if they perform the behavior of interest, with each *behavioral belief* weighted by the value the person attaches to the outcome (i.e., *outcome evaluation*). For example, a truck driver may believe that taking a particular medication is very likely to cause drowsiness (i.e., a behavioral belief) and that this side-effect is very undesirable (i.e., the associated *outcome evaluation*). These factors would have a negative effect on the truck driver's attitude toward using the medication. However, in most cases, attitudes are influenced by multiple salient beliefs. Thus, the same truck driver may also believe that the medication will alleviate bothersome symptoms and that this is more important than the possibility of experiencing drowsiness. Thus, the truck driver may take the medication despite his concerns about experiencing drowsiness.

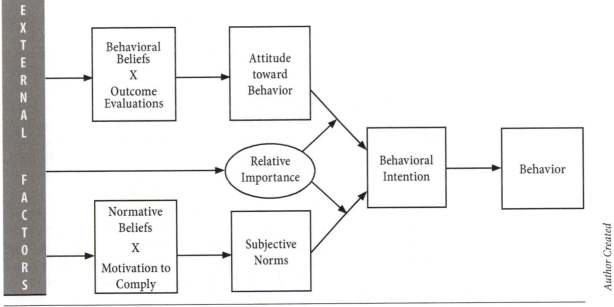

Author Created

FIGURE 3-1: THEORY OF REASONED ACTION

The second factor that has a direct effect on behavioral intention is *subjective norms*, which reflect the extent to which an individual perceives social pressure to perform the behavior of interest. *Subjective norms* are influenced by a set of *normative beliefs*, each indexing an individual's perception that a specific other person (or group of people) believe the individual should perform the behavior, with each normative belief weighted by *motivation to comply* (i.e., the extent to which the individual believes he should comply with the wishes of these other people or groups). For example, the truck driver introduced above is likely to believe that his doctor thinks he should take the prescribed medication. Assuming that he also believes he should follow his doctor's wishes, his *subjective norm* will favor taking the medication. However, in the same way that *attitude toward the behavior* is influenced by multiple salient beliefs, subjective norms are influenced by multiple normative beliefs. Thus, the truck driver may also believe that family members, friends, and co-workers think he either should or should not take the medication. *Subjective norms* reflect the integration of perceived social pressure from all people (or groups of people) who are important to the individual.

According to the TRA, *behavioral intention* is influenced directly only by *attitude toward the behavior* and *subjective norms*. All other factors (e.g., gender, race, age, education, health status), labeled *external factors* in Figure 3-1, exert their effect on *behavioral intention* through their effects on *attitudes* and *subjective norms*. In some cases, attitudes will have the greatest effect on intention; whereas, in other cases, subjective norms will have a greater effect. Thus, it is important to determine, in any particular instance, the extent to which behavior is under attitudinal or normative control.

The Theory of Planned Behavior (TPB) is an extension of the TRA.[21] As shown in Figure 3-2, the TPB identifies a third variable, *perceived behavioral control*, which can have a direct effect on both *behavioral intention* and *behavior*. *Perceived behavioral control* is a person's overall perception of how easy or difficult it is for him/her to perform a behavior. *Perceived behavioral control* is influenced by a set of salient *control beliefs*, reflecting the presence of factors that either facilitate or interfere with performance of the behavior of interest, with each *control belief* weighted by the extent to which the person believes the factor makes performing the behavior either easier or more difficult (i.e., *perceived power*). To continue with the earlier example, the truck driver may believe that it is difficult to remember to take the medication multiple times a day. As a result, he may decide not to even try to take the medication as directed—assuming that he would fail. Moreover, to the extent that his belief is accurate (i.e., he really does experience difficulty remembering to take the medication throughout the day), he will be unlikely to be successful in taking the medication as directed even if he intends to do so. This suggests that, if *perceptions of behavioral control* are accurate, they may have a direct effect on *behavior*, in addition to the indirect effect that is mediated by *behavioral intention*.

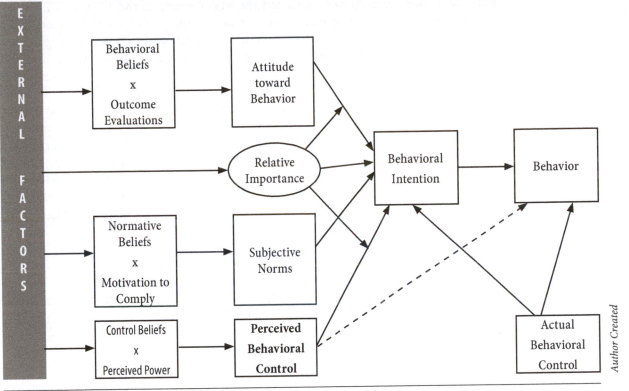

FIGURE 3-2: THEORY OF PLANNED BEHAVIOR

In practice, individuals who wish to use the TRA or TPB must begin by identifying the salient *behavioral, normative,* and *control beliefs* that underlie the behavior of interest. For example, if one is interested in better understanding the factors that predict adherence to a particular medication, members of the target population (i.e., individuals who are either users or potential users of the medication) should be interviewed to assess their *behavioral, normative* and *control beliefs* regarding use of the medication. For those interested in learning more about how to conduct elicitation interviews, Fishbein and Ajzen provide detailed guidelines.[20, 22]

The TRA and TPB have been used to investigate a number of medication use issues. These include: medication adherence [23-29]; duration of benzodiazepine therapy[30]; utilization of postoperative analgesics[31]; utilization of herbal remedies[32, 33] ; intention to use a medication within the context of a hypothetical scenario[34]; patient-pharmacist communication about antibiotics and antibiotic resistance[35]; pharmacist recommendations concerning the treatment of vaginal candidiasis with non-prescription medications[36]; pharmacist intention to provide Medicare medication therapy management services[37] ; and physician use of different sources of drug information[38, 39]. For the most part, this research has supported the major tenets of the TRA and TPB. An interesting exception, however, involved a study of analgesia use following orthopedic surgery in which actual analgesia use was not related to patients' presurgery ratings of the amount of analgesia they intended to use (rating scale ranged from 0=*No medication* to 10=*The most that I am allowed*).[31] This study is highlighted because it illustrates an important limitation of the TRA and TPB. That is, the link between *intention* and *behavior* will be strongest when *intentions* are based on a good understanding of relevant issues and little new information is subsequently encountered. Obviously, as new information is obtained, *intentions* may change. In the analgesia study, for example, individuals exhibited a limited understanding of the amount of post-surgical pain they were likely to experience, as evidenced by only a modest correlation between anticipated and actual pain reports. Thus, the lack of a relationship between preoperative intentions and subsequent behavior is understandable.

HEALTH BELIEF MODEL

The Health Belief Model (HBM) is one of the oldest and most widely-recognized individual-level theories of health behavior. Unlike the other theories mentioned to this point in the chapter, the HBM was developed to specifically explain health behavior. The HBM was originally developed in the 1950s by researchers with the United States Public Health Service to better understand poor rates of participation in a community-based tuberculosis screening program.[40] As shown in Figure 3-3, the model posits that *perceived susceptibility* to a particular health problem and the *perceived severity* of that health problem combine to determine *perceived health threat*. According to the model, *perceived health threat* motivates action to prevent the health problem, but it does not determine the specific actions that will be taken. For example, to reduce one's chances of developing complications as a result of having hypertension, one might: take medications, lose weight, begin an exercise program, or restrict salt intake. To determine the specific action(s) to adopt, the model posits that people consider the *perceived benefits* associated with different actions as well as the *perceived barriers* associated with those actions. They then tend to adopt behavior(s) where the anticipated benefits outweigh the anticipated barriers. For example, an individual with hypertension may take medications to control his hypertension because he believes that (1) it will reduce the risk of long-term complications and (2) there are few barriers to incorporating medication-taking into his daily routine. However, he may not increase his exercise level, despite believing that it would be beneficial to do so, because he believes that exercising on a regular basis is too time-consuming. The HBM also posits that *perceived health threat* can be increased by exposure to *cues to action*, which can be either internal (e.g., experience of physical symptoms) or external (e.g., exposure to a direct-to-consumer commercial about a medication to reduce disease risk). Finally, in Figure 3-3, the HBM also posits that perceived *susceptibility, perceived severity, perceived threat, perceived benefits,* and *perceived barriers* can be influenced by demographic factors (e.g., age, gender, race, ethnicity), psychosocial factors (e.g., personality, peer pressure), and structural factors (e.g., knowledge of the disease, access to resources).[41]

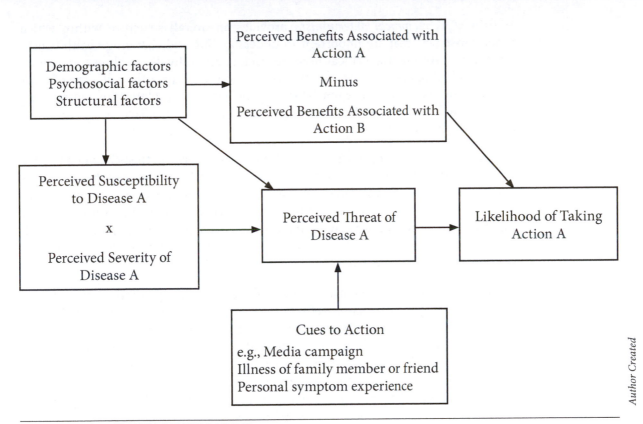

FIGURE 3-3: HEALTH BELIEF MODEL

The HBM has been used to better understand the determinants of medication adherence in a variety of different therapeutic areas, including heart failure[6], malaria chemoprophylaxis[27,29], hypertension[42,43], human immunodeficiency virus (HIV)[44,45], mental illness[46-50], kidney transplant[51], epilespy[52,53], diabetes mellitus[54], sickle cell disease[55], a combination of chronic diseases[56], and following a pediatric emergency room visit[57]. The HBM also has been used to better understand the determinants of using medications to treat or prevent osteoporosis.[58,59] In general, the findings from these studies provide support for the importance of HBM variables in influencing medication adherence and use. However, the specific factors that emerge as significant vary across studies and reasons for this variability remain poorly understood.

BANDURA'S SOCIAL COGNITIVE THEORY

Social Cognitive Theory (SCT) is a dynamic theory addressing both individual and interpersonal factors of human behavior. SCT views behavior as the result of the triadic, reciprocal interaction of personal factors, behavioral patterns and the environment.[60] Personal factors relate to the cognitive, affective, and biological characteristics of the individual. Environment refers to objective factors external to the person that affect behavior including the social environment (family, friends, coworkers) and the physical environment (facilities, temperature, geography). The interaction of person, behavior, and environment is termed *reciprocal determinism* and it implies that the three components are constantly influencing one another, with change in one component effecting change in the other components.

Within SCT, *reciprocal determinism* provides an overall structure within which other constructs that are important to understanding and changing health behavior operate. Among the critical personal factors are individuals' ability to acquire behavioral competence, learn by observing others, anticipate the outcome of one's behavior, develop confidence in performing the behavior of interest (including overcoming performance barriers), self-regulate behavior, and reflect on and evaluate one's performance.[61]

To perform any behavior, a person must know how to perform the behavior and have the required skills. Thus, behavioral competence, or *behavioral capability*, reflects both knowledge and skill. However, even with the requisite knowledge and skills, SCT posits that individuals will not perform a behavior unless (1) they are confident that they can perform the behavior and (2) believe that performing the behavior will result in valued outcomes. These two types of beliefs are called *self-efficacy* and *outcome expectations*, respectively.

Self-efficacy is perhaps the most powerful SCT construct in predicting and explaining behavioral performance. It reflects the level of confidence individuals have in their ability to perform a specific behavior, including their ability to overcome performance barriers. Results of numerous studies of diverse health behaviors reveal that the effects of behavior change interventions are often mediated, at least in part, by their effects on *self-efficacy*. The stronger the *self-efficacy* beliefs that a program instills, the more likely program participants are to initiate behavior change efforts and sustain the effort needed to maintain beneficial health behaviors.[62]

Self-efficacy has three dimensions: strength, magnitude, and generality. Strength reflects how confidant individuals are that they can perform a specific behavior. Magnitude reflects the level of difficulty associated with performing the behavior. Generality reflects the extent to which *self-efficacy* developed in one situation carries over to other situations. For example, a patient with hypertension and chronic obstructive pulmonary disease may be prescribed both oral tablets and medications delivered via inhalers. The magnitude of difficulty associated with taking the medications prescribed is probably greater for the inhalers than for the oral tablets. Thus, the patient may be very confident that he can take his oral medications correctly when at home, but may be less confident of his ability to use his inhalers correctly in this same situation. In this example, the strength of the patient's self-efficacy beliefs (i.e., level of confidence) varies as a function of the magnitude of task difficulty. The strength of the patient's self-efficacy beliefs may also vary across situations (e.g., taking oral tablets as prescribed when at home versus when on a trip), an issue of generality.

Self-efficacy is influenced by four sources of information: verbal persuasion, vicarious experience, direct experience, and emotional arousal.[63] Verbal persuasion, which involves telling a person that he/she has the ability to perform a behavior, is the weakest source of efficacy information. Vicarious experience, which is considerably more potent, involves observing others perform the behavior. Through this type of observational learning, individuals can come to better understand how to perform the behavior, the skills that are required for success, and the outcomes that accompany success and failure. Self-efficacy is most likely to be enhanced by observing similar others successfully perform the behavior—the inference being, "If that person can do it, I can too." Many health education interventions include strategies designed to take advantage of learning through vicarious experience. For example, a video on childhood asthma might show a child using his inhaler and subsequently experiencing symptom relief. Direct experience, which involves performing the behavior oneself, is also often incorporated into health education programs and is the most potent source of information about self-efficacy. Typically, individuals are given an opportunity to practice the behavior in a supportive environment with supervision. In this type of program, complex behaviors might be broken into component steps to facilitate the acquisition of both behavioral capability and self-efficacy. Finally, emotional arousal can have either positive or negative effects on self-efficacy. For example, heightened anxiety may undermine self-efficacy, whereas positive affect may enhance it.

The four sources of efficacy information described above also provide information about the outcomes that are most likely to follow performance of a behavior. As an example, if an individual experiencing a migraine takes a medication that relieves the migraine, he/she will come to expect that, in the future if another migraine is experienced, taking the medication will once again produce relief. Similarly, beliefs concerning the link between behavior and outcomes may be learned by seeing an advertisement on television for a migraine medication that promises symptom relief.

Like Rotter's Social Learning Theory, SCT posits that individuals will tend to engage in behaviors that are likely to result in valued outcomes. In SCT, individuals' beliefs that performance of a specific behavior will lead to given outcomes are called *outcome expectations* and the value attached to those outcomes are called *outcome expectancies*.[64] These beliefs correspond to the expectations and reinforcement values captured, respectively, in the "E" and "RV" terms in Rotter's Social Learning Theory.

Outcomes that increase the likelihood that a behavior will be repeated are called *reinforcements*. SCT distinguishes between three types of reinforcements: direct reinforcement (e.g., decrease in symptoms after taking a migraine medication), vicarious reinforcement (e.g., observing another person appear to experience symptom relief after taking a migraine medication), and self-reinforcement (e.g., feeling good about oneself after successfully managing a migraine).[64] The mechanisms that underlie self-reinforcement play a central role in SCT, because they allow individuals to exercise self-control of behavior. To exercise self-control, individuals must monitor their behavior and its effects, compare their performance to a personal standard or goal, and reward oneself when goals are achieved.[62] Providing people with opportunities for decision-making, goal setting, problem-solving, and self-reward have all been shown to encourage personal control of behavior.[64]

The final factor that plays an important role in SCT involves *emotional coping responses*. Attempting to learn and enact a new behavior can be emotionally arousing and negative emotions can inhibit learning and performance of desired behaviors.[61] To be successful, individuals must manage these negative emotions and foster positive ones. *Emotional coping responses* are the tactics people use to deal with emotional stimuli. Providing people with training and opportunities to practice target behaviors in emotionally challenging circumstances can reduce emotional distress and increase self-efficacy.

SCT has been used to examine adherence to treatment regimens within the context of several chronic diseases. These studies have found high self-efficacy to be associated with greater treatment adherence in diabetes[65,66], cardiovascular disease[67,68], HIV/AIDS[69,70], and rheumatoid arthritis.[71] Interventions using SCT principles have been designed to increase knowledge, expectancies, skills, and environmental support, as well as foster self-regulation, self-monitoring, goal setting, self-incentives, and social support. Results of randomized controlled trials employing SCT constructs have shown marked improvement in outcomes for the intervention group in adherence to treatment for cardiovascular disease[67] and HIV/AIDS.[70]

STAGE THEORIES

Most of the theories that have been reviewed to this point suggest that simple, linear equations can be used to predict behavior and behavior change. For example, Rotter's Social Learning Theory suggests that the likelihood that patients will adopt a recommended behavior can be increased by strengthening their beliefs that valued outcomes will result from adoption of the behavior. Stage theories suggest that it is not that simple. Stage theories view behavior change from a process perspective. These theories suggest that, at any one point in time, individuals will be in one stage of the behavior change process and that, over time, they may move across stages. Moreover, stages theories posit that the factors that influence stage transitions depend on one's current stage in the behavior change process. Stage theorists argue that attempting to apply a simple prediction equation to people in different stages of change is an oversimplification of the behavior change process.[72]

Stage theories include four essential elements:

1. *A classification scheme to define the stages.* Stage theories include rules that allow classification of individuals into different stages of change. These rules must identify boundaries between stages so that, at any one point in time, an individual can be classified into a specific stage of change and, over time, it is possible to determine when the individual moves to other stages.

2. *An ordering of the stages.* Stages should be ordered in such a way that it is possible to differentiate between people in the early and latter stages of change. The earliest stage of change usually includes people who are not considering adopting the target behavior and the latter stages usually include people who are currently performing the behavior. Despite the ordering of stages, progress through the stages is not assumed to be linear as people may cycle back through stages, skip stages, or remain in one stage indefinitely.

3. *Within stages, assumption of common barriers to change.* Stage theories assume that individuals in the same stage face similar barriers to change. This assumption allows researchers to deliver stage-specific interventions to help people move across stages.

4. *Across stages, assumption of different barriers to change.* Stage theories assume that individuals in different stages face different barriers to change. Thus, different types of interventions are needed by people in different stages to help them progress through the behavior change process.[72]

Completely specified stage theories identify both the criteria that define stages and the stage-specific barriers to change. Although the stage definitions will apply across diverse behaviors, the barriers to change may be behavior-specific. For example, barriers relevant to adherence to asthma medications delivered via inhalers probably differ from the barriers relevant to adherence to oral asthma medications. Further, barriers associated with different oral medications may vary depending on their side-effect profiles.

Two of the most widely used stage models are the Transtheoretical Model of Change and the Precaution Adoption Process Model. These models are described next.

THE TRANSTHEORETICAL MODEL OF CHANGE (TTMC)

The TTMC was developed in the 1970s, within the context of addictive disorders, in an effort to produce a comprehensive model of behavior change.[73] Developers of the TTMC drew on concepts from over 300 leading theories of psychotherapy to support one overarching idea—that behavioral change occurs in stages.[74]

As shown in Table 3-1, the TTMC identifies five stages of change: precontemplation, contemplation, preparation, action, and maintenance. A final stage, termination, has been proposed but is not generally emphasized because it is difficult (if not impossible) to achieve.[74]

TABLE 3-1: STAGES OF CHANGE FROM TRANSTHEORETICAL MODEL OF CHANGE

STAGES OF CHANGE	DESCRIPTION
Precontemplation	Have no intention to act within the next 6 months. May be uninformed about or unaware of the consequences of their behavior.
Contemplation	Plans to change within the next 6 months. Aware of the pros and cons of their behavior. Some may reach a point of "behavioral procrastination" (not ready for action) and could be stuck in this stage for prolonged periods.
Preparation	Intend to act in the immediate future (next month). Has taken some significant action in the previous year. Has a plan and would be a good candidate for an action-oriented program/intervention.
Action	Overt lifestyle change in the past 6 months. Sometimes could be considered behavioral change.
Maintenance	Active relapse prevention and relapse temptation reduction. Individuals have increasing confidence in their ability to continue changes.

In addition to the stages of change, the TTMC emphasizes three key constructs that play critical roles in the behavior change process: decisional balance, self-efficacy, and the processes of change.[74] Decisional balance is based on the value-expectancy framework and concerns how individuals weigh the pros and cons of changing.[75] As suggested by value-expectancy theories, individuals are more likely to engage in behaviors if they believe that the pros associated with the behavior outweigh the cons. Moreover, in the behavior change process, research suggests that increases in the perceived pros associated with a target behavior prompt individuals to contemplate behavior change, but that actual behavior change is unlikely to occur as long as perceived cons remain high.[73] In the TTMC, self-efficacy, drawn from Bandura's SCT, plays a critical role in predicting relapse following behavior change—especially when dealing with addictive behaviors such as alcohol abuse or smoking.[76] Lower self-efficacy is generally associated with a greater risk of relapse. Finally, the TTMC identifies ten processes of change. As shown in Table 3-2, these processes can be aggregated into two higher order factors: cognitive-affective processes and behavioral processes.[77,78] The processes of change reflect the strategies that people use during the behavior change process. Research suggests that people tend to use cognitive-affective strategies early in the behavioral change process and behavioral strategies in later stages.[79] It is also important to avoid action-oriented behavioral interventions until an individual is ready for change such as in preparation stage. Applying action-oriented interventions too early can be met with resistance/avoidance and thwart desired change.

TABLE 3-2: PROCESSES OF CHANGE FROM TRANSTHEORETICAL MODEL OF CHANGE

STAGES OF CHANGE	DESCRIPTION
Cognitive-Affective	
Consciousness Raising	Gathering information about the behavior.
Self-Reevaluation	Evaluating the personal consequences for continuing or stopping the behavior.
Dramatic Relief	Expressing and experiencing emotional arousal related to the behavior.
Environmental Reevaluation	Evaluating the consequences on others for continuing or stopping the behavior.
Social Liberation	Evaluating the social norms related to the behavior.
Behavioral	
Counter-Conditioning	Replacing undesirable behaviors with desirable ones.
Stimulus Control	Replacing environmental cues to encourage resisting the behavior.
Reinforcement Management	Introducing rewards for resisting the undesirable behavior.
Helping Relationships	Using social support to reinforce behavioral change.
Self-Liberation	Committing to permanent behavioral change.

Ficke and Farris reviewed papers published from 1995–2004 that used the TTMC to study medication use issues.[80] Two of these papers focused on developing psychometrically-sound measures of the stages of change concept.[81,82] The remaining studies used the model to examine adherence to oral contraceptives[83], discontinuation of therapy with interferon beta-1a[84], and pharmacists' readiness to provide pharmaceutical care.[85] In addition to these empirical papers, Ficke and Farris identified six conceptual papers that used the TTMC to discuss medication management issues in the context of diabetes[86], hypertension[87, 88], HIV/AIDS[89], organ transplant[90], and pharmaceutical policy.[91] Berger and colleagues reported positive findings for a TTMC-based intervention designed to decrease discontinuation of therapy with interferon beta-1a.[92] The TTMC also guided a study that involved training pharmacists and pharmacy technicians to identify pharmacy customer's stage-of-change for smoking cessation in an attempt to improve counseling and nicotine replacement therapy use.[93] Although smoking cessation rates did not differ between the intervention and control groups, TTMC-trained pharmacists were more likely than untrained pharmacists to talk with their customers about smoking cessation. Thus, the limited evidence available suggests that the TTMC provides a useful framework for studying medication use issues. More work is needed, however, to determine the extent to which interventions based on the TTMC are more effective than non-stage based interventions in prompting and sustaining behavior change efforts.

PRECAUTION ADOPTION PROCESS MODEL (PAPM)

The PAPM was introduced in 1988 to better describe the processes through which individuals adopt behaviors recommended to reduce the risk associated with potential health threats. The model is similar to the TTMC in many respects, however, a major difference between the two models is the definition of the early stages of change. In the TTMC, all individuals who are not currently either thinking about adopting a recommended behavior or actively involved in the behavior change process are classified together as *precontemplators*. In contrast, the PAPM essentially subdivides the TTMC *Precontemplation Stage* into three distinct stages. Thus, as shown in Figure 3-4, in PAPM Stage 1, individuals have never heard of the health threat of interest or precautions recommended to reduce risks associated with the threat. In PAPM Stage 2, individuals have heard of the threat, but have never considered adopting the precaution(s) recommended to reduce risk. In PAPM Stage 3, individuals have thought about adopting the precaution(s), but have decided against it. The value of distinguishing among people in these three different early PAPM stages is probably greatest in situations where information concerning the health threat or available precautions is actively evolving. For example, the PAPM may be particularly appropriate to study the behavior change process in relation to vaccination against cervical cancer. Many women may be unaware that the vaccine exists or have had little opportunity to consider obtaining it. The PAPM also suggests that individuals who have decided against adopting a particular precaution may be especially difficult to engage in behavior change efforts. Research suggests that individuals in this stage (i.e., Stage 3) can be quite well informed[94] and that they will tend to reject information that is inconsistent with their decision.[95]

Stage 1	Stage 1	Stage 3	Stage 5	Stage 6	Stage 7
Not Aware of the Issue	Unengaged by the Issue	Deciding About Acting	Decided to Act	Acting	Maintaining Behavior Change
		Stage 4			
		Decided Not to Act			

Author Created

FIGURE 3-4: PRECAUTION ADOPTION PROCESS MODEL

The PAPM has been used to study receipt of hepatitis B vaccination[96] and has been used in a series of studies to examine adoption of precautions recommended to prevent osteoporosis.[94, 97-99] In general, this research supports the basic stage model assumption that individuals in different stages face different barriers to change. However, it is too early to determine if interventions based on the PAPM are superior to non-stage based interventions in terms of facilitating behavior change efforts.

THEORIES INTEGRATING EMOTION AND TEMPORAL CHANGES IN OUTCOMES AND EXPECTATIONS

LEARNED HELPLESSNESS AND LEARNED RESOURCEFULNESS

Related to Rotter's control beliefs involving things that happen by chance, Abramson and colleagues postulated that exposure to uncontrollable, unpredictable, aversive events resulted in a condition consisting of motivational, cognitive, and emotional deficits (known as "learned helplessness").[100] The theory provided additional attention to how patients perceived and to what they attributed the cause of a negative/positive event. Specifically, there are three dimensions that contribute to the development of learned helplessness: (1) internal versus external causal explanation (equivalent to the internal/external locus of control mentioned in the previous section), (2) stable versus unstable causal explanation, and (3) global versus specific causal attribution. Patients are predisposed to learned helplessness if they adopt a pessimistic explanatory style that involves attributing negative events to internal, stable, and global causes and positive events to external, unstable, and specific causes.

Learned helplessness is a useful model to describe medication nonadherence in chronic illnesses. Medications for chronic illnesses are typically taken to provide relief of daily symptoms and/or to slow the progression of disease; chronic medication use typically does not afford the patient an eventual cure. Therefore, chronic illnesses often involve symptom exacerbations that are unpredictable and uncontrollable. It is conceivable that a patient with a poorly controlled illness would become discouraged with continuous and seemingly noncontingent exacerbation of symptoms.[101-104] A patient with epilepsy might experience learned helplessness and form attributions that she has no control over her condition (external locus of control), that the lack of adequate seizure control will be a chronic occurrence (stable attribution), and that her inability to maintain a stable job or friendship as indicative of epilepsy's impact on many domains of her life (global attribution). This patient may question the utility of medication adherence as she senses that her recovery is not contingent on proper medication use. It is important to note that medication nonadherence may also reflect a patient's effort to control his or her medical situation. Despite the above theoretical connections, there has been little experimental research associating learned helplessness with medication nonadherence.

All of the above learned helplessness studies suggest that a learned helplessness response (pessimistic explanatory style) can result from a chronic illness trajectory that is unpredictable and uncontrollable. It is important to note that these studies used different measures of learned helplessness and thus the consistency between findings is questionable. It is still unknown whether there is a direct link between a patient's pessimistic explanatory style and his or her decision toward medication nonadherence. Depression is often associated with a pessimistic explanatory style and it is now known that depression is an independent risk factor for medication non-adherence.[105] Perhaps we will come to learn that depression exerts its role as an independent risk factor for non-adherence through individuals possessing a pessimistic explanatory style.

There is some research connecting learned resourcefulness (LR), a concept that contrasts with learned helplessness, and treatment adherence. LR is a collection of behavioral and cognitive skills used to self-regulate internal responses that interfere with an individual's ongoing actions.[106] Specific LR strategies include the following: (1) using cognitions to control emotions, (2) using problem-solving strategies, (3) delaying immediate gratification, and (4) self-regulating internal events. These strategies have been shown to yield positive health outcomes in epilepsy, seasickness, and chronic headaches.[107] White and colleagues conducted a study that showed that LR both reduced the number of negative episodes in insulin-dependent diabetes and improved the patients' perceived control over their treatment.[108] There is mixed evidence that LR may help preserve treatment adherence.[109,110]

Emotion often has profound effects on health and illness behavior. For example, fear of needles may prevent individuals from obtaining immunizations that they know they need.[111] As another example, depression may interfere with individuals engaging in a broad range of self-care activities, including adhering to prescribed medications.[112] Emotion plays a more integral role in two other theories that were not reviewed in this chapter due to space limitations. These are the dual process model of self-regulation, developed by Leventhal and colleagues[113], and the transactional model of stress and coping developed by Lazarus and colleagues.[114,115] Interested readers may refer to the references provided for additional information about these models.

DYNAMIC EXCHANGE MODEL FOR MEDICATION ADHERENCE LEVELS AND COMPARISON OF OUTCOMES

In 2010, Rickles developed a multi-level explanatory model called the Dynamic Exchange Model for Medication Adherence Levels and Comparison of Outcomes (DEMMALCO).[116] This model is intended for explaining how patients attribute medication use outcomes to their current medication adherence behaviors and choose future actions based on expectations and available alternatives. DEMMALCO indicates that patients make initial attributions of their control over their illness which affects subsequent medication adherence. Patients are actively comparing their treatment outcomes with their expectations for outcomes and what might result from other available alternatives. Further, DEMMALCO postulates individuals reassess how their control in treatment was related to desired outcomes and subsequently modify their adherence behavior based on the presence or absence of resources. The model needs to be tested for validation, but offers researchers and clinicians a different perspective on how patients attribute adherence outcomes to themselves given alternatives and expectations.

LIMITATIONS OF THE THEORIES REVIEWED

The theories reviewed in this chapter provide considerable insight into individual and interpersonal factors that influence health and illness behavior. However, two important limitations of the theories should also be noted. First, most of the theories assume that behavior is volitional. Thus, individuals are viewed as consciously deciding whether or not to engage in different behaviors. Because of the heavy emphasis placed on individual perceptions (e.g., *perceived benefits, perceived barriers, subjective norms*), most of the theories reviewed pay little attention to the effects that objective social and political factors may have on health behavior. However, Bandura's Social Cognitive Theory and The Theory of Planned Behavior explicitly recognize the influence of environmental factors on individual health behaviors.

Second, the theories reviewed tend to assume that individuals consciously consider the advantages and disadvantages associated with different courses of action and choose to enact behaviors that optimize their outcomes. However, behavior often appears less deliberate than this conceptualization would suggest. For example, while picking up a prescription at a pharmacy, a person may notice an attractive display of vitamin and mineral preparations and be prompted to make a purchase with little consideration of the advantages and disadvantages. In the Health Belief Model, this type of store display would be considered a *cue to action*. However, none of the other theories reviewed recognize the important role that such environmental cues may have on behavior. In addition, recent work in the area of judgment and decision making suggests that adults often make decisions based on intuitive principles, rather than a careful balancing of the advantages and disadvantages of different courses of action.[117,118] Additional research is needed to fully understand the practical implications of these recent findings.

SUMMARY

In this chapter, we reviewed several individual and interpersonal theories of health and illness behavior. We also noted that these models only address a relatively small number of factors that influence health behavior. Other chapters in this book address factors at other levels of the social ecological framework. We also discussed limitations of the various models reviewed. As new findings emerge, current theories are likely to be adapted or replaced by newer theories. A major weakness of the literature on medication use and pharmacy practice is that often investigators do not use any theoretical framework to guide their work. Given that most of the theories reviewed in this chapter have been widely used to guide research on other health behaviors, it is surprising that they have not been used more often to study issues related to medication use and pharmacy practice. As described in the introduction, theories provide a vehicle for summarizing and communicating empirical findings. They provide a mechanism through which the knowledge base in a particular area can be built and organized. As a consequence of the relative dearth of theoretically-informed research in our area, it is often difficult to synthesize empirical findings across studies in a meaningful way. Pharmacy practitioners developing interventions to improve adherence and treatment outcomes often do so with little consideration given to the existing theoretical literature. Thus, they often end up reinventing the wheel with each new intervention. Hopefully, the information provided in this chapter will increase awareness of the theoretical frameworks that can be used to guide intervention efforts and will stimulate interest in the development of interventions that are both theoretically-informed and evidence-based.

Acknowledgments: The authors would like to acknowledge the contributions of two prior authors, Drs. Ashley J. Beard and Stacie B. Dusetzina, of this chapter previously published in 2009 under the title "Social and Behavioral Aspects of Pharmaceutical Care." Although the present chapter has been revised and updated, it is partially based on the 2009 chapter.

REFERENCES

1. Cohen, D.A., Scribner, R.A., & Farley TA. (2003). A structural model of health behavior: A pragmatic approach to explain and influence health behaviors at the population level. *Prev. Med.* 30(2):146–54.

2. Kerlinger, F.N.(1986). *Foundations of behavioral research.* 3rd ed New York: Holt, Rinehart and Winston.

3. Glanz, K., Rimer, B.K., & Lewis, F.M. (2002). *Health behavior and health education: Theory, research, and practice.* 3rd ed San Francisco: Jossey-Bass.

4. Rotter, J.B. (1966). Generalized expectancies for internal versus external control of reinforcement. *Psychol. Monogr.* 80(1):1–28.

5. Wallston, K.A., Wallston, B.S., DeVellis, R.F. (1978). Development of the multidimensional health locus of control scales (MHLC). *Health Educ. Monogr.* 6:160–70.

6. George, J. & Shalansky, S.J. (2007). Predictors of refill non-adherence in patients with heart failure. *Br. J. Clin. Pharmacol.* 63(4):488–93.

7. Bane, C., Hughes, C.M., & McElnay, J.C. (2006). The impact of depressive symptoms and psychosocial factors on medication adherence in cardiovascular disease. *Patient Educ. Couns.* 60(2):187–93.

8. Apter, A.J., Reisine, S.T., Affleck, G., Barrows, E., & ZuWallack, R.L. (1998). Adherence with twice-daily dosing of inhaled steroids. Socioeconomic and health-belief differences. *Am. J. Respir. Crit. Care Med.* 157(6 Pt 1):1810–7.

9. Weng, F.L., Israni, A.K., Joffe, M.M., et al. (2005). Race and electronically measured adherence to immunosuppressive medications after deceased donor renal transplantation. *J. Am. Soc. Nephrol.* 16(6):1839–48.

10. Frazier, P.A., Davis-Ali, S.H., & Dahl, K.E. (1994). Correlates of noncompliance among renal transplant recipients. *Clin. Transplant* 8(6):550–7.

11. Tamaroff, M.H., Festa, R.S., Adesman, A.R., & Walco, G.A. (1992). Therapeutic adherence to oral medication regimens by adolescents with cancer. II. Clinical and psychologic correlates. *J. Pediatr* 120(5):812–7.

12. Atkins, L. & Fallowfield, L. (2006). Intentional and non-intentional non-adherence to medication amongst breast cancer patients. *Eur. J. Cancer* 42(14):2271–6.

13. McDonough, E.M., Boyd, J.H., Varvares, M.A., & Maves, M.D. (1996). Relationship between psychological status and compliance in a sample of patients treated for cancer of the head and neck. *Head Neck* 18(3):269–76.

14. Haley, C.J., Drake, R.J., Bentall, R.P., & Lewis, S.W. (2003). Health beliefs link to duration of untreated psychosis and attitudes to later treatment in early psychosis. *Soc. Psychiatry Psychiatr. Epidemiol* 38(6):311–6.

15. Budd, R.J., Hughes, I.C., & Smith, J.A. (1996). Health beliefs and compliance with antipsychotic medication. *Br. J. Clin. Psychol* 35 (Pt 3):393–7.

16. Molassiotis, A., Nahas-Lopez, V., Chung, W.Y., Lam, S.W., Li, C.K., & Lau, T.F. (2002). Factors associated with adherence to antiretroviral medication in HIV-infected patients. *Int. J. STD AIDS* 13(5):301–10.

17. Altice, F.L., Mostashari, F., & Friedland, G.H. (2001). Trust and the acceptance of and adherence to antiretroviral therapy. *J. Acquir. Immune Defic. Syndr* 28(1):47–58.

18. Wallston, K.A. (1992). Hocus-pocus, the focus isn't strictly on locus: Rotter's social learning theory modified for health. *Cognit. Ther. Res* 16(2):183–99.

19. Oberle, K. (1991). A decade of research in locus of control: What have we learned? *J. Adv. Nurs* 16(7):800–6.

20. Fishbein, M. & Ajzen I. (1975). *Belief, attitude, intention and behavior: An introduction to theory and research.* Boston: Addison-Wesley.

21. Ajzen, I. (1985). From intentions to actions: A theory of planned behavior. In Kuhl, J. & Beckman, J. (Eds.), *Action-contol: From cognition to behavior.* Heidelberg: Springer, 11–39.

22. Ajzen, I. Constructing a tpb questionnaire: Conceptual and methodological considerations [pdf file on Internet]. [updated 2006, January; cited 2007, April 2]. Available from: Http://www-unix.Oit.Umass.Edu/~aizen/pdf/tpb. Measurement.Pdf. Accessed at http://www-unix.oit.umass.edu/~aizen/pdf/tpb.measurement.pdf on April 2. Last updated on January 2006.

23. Ried, L.D. & Christensen, D.B. (1988). A psychosocial perspective in the explanation of patients' drug-taking behavior. *Soc. Sci. Med* 27(3):277–85.

24. Austin, J.K. (1989). Predicting parental anticonvulsant medication compliance using the theory of reasoned action. *J. Pediatr. Nurs.* 4(2):88–95.

25. Jackson, C. (2006). Promoting adherence to antibiotics: A test of implementation intentions. *Patient Educ. Couns* 61(2):212–8.

26. de Bruin, M., Hospers, H.J., van den Borne, H.W., Kok ,G., & Prins, J.M. (2005). Theory- and evidence-based intervention to improve adherence to antiretroviral therapy among HIV-infected patients in the Netherlands: A pilot study. *Aids Patient Care STDS* 19(6):384–94.

27. Abraham, C., Clift, S., & Grabowski, P. (1999). Cognitive predictors of adherence to malaria prophylaxis regimens on return from a malarious region: A prospective study. *Soc. Sci. Med.* 48(11):1641–54.

28. Miller, P., Wikoff, R., & Hiatt, A. (1992). Fishbein's model of reasoned action and compliance behavior of hypertensive patients. *Nurs. Res.* 41(2):104–9.

29. Farquharson, L., Noble, L.M., Barker, C., & Behrens, R.H. (2004). Health beliefs and communication in the travel clinic consultation as predictors of adherence to malaria chemoprophylaxis. *Br. J. Health Psychol.* 9(Pt 2):201–17.

30. van Hulten, R., Bakker, A.B., Lodder, A.C., Teeuw, K.B., Bakker, A., & Leufkens, H.G. (2003). The impact of attitudes and beliefs on length of benzodiazepine use: A study among inexperienced and experienced benzodiazepine users. *Soc. Sci. Med.* 56(6):1345–54.

31. Pellino, T.A. (1997). Relationships between patient attitudes, subjective norms, perceived control, and analgesic use following elective orthopedic surgery. *Res. Nurs. Health.* 20(2):97–105.

32. Gupchup, G.V., Abhyankar, U.L., Worley, M.M., Raisch, D.W., Marfatia, A.A., & Namdar, R. (2006). Relationships between hispanic ethnicity and attitudes and beliefs toward herbal medicine use among older adults. *Res. Social Adm. Pharm.* 2(2):266–79.

33. Bharucha, D.X., Morling, B.A., & Niesenbaum, R.A. (2003). Use and definition of herbal medicines differ by ethnicity. *Ann. Pharmacother.* 37(10):1409–13.

34. Bersellini, E., & Berry, D. (2007). The benefits of providing benefit information: Examining the effectiveness of provision of simple benefit statements on people's judgments about a medicine. *Psychol. Health* 22(1):61–82.

35. Coleman, C.L. (2003). Examining influences of pharmacists' communication with consumers about antibiotics. *Health Commun.* 15(1):79–99.

36. Walker, A., Watson, M., Grimshar, J., & Bond, C. (2004). Applying the theory of planned behavior to pharmacists' beliefs and intentions about the treatment of vaginal candidiasis with non-prescription medicines. *Fam. Pract.* 21(6):670–6.

37. Herbert, K.E., Urmie, J.M., Newland, B.A., & Farris, K.B. (2006). Prediction of pharmacist intention to provide Medicare medication therapy management services using the theory of planned behavior. *Res. Social Adm. Pharm.* 2(3):299–314.

38. Gaither, C.A., Bagozzi, R.P., Ascione, F.J., & Kirking, D.M. (1996). A reasoned action approach to physicians' utilization of drug information sources. *Pharm. Res.* 13(9):1291–8.

39. Gaither, C.A., Bagozzi, R.P., Ascione, F.J., & Kirking, D.M. (1997). The determinants of physician attitudes and subjective norms toward drug information sources: Modification and test of the theory of reasoned action. *Pharm. Res.* 14(10):1298–308.

40. Hochbaum, G.M. (1958). *Public participation in medical screening programs; a socio-psychological study.* Washington: U.S. Department of Health, Education, and Welfare, Public Health Service, Bureau of State Services, Division of Special Health Services, Tuberculosis Program.

41. Janz, N.K. & Becker, M.H. (1984). *The health belief model: A decade later.* Health Educ. Q. 11(1):1–47.

42. Hershey, J.C., Morton, B.G., Davis, J.B., & Reichgott, M.J. (1980). Patient compliance with antihypertensive medication. *Am. J. Public Health.* 70(10):1081–9.

43. Brown, C.M. & Segal, R. (1996). The effects of health and treatment perceptions on the use of prescribed medication and home remedies among African American and white American hypertensives. *Soc. Sci. Med.* 43(6):903–17.

44. Wutoh, A.K., Brown, C.M., Dutta, A.P., Kumoji, E.K., Clarke-Tasker V., & Xue, Z. (2005). Treatment perceptions and attitudes of older human immunodeficiency virus-infected adults. *Res. Social Adm. Pharm.* 1(1):60–76.

45. Muma, R.D., Ross, M.W., Parcel, G.S., & Pollard, R.B. (1995). Zidovudine adherence among individuals with HIV infection. *AIDS Care.* 7(4):439–47.

46. Kelly, G.R., Mamon, J.A., & Scott, J.E. (1987). Utility of the health belief model in examining medication compliance among psychiatric outpatients. *Soc. Sci. Med.* 25(11):1205–11.

47. Adams, J. & Scott, J. (2000). Predicting medication adherence in severe mental disorders. *Acta Psychiatr. Scand.* 101(2):119–24.

48. Mulaik, J.S. (1992). Noncompliance with medication regimens in severely and persistently mentally ill schizophrenic patients. *Issues Ment. Health Nurs.* 13(3):219–37.

49. Seo, M.A. & Min, S.K. (2005). Development of a structural model explaining medication compliance of persons with schizophrenia. *Yonsei Med. J.* 46(3):331–40.

50. Nageotte, C., Sullivan, G., Duan, N., & Camp, P.L. (1997). Medication compliance among the seriously mentally ill in a public mental health system. *Soc. Psychiatry Psychiatr. Epidemiol.* 32(2):49–56.

51. Kiley, D.J., Lam, C.S., & Pollak, R. (1993). A study of treatment compliance following kidney transplantation. *Transplantation* 55(1):51–6.

52. Shope, J.T. (1988). Compliance in children and adults: Review of studies. *Epilepsy Res. Suppl.* 1:23–47.

53. Al-Faris, E.A., Abdulghani, H.M., Mahdi, A.H., Salih, M.A., & Al-Kordi, A.G. (2002). Compliance with appointments and medications in a pediatric neurology clinic at a university hospital in Riyadh, Saudi Arabia. *Saudi Med J.* 23(8):969–74.

54. Polly, R.K. (1992). Diabetes health beliefs, self-care behaviors, and glycemic control among older adults with non-insulin-dependent diabetes mellitus. *Diabetes Educ.* 18(4):321–7.

55. Elliott, V., Morgan, S., Day, S., Mollerup, L.S., & Wang, W. (2001). Parental health beliefs and compliance with prophylactic penicillin administration in children with sickle cell disease. *J. Pediatr. Hematol. Oncol.* 23(2):112–6.

56. Nagy, V.T. & Wolfe, G.R. (1984). Cognitive predictors of compliance in chronic disease patients. *Med. Care.* 22(10):912–21.

57. Soliday, E. & Hoeksel, R. (2000). Health beliefs and pediatric emergency department after-care adherence. *Ann. Behav. Med.* 22(4):299–306.

58. Unson, C.G., Fortinsky, R., Prestwood, K., & Reisine, S. (2005). Osteoporosis medications used by older African American women: Effects of socioeconomic status and psychosocial factors. *J. Community Health.* 30(4):281–97.

59. Cline, R.R., Farley, J.F., Hansen, R.A., & Schommer, J.C. (2005). Osteoporosis beliefs and antiresorptive medication use. *Maturitas* 50(3):196–208.

60. Bandura, A. (1999). Social cognitive theory: An agentic perspective. *Asian J. Social Psychol.* 2(1):21–41.

61. Bandura, A. (1977). Self-efficacy: Toward a unifying theory of behavioral change. *Psychol. Rev.* 84(2):191–215.

62. Bandura, A. (1994). Social cognitive theory and exercise of control over HIV infection. In: DiClemente CC, Peterson JL, eds. *Preventing aids: Theories and methods of behavioral interventions.* New York: Plenum Press, 336.

63. Bandura, A. (1986). *Social foundations of thought and action: A social cognitive theory.* Englewood Cliffs, NJ: Prentice-Hall.

64. Baranowski, T., Perry, C.L., & Parcel, G.S. (2002). How individuals, environments, and health behavior interact. In Glanz, K., Rimer, B.K., & Lewis, F.M. (Eds.), *Health behavior and health education: Theory, research, and practice.* San Francisco: Jossey-Bass, 165–84.

65. Kavanagh, D.J., Gooley, S., & Wilson, P.H. (1993). Prediction of adherence and control in diabetes. *J. Behav. Med.* 16(5):509–22.

66. McCaul, K.D., Glasgow, R.E., & Schafer, L.C. (1987). Diabetes regimen behaviors. Predicting adherence. *Med. Care.* 25(9):868–81.

67. DeBusk, R.F., Miller, N.H., Superko, H.R., et al. (1994). A case-management system for coronary risk factor modification after acute myocardial infarction. *Ann. Intern. Med.* 120(9):721–9.

68. Haskell, W.L., Alderman, E.L., Fair, J.M., et al. (1994). Effects of intensive multiple risk factor reduction on coronary atherosclerosis and clinical cardiac events in men and women with coronary artery disease. The Stanford coronary risk intervention project (scrip). *Circulation* 89(3):975–90.

69. Gifford, A.L., Bormann, J.E., Shively, M.J., Wright, B.C., Richman, D.D., & Bozzette, S.A. (2000). Predictors of self-reported adherence and plasma HIV concentrations in patients on multidrug antiretroviral regimens. *J. Acquir. Immune Defic. Syndr.* 23(5):386–95.

70. Smith, S.R., Rublein, J.C., Marcus, C., Brock, T.P., & Chesney, M.A. (2003). A medication self-management program to improve adherence to HIV therapy regimens. *Patient Educ. Couns.* 50(2):187–99.

71. Taal, E., Rasker, J.J., Seydel, E.R., & Wiegman, O. (1993). Health status, adherence with health recommendations, self-efficacy and social support in patients with rheumatoid arthritis. *Patient Educ. Couns.* 20(2-3):63–76.

72. Weinstein, N,D,, Sutton, S,R., & Rothman, A.J. (1998). Stage theories of health behavior: Conceptual and methodological issues. *Health Psychol.* 17(3):290–9.

73. Prochaska, J.O., Velicer, W.F., Rossi, J.S., et al. (1994). Stages of change and decisional balance for 12 problem behaviors. *Health Psychol.* 13(1):39–46.

74. Prochaska, J.O., Redding, C.A., & Evers, K.E. (2002). The transtheoretical model and stages of change. In: Glanz K, Rimer BK, Lewis FM, eds. *Health behavior and health education: Theory, research, and practice.* San Francisco: Jossey Bass, 99–116.

75. Janis, I. & Mann, L. (1977). *Decision making: A psychological analysis of conflict, choice and commitment.* New York: The Free Press.

76. DiClemente, C.C., Fairhurst, S.K., & Piotrowski, N.A. (1995). The role of self-efficacy in the addictive behaviors. In: Maddux J, ed. *Self-efficacy, adaptation and adjustment: Theory, research and application.* New York: Plenum, 109–41.

77. Prochaska, J.O. & DiClemente, C.C. (1982). Transtheoretical therapy: Toward a more integrative model of change. *Psychotherapy: Theory, Research, and Practice* 19:276–88.

78. Rosen, C.S. (2000). Is the sequencing of change processes by stage consistent across health problems? A meta-analysis. *Health Psychol.* 19(6):593–604.

79. Prochaska, J.O., DiClemente, C.C., & Norcross, J.C. (1992). In search of how people change: Applications to addictive behaviors. *Am. Psychol.* 47(9):1102–14.

80. Ficke, D.L. & Farris, K.B. (2005). Use of the transtheoretical model in the medication use process. *Ann. Pharmacother.* 39(7-8):1325–30.

81. Cook, C.L. & Perri, M, 3rd. (2004). Single-item vs multiple-item measures of stage of change in compliance with prescribed medications. *Psychol. Rep.* 94(1):115–24.

82. Willey, C., Redding, C., Stafford, J., et al. (2000). Stages of change for adherence with medication regimens for chronic disease: Development and validation of a measure. *Clin. Therapeutics* 22(7):858–71.

83. Johnson, S.S., Grimley, D.M., & Prochaska, J.O. (1998). Prediction of adherence using the transtheoretical model: Implications for pharmacy care practice. *J. Social Adm. Pharm.* 15:135–48.

84. Berger, B.A., Hudmon, K.S., & Liang, H. (2004). Predicting treatment discontinuation among patients with multiple sclerosis: Application of the transtheoretical model of change. *J Am Pharm Assoc* (Wash DC).44(4):445–54.

85. Berger, B.A. & Grimley, D. (1997). Pharmacists' readiness for rendering pharmaceutical care. *J Am Pharm Assoc (Wash)* NS37(5):535–42.

86. Corelli, R.L. & Hudmon, K.S. (1999, Sept/Oct). Promoting treatment adherence in diabetes: A practical strategy for pharmacists. *Calif. J. Health Syst. Pharm* 6.

87. Sher, T.G., Bellg, A.J., Braun, L., Domas, A., Rosenson, R., & Canar, W.J. (2002). Partners for life: A theoretical approach to developing an intervention for cardiac risk reduction. *Health Educ. Res.* 17(5):597–605.

88. Willey, C. (1999). Behavior-changing methods for improving adherence to medication. *Curr. Hypertension Rep.* 1(6):477–81.

89. Tuldra, A. & Wu, A.W. (2002). Interventions to improve adherence to antiretroviral therapy. *J. Acquir. Immune Defic. Syndr.* 31(Suppl 3):S154–7.

90. Robbins, M.L. (1999). Medication adherence and the transplant recipient: Helping patients at each stage of change. *Transplant Proc.* 31(4A):29S–30S.

91. Roughead, E.E., Gilbert, A.L., & Primrose, J.G. (1999). Improving drug use: A case study of events which led to changes in use of flucloxacillin in Australia. *Soc. Sci. Med.* 48(6):845–53.

92. Berger, B.A., Liang, H., & Hudmon, K.S. (2005). Evaluation of software-based telephone counseling to enhance medication persistency among patients with multiple sclerosis. *J Am Pharm Assoc (Wash DC)* 45(4):466–72.

93. Sinclair, H.K., Bond, C.M., Lennox, A.S., et al. (1998). Training pharmacists and pharmacy assistants in the stage-of-change model of smoking cessation: A randomised controlled trial in Scotland. *Tob. Control.* 7(3):253–61.

94. Blalock, S.J., DeVellis, R.F., & Giorgino, K.B., et al. (1996). Osteoporosis prevention in premenopausal women: Using a stage model approach to examine the predictors of behavior. *Health Psychol.* 15:84–93.

95. Weinstein, N.D., & Sandman, P.M. (1992). A model of the precaution adoption process: Evidence from home radon testing. *Health Psychol.* 11(3):170–80.

96. Hammer, G.P. (1997). *Hepatitis b vaccine acceptance among nursing home workers* [Doctoral dissertation].

97. Blalock, S.J. (2007). Predictors of calcium intake patterns: A longitudinal analysis. *Health Psychol.* 26(3):251–258.

98. Blalock, S.J., Currey, S.S., DeVellis, R.F., et al. (2000). Effects of educational materials concerning osteoporosis on women's knowledge, beliefs, and behavior. *Am. J. Health Promot.* 14:161–9.

99. Blalock, S.J., DeVellis, B.M., Patterson, C.C., Campbell, M.K., Orenstein, D.R., & Dooley, M.A. (2002). Effects of osteoporosis prevention program incorporating tailored educational materials. *Am. J. Health Promot.* 16:146–56.

100. Abramson, L.Y., Seligman, M.E.P., & Teasdale, J.D. (1978). Learned helplessness in humans: critique and reformulation. *J Abnorm Psychol* 87:49–74.

101. Smith, T.W., Peck, J.R., & Ward, J.R. (1990). Helplessness and depression in rheumatoid arthritis. *Health Psychol* 9(4):377–389.

102. Gehlert, S. (1996). Perceptions of control in adults with epilepsy. *Epilepsia* 35(1):81–88.

103. McGuiness, S. (1996). Learned helplessness in the multiple sclerosis population. *J Neurosci Nurs* 23(3):163–170.

104. Hermann, B.P., Trenerry, M.R., & Colligan, R.C. (1996). Learned helplessness, attributional style, and depression in epilepsy: Bozeman Epilepsy Surgery Consortium. *Epilepsia* 37(7):680–686.

105. DiMatteo, M.R., Lepper, H.S., & Croghan, T.W. (2000). Depression is a risk factor for noncompliance with medical treatment. *Arch Intern Med* 160:2101–07.

106. Rosenbaum, M. (1980). A schedule for assessing self-control behaviors: preliminary findings. *Behav Therapy* 11:109–124.

107. Rosenbaum, M. (1988). Learned resourcefulness, stress, and self-regulation. In Fisher, S., & Reason, J. (Eds.), *Handbook of life stress, cognition, and health.* New York:Wiley, 483–496.

108. White, R., Tata, P., & Burns, T. (1996). Mood, learned resourcefulness and perceptions of control in type I diabetes mellitus. *J Psychosomatic Res* 40(2):205–212.

109. Rosenbaum, M. & Smira, K. (1986). Cognitive and personality factors in the delay of gratification of hemodialysis patients. *J Personality Soc Psychol* 51(2):357–364.

110. Aikens, J.E., Wallender, J.L., Bell, D.S.H., & Cole, S.A. (1992). Daily stress variability, learned resourcefulness, regimen adherence and metabolic control in Type I diabetes mellitus: evaluation of a path model. *J Consult Clin Psych* 60(1):113–118.

111. Crockett, M. & Keystone, J. (2005). "I hate needles" and other factors impacting on travel vaccine uptake. *J. Travel Med.* 12 Suppl 1:S41–6.

112. Rubin, R,R. (2005). Adherence to pharmacologic therapy in patients with type 2 diabetes mellitus. *Am. J. Med.* 118 Suppl 5A:27S–34S.

113. Leventhal, H., Leventhal, E.A., & Cameron, L.D. (2001). Representations, procedures, and affect in illness self-regulation: A perceptual-cognitive model. In Baum, A., Revenson, T.A., & Singer, J.E. (Eds.), *Handbook of health psychology.* Mahway, NJ: Erlbaum, 19–47.

114. Lazarus, R.S. & Folkman, S. (1984). *Stress, appraisal, and coping* New York: Springer Publishing.

115. Lazarus, R.S. (1998). *Fifty years of research and theory by r.S. Lazarus: An analysis of historical and perennial issues* Mahwah, NJ: Lawrence Erlbaum Associates.

116. Rickles, N.M. (2010). A multi-theoretical approach to linking medication adherence levels and the comparison of outcomes. *Res Soc Admin Pharm* 6:49–62.

117. Blalock, S.J. & Reyna, V.F. (n.d.) Using fuzzy-trace theory to understand and improve health judgments, decisions, and behaviors: A literature review. *Health Psychol*, in press

118. Reyna, V.F., Lloyd, F.J., & Brainerd, C.J. (2003). Memory development, and rationality: An integrative theory of judgment and decision making. In Schneider, S.l., & Shanteau, J. (Eds.), *Emerging perspectives on judgment and decision research.* Cambridge: Cambridge University Press.

SUGGESTED READINGS

Ajzen, I. (1985). From intentions to actions: A theory of planned behavior. In Kuhl, J. & Beckman, J., (Eds.) *Action-contol: From cognition to behavior.* Heidelberg: Springer, 11–39.

Bandura, A. (1986). *Social foundations of thought and action: A social cognitive theory.* Englewood Cliffs, NJ: Prentice-Hall.

Ficke, D.L. & Farris, K.B. (2005). Use of the transtheoretical model in the medication use process. *Ann. Pharmacother.* 39(7–8):1325–30.

Glanz, K., Rimer, B.K., & Lewis, F.M. (2002). *Health behavior and health education: Theory, research, and practice.* 3rd ed San Francisco: Jossey-Bass; 2002.

Janz, N.K. & Becker, M.H. (1984). The health belief model: A decade later. *Health Educ. Q.* 11(1):1–47.

Lazarus, R.S. (1998). *Fifty years of research and theory by r.S. Lazarus: An analysis of historical and perennial issues* Mahwah, NJ: Lawrence Erlbaum Associates.

Lazarus, R.S. & Folkman, S. (1984). *Stress, appraisal, and coping* New York: Springer Publishing.

Leventhal, H., Leventhal, E.A., & Cameron, L.D. (2001). Representations, procedures, and affect in illness self-regulation: A perceptual-cognitive model. In: Baum A, Revenson TA, Singer JE, eds. *Handbook of health psychology.* Mahway, NJ: Erlbaum, 19–47.

Reyna, V.F., Lloyd, F.J., & Brainerd, C.J. (2003). Memory development, and rationality: An integrative theory of judgment and decision making. In Schneider, S.l., Shanteau, J., (Eds.), *Emerging perspectives on judgment and decision research.* Cambridge: Cambridge University Press.

Weinstein, N.D., Sutton, S.R., & Rothman, A.J. (1998). Stage theories of health behavior: Conceptual and methodological issues. *Health Psychol.* 17(3):290–9.

CHAPTER 4

HEALTH SERVICES PROGRAMS: PLANNING AND EVALUATION

Jon C. Schommer, Ph.D.

LEARNING OBJECTIVES:

1. Describe the PRECEDE-PROCEED framework for program planning and assessment.
2. Describe the Intervention Mapping framework for program planning and assessment.
3. Describe the RE-AIM framework for program planning and assessment.
4. Outline an eight (8) - step process for program evaluation.
5. Describe the four standards for effective program evaluation.

KEY TERMS

Program Planning

Program Assessment

Program Evaluation

Standards

Validity

Program planning and evaluation have a reciprocal relationship in which planning informs evaluation and evaluation informs subsequent planning. Too often, health services programs are evaluated by simply measuring outcomes that were achieved from various strategies and techniques (what was obtained from what was done). A reciprocal approach to planning and evaluation allows organizations and programs to evaluate more deeply and reframe goals and values to also address the question "why we do what we do." This approach allows for reassessment of goals, which may lead to improvements in methods. This approach may be used internally to help organizations and programs plan, conduct self-assessment, and continuously improve. In addition, external parties may wish to determine the value of programs for translation to other settings and situations. With this reciprocal process in mind, the purpose of this chapter is to describe program planning and evaluation frameworks that can be applied to health services programs both internally and externally.

PROGRAM PLANNING

Regarding program planning, Hudmon[1] presented three relevant frameworks that are commonly used to facilitate program planning and self-assessment:

1. PRECEDE-PROCEED[2]
2. Intervention Mapping[3]
3. RE-AIM[4, 5]

THE PRECEDE-PROCEED PLANNING MODEL

In this framework, health behavior is regarded as being influenced by both individual and environmental factors, and hence has two distinct parts. First is an "educational diagnosis"—PRECEDE, an acronym for **P**redisposing, **R**einforcing and **E**nabling **C**onstructs in **E**ducational **D**iagnosis and **E**valuation. Second is an "ecological diagnosis"—PROCEED, for **P**olicy, **R**egulatory, and **O**rganizational **C**onstructs in **E**ducational and **E**nvironmental **D**evelopment.

The PRECEDE-PROCEED model necessitates careful assessment of *(a)* the social environment, *(b)* the epidemiology of the problem, *(c)* the behavior(s) that are impacting the health problem in question, *(d)* educational and ecological factors, and *(e)* administrative and policy factors. Each of these is paramount to the planning process and informs intervention development. Below, we describe each component as described by Hudmon[1] and by Green and Kreuter.[2,6]

PHASES OF THE PRECEDE-PROCEED FRAMEWORK FOR PROGRAM PLANNING

PHASE 1: SOCIAL ASSESSMENT

The social assessment phase focuses on characterizing a population's perceived needs and quality of life, as opposed to simply assessing disease-related outcomes. There are many ways to assess different aspects of quality of life, but in general all of these assessments attempt to ascribe a number or set of numbers to quantify "the perception of individuals or groups that their needs are being satisfied and that they are not being denied opportunities to pursue happiness and fulfillment"[6] (p. 54). Objective social indicators (e.g., unemployment rates, air quality, health-care insurance coverage) or subjective assessments of perceptions, provided by community members can be used. These assessments are important because quality of life and health are closely connected—quality of life impacts health, and health impacts quality of life. If a health program aims to meet patient needs, one must first understand what those needs are. A clear understanding of the capacity of the population is needed—strengths and weaknesses, and how these impact receptivity to an intervention.[1]

Immersion in the community fosters an enhanced understanding of the problem. Specifically, planners should observe the population, conduct in-depth interviews with key informants (e.g., community leaders, opinion leaders), conduct focus groups, host community forums, and/or administer surveys to representative members of the broader community population. The goal in this phase is to gain a complete understanding of quality of life concerns, from the community's perspective. This is best achieved with full, active participation of community members.[1]

PHASE 2: EPIDEMIOLOGIC ASSESSMENT

The epidemiologic assessment phase aims to identify all health-related factors contributing to the societal problems defined in Phase I. Specifically, the assessment attempts to obtain objective measures that pinpoint which health-related conditions are important and identify the behavioral and environmental factors contributing to the incidence of those conditions.

Epidemiologic data are available through national databases maintained by the National Centers for Health Statistics, the Centers for Disease Control and Prevention, Health and Human Services, the Census Bureau, state and local health departments, and other organizations. Typically, an epidemiologic assessment examines morbidity, mortality, and disability in a population. Statistics can include prevalence (the *proportion* of a population that possesses the characteristic at a give point in time) or incidence (the *rate* at which members of a population convert status (e.g., from nondiseased to diseased, creating "new cases").[1]

Green and Kreuter[2] provide guidelines to assist planners in setting priorities for health programs:

1. Which health problem has the greatest impact? (e.g., death, disease, disability, absenteeism, cost, etc.)
2. Are any subpopulations (e.g., children, mothers, racial/ethnic groups) at an elevated risk?
3. Which problems would be most susceptible to intervention?
4. Which problems are not being addressed by other agencies or programs?
5. Which problems have the greatest potential for achieving a significant intervention impact?
6. Are any of the health problems ranked high at the nation or local level?

After these six questions have been answered and priorities are aligned, objectives must be delineated. This is achieved by asking four questions:[2]

1. Who will receive the program?
2. What health benefit should the population receive?
3. How much of that benefit should be achieved?
4. By when should it be achieved, and for how long will the program run?

These objectives must be carefully operationalized—as an example, "the prevalence of smoking in African American women in Los Angeles will be reduced by 5 percentage points in the next 12 months, and by an additional 3 percentage points in the following 24 months." Defining measurable program objectives enables evaluators to gauge the overall success of a program and facilitates associated resource allocation.[1]

PHASE 3: BEHAVIORAL AND ENVIRONMENTAL ASSESSMENT

This phase aims to assess the myriad of factors that are known or hypothesized contributors to the negative health outcome under investigation. *Behavioral factors* are the specific behaviors and/or lifestyle choices that manifest in the target population and contribute to incidence or severity. In contrast, *environmental factors* include social and physical forces that are external to an individual and often not under his or her control. Ideally, many of these factors will be modifiable through intervention. Factors that are not modifiable, such as genetic predisposition, might be useful however in identifying specific subgroups of a population that are at an elevated risk.[1]

A series of steps comprise the **behavioral assessment**:

1. *Differentiate behavioral and nonbehavioral determinants of the health problem.* As an example, if acute myocardial infarction is the health problem of interest, smoking would be the primary behavioral determinant. Some related but nonbehavioral determinants would include lipid panel indicators of atherosclerosis, high blood pressure, and elevated body mass index.
2. *Develop an inventory of behaviors.* This involves refining the list of behavioral factors to specify preventive behaviors (e.g., smoking cessation, regular exercise, mammography screening, stress reduction) versus associated actions

or treatment/interventions (e.g., adherence with medical regimens, smoking cessation, weight reduction). Note that some behaviors might be classified in both categories. For example, smoking cessation is a preventive behavior (e.g., in an adolescent patient), but it also might be a treatment (e.g., in a patient with emphysema).

3. *Rate the behaviors based on importance.* Any behavior that is closely correlated with the outcome of interest is considered important. In this step, the goal is to reduce the list of behaviors to include only those that are most important, whereby importance is gauged by the behavior's frequency and level of relatedness to the health problem.

4. *Rate the behaviors based on extent of changeability.* Behaviors that are closely associated with the outcome of interest but offer little opportunity for change typically are not ideal targets for program planning. In estimating changeability, it is important to consider anticipated timelines for change—how long will it take for the change to occur? High changeability typically is more likely when behaviors are in the developmental stages or have recently been established (e.g., smoking initiation among adolescents or young adults) than when the behavior is well established. Behaviors with high relapse rates tend to be more difficult to change and often require more intensive interventions.

5. *Choose behavioral targets.* Based on information gathered and processed in steps 1–4, the focus of the intervention is chosen.

The behavioral assessment process requires careful specification of behavioral objectives. Objectives should be stated and address the following: Who is the target population? What is the desired change to be achieved? How much of the condition/outcome is to be achieved? In what time frame is the change expected to occur?

The **environmental assessment** follows the same methodology, with a focus on environmental influences. If the scope of environmental factors gets unmanageable, consider limiting the list to environmental aspects that are more social than physical (e.g., organizational and economic), interactive with behavior in its impact on health, and has the potential to be changed through social action or health policy.[6]

PHASE 4: EDUCATIONAL AND ECOLOGICAL ASSESSMENT

Three categories of factors impact individual or group behavior, and these are targeted in phase 4 of *PRECEDE*:

Predisposing factors: antecedents to behavior that provide the rationale or motivation for the behavior. Examples: knowledge, awareness, attitudes, beliefs, perceived needs, self-efficacy, and existing skills.

Enabling factors: factors that facilitate the performance or enactment of a behavior. Examples: availability, accessibility or convenience, affordability, new skills, and environmental conditions. Some enabling factors might exert a negative impact on change.

Reinforcing factors: consequences of action that provide either positive or negative feedback for the action. Examples: physical response, reactions of peers or coworkers, social support, advice from a clinician.

Phase 4 is the assessment step for which behavioral theory tends to be most relevant. This step focuses on the delineation of factors that impact behavioral and environmental factors.[1] Constructs from existing behavioral theories, such as the Health Belief Model,[7-10] the Transtheoretical Model of Change,[11-12] the Theory of Reasoned Action or Planned Behavior,[13-14] or Social Cognitive Theory[15] can help us to understand the target behavior.

Selecting factors to be targeted and setting priorities is achieved by identifying all the causal factors and categorizing them based on whether they exhibit predisposing, enabling, or reinforcing properties. Among the three categories, the constituent factors should be prioritized. Finally, the planners must determine which factors in each category are to be targeted first. Characteristics to consider are importance (frequency and extent of relatedness to the outcome of interest) and changeability. As a final step in the PRECEDE component of the model, one must write learning and resource objectives that (a) define the predisposing factors and skills that will be targeted by the new intervention (b) provide measurable criteria by which the program can be evaluated, and (c) specify what resources or conditions will be present at the conclusion of the program.

PHASE 5: ADMINISTRATIVE AND POLICY ASSESSMENT

Phase 5 involves the delineation of intervention strategies and outlining the logistics of program implementation. A planner must clarify the resources needed for program implementation, any organizational barriers and facilitators for implementation, and any policies that are relevant to the success of the program. This information is used to establish project timelines, allocate resources, and develop a working budget.

ADMINISTRATIVE ASSESSMENT

1. *Assessment of necessary resources.* What resources are needed to implement the proposed program? Items to consider include time, personnel, and budget.

2. *Assessment of available resources.* What resources does the planning team have available to support the program? A primary focus here is on identifying personnel to accept responsibility for the various duties. Are new employees needed, or can existing employees be retrained? What level of funding is available, and what are the budgetary constraints? Lack of funding might necessitate modifications to the program components or its reach.

3. *Assessment of factors influencing implementation.* Investigation of potential factors influencing program implementation might reveal barriers that can be circumvented up front, or might identify positive facilitators—such as program champions that might otherwise have gone unnoticed. At this step,

planners should assess staff commitment and attitudes, revisit the programmatic goals (adjust as necessary), consider the anticipated rate of change (might it be prudent to take smaller, more manageable steps?), promote familiarity of the new procedures among staff through training, attempt to reduce complexity where possible, ensure that appropriate space is available, and anticipate resistance that might be encountered from community members. Also at this step, planners should make certain that program personnel have received adequate training and that a plan for ongoing supervision is in place. This promotes quality assurance.

POLICY ASSESSMENT

Does your proposed program "fit" within the existing polices, regulations and organizational structure and values? Are there any political forces that must be reconciled before the program is launched? There are several approaches for examining the policy environment within an organization or system. The interested reader is referred to Green and Kreuter for a more detailed discussion.[2]

PHASES 6 TO 9: IMPLEMENTATION AND INTERNAL ASSESSMENT

Moving from the PRECEDE (assessment/diagnostic steps) to the PROCEED component of the model, Phase 6 is where the program is actually developed and implemented. All necessary resources are in place, and the program launch is imminent. In Phase 7, the team conducts an ongoing self-assessment of the program processes, to estimate the extent to which the program was implemented according to plan. This *process evaluation* is a necessary component of all program evaluations because it enables the team to more fully interpret the results from the impact and outcome evaluations (Phases 8 and 9). According to the model, impact measures capture changes in the behavioral and environmental factors as well as the predisposing, enabling, and reinforcing factors. Outcome measures estimate the effect of the program on health and quality of life.[1]

In summary, the PRECEDE component begins with analysis of quality of life, health, behavioral and environmental factors, and predisposing, enabling, and reinforcing determinants of the health problem under investigation and its associated environmental factors. In the PROCEED component, a health promotion program is developed, implemented in the defined setting, and internally assessed using process, impact, and outcome measures. This comprehensive approach is achieved through collaboration between planners and the target community.[1] The PRECEDE-PROCEED model has been used as an intervention framework and is an integral component of training for public health advocates. Its underlying principles are germane to the next framework, *Intervention Mapping*.

INTERVENTION MAPPING

Intervention Mapping, developed by Bartholomew and colleagues, provides a protocol for the development of theory-based health promotion programs. The six-step protocol enables the effective translation of knowledge about behavioral determinants into specific change goals, and subsequently into theory-based intervention methods and strategies.[3, 16-24]

Intervention Mapping builds upon the work achieved in a *PRECEDE-PROCEED* phase and facilitates the development of proximal program objectives, the selection of theory-based intervention methods and practical strategies to promote change, the delineation of program components, the anticipation of program dissemination and adoption, and the anticipation of process and outcome evaluations. This process is assisted by the creation of intervention matrices—the matrices collectively create an "intervention map" that guides the translation of objectives to change strategies and intervention activities. The approach, which builds on existing frameworks and applies behavioral theories in the planning process, is a tool that "maps the path from recognition of a need or problem to the identification of a solution." [20] (p. 87).

Although Intervention Mapping is presented as a series of steps, the planning process is more iterative and cumulative than linear.[3] Several core processes are integral to Intervention Mapping; these are applied through group process, with interactive discussion. The mapping process, which operationalizes the theory-based intervention, begins after the needs assessment (e.g., the PRECEDE-PROCEED component, Step 1) has been completed. The mapping process is labor intensive, but is comprehensive in approach.[1, 3]

In Step 2, planners specify *who* and *what* will be the target of the intervention. Toward this goal, a set of matrices is created for each of the relevant ecological levels (e.g., individual, group, organization, societal) that integrate performance objectives for each ecological level with behavioral determinants to produce change objectives. In Step 3, the team identifies evidence-based theories and methods and strategies that are hypothesized to be effective in promoting change at the relevant ecological levels. The end-products of Step 4 include a defined scope and sequence of the intervention components, a complete set of program materials, and carefully operationalized program implementation protocols. All materials and protocols should have undergone pilot testing with the personnel who are responsible for implementing the program as well as the recipients of the program. The emphasis in Step 5 is program adoption, implementation, and maintenance of implementation over time. In Step 6, the team finalizes an evaluation plan that is designed to parallel the intervention map. The focus is on both process and impact/outcome measures, as described previously.[1]

In summary, Intervention Mapping is a tool to aid health planners in applying behavioral science theories to program development and evaluation. It is a practical approach, and while it does not offer new theories or strategies *per se*, it increases the likelihood that new interventions are theoretically solid and are directly linked to the programmatic objectives.[1]

RE-AIM

The RE-AIM framework (Reach Effectiveness Adoption Implementation Maintenance) was designed in response to an identified need to expand the number of "dimensions of quality" that are addressed in the evaluation of health promotion programs.[1] According to the RE-AIM framework, the impact of a health promotion program is a function of five key factors, and each of these can be expressed on a scale that ranges from 0 to 1 (or as a percentage, from 0% to 100%). The factors are described in greater detail next.[4, 5, 25]

Reach. The *reach* of a program describes the proportion of at-risk persons who are exposed to the impact of a policy or program. Careful consideration is given to defining both the numerator and the denominator comprising the proportion—examples of denominators could include the total number of patients serviced at a specific inpatient or outpatient clinic, the number of employees at a specific worksite, or census data. In estimating the extent to which a program is reaching its intended target population, it is important to define the target population and to identify both over-inclusion (did some individuals who received the program not need it?) and under-inclusion (were there individuals in need who did not receive the program?). Under-inclusion can lead to increased health-care costs and over-inclusion can result in wasted resources.[1]

Effectiveness. When evaluating a health services program—it is important to capture both positive and negative outcomes of the program.[1] In addition, evaluators should assess changes in clinical outcomes, behavioral outcomes, and quality of life. The impact of the intervention should be estimated using sound study designs that are able to capture changes over time. Prospective designs are best in most cases, and these should include baseline measures and either a control group or a comparison group so as to protect the internal validity of study results.[1]

Adoption. The third component of the RE-AIM model is *adoption*, and this answers the question, "What is the proportion and representativeness of settings that adopt the program?" While some programs might target only one setting, others are designed for more broad-scale dissemination. Some change agents or sites will be early adopters, some will be late adopters, and some will not adopt at all. It is important to examine a representative sample of all persons or settings, regardless of adoption status. Sometimes the most useful information comes from those that do not choose to adopt. Extent of adoption can be assessed through direct observation, interviews, or surveys.[1]

Implementation. The *implementation* factor is essential in understanding the extent to which the program adhered to the specified protocol. Was the program delivered as intended? If not, how did it deviate? Deviations can occur at the individual and the setting level. At the individual level, some patients might not have participated fully in the program—for example, some might have attended only three of five scheduled group sessions. Or some might not have taken their medication as prescribed. At the setting level, some staff might have implemented the intervention with 100% of patients who met the inclusion criteria while other staff members might have applied the intervention intermittently when time was limited. Implementation is assessed by computing the percentage of process objectives that were achieved—for example, what proportion of brochures were distributed, how many of the planned training sessions were taught, or what proportion of the prescribed medication was consumed? Other process measures that are important and can inform future work include costs of staff time and other resources expended during implementations.[1]

Maintenance. Many program evaluations examine adoption but fail to examine ongoing maintenance of the program. At the individual level, program evaluators might want to assess relapse (e.g., recidivism back to smoking, for a cessation program). At the setting level, once a program has been disseminated, what are the predictors of ongoing institutionalization?[1]

In summary, the RE-AIM model provides a structure for designing interventions and planning internal assessments.[1,25] Each of the five elements is paramount for evaluations of programs that are designed for broad-scale dissemination. RE-AIM draws upon previous work in several areas including Rogers' Diffusion of Innovations theory[26] and the PRECEDE-PROCEED approach.[2] RE-AIM differs from existing models in that it was designed to facilitate translation of research into practice.[1] It places equal emphasis on internal and external validity and emphasizes representativeness of individuals as well as settings, and it outlines standard methods to guide assessment of key factors involved in evaluating potential for public health impact and dissemination.

SECTION SUMMARY

So far, this chapter described three relevant frameworks that are commonly used to facilitate program planning and self-assessment: (1) PRECEDE-PROCEED, (2) Intervention Mapping, and (3) RE-AIM. They are useful for: planning health services programs that meet genuine needs, measuring outcomes that are achieved from various strategies and techniques (what was obtained from what was done), and self-assessment that can help reframe goals and values and address the question "why we do what we do." These frameworks are useful for helping organizations and programs plan, self-assess, and continuously improve.

In addition, external parties may wish to determine the value of programs for translation to other settings and situations. Thus, in addition to planning and self-assessment for health services programs, there is also the need to conduct program evaluation by external parties who may wish to determine the value of the programs for translation to other settings and situations. According to McNamara[27], program evaluation is helpful to:

1. Understand, verify, or increase the impact of products or services on customers, clients, or patients.
2. Improve delivery mechanisms to be more efficient and reduce waste.
3. Verify that the organization is implementing programs as originally planned.
4. Facilitate managerial decision-making regarding goals, how to meet goals, and how to determine if goals are being met.

5. Produce information that can be used to verify desired outcomes and be used for public relations and promoting programs in the community and to sponsors.

6. Produce valid comparisons between programs to help decide which should be retained or expanded.

7. Fully examine and describe effective programs for replication elsewhere.

PROGRAM EVALUATION

STEPS FOR PROGRAM EVALUATION

In this section, a step-by-step approach for program evaluation is presented that can be used for both self-assessments and also for external evaluations. It should be noted that each step builds upon decisions made at previous steps and that the approach is an iterative process in which adjustments will be made to previous steps before the final process is set.[28]

STEP 1: CONSIDER GOALS-BASED, PROCESS-BASED, AND OUTCOMES-BASED EVALUATIONS

The program planning frameworks described earlier (PRECEDE-PROCEED; Intervention Mapping; RE-AIM) engage stakeholders who would make decisions based on the planning and self-assessment processes utilized. As external evaluation is conducted, stakeholders and researchers should address whether the program evaluation would best be designed as a (1) goals-based evaluation, (2) process-based evaluation, or (3) outcomes-based evaluation.[27] For some evaluations, **goals-based evaluation** may be most relevant. Such an evaluation would study the extent to which programs are meeting predetermined goals or objectives. Alternatively, decision makers might be most interested in making decisions related to how a program works. **Process-based evaluations** are geared to fully understand how a program produces the results that it does. Finally, **outcomes-based evaluations** help understand if an organization is accomplishing the outcomes that are needed by its clients. Taking time to consider the nature of the decision problem being addressed in terms of being goals-based, process-based, or outcomes-based can help initial discussions with stakeholders be more fruitful and lead to consensus about the true nature of the decision problem and resultant research problem to be addressed in the program evaluation.[28]

STEP 2: USE OF THEORIES FOR GUIDING EVALUATIONS

The next step would be to conduct a systematic literature review to (1) define the domain being addressed, (2) identify previous research conducted in that domain, and (3) identify useful frameworks or theories that could help guide the evaluation. A systematic literature review not only can help "frame the decisions and issues" stakeholders are facing, but also can uncover previous work that already has addressed and, in some cases, answered the questions set before the decision makers.[28]

STEP 3: FORMULATE PROBLEM

With careful and thorough background work, the problem formulation process can be accomplished through a transparent and consensual manner. Only when the problem is carefully and precisely defined, can research be designed to provide pertinent information.[28] The importance of writing down the research problem and specific objectives for the project(s) being undertaken cannot be overstated.

When developing a program evaluation, decision makers often want to know everything they can about their products, services, or programs. They say in effect, "Here are some things I don't know. When the results come in, I'll know more. And when I know more, then I can figure out what to do." Such an approach can provide findings that turn out to be interesting, but not very actionable.[29] The findings might reduce levels of uncertainty about the health care program being studied, but provide little understanding of the true decision problem that is facing the decision makers. Thus, the research must reflect decision makers' priorities and concerns, for "It is far better to resolve the right decision problem partially than to resolve the wrong problem fully."[30]

An old adage says, "A problem well defined is half-solved."[29] This is especially true for program evaluation; for it is only when the problem has been clearly defined and the objectives of the evaluation research precisely stated that the evaluation can be designed to generate the information needed in an efficient manner. A research problem is essentially a restatement of the decision problem in research terms.

In developing the research problem, the researcher must make certain the real decision problem, not just the symptoms, is being addressed.[29] One way to make sure that the true decision problem will be addressed by the research is to execute a "**research request step**."[29] This step requires that the decision maker and the researcher have a meeting in which the decision maker describes the problem and the information that is needed. The researcher then drafts a statement describing his or her understanding of the problem. This written statement should be submitted to the decision maker in writing for his or her approval, including signature and date. This step will help assure that the purpose of the evaluation research is agreed on before the research is designed.

Getting to this point in a program evaluation is not easy. Decision makers who will be using information from the evaluation and researchers who will be conducting the evaluation often have different training, priorities, and viewpoints. In order to facilitate communication regarding identification of the decision problem and translating it into a research problem for a program evaluation, spending time with stakeholders to describe the program being evaluated can be useful.[28]

STEP 4: DETERMINE RESEARCH DESIGN

Research design depends upon how much already is known about the problem. If previous steps reveal that relatively little is known about the phenomenon to be investigated, exploratory research will be warranted. Exploratory research may involve review of available existing data, interviewing knowledgeable people, conducting focus groups, conducting in-depth interviews, or investigating literature that discusses similar cases. One of the benefits of exploratory research is its flexibility. It allows the researcher to follow leads that may develop during the process.[28]

If the problem is precisely and unambiguously formulated, then descriptive or causal (experimental or quasi-experimental) research is better suited for program evaluation. In these research designs, data collection is rigidly specified, with respect to both data collection forms and the sample design. The advantage of these methods is that they allow testing hypotheses, making population estimations, and testing cause-effect relationships.[28]

STEP 5: DESIGN DATA COLLECTION AND FORMS

Quite often, the information needed for a program evaluation can be obtained from an organization's own databases or internal records, or in published documents such as government reports or publicly available databases. However, some evaluations must depend on primary data, which are collected specifically for the study. At this point, a number of decisions must be made for the evaluation research. For example, should the data be collected by observation or questionnaire? Should the form be structured as a fixed set of answers or should they be open-ended? Should the purpose of the study be made clear to the respondent, or should the study objectives be disguised? Each decision will depend upon the research problem and study objectives as well as the time and resources available for conducting the study.

Sometimes a new measure must be developed for research. Because the meaning attributed to a measure by the investigator may not be the same as the meaning imputed to it by the respondents, a systematic process for developing measures should be followed that includes: (1) specify the domain of the construct, (2) generate a pool of items and determine the format of the measure, (3) have the initial pool of items reviewed by experts, (4) consider inclusion of validation items, (5) administer items to a development sample, (6) purify the measure, and (7) optimize the practicality of the measure (see DeVellis, 2003 for a useful summary of this process.[31])

STEP 6: DESIGN SAMPLE AND COLLECT DATA

In designing the study sample, the researcher must specify the sampling frame, the sample selection process, and the size of the sample. The sampling frame is the list of population elements from which the sample will be chosen. After the sampling frame is specified, the sample selection process entails decisions about using a probability sample, in which each population element has a known chance of being selected, or about using a non-probability sample such as a convenience, judgment, or quota sample. Finally, the decision on sample size involves decisions about the number of sample elements that will be chosen for the study. Sample size requirements depend upon sizes need for analysis, and the time and resources available for the study.

Dillman[32] provides useful guidance for designing and implementing self-administered surveys. His approach uses a social exchange perspective in which the researcher designs surveys to create trust and influence the respondent's expectations for increasing rewards and reducing social costs for completing the survey.

STEP 7: ANALYZE AND INTERPRET DATA

Researchers may amass a mountain of data, but these data are useless unless the findings are analyzed and the results interpreted in light of the problem at hand.[28] Data analysis involves multiple steps. First, data collection forms must be reviewed to be sure that they are complete and consistent with instructions in the forms. Editing of forms may be needed to correct errors, convert responses into the units specified in the instructions, and to address item non-responses. The next step after editing is coding, which involves assigning numbers (or other interpretable values such as text) to each of the answers so that they may be analyzed, typically by computer. The final step in analyzing data is tabulation. This refers to the orderly arrangement of data in a table or other summary format by counting the frequency of responses to each question and by conducting statistical analysis for testing hypothesized differences or relationships. The statistical tests applied to the data, if any, are somewhat unique to the particular sampling procedures and data collection instruments used in the research. Statistical tests should be anticipated before data collection begins so that the data and analyses will be germane to the problem as specified for the study. It should be noted that data analysis in program evaluation can pose challenges. Some of the common challenges include: (1) cluster bias, (2) non-linear relationships, (3) case-mix, (4) mediating/moderating effects, (5) time effects (recall bias, time-to-event, longitudinal effects), and (6) acquiescent response.[28,32-38]

STEP 8: PREPARE THE RESEARCH REPORT

Interpretations of findings into actionable conclusions are justified when they are linked to the evidence gathered and judged against agreed-upon standards set by the stakeholders. Stakeholders must agree that conclusions are justified before they will use the evaluation results with confidence. A **research report** is a useful communication tool for sharing findings with stakeholders, for obtaining feedback on draft versions, and developing a final version that can be agreed upon by stakeholders. In some cases, alternative views and interpretations may be included in the report to help maintain transparency and fair balance.

The research report is all that most stakeholders will see of the program evaluation, and it becomes the standard by which the research is judged. Thus, it is imperative that the research report be complete, clear, accurate, and concise since no matter how well all previous steps have been completed, the project will be no more successful than the research report.[28] A general outline for research reports consists of (1) title page, (2) table of contents, (3) executive summary, (4) introduction, (5) methods, (6) results, (7) discussion of results within the context of the purpose of the study, (8) conclusions and recommendation, and (9) appendices (e.g. copies of data collection forms, detailed calculations used for analysis, tables not included in the main part of the report, bibliography).

STANDARDS FOR EFFECTIVE PROGRAM EVALUATION

External program evaluation should be blended with program planning and self-assessment as well. This helps program evaluation research become a practical tool that stakeholders and decision makers can use to inform program's efforts and assess their impact. Thus, these evaluations need to be integrated into day-to-day planning, implementation, and management for programs.[1, 28, 38–40]

The following standards are proposed for making sound and fair evaluations practical. They are (1) utility, (2) feasibility, (3) propriety, and (4) accuracy. The standards provide guidelines to follow when having to decide among evaluation options and help avoid creating imbalanced action plans (e.g. pursuit of a plan that is accurate and feasible but not useful; or one that is useful and accurate but is infeasible). The standards are guiding principles, not mechanical rules. Thus, whether a given standard has been addressed adequately in a particular situation is a matter of judgment.[39,40] The four standards are described next.

UTILITY

Utility standards ensure that information needs of evaluation users are satisfied. Seven specific utility standards include:[39,40]

1. *Stakeholder identification—persons involved in or affected by the evaluation should be identified so that their needs can be addressed.*
2. *Evaluator credibility—persons conducting the evaluation should be trustworthy and competent in performing the evaluation.*
3. *Information scope and selection—information collected should address pertinent questions regarding the program and be responsive to the needs and interests of clients and other specified stakeholder.*
4. *Values identification—perspectives, procedures, and rationale used to interpret findings should be described.*
5. *Report clarity—reports should clearly describe the program being evaluated, including its context and purposes, procedures, and findings of the evaluation.*
6. *Report timeliness and dissemination—substantial interim findings and evaluation reports should be disseminated to intended users.*
7. *Evaluation impact—evaluations should be planned, conducted, and reported in ways that encourage follow-through by stakeholders.*

FEASIBILITY

Feasibility standards ensure that the evaluation is viable and pragmatic. Three specific feasibility standards include:[39,40]

1. *Practical procedures—evaluation procedures should be practical while needed information is being obtained to keep program disruption to a minimum.*

2. *Political viability—consideration should be given to the varied positions of interest groups so that their cooperation can be obtained and maintained.*

3. *Cost-effectiveness—the evaluation should be efficient and produce valuable information to justify expended resources.*

PROPRIETY

Propriety standards ensure that the evaluation is conducted with regard for the rights and interests of those involved and affected. Eight propriety standards include:[39,40]

1. *Service orientation—the evaluation should be designed to assist organizations in addressing and serving the needs of the target participants.*

2. *Formal agreements—principal parties for the evaluation should agree in writing to their obligations.*

3. *Rights of human subjects—the rights and welfare of human subjects must be respected and protected.*

4. *Human interactions—interactions with other persons associated with an evaluation should be respectful so that participants are not threatened or harmed.*

5. *Complete and fair assessment—the evaluation should record strengths and weaknesses of the program completely and fairly so that strengths can be enhances and problem areas addressed.*

6. *Disclosure of findings—full evaluation findings with pertinent limitations should be made accessible to persons affected by the evaluation and any others with expressed legal rights to receive the results.*

7. *Conflict of interest—conflict of interest should be handled open and honestly.*

8. *Fiscal responsibility—allocation and expenditure of resources should reflect sound accountability procedures.*

ACCURACY

Accuracy standards ensure that the evaluation produces findings that are considered correct. Twelve accuracy standards include:[39,40]

1. *Program documentation—the program being evaluated should be described clearly and accurately.*

2. *Context analysis—the context in which the program exists should be examined in enough detail to identify probable influences on the program.*

3. *Purposes and procedures—purposes and procedures for the documentation should be described in sufficient detail so that they can be monitored and audited.*

4. *Defensible information sources—sources of information should be described in enough detail to assess the adequacy of the data.*

5. *Valid information—information gathering procedures should be described to ensure valid interpretations.*

6. *Reliable information—information gathering procedures should be described to ensure sufficiently reliable information for intended use.*

7. *Systematic information—information collected, processed, and reported should by systematically reviewed and any errors corrected.*

8. *Analysis of quantitative information—quantitative analysis techniques should be described so that others can replicate the work.*

9. *Analysis of qualitative information—qualitative analysis techniques should be described so that others can replicate the work.*

10. *Justified conclusions—conclusions should be explicitly justified for stakeholders' assessment.*

11. *Impartial reporting—reporting procedures should guard against distortion caused by personal feelings and biases of any party.*

12. *Meta-evaluation—the evaluation should be formatively and summatively assessed against these and other pertinent standards so that upon completion, enable close examination of its strengths and weaknesses by stakeholders.*

SUMMARY

The purpose of this chapter was to describe program planning and evaluation frameworks that can be applied to health services programs. Health care resources are limited, and as such one cannot overstate the need for effective program planning and evaluation in our public health efforts. The frameworks presented should be used in tandem with sound research designs, psychometrically solid study measures, and carefully operationalized protocols for program implementation, data collection, data management, and data analysis.

Program planning and evaluation have a reciprocal relationship in which planning informs evaluation and evaluation informs subsequent planning. The goal of this chapter was to not only provide suggestions for how to assess "what was obtained from what was done" but also to help address the question of "why we do what we do." The approaches outlined in this chapter can be used internally to help organizations and programs conduct self-assessment and to help them continuously improve. In addition, the approaches can be used to meet the needs of external parties who may wish to determine the value of programs for translation to other settings and situations. The "real world" of program planning and evaluation is challenging, but also rewarding. There is no doubt that successful programs have the potential to substantially alter the landscape of public health.

Acknowledgements: The author gratefully acknowledges Karen S. Hudmon, Dr PH, MS, RPh for her insights on this chapter. Portions of this chapter are based upon her work "Health Promotion—Program Planning and Evaluation" in *Social and Behavioral Aspects of Pharmaceutical Care*, Second Edition, 2010.

Some portions of this chapter are based upon a chapter written by Jon C. Schommer, PhD, MS, RPh titled "Program Evaluation" in Aparasu, R (ed) (2011). *Research Methods for Pharmaceutical Practice and Policy*. Pharmaceutical Press, London. Used with permission from Pharmaceutical Press.

REFERENCES

1. Hudmon, K.S. (2010). In Rickles, Wertheimer, Smith (Eds.), *Health promotion: program planning and evaluation. social and behavioral aspects of pharmaceutical care.* Boston: Jones and Bartlett Publishers.

2. Green, L.W. & Kreuter M.W. (2005). Health program planning: An educational and ecological approach. New York, NY: McGraw-Hill.

3. Bartholomew, L.K., Parcel, G.S., Kok, G.,& Gottlieb (2006). *N.H. planning health promotion programs: an intervention mapping approach.* San Francisco, CA: Wiley & Sons, Inc.

4. Glasgow, R.E., Vogt, T.M., & Boles, S.M. (1999). Evaluating the public health impact of health promotion interventions: the RE-AIM framework. *Am J Public Health* 89(9):1322–1327.

5. Re-AIM. http://www.re-aim.org/. Accessed October 15, 2007.

6. Green, L.W. & Kreuter, M.W. (1999). *Health promotion planning: An educational and ecological approach* 3rd ed. Mountain View, CA: Mayfield Publishing Company.

7. Becker, M.H. & Maiman, L.A. (1975). Sociobehavioral determinants of compliance with health and medical care recommendations. *Med Care.* 13:10–24.

8. Becker, M.H., Maiman, L.A., Kirscht, J.P., Haefner, D.P., Drachman, R.H., & Taylor, D.W. (1979). Patient perceptions and compliance: Recent studies of the health belief model. In: Haynes, R.B., Taylor, D.W., & Sackett, D.L., (Eds.), *Compliance in health care.* Baltimore: The Johns Hopkins University Press: 78–109.

9. Janz, N.K. & Becker, M.H. (1984). The health belief model: A decade later. *Health Education Quarterly* 11:1–47.

10. Rosenstock, I.M. (1974). The health belief model and preventive health behavior. *Health Education Monographs* 2:354–386.

11. Prochaska, J.O. (1979). *Systems of psychotherapy: A transtheoretical approach.* Homewood, IL: Dorsey Press.

12. Prochaska, J.O. & DiClemente, C.C. (1984). *The transtheoretical approach: Crossing traditional boundaries of therapy.* Homewood, IL: Dow Jones-Irwin.

13. Ajzen, I. & Fishbein, M. (1980). *Understanding attitudes and predicting social behavior.* Englewood Cliffs, N.J.: Prentice-Hall.

14. Ajzen I. (1991). The theory of planned behavior. *Organizational Behavior and Human Decision Processes* 50:179–211.

15. Bandura A. (1986). *Social foundations of thought and action.* New Jersey: Prentice Hall.

16. Abbema, E.A., Van Assema, P., Kok, G.J., De Leeuw, E., & De Vries, N.K. (2004). Effect evaluation of a comprehensive community intervention aimed at reducing socioeconomic health inequalities in The Netherlands. *Health Promot Int.* 19(2):141–156.

17. Bartholomew, L.K., Parcel, G.S., Kok, G. (1998). Intervention mapping: A process for developing theory- and evidence-based health education programs. *Health Educ Behav.* 25(5):545–563.

18. Fernandez, M.E., Gonzales, A,. Tortolero-Luna, G., Partida, S., & Bartholomew, L.K. (2005). Using intervention mapping to develop a breast and cervical cancer screening program for Hispanic farmworkers: Cultivando La Salud. *Health Promot Pract.* 6(4):394–404.

19. Heinen, M.M., Bartholomew, L.K., Wensing , M., van de Kerkhof, P., & van Achterberg, T. (2006). Supporting adherence and healthy lifestyles in leg ulcer patients: Systematic development of the Lively Legs program for dermatology outpatient clinics. *Patient Educ Couns.* 61(2):279–291.

20. Kok, G., Schaalma, H., Ruiter, R.A., van Empelen, P., & Brug, J. (2004). Intervention mapping: Protocol for applying health psychology theory to prevention programmes. *J Health Psychol.* 9(1):85–98.

21. Kwak, L., Kremers ,S.P., Werkman, A., Visscher, T.L., van Baak, M.A.,& Brug, J. (2007). The NHF-NRG In Balance-project: The application of Intervention Mapping in the development, implementation and evaluation of weight gain prevention at the worksite. *Obes Rev.* 8(4):347–361.

22. Van Empelen, P,. Kok, G., Schaalma ,H.P., Bartholomew, L.K. (2003). An AIDS risk reduction program for Dutch drug users: An intervention mapping approach to planning. *Health Promot Pract.* 4(4):402–412.

23. Van Kesteren, N.M., Kok, G., Hospers, H.J., Schippers, J., & De Wildt, W. (2006). Systematic development of a self-help and motivational enhancement intervention to promote sexual health in HIV-positive men who have sex with men. *AIDS Patient Care STDS.* 20(12):858–875.

24. Van Oostrom, S.H., Anema, J.R., Terluin, B., Venema, A., de Vet, H.C., & van Mechelen, W. (2007). Development of a workplace intervention for sick-listed employees with stress-related mental disorders: Intervention Mapping as a useful tool. *BMC Health Serv Res.* 7:127.

25. Glasgow, R.E., Toobert, D.J., Hampson, S.E., & Strycker, L.A. (2002). Implementation, generalization and long-term results of the "choosing well" diabetes self-management intervention. *Patient Educ Couns.* 48(2):115–122.

26. Rogers, E.M.(2003). *Diffusion of innovations.* 5th ed. New York, NY: Free Press.

27. McNamara, C. (2006). *Field guide to nonprofit program design, marketing and evaluation, 4th Edition.* Minneapolis: Authenticity Consulting,

28. Schommer, Jon C. (2011). Program Evaluation. In Rajender Aparasu (Ed.), *Research methods for pharmaceutical practice and policy.* London: Pharmaceutical Press, 261–274.

29. Churchill, G.A. (1995). *Marketing research, methodological foundations*, 6th Edition. New York: The Dryden Press, New York.

30. O'Dell, W., Ruppel, A.C., Trent, R.H., & Kehoe, W.J. (1988) *Marketing decision-making: Analytic framework and cases*, 4th Edition.Cincinnati: South-Western Publishing Company.

31. DeVellis, R.F. (2003) *Scale development, theory and applications, second edition, applied social research methods series*, Volume 26. Thousand Oaks, CA: SAGE Publications.

32. Dillman, D.A. (2000). *Mail and internet surveys, second edition.* New York: John Wiley & Sons.

33. Bieler, G.S. & Williams, R.L. (1997). *Application of the SUDAAN software package to clustered data problems in pharmaceutical research.* Research Triangle Park: NC Research Triangle Institute.

34. Bryk, A.S. & Raudenbush, S.W. (1992.) *Hierarchical linear models, advanced quantitative techniques in the social sciences series*, Volume 1. Newbury Park, CA: SAGE Publications.

35. Johnson, J.A. (1997) Patient Satisfaction. In pharmacoeconomics and outcomes: Applications for patient care, *American College of Clinical Pharmacy:* 111–154.

36. Lobo, F.S. (2003). Assessment of channeling bias and its impact on interpretation of outcomes in observational studies: The case of the cyclooxygenase-2 (cox-2) inhibitors. Unpublished Doctoral Dissertation, University of Minnesota.

37. Baron, R.M. & Kenny, D.A. (1986). The moderator-mediator variable distinction in social psychological research: Conceptual, strategic, and statistical considerations. *Journal of Personality and Social Psychology*, 51(6): 1173–1182.

38. Babar, Z. (2015). *Pharmacy Practice Research Methods.* Switzerland: Adis, Springer International Publishing

39. Centers for Disease Control and Prevention. (1999). Framework for Program Evaluation in Public Health. *Morbidity and Mortality Weekly Report* 48 (RR11): 1–40.

40. U.S. Department of Health and Human Services. Centers for Disease Control and Prevention. Office of the Director, Office of Strategy and Innovation. (2005). *Introduction to program evaluation for public health programs: A self-study guide.* Atlanta, GA: Centers for Disease Control and Prevention.

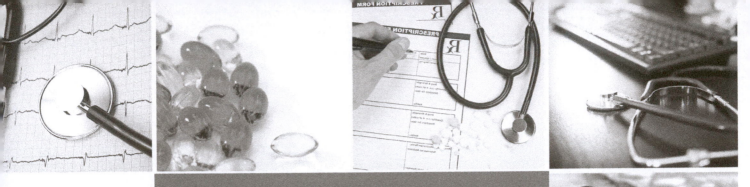

PART II APPROACHES TO RESOLVE HEALTH PROBLEMS

SECTION A

BEHAVIORAL MEDICINE

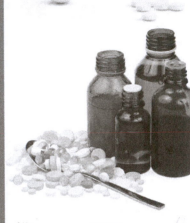
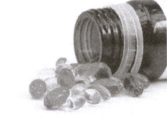
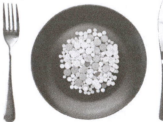
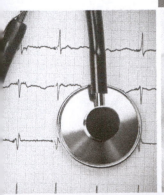
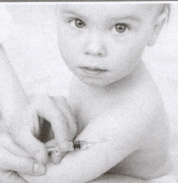
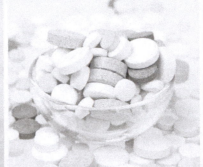
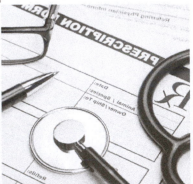

CHAPTER 5

BEHAVIORAL MEDICINE

John M. Lonie, RPh, EdD, Karishma Desai, PhD, M.S., B.Pharm, Cherie Tsingos-Lucas, PhD, Gina Paola Torres Rubiano, MD

LEARNING OBJECTIVES:

1. Summarize the theoretical basis of behavioral medicine practices.
2. Explain the role of the human stress response and how behavioral strategies can mitigate stress.
3. Describe how patient's decision-making processes affect their choices regarding behavioral medicine practices.
4. Compare and contrast the most commonly used behavioral approaches to health and illness.
5. Describe the role of the pharmacist in helping guide patients toward appropriate behavioral health treatments.

KEY TERMS

Behavioral medicine

Behavioral therapeutic interventions

Decision-making and behavioral medicine

Health and learning theories

Health belief model

Placebo effect

Stress and pharmacists

OVERVIEW

Over the past several decades, the behavioral sciences have become a well-recognized resource for healthcare professionals.[1] This may be due to the fact that many chronic health conditions require behavioral lifestyle changes.[2] Today, few healthcare professionals can argue against the role that the mind (and its impact on behavior) plays on behavior, health and illness. Dolinsky, using Shunichi's definition of behavioral medicine, noted that, "behavioral medicine is an interdisciplinary applied science concerned with the development and integration of behavioral and biomedical science, knowledge and techniques related to health and illness, and the application of this knowledge and these techniques to prevention, diagnosis, treatment and rehabilitation." [3,4]

This chapter will focus on the primary areas in which evidence-based contributions from the behavioral sciences have affected the health professions and will be organized around six major topic areas: (1) An overview of the theoretical basis of behavioral medicine; (2) The human stress response; (3) The placebo response; (4) How patients make decisions regarding the use of behavioral medicine modalities; (5) Commonly accepted behavioral medicine modalities and (6) Pharmacist's role in Behavioral Medicine.

As the definition reads, behavioral medicine is an adaptation and application of many concepts, principles, and theories of a number of scientific disciplines. These include psychology, sociology, epidemiology, anthropology, physiology, nutrition, endocrinology, pharmacology, and immunology.[5] The disciplines of social psychology, health psychology and cognitive psychology have contributed the most to the development of behavioral medicine treatments.[3,6] For that reason, this chapter will begin with a focus on the theories within each of these disciplines that have advanced the understanding of how behavioral medicine has affected patient care.

THE THEORETICAL BASIS OF BEHAVIORAL MEDICINE

As mentioned, the theoretical basis of behavioral medicine extends to a number of disciplines.[7] However, a question that often arises in pharmacy practice and education is whether or not students (and pharmacists) are able and motivated to apply theories from other disciplines (i.e. psychology, sociology) to real-life professional practice problems. In seeking an answer to this problem, Sleath sought to determine whether or not pharmacy students would be able to apply social psychological theories to the solution of real-life pharmacy practice situations. She found that students are able to make connections and apply these theories in order to solve patient care problems.[8] Despite some reluctance, pharmacists are in a unique position to effect behavior change through the application of social science theories.[9,10] Many behavioral interventions require reinforcement. Since pharmacists see their patients frequently, opportunities exist for pharmacists to help the behavioral reinforcement process.

However, just what are these theories, and which may be used with the greatest practicality by pharmacists? The discipline of health psychology is an area that has guided conceptual models into behavioral medicine practices. Health psychology is primarily concerned with the understanding, prevention, and treatment of illnesses using a psychosocial framework. This understanding, prevention, and treatment occur from within the biopsychosocial model of health and illness.[3,6] That is, health psychologists operate from the framework that physical illness can best be explained and treated if the illness is viewed from its biological, psychological and sociological components.[3]

HEALTH BELIEF MODEL

Within the field of health psychology, the Health Belief Model (HBM) is has been one of the most widely used theories in behavioral medicine. As noted in a previous chapter, the purpose of the HBM is to explain and predict why people make specific health-related decisions.[8] The HBM is predicated on several key assumptions: individuals will take or not take action based upon (i) their perceived susceptibility to a particular illness; (ii) the perceived severity of the illness; (iii) the perceived costs (barriers) of taking action; and (iv) the perceived benefits of taking action. The HBM has been used with success in a number of areas including predicting and explaining adherence to medical regimens.[11] For example, a patient visits his physician and it is determined that the patient has elevated cholesterol levels. The physician prescribes a modification in the patient's diet as well as an exercise program for the patient to follow. According to the HBM, the patient will or will not follow the advice of his physician based upon their own perceptions of susceptibility, severity, costs, and benefits of following through. The patient may ask himself, "How susceptible am I to the medical effects of having high cholesterol? How severe are these effects? What are the costs versus the benefits of me adhering to my physician's advice? Will I have to substantially change my lifestyle? How important is it for me to change my lifestyle? How the patient decides (i.e. cognition) to answer these questions will determine adherence or non-adherence (i.e. behavior) to his physician's advice.

In the past, research using the HBM on issues related to the profession of pharmacy included the cognitive predictors of adherence to medication regimens,[12,13,14] especially in chronic conditions[15,16,17] and the decision to use different education/pharmacy services.[18] The HBM has consistently shown to have strong predictive power in terms of health behaviors, particularly the cost /benefit constructs.[19] HBM has also widely been used to guide the development of pharmacist-led intervention in pharmacies.[19] Despite its frequent use, a recent review identified intervention studies using HBM geared to improve adherence. The author's reported that the success of the intervention was not linked to the HBM constructs. However, the same study also reported only six of the studies included in the review used all constructs of the HBM.[20] More discussion of HBM and some of the other theories presented below are also presented in additional details in Chapter 3 on individual and interpersonal theories of health behavior.

LEARNING THEORIES AND HEALTH BEHAVIOR

Learning theorists believe that behavior change is based not only upon the decisions an individual makes, but also on the external environment in which the decision is made. In addition, learning theorists place a great deal of importance on the consequences that decisions have on the individual (i.e. rewards, punishments, etc).[21] This section will examine the following learning theories as they relate to health behavior change: Operant conditioning; Observational learning; and Self-efficacy.

OPERANT CONDITIONING

Operant conditioning is based on the premise that positive behavioral responses will occur if the person is rewarded for their behavior.[22] Essentially, the reward feels good to the individual and people tend to repeat behaviors that make them feel good.[22] An aspect of the principle of operant conditioning that has important implications for health behaviors is the gradient of reinforcement, which implies that immediate rewards are more effective than delayed rewards.[5]

For example, patients suffering from chronic pain may find immediate relief after using an analgesic, which leads them to sometimes over use pain medications without considering the side effects or adverse events that could result from overdosing. Similarly, if a patient were to face a side effect in the first instance of using a drug, they may be less likely to adhere to their medication regimes.

An example of research utilizing operant conditioning as a theoretical approach was conducted by Heapy.[23] She studied diabetic patients' adherence to treatment regimens using the Inherent Consequences Model (ICM). This model is based upon operant conditioning principles. Heapy found that the ICM has significant predictive power and may be useful in determining adherence issues using the principles of operant conditioning. Operant conditioning has mainly been used to help pain management.[24] Although there have been a number of experimental studies to support its use in pain behaviors,[25] it is much harder to implement such environmental triggered behavior learning beyond an experimental setting. However, use of operant conditioning has shown to help reduce pain perception and pain related interferences.[26]

The use of operant conditioning is not limited to changing behavior amongst patients. In recent years there has been increasing importance towards improving the quality of healthcare. In order to improve quality, the Center for Medicare and Medicaid Services (CMS) has started shifting to pay-for-performance framework. According to this framework, health professionals and hospitals are incentivized or rewarded financially according to set quality standards. Although much of this initially started with physicians and hospitals, the focus now has also included pharmacies and pharmacists to improve the quality of medication use.[27,28]

OBSERVATIONAL LEARNING

Some patients learn to change behavior by observing the actions and consequences of others. As opposed to individual learning, observational learning is not based on directly experienced outcome prediction errors.[29] Observational learning as defined by Bandura is any learning that occurs through observing the behavior of others.[30] This learning can manifest in a number of ways, including the imitation of the learned behaviors. Observational learning depends on the capability to correctly interpret the actions of others, and to understand connections between these behaviors and their associated consequences.[31]

Research also supports the notion that individuals who operate at various cognitive development levels respond differently to observed events than they would respond to verbal or written instructions.[30] For example, a graphic television commercial which features the adverse health effects of smoking may be a more powerful stimulus to stop smoking for some individuals than would the verbal advice of a physician. It appears that, for some individuals, the act of observing is a powerful cognitive influence. Participating in proactive actions, such as joining and imitating the behavior of others, and taking part in responses that implicate attention to instructions could simplify observational learning.[31] This has important implications for individuals practicing any form of behavioral modification. If cognitive developmental levels are assessed appropriately, the desired behavioral modification can be delivered more efficiently.[32] Additionally, observational learning has shown to be useful mechanism to improve training. This included training patients, particularly in conditions that require use of devices like asthma[35] as well as training pharmacists through the mandatory experiential learning program. One of the key features of the experiential or clerkship program is to visit multiple sites over the course of time and learn through observing different settings of practice.

SELF-EFFICACY

Self-efficacy implies the influence of people's beliefs in their ability to organize and perform the action required to achieve expected results.[34] Perhaps more influential than his theory of observational learning was Bandura's social cognitive theory of self-efficacy.[30] The social cognitive theory has been used to understand the motivational determinants of human behavior. The theory is based on the term "triadic reciprocity," which means that a person's behavior is frequently influenced by the environment and personal perceptions, known as his or her predetermined goals.[35] Bandura noted that people regularly monitor (self-regulate) their actions in line with predetermined goals. Central to the self-efficacy theory is the idea that a person's beliefs about the successful attainment of those goals will influence their ability to attain those goals. For example, if an individual wants to lose 20 pounds, their level of self-efficacy (their belief that they can lose 20 pounds) will be affected by the magnitude of the goal itself as well as their ability to self-regulate their behavior (i.e., exercise) in order to meet that goal.[36] The same situation could be applied to such areas as academic performance. This theory proposes that the academic performance (behavior) is influenced by the student's beliefs (cognitions) and also by the attention provided by his or her parents, teachers, and peers (the environment).[37]

Self-efficacy theory has been used in a myriad of health-related research projects. In the context of pharmacy, most of these projects can be grouped into 1) intervention evaluation studies and 2) assessment of ability to self-manage chronic conditions/adherence to medication regimens.[36,38,39] Since the importance of self-efficacy has already been established in terms of improving health,[40] self-efficacy is often used to assess improvement in self-efficacy after particular interventions. Improvement in self-efficacy scores may suggest the intervention could in turn help improve health.[41,42,43] Similarly, self-efficacy has been used to assess how well patients feel they can manage their health conditions or adhere to regimens.[44,45] Self-efficacy has been also associated with motivational concepts such as self-esteem, optimism, goal orientation, academic help-seeking, and anxiety.[37]

THE HUMAN STRESS RESPONSE

WHAT IS STRESS?

Stress results when an organism is required to change or adapt to its environment.[46] From this definition, stress can result from anything. For example, just getting up from a seated position can be stressful because of the physical demand that gravity exerts on the body. Stress can be either useful or damaging to both the physical body and an individual's psychological state. Stress that is helpful to individuals is known by the term eustress.[47] Examples of eustress could be seen when an individual has a small amount of anxiety before speaking in public, or when an athlete is about to take the field in a big game. In both of these instances, the stress experienced is not debilitating and can actually lead to better performances by the speaker and the athlete. Stress becomes problematic and debilitating when it leads to some form of alteration of normal activities in an individual.

Stress can be acute (short term) or chronic (long-term). Acute stress is the response to an abrupt threat and often manifests physiologically as the fight or flight response. The threat can be any situation that is interpreted consciously or unconsciously as possibly causing harm to the individual. Common acute stressors include noise pollution, crowded settings, sudden danger, and certain illnesses.[48] Common forms of chronic stressors are prolonged tensions in work environments, problems in interpersonal relationships, and various social, economic, and cultural adaptations.[48]

STRESS AND HUMAN PHYSIOLOGY

A number of biochemical and neuro-chemical changes occur in response to stress. The hypothalamic-pituitary-adrenal (HPA) system becomes activated in the brain. The HPA system activates the production and release of the steroid hormones and neurotransmitters.[49] A wide range of biological functions within the human body including the immune system, integumentary system, and metabolic system are affected. Both the cardiovascular and respiratory systems respond to the stress by means of adaptation. For example, the heart rate and blood pressure increase in response to perceived threats. Prolonged elevation of heart rate and blood pressure has detrimental effects on the body.[47,49] Prolonged and severe stress can alter the neurophysiology, causing depression and anxiety.[47,49] Additional findings suggest that the repeated release of cortisol produces hyperactivity in the hypothalamic-pituitary-adrenal axis, which disrupts the normal levels of serotonin, which is responsible for feelings of well-being.[49] Prolonged psychological stress has been shown to cause injury to the inner lining of blood vessels leading to hypertension.[50] There is also evidence that stress contributes to changes in the immune system. Chronic stress hinders the immune response and poses a greater risk for infections.[51] Patients with chronic stress often present with below normal levels of white blood cells, making these patients more susceptible to cold and flu viruses.[52]

There is evidence that shows relationships between various types of headaches, muscular and joint pain and stress.[49,52] Other studies relate stress to a vast number of other conditions including, insomnia, external pollutants that cause allergies, skin disorders, hair lose, premature teeth lose, gum disease, sexual and reproductive dysfunction, premenstrual syndrome, fertility, and pregnancy conditions leading to miscarriages and premature births.[49]

Stress also impairs memory, concentration and learning. Research focusing on the effects of acute stress on short-term memory found that increased cortisol levels impaired the ability of the participants to memorize. Enduring chronic stress, such as post-traumatic stress has been shown to shrink the gray matter volume (GMV) in fear regulatory areas like the ventromedial prefrontal cortex (vmPFC) and hippocampus.[53] Furthermore, research has confirmed the negative effects of stress on psychological and biological systems of the human body.[54]

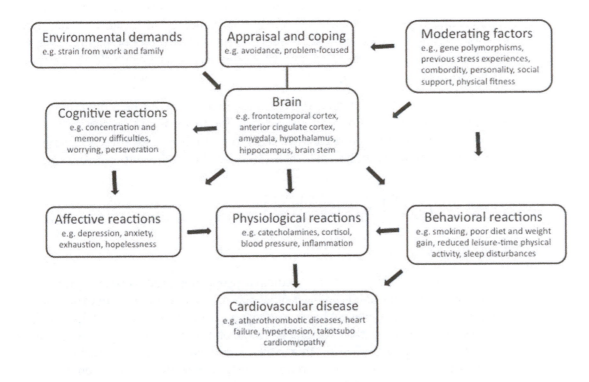

FIGURE 5-1: STRESS MODEL AND ITS INFLUENCE IN THE HUMAN BODY

Adapted from: von Känel, R. Psychosocial stress and cardiovascular risk – current opinion. Swiss Med Wkly. 2012;142:w13502

IMPACT OF STRESS ON PHARMACISTS

Stress is a common phenomenon among pharmacists and other health care professionals.[55] A study examining community pharmacists' job satisfaction found, that among other factors, the routine stressors of pharmacy practice led in some cases to negative evaluations of their job satisfaction.[56] Research has shown that prolonged stress can be a causative factor in many medication errors,[57] especially among pharmacists[58] (see Figure 5-1).

Gaither conducted a cross-sectional mail survey of 1,088 licensed pharmacists in the United States practicing in chain, independent, or hospital pharmacies. The objective of this study was to determine whether career commitment mediates the effects of job stress on pharmacists. The research examined the effects of job stress, career commitment, job satisfaction, and other variables on job turnover intention.[59] The results indicated that more than 65% of the respondents were satisfied with their present job and 50% indicated that they would choose pharmacy again as a career. Seventy percent of pharmacists indicated that their work was creative and important. The results suggest that career commitment and other factors can mediate the effects of job stress. The author suggested that strategies should be developed to increase the career commitment of pharmacists through career planning and the use of mentors.[60]

Researchers also investigated the levels of job satisfaction and job stress among consulting and community pharmacists. The results of this study showed that the majority of pharmacists surveyed would choose to be pharmacists again despite the stressors that they experienced.[61] The most common stressors among pharmacists included personal obligations, which were difficult to carry out because of long hours at work, overload of work as a result of short staffing, and the lack of opportunities for job advancement. The most common stressor experienced by one-third of respondents was the fear of making a mistake when filling a prescription.[61]

Stress is a natural phenomenon which in moderate levels can be motivating. However, in high levels and under prolonged conditions stress can be debilitating and lead to physical and psychological damage. The practice of pharmacy is stressful. However, research has shown that stress can be mediated through various factors.

THE PLACEBO EFFECT

WHAT ARE PLACEBOS?

A placebo is a substance with no medicinal properties used to treat a physical or psychological condition. it is an inert substance used as a control in an experiment.[62] The origin of the placebo effect began among physicians who intended to please their patients with medicines that instilled the hope of a speedy recovery when in reality the medicinal substance had no therapeutic significance to the medical condition. Placebos that are administered through ingestion, injection, or incision, often are considered more powerful than non-invasive placebo methods.[63]

Placebos, when administered by healthcare providers, can have beneficial effects on various physical and psychological disease processes. These beneficial effects are due to the beliefs and expectations of the person receiving the placebo treatment. Whether or not a placebo will work depends a great deal on the amount of faith the patient has in the treatment itself and the practitioner administering the placebo. It is understood the more a patient believes in the benefits of treatment, the more likely it is that the patient will experience a positive medical benefit from the placebo treatment.[64] Research conducted on patients with illnesses ranging from arthritis to depression showed a 30–60% substantial improvement in their symptoms after receiving placebo treatments.[65,66] Also, it has been demonstrated that psychological factors, especially the patient's attitude towards their healthcare provider or the patient-provider relationship during a treatment, can affect the impact of the treatment of an illness.[67]

There is a unique and intimate connection between the mind and the body.[65] Suggestion is the term used to describe the process by which a physical or mental state is created by a thought or idea.[68] Placebo effects frequently demonstrate an influence of suggestion or how the body is frequently influenced by the mind. A person's psychological state when influenced by suggestion can trigger neurochemical release, which then can affect that person's physiology.[69]

Other examples of the effects of placebo treatment include a study conducted by the Coronary Drug Project where researchers set out to find the safety and effectiveness of drugs used for long-term treatment among males with coronary heart disease. The results showed those who were adherent to the placebo treatment demonstrated nearly half the mortality rate as those who were not.[70] Placebo treatments have been used to alter immune responses in cancer patients and in patients suffering from rheumatoid arthritis as well as in treating patients with depression.[71]

HOW PATIENTS MAKE DECISIONS ABOUT BEHAVIORAL MEDICINE MODALITIES

Patients expect that the decisions made by health care providers should be guided through evidence-based science. However, patients themselves do not always make health care decisions for themselves that are evidence based.

There is broad access of medical information through internet, public libraries, and in the media.[72] This has made individuals much better-informed patients, and in some ways, more active participants of their own care.[73] This access of medical information has given patients the ability to explore treatments that go beyond the information transmitted by healthcare providers and has allowed patients to choose additional resources. What are the factors that influence a patient's decision-making? A different chapter will focus more specifically on patient decision-making.

Considering how complex the answer is, we shall only be discussing the decision-process method used by patients to decide whether or not to use complementary and alternative medicines (CAM), which are closely related to Behavioral Medicine Modalities. The National Center for Complementary and Alternative Medicine (NCCAM), the lead agency for scientific research on complementary and alternative medicine in the United States, defines CAM as "a group of diverse medical and health care systems, practices, and products that are not generally considered part of conventional medicine…"[74] There is a pattern that patients usually follow when they decide to choose CAM after being diagnosed with an illness or just as an aid for well-being, and is briefly illustrated in the following scheme.[75]

Exploratory studies have suggested a number of factors affecting a patient's decision to use CAM. These can be divided into 3 categories: 1) Provider characteristics, Patient characteristics, and 3) Practice characteristics.[76]

PROVIDER CHARACTERISTICS:

This is perhaps, one of the predominant reasons patients decide to use CAM. Patients usually describe the "welcoming" feeling that they receive when they visit a CAM provider as compared to the "cold" feeling when they opt for conventional medicine.[77]

Many CAM practitioners seem to effectively rely on and utilize communication skills, allowing patients to feel safe and comfortable.[77] For example, they use a variety of active listening skills that demonstrate their interest and concern for the patient.[78]

PRACTICE CHARACTERISTICS:

Patients usually feel comfortable with a more suitable, calm, and attractive physical space that is often used by CAM providers.[79] Additionally, patients prefer the relaxing environment and the importance that CAM providers place on a patient's overall well-being.[80]

Another interesting practice characteristic is that consultations made for CAM modalities are usually more detailed, which appears to be very satisfying for patients.[81] The CAM holistic approach to patient care seems to provide a better patient experience.[81] Research has suggested that patients often seek second opinions (leading to CAM practitioners) due to lack of information provided from their initial evaluation.[82]

PATIENT CHARACTERISTICS:

Some of the most significant predictors why patients choose CAM modalities are the patient's level of educational and current health status.[83] Patients with at least some college background are more likely to seek out CAM modalities.[84] In addition, patients with poor overall health status, particularly those suffering from chronic anxiety or pain are more likely to seek out CAM modalities.[84] Patients also seem to be attracted to the CAM modalities that provide faster and more affordable alternatives[85] (see Table 5-1).

Furthermore, many patients perceive CAM as being highly effective[86] more "natural," and less toxic to the body.[87] Patients are becoming increasingly concerned about the side-effects of conventional medical treatments, and believe CAM alternatives to pose as a better option to other conventional drugs.[88] Another contributing factor to CAM use is the risk of iatrogenic disease. Iatrogenic diseases are those believed to be caused by obtaining treatment or seeking advice for health conditions[89,90] (see Figure 5-2).

TABLE 5-1: REASONS WHY PATIENTS USE CAM MODALITIES

USER	REASON FOR USING CAM OR USER CHARACTERISTICS
Experimenter open to new experience or skeptical to CAM	Try and see, nothing to lose, even when user does not have positive expectations.
Those heavily influenced by the commodification of health	Responds to the health claims of CAM no differently from the response to other health products; consumes health products in order to stay healthy
Heavy users of all systems of medicine and types of practitioners	Is either very health conscious or derives secondary gain from seeking help, or may use care-seeking as an idiom of distress or as a way of mobilizing support
Enlightened users of CAM, interested in promoting wellness or prevent illness	The ideology of the CAM system may be embraced as a form of spiritual practice or as a philosophy or as preventive health aid
Seekers of new cure for an old problem that persists or those afflicted with a chronic illness, disease or disability	CAM enables the patient to play a more active and participatory role in care, assume greater responsibility; the patient is looking for other ways to understand illness to make the experience more coherent.
Those who mistrust the health care system	Health care system has not met expectations
Those dissatisfied by traditional doctor-patient relationship	Looking for more patient-centered approach to the treatment of illness which fits the treatment to the patient's life and what is valued by the patient
Those who have limited access to conventional medicine and who cannot afford it except for cases of severe illness	CAM serves as a stop-gap function and is used as just another form of over-the counter medicine
Those encouraged by friends or family to try CAM	Direct and indirect influence by people who have heard that the CAM modality can help

Adapted from: Committee on the Use of Complementary and Alternative Medicine by the American Public Board on Health Promotion and Disease Prevention. Complementary and Alternative Medicine in the United States. 2005. http://www.ncbi.nlm.nih.gov/books/NBK83794/

COMMONLY ACCEPTED BEHAVIORAL MEDICINE THERAPEUTIC INTERVENTIONS

There are many different forms of behavioral medicine (CAM) interventions. Even though they are usually grouped together, complementary and alternative medicine are actually two different behavioral medicine interventions: complementary medicine ,which can be used in addition to traditional forms of medicine, and alternative medicine used primarily in place of traditional or conventional medicine.[91] Despite the fact that most CAM modalities have been in use for thousands of years, it was only recently that they have become part of research and Evidence-Based Medicine (EBM).[92] Recent research has demonstrated the effectiveness of many CAM modalities for the treatment of a wide range of ailments and disorders.[93,94,96]

THE MIND-BODY CONNECTION

The belief that the mind and body are connected goes back to antiquity. Although different cultures have had various understandings of the mind-body connection, most considered the mind-body as one element.[95] The ancient Greek and Chinese societies first conceptualized health and disease as being due to natural (as opposed to supernatural) causes. Although both of these cultures developed a more sophisticated understanding of illness, the idea that the mind and body were intimately connected was still viable. During this time, it was understood that physical illness might be caused by a malady within the blood or nervous system, but it was also understood and accepted that the person's mental state played a key role in the outcome of the illness.[96] However, throughout the Middle Ages there was an emphasis back toward the view that health and illness were solely spiritually mediated. This was due more to the influence and control of the Christian Church than a widespread change in core belief systems. It was during the Renaissance and the Scientific Revolution that a systematic theory of health and illness took hold. The biomedical model became the commonly-used theory that guided thinking around the determinants of health and illness. As useful as this conception has been, it has also received some criticism. For example, the biomedical model breaks all physical illness down into its component parts. By doing this, it does not take into account the myriad of psychological and social factors that contribute to health and illness. As a result of this, a biopsychosocial approach to health and illness emerged. As the name suggests, the biopsychosocial approach takes into account the biomedical, psychological and social factors that contribute to health and illness.[97]

Research has shown that the mind can influence the perception of many different physical and psychological illnesses. A large percentage of patient visits to primary healthcare providers are the result of psychological issues.[98] Researchers have examined the role that family practitioners and primary care physicians had in treating patients with psychosomatic complaints. They determined that over half of all patient visits to these healthcare practitioners were the result of psychosocial problems which present as somatic complaints.[97,98] Psychological stress may be the most common inducer of psychosomatic complaints.[99] The use of mind-body treatments have been used with varying success in many physical and psychological disorders.[95,97–102] The most well-known and commonly accepted mind-body treatments used have been relaxation/controlled breathing techniques, meditation/prayer, yoga/movement therapy and biofeedback.

RELAXATION / CONTROLLED BREATHING TECHNIQUES

Relaxation techniques have been used with great success in combating various physical and psychological disorders like hypertension, migraine headaches, and stress disorders. In traditional medical practices relaxation techniques often combined with controlled breathing techniques have been used to combat stress and anxiety. Examples include the tense-release method and deep breathing.[103-105]

The tense-release relaxation method involves tensing different muscle groups in the body then releasing them completely and relaxing. This technique usually requires individuals to begin at the feet and then systematically move through the body. This method can be done several times per day and is popular because it can be done in two to three minutes.[105]

The deep breathing technique is also a popular relaxation technique because it can be done in a relatively short period of time in almost any space. Deep breathing is thought to reduce stress through both physiological and psychological mechanisms. The act of taking in oxygen at a slow rate, gently holding the breath, and then slowly releasing the breath has positive effects on the central nervous system, cardiovascular system, and gastrointestinal system.[105]

MEDITATION/PRAYER

Meditation involves a variety of methods, which allow individuals to learn to "disconnect" their attention from the outside in order to gain awareness about themselves and their environment.[106] Meditation has been used for centuries by many different cultures and religions with the goal of centering the mind and body. There are many different forms of meditation; all of them can be classified into two categories: mindfulness meditation and concentrative meditation.[107]

One of the most popular forms of meditation is mindfulness meditation. Mindfulness meditation involves focusing the consciousness on what one is doing in the present moment. This involves gently pushing aside random and often upsetting thoughts that appear in a person's consciousness. For many, this is a difficult process to learn. However, proponents of various meditative practices claim that a steady meditation practice can increase self-awareness, self-trust, and self-acceptance. Many claim that meditation enhances appreciation of life and provides serenity.[109] There is also evidence that meditation provides long-term decreases in stress-related physical and psychological health problems.[108] Meditation is a modality that has been incorporated into many traditional healthcare therapies.[109,110]

YOGA / MOVEMENT THERAPY

Yoga, a form of movement therapy, has been practiced for thousands of years and consists of many different varieties. Generally, yoga is a method of relaxing the physical body, which enhances the balance of the mind, body, and the spirit.[111] It includes a myriad of techniques such as breathing exercises, meditation, concentration, and physical postures, with the aim to increase strength and flexibility and concentration.[112] There are several forms of yoga such as Ananda, Anusara, Ashtanga, Bikram, Hatha, Kundalini, Vinasha and Viniyoga.[111] Research has shown that yoga is effective at treating anxiety, depression, and chronic pain.[112,113]

BIOFEEDBACK

Biofeedback is a modality that teaches patients how to modify their physiological activity in order to improve health and performance.[114] Research has shown biofeedback to be effective in the treatment of pain, depression, ADHD, and headaches.[115-117]

PHARMACISTS' ROLE IN BEHAVIORAL MEDICINE

In recent years there has been an impetus for pharmacists to provide cognitive services and other interventions directly related to behavioral modalities. Two important areas that directly affect patient behavior where pharmacists can play an impactful role include 1) Patient Education and 2) Preventive Medicine.

1. Patient Education

Patient education regarding disease state and the impact of interactions between a prescription, over-the counter, and herbal medicines on health are very important predictors for adherence to lifestyle modification and medications.[118-119] This is probably one of the most important areas for pharmacists to make a difference as they are the most-accessible health care providers. Their wide-spread knowledge of pharmacology and interactions of prescription, over-the counter, and herbal medications along with their expertise in evaluating the appropriateness of these medications for various health conditions, places them in a powerful position to have a profound effect on positive health outcomes.[120] There has been tremendous amount of research on the importance of pharmacist-led counseling in improving adherence and in turn health outcomes for various chronic conditions such as high blood pressure, HIV, asthma, and diabetes.[121-122] Pharmacists are in a unique position to meet patients, their families, and get to know them on a more personal level. An exchange of conversation between a pharmacist and a patient may not only be about medications, but may also explore insights into their assumptions, approaches, attitudes, and beliefs towards medicines and lifestyle issues.[123] This interaction between a pharmacist and a patient has the potential to contribute to patient health outcomes. Through reflective processes, a pharmacist's role looks beyond the mechanics of dispensing by conceptualizing clinical practice, "taking account of other crucial elements, perspectives, biases and assumptions by drawing on a person's awareness of self and others."[123] Pharmacists have the opportunity to discuss a multitude of topics ranging from health conditions, medications, side effects, to family or personal issues, lifestyle choices, and adherence issues or concerns. As part of pharmacist-patient communication in the form of patient counseling, it is important for the pharmacist to recognize when it is appropriate to integrate a specific behavioral modality into a patient's treatment or to persuade the patient against the modality in practice when is necessary.

Another area where pharmacists have been targeted for identifying needs and implementing interventions is in preventative medicine. Pharmacists have always shown an interest in taking on an active role in preventative medicine while also acknowledging the limitations in the current system, making it difficult to implement in practice.[126-127] Some of the barriers to providing preventative services noted include time constraints, lack of private space for counseling, and insufficient training.[128] However, despite the hurdles, pharmacists have been found to help promote a number of preventative services. Some of the areas in which pharmacists have an important role in preventative interventions include weight management,[129] smoking cessation,[130] cardiovascular diseases[131] and alcohol misuse.[132] Additionally, the pharmacist's involvement in immunization has been found to increase the rate and uptake of adult vaccinations, further depicting their influence on patient behavior.[133,134,135] All this points towards the increase in roles played by pharmacists. In today's world, pharmacists are not only acting as drug experts, but also participating in public health endeavors. Much of this work to accomplish better results, be it changing behaviors or improving patient knowledge, could be facilitated by applying different psychosocial theories and strategies.

SUMMARY

Behavioral medicine came into its own in the 1970s. Since then behavioral medicine has a number of proponents as well as skeptics. There are several areas where behavioral medicine has experienced great successes: cardiovascular disease, epilepsy, infertility, menopause, psychiatric diseases, and cancer, to name a few. Research in these areas now focuses on modifiable risk factors associated with these diseases. However, despite some advances in behavioral medicine, there are still challenges that exist in the field that hinder its full integration into mainstream medical practice. Such hindrances include concerns about the validity and reliability of behavioral medicine research. Some scientists dispute the quality of the data that support the efficacy of various interventions. Healthcare decision makers also question how best to integrate theory and concepts of behavioral medicine into the current health care system.

Despite these proposed limitations, it appears that the amount of research in behavioral medicine will continue to grow well in the near future. Perhaps the biggest challenge facing behavioral medicine is communicating its value to skeptics.

REFERENCES

1. Larzelere, M.M., Campbell, J.S., et al. (2010, June). Complementary and alternative medicine usage for behavioral health indications. *Prim Care:* 213–36.

2. Bholat, M.A., Ray, L, et al. (2012, Dec.). Integration of behavioral medicine in primary care. *Prim Care* 39(4):605–14.

3. Dolinsky, D. (1996). Recent developments in behavioral medicine. In: Smith, M.C., & Wertheimer, AI (Eds.), *Social and behavioral Aspects of pharmaceutical care.* Binghamton, New York: Haworth Press.

4. Shunichi, A. (Ed.). (1992). *An integrated behavioral approach to health and illness.* Amsterdam: Elsevier.

5. Miller, N.E. (1983). Behavioral medicine: symbiosis between laboratory and clinic. *Annu Rev Psychol.* 34:1–31.

6. Engel, G.L. (1977, April 8). The need for a new medical model: A challenge for biomedicine. *Science* 196(4286):129–36.

7. Matarazzo, J.D. (1980, Sept.). Behavioral health and behavioral medicine: Frontiers for a new health psychology. *Am Psychol.* 35(9):807–17.

8. Sleath, B. (1997). Teaching pharmacy students how to use social psychological theories when monitoring chronic disease patients. *J Soc Admin Phar* 14(1)16–25.

9. Johnson, J.A. (1996, May June). Self-efficacy theory as a framework for community pharmacy-based diabetes education programs. *Diabetes Educ.* 22(3):237–41.

10. Elliott, R.A., Barber, N., et al. (2008, Jan). The cost effectiveness of a telephone-based pharmacy advisory service to improve adherence to newly prescribed medicines. *Pharm World Sci.* 30(1):17–23.

11. Wallston, B.S., Wallston, K.A., et al. (1984). Social psychological models of health behavior: An examination and integration. In: A. Baum, S.E., Taylor & J.E. Singer (Eds.) *Handbook of psychology and health.* Hillsdale, NJ: Erlbaum.

12. Abraham, C., Clift ,S., et al. (1999). Cognitive predictors of adherence to malaria prophylaxis regimens on return from a malarias region: protective study. *Soc Sc Med* 48(11) 1641–1654.

13. Van Hulten, R., Bakker, A.B., et al. (2003). The impact of attitudes and beliefs on length of benzodiazepine use: A study among inexperienced and experienced benzodiazepine users. *Soc Sc Med* 56(6):1345–1354.

14. Orensky, I.A., Holdford, D.A, et al. (2005). Predictors of noncompliance with warfarin therapy in an outpatient anticoagulation clinic. *Pharmacotherapy* 25(12):1801–1808.

15. Gao, X., Nau, D.P., et al. (2000). The relationship of disease severity, health beliefs and medication adherence among HIV patients. *AIDS Care* 12(4): 387–398.

16. Pham, D.T., Fortin, F., et al. (1996, Mar-Apr.). The role of the Health Belief Model in amputees' self-evaluation of adherence to diabetes self-care behaviors. *Diabetes Educ.* 22(2):126–32.

17. DiMatteo, M.R.1., Haskard ,K.B., et al. (2007, Jun.) Health beliefs, disease severity, and patient adherence: a meta-analysis. *Med Care* 45(6):521–8.

18. Pinto, S. L., Lively, B. T., et al. (2006). Using the Health Belief Model to test factors affecting patient retention in diabetes-related pharmaceutical care services. *Research in social & administrative pharmacy* (RSAP) 2(1):38–58.

19. Carpenter, C. J. (2010). A meta-analysis of the effectiveness of health belief model variables in predicting behavior. *Health communication* 25(8):661–669.

20. Jones, C. J., Smith, H., et al. (2013). Evaluating the effectiveness of health belief model interventions in improving adherence: a systematic review. *Health Psychology Review* 1–17.

21. Lonie, J.M. (2006, Dec.). From counting and pouring to caring: the empathic developmental process of community pharmacists. *Res Social Adm Pharm* 2(4):439–57

22. Chesney, M.A. (1984). Behavior modification and health enhancement, In: J.D. Matarazzo, S.M. Weiss, J.A. Herd, N.E. Miller, & S.M. Weiss, (Eds.). *Behavioral health: A handbook of health enhancement and disease prevention.* New York: Wiley.

23. Heapy, A.A. (2004). *The inherent consequences and prediction of diabetic regimen adherence* (Dissertation). Purdue University.

24. Fawzy, F.I., Fawzy N.W., et al. (1995) Critical review of psychosocial interventions in cancer care. *Arch Gen Psychiatry.* 52:100–13.

25. Gatzounis, R., Schrooten, M.G., et al. (2012, April) Operant learning theory in pain and chronic pain rehabilitation. *Curr Pain Headache Rep.* 16(2):117–26.

26. Thieme, K. & Turk, D. (2012). Cognitive-behavioral and operant-behavioral therapy for people with fibromyalgia. *Reumatismo* 64(4):275–85.

27. Nau, D.P. (2003.) Quality measurement: Time to get serious. *J Am Pharm Assoc* 2006 Nov-Dec;46(6):668, 671–2.

28. Koenigsfeld, C.F., Horning, K.K., et al. (2012, Feb.). Medication therapy management in the primary care setting: a pharmacist-based pay-for-performance project. *J Pharm Pract.* (1):89–95.

29. Burke, C.J., Tobler, P.N., et al. (2010). Neural mechanisms of observational learning. *Proc Natl Acad Sci U S A.*; 107:14431–14436.

30. Bandura, A. (1977 Mar). Self-efficacy: toward a unifying theory of behavioral change. *Psychol Rev.* 84(2):191–215.

31. Monfardini, E., Gazzola, V, et al. (2013). Vicarious neural processing of outcomes during observational learning. *PLoS ONE* 8(9): e73879.

32. Taylor, B.A. & DeQuinzio, J.A. (2012 May). Observational learning and children with autism. *Behav Modif.* 36(3):341–60.

33. Sleath, B., Carpenter, D.M., et al. (2012 Nov). Communication during pediatric asthma visits and child asthma medication device technique 1 month later. *J Asthma* 49(9):918–25.

34. Bandura, A. (1997). Self-Efficacy: The exercise of control. New York: WH Freeman.

35. Bandura, A. (2001). Social cognitive theory: An agentic perspective. *Annu Rev Psychol.* 52:1–26.

36. Ngo, A. & Murphy, S. (2005 May June). A theory-based intervention to improve nurses' knowledge, self-efficacy, and skills to reduce PICC occlusion. *J Infus Nurs.* (3):173–81.

37. Tsang, S.K., Hui, E.K., et al. (2012). Self-efficacy as a positive youth development construct: A conceptual review. *ScientificWorldJournal* 452327.

38. Do, C. (2004, Feb. 15). Applying social learning theory to children with dental anxiety. *J Contemp Dent Pract.* 5(1):126–35.

39. Ngoh, L.N. & Shepherd, M.D. (1997). Design, development, and evaluation of visual aids for communicating prescription drug instructions to nonliterate patients in rural Cameroon. *Patient Educ Couns.* (3):245–61.

40. Lev, E.L., Kolassa, J., & Bakken, L.L. (2010). Faculty mentors' and students' perceptions of students' research self-efficacy. *Nurse Educ Today* 30(2):169–74.

41. Lorig, K.R., & Ritter, P. (2001). Chronic disease self-management program: 2-year health status and health care utilization outcomes. *Med Care.* 39(11):1217–23.

42. Marks, R. & Allegrante, J.P. (2005). A review and synthesis of research evidence for self-efficacy-enhancing interventions for reducing chronic disability: implications for health education practice (part II). *Health Promot Pract.* 6(2):148–56.

43. Johnson, J.A. (1996). Self-efficacy theory as a framework for community pharmacy-based diabetes education programs. *Diabetes Educ.* 22(3):237–41.

44. Wolf, M.S., Davis, T.C., et al. (2007). Literacy, self-efficacy, and HIV medication adherence. *Patient Educ Couns.* 65(2):253–60.

45. Johnson, M.O., Chesney, M.A., et al. (2006). Positive provider interactions, adherence self-efficacy, and adherence to antiretroviral medications among HIV-infected adults: A mediation model. *AIDS Patient Care STDS.* 20(4):258–68.

46. National Institute of Mental Health. [accessed on November 15th 2014]; Adult Stress-Frequently Asked Questions. http://www.nimh.nih.gov/health/publications/stress/Stress_Factsheet_LN_142898.pdf

47. Le Fevre, M., Matheny, J., et al.(2003). Eustress, distress, and interpretation in occupational stress. *J Manag Psychol.* 18:7,726–744

48. Lyle, H.M., Alma, D.S., et al. (1994). The stress solution: An action plan to manage the stress in your life. Pocket Books.

49. Everly, Jr., G.S. & Lating, J.M. (2013). A clinical guide to the treatment of the human stress response. Springer Science & Business Media.

50. Bercovich, E., Keinan-Boker, L., et al. (2014).Long-term health effects in adults born during the Holocaust. *Isr Med Assoc J.* 16(4):203–7.

51. Qin, H.Y., Cheng, C.W, et al. (2014). Impact of psychological stress on irritable bowel syndrome. *World J Gastroenterol.* 20(39):14126–14131.

52. Ortiz, M.S., Willey, J.F., et al. (2014). How stress gets under the skin. *Rev Med Chil.* 142(6):767–74.

53. Keding, T.J. & Herringa, R.J. (2014, Sept). Abnormal structure of fear circuitry in pediatric post-traumatic stress disorder. Neuropsychopharmacology. 12.

54. Maeda, E. & Iwata, T. (2014, Nov. 8). Effects of work stress and home stress on autonomic nervous function in Japanese male workers. *Ind Health.*

55. Schmid, A. Work stress in the second half of adult life. (2014 Aug 20). *Praxis* 103(17):1017–21.

56. Longshaw, R.N. & Asghar, M.N. (1999). Where the grass is not greener. *Pharmacy in Practice* (England) 9:276

57. Wick, J.Y. & Zanni, G.R. (2002 Jan-Feb). Stress in the pharmacy: changing the experience. *Am Pharm Assoc* (Wash) 42(1):16–20.

58. Buckley, J. (2002). Daily life stresses of pharmacists can contribute to medication errors. *Pharm Prac News.* 29(7):21–2

59. Gaither, C.A. (1999). Career commitment: a mediator of the effects of job stress on pharmacists' work-related attitudes. *J Am Pharm Assoc* (Wash)39(3):353–61.

60. Gaither, C.A., Kahaleh, A.A., et al. (2008, Sep). A modified model of pharmacists' job stress: the role of organizational, extra-role, and individual factors on work-related outcomes. *Res Social Adm Pharm.* 4(3):231–43.

61. Lapane, K.L. & Hughes, C.M. (2004 Nov). Baseline job satisfaction and stress among pharmacists and pharmacy technicians participating in the Fleetwood Phase III Study. *Consult Pharm.*; 19(11):1029–37.

62. Andreou, Ch., Bozikas, V,P. (2008 Apr). The PLACEBO effect: Definition, theories of action, ethical considerations. *Psychiatriki.*; 19(2):153–64.

63. Lichtenberg, P., Heresco-Levy, U., et al. (2004 Dec).The ethics of the placebo in clinical practice. *J Med Ethics.*; 30(6):551–4.

64. Fässler, M., Gnädinger, M., et al. (2011 Feb). Placebo interventions in practice: a questionnaire survey on the attitudes of patients and physicians. *Br J Gen Pract.*; 61(583):101–7.

65. Santiago, T,. Geenen, R., et al. (2014 Aug). Psychological factors associated with response to treatment in rheumatoid arthritis. Curr Pharm Des. 25.

66. Leuchter, A.F., Morgan, M., et al. (2004).Pretreatment neurophysiological and clinical characteristics of placebo responders in treatment trials for major depression. *Psychopharmacology* (Berl);177(1-2):15–22.

67. Colloca. L. & Jonas, W.B.(2014). Reevaluating the placebo effect in medical practice. *Z Psychol.* 222(3):124–127.

68. Wehrli, H. (2014 Jul 2). Hypnotic communication and hypnosis in clinical practice. *Praxis* (Bern 1994).;103(14):833–9.

69. Hyland, M.E. (2003). Using the placebo response in clinical practice. *Clin Med.*; 3(4):349.

70. [No authors listed]. (1980). Influence of adherence to treatment and response of cholesterol on mortality in the coronary drug project. *N Engl J Med.*; 303(18):1038–41.

71. Dworkin, R.H.1., Katz ,J,. et al. (2005 Dec 29). Placebo response in clinical trials of depression and its implications for research on chronic neuropathic pain. *Neurology*; 65(12 Suppl 4):S7–19.

72. Elolemy, A.T. & Albedah, A.M. (2012 Jan). Public knowledge, attitude and practice of complementary and alternative medicine in Riyadh region, Saudi Arabia. *Oman Med J.*; 27(1):20–6.

73. De Las Cuevas, C. & Peñate, W. (2014 Oct). To what extent psychiatric patients feel involved in decision making about their mental health care? Relationships with socio-demographic, clinical, and psychological variables. *Acta Neuropsychiatr.* 7:1–10.

74. National Center for Complementary and Alternative Medicine. (2014.) [accessed on November 15th 2014]; Complementary, Alternative, or integrative health: What's in a name? http://nccam.nih.gov/health/whatiscam.

75. Weeks, L. & Balneaves, L.G. (2014). Decision-making about complementary and alternative medicine by cancer patients: integrative literature review. *Open Medicine.* Vol 8, No.2.

76. Astin, J.A. (1998 May 20). Why patients use alternative medicine: results of a national study. *JAMA*; 279(19):1548–53.

77. Hoerster, K.D., Butler, D.A., et al. (2012 Jan). Use of conventional care and complementary/alternative medicine among US adults with arthritis. *Prev Med.*; 54(1):13–7.

78. Singer, J. & Adams, J. (2014 May 22). Integrating complementary and alternative medicine into mainstream healthcare services: The perspectives of health service managers. *BMC Complement Altern Med.* 14:167.

79. NCCAM and the Royal College of Physicians. (January 23–24, 2001). Report: *Can alternative medicine be integrated into mainstream care?* London, England.

80. Maha, N. & Shaw, A. (2007 May). Academic doctors' views of complementary and alternative medicine (CAM) and its role within the NHS: an exploratory qualitative study. *BMC Complement Altern Med.* 30;7:17.

81. O'Reilly, E. & Sevigny ,M. (2014 Oct 14). Perspectives of complementary and alternative medicine (CAM) practitioners in the support and treatment of infertility. *BMC Complement Altern Med.*; 14(1):394.

82. Shumay, D.M., Maskarinec, G., et al. (2001 Dec). Why some cancer patients choose complementary and alternative medicine instead of conventional treatment. *J Fam Pract.*;50(12):1067

83. Huebner J, Prott, F.J., et al. (2014). Online survey of cancer patients on complementary and alternative medicine. *Oncol Res Treat.* 37(6):304–8.

84. Laiyemo, M.A., Nunlee-Bland, G., et al. (2014 Nov 6). Characteristics and health, perceptions of complementary and alternative medicine users in the United States. *Am J Med Sci.*

85. Barnes, P.M., Bloom, B., et al. (2008 Dec 10). Complementary and alternative medicine use among adults and children: United States, 2007. *Natl Health Stat Report.*;(12):1–23.

86. Buhling, K.J. & Daniels, B.V. (2014 Feb). The use of complementary and alternative medicine by women transitioning through menopause in Germany: results of a survey of women aged 45-60 years. *Complement Ther Med.*;22(1):94–8.

87. Kretchy, I.A., Owusu-Daaku, F. et al. (2014 Feb 4). Patterns and determinants of the use of complementary and alternative medicine: a cross-sectional study of hypertensive patients in Ghana. *BMC Complement Altern Med.*;14:44

88. Dalla Libera, D., Colombo, B, et al. (2014 May). Complementary and alternative medicine (CAM) use in an Italian cohort of pediatric headache patients: The tip of the iceberg. *Neurol Sci.*;35 Suppl 1:145–8.

89. Evans, M. & Shaw, A., et al. (2007 Aug 4). Decisions to use complementary and alternative medicine (CAM) by male cancer patients: information-seeking roles and types of evidence used. *BMC Complement Altern Med.* 7:25.

90. White, M.A. & Verhoef, M.J. (2007 Aug 4). Seeking mind, body and spirit healing-Why some men with prostate cancer choose CAM (Complementary and Alternative Medicine) over conventional cancer treatments. Med.;7:25. *Integr Med Insights.* 2008;3:1–11.

91. Zwickey, H. & Schiffke, H. (2014 Nov 7). Teaching evidence-based medicine at complementary and alternative medicine institutions: Strategies, competencies, and evaluation. *J Altern Complement Med.*

92. Kozasa, E.H. & Tanaka, L.H. (2012 Oct). The effects of meditation-based interventions on the treatment of fibromyalgia. *Curr Pain Headache Rep.* 16(5):383–7.

93. Marc, I. & Toureche, N. (2011 Jul). Mind-body interventions during pregnancy for preventing or treating women's anxiety. *Cochrane Database Syst Rev.* 6;(7):CD007559.

94. Kaplan, H.I. (1975) (DATE). Current psychodynamic concepts in psychosomatic medicine. In R.O. Pasnau (ed.) *Consultation—Liaison Psychiatry.* New York: Grune & Stratton.

95. Chambers, J.B. & Marks, E.M. (2014 Oct 31). A multidisciplinary, biopsychosocial treatment for non-cardiac chest pain. *Int J Clin Pract.*

96. Yoeli-Tlalim, R. (2010 Dec). Tibetan 'wind' and 'wind' illnesses: towards a multicultural approach to health and illness. *Stud Hist Philos Biol Biomed Sci.*;41(4):318–24.

97. Sternlieb, J.L. (2014). The unique contribution of behavioral scientists to medical education: The top ten competencies. *Int J Psychiatry Med.*;47(4):317–26.

98. McGrady, A.V. & Andrasik, F. (1999 Aug). *Psychophysiologic therapy for chronic headache in primary care.* Prim Care Companion J Clin Psychiatry.;1(4):96–102.

99. Wu, T., Bian, Z.X, et al. (2014). Complementary and alternative medicine for respiratory tract infectious diseases: prevention and treatments. *Evid Based Complement Alternat Med.*;2014:913095.

100. Tomiyama, A.J., Ahlstrom, B., et al. (2014 Jan). Evaluating eating behavior treatments by FDA standards. *Front Psychol.* 3;4:1009.

101. Kligler, B. & Lynch ,D. (2003 Nov-Dec). An integrative approach to the management of type 2 diabetes mellitus. *Altern Ther Health Med.*;9(6):24–32; quiz 33.

102. Terathongkum, S. & Pickler, R.H. (2004 Sep). Relationships among heart rate variability, hypertension, and relaxation techniques. *J Vasc Nurs.*;22(3):78–82; quiz 83–4.

103. Chaudhuri, A. & Ray, M. (2014 Sep). Effect of progressive muscle relaxation in female health care professionals. *Ann Med Health Sci Res.*;4(5):791–5.

104. Minen, M.T. & Seng, E.K. (2014 Mar). Influence of family psychiatric and headache history on migraine-related health care utilization. *Headache.*; 54(3):485–92.

105. National Center for Complementary and Alternative Medicine. (2013). [accessed on November 15th 2014]; Relaxation techniques for Heath: An introduction. 2013 http://nccam.nih.gov/health/stress/relaxation.

106. Duke Center for Integrative Medicine (DCIM). (2006). *The Duke encyclopedia of new medicine: Conventional & alternative medicine for all ages.* London, UK: Rodale Books International.

107. National Center for Complementary and Alternative Medicine. (2010). [accessed on November 15th 2014]; *Meditation: An introduction.* http://nccam.nih.gov/health/meditation/overview.

108. Serpa, J.G. & Taylor, S. (2014 Dec). Mindfulness-based Stress Reduction (MBSR) Reduces Anxiety, Depression, and Suicidal Ideation in Veterans. *Med Care.*;52 Suppl 5, Building the evidence base for complementary and integrative medicine use among veterans and military personnel:S19–S24.

109. Grossman, P., Niemann, L., et al. (2004). Mindfulness-based stress reduction and health benefits. A meta-analysis. *J Psychosom Res.*;57(1):35–43.

110. Rainforth, M.V., Schneider, R.H., et al. (2007 Dec), Stress reduction programs in patients with elevated blood pressure: a systematic review and meta-analysis. *Curr Hypertens Rep.* 9(6):520–8.

111. *National Center for Complementary and Alternative Medicine.* (2013). [accessed on November 15th 2014]; Yoga for Heath. http://nccam.nih.gov/health/yoga/introduction.

112. Khalsa, S.B., Shorter, S.M,. et al. (2009 Dec). Yoga ameliorates performance anxiety and mood disturbance in young professional musicians. *Appl Psychophysiol Biofeedback* 34(4):279–89. doi: 10.1007/s10484-009-9103-4

113. Verrastro, G. (2014). *Yoga as therapy: When is it helpful?* J Fam Pract. 63(9):E1–6.

114. Association for Applied Psychophysiology and Biofeedback (AAPB). (2011). [accessed on November 15th 2014]; about biofeedback. http://www.aapb.org/i4a/pages/index.cfm?pageid=3463

115. Karavidas, M.K., Lehrer, P.M., et al. (2007 Mar). Preliminary results of an open label study of heart rate variability biofeedback for the treatment of major depression. *Appl Psychophysiol Biofeedback*;32(1):19–30.

116. Hawkins, R.S. & Hart, A.D. (2003 Dec), The use of thermal biofeedback in the treatment of pain associated with endometriosis: preliminary findings. *Appl Psychophysiol Biofeedback* 28(4):279–89.

117. Fuchs, T., Birbaumer, N., et al. (2003 Mar). Neurofeedback treatment for attention-deficit/hyperactivity disorder in children: a comparison with methylphenidate. *Appl Psychophysiol Biofeedback* 28(1):1–12.

118. Alm-Roijer, C., Stagmo, M., et al. (2004 Dec). Better knowledge improves adherence to lifestyle changes and medication in patients with coronary heart disease. *Eur J Cardiovasc Nurs* 3(4):321–30.

119. Burge, S., White, D., et al. (2005 Nov-Dec). Correlates of medication knowledge and adherence: findings from the residency research network of South Texas. *Fam Med* 37(10):712–8.

120. Murphy, C., DeBellis. R.J. (2012 Nov). Pharmacology in lifestyle medicine and the role of the pharmacist. *Am J Lifestyle Med* 6(6): 479–88. Doi: 10.1177/1559827612444519

121. Cocohoba, J.M., Althoff, K.N. et al. (2012). Pharmacist counseling in a cohort of women with HIV and women at risk for HIV. *Patient Prefer Adherence* 6:457–63.

122. Wang, K.Y., Chian, C.F, et al. (2010 Dec). Clinical pharmacist counseling improves outcomes for Taiwanese asthma patients. *Pharm World Sci.* 32(6):721–9.

123. Tsingos, C., Bosnic-Anticevich, S., & Smith, L. (2014 Feb). Reflective practice and its implications for pharmacy education. *Am J Pharm Educ.* 78(1). Article 18.

124. Shah, M., Norwood, C.A., et al. (2013 Apr). Diabetes transitional care from inpatient to outpatient setting: pharmacist discharge counseling. *J Pharm Pract.* 26(2):120–4.

125. Santschi, V., Chiolero, A. et al. (2014 Apr). 10Improving blood pressure control through pharmacist interventions: A meta-analysis of randomized controlled trials. *J Am Heart Assoc* 3(2):e000718.

126. O'Loughlin, J., Masson, P., et al. (1999 Mar). The role of community pharmacists in health education and disease prevention: A survey of their interests and needs in relation to cardiovascular disease. *Prev Med* 28(3):324–31.

127. Zaller, N., Jeronimo, A, et al. (2010 Dec). Pharmacist and pharmacy staff experiences with non-prescription (NP) sale of syringes and attitudes toward providing HIV prevention services for injection drug users (IDUs) in Providence, RI. *J Urban Health* 87(6):942–53.

128. Watson, L., Bond, C. et al. (2003 Mar). A survey of community pharmacists on prevention of HIV and hepatitis B and C: Vurrent practice and attitudes in Grampian. *J Public Health Med* 25(1):13–8.

129. Conrad, A.O., Dubin, R.L., et al. (2013 Feb). Clinical pharmacist services in a multidisciplinary weight management clinic. *J Health Care Poor Underserved* 24(1 Suppl):29–35.

130. Sinclair, H.K., Bond, C.M., et al. (2004). Community pharmacy personnel interventions for smoking cessation. *Cochrane Database Syst Rev.* (1):CD003698

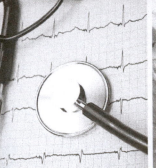
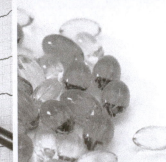
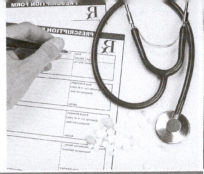
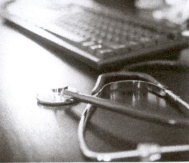

SECTION B

MEDICATION USE SERVICES AND CARE

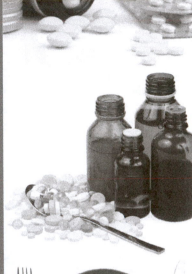
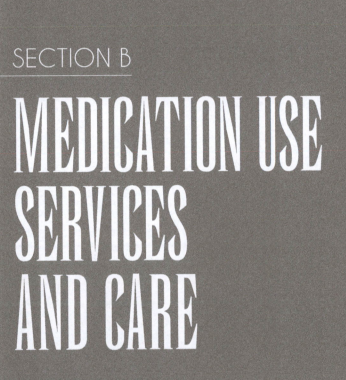
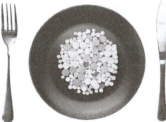
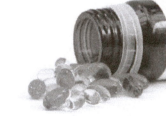
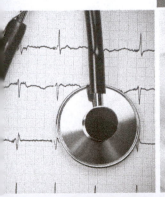
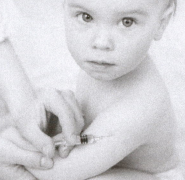
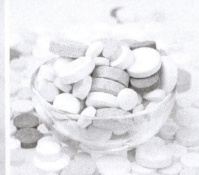
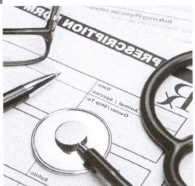

CHAPTER 6

PROFESSIONAL SOCIALIZATION OF PHARMACISTS

Gregory F. Higby, PhD, Andrew P. Traynor, Pharm.D., BCPS

LEARNING OBJECTIVES:

1. Define and distinguish between the terms profession, professional, professionalism, and professional socialization.
2. Describe to a layperson why and how pharmacy is a profession.
3. Summarize the historical and present day challenges relating to professional socialization in pharmacy.
4. Outline strategies to achieve the goal of professional socialization.
5. Identify ways in which an individual can take responsibility for their professional socialization and why this is important.

KEY TERMS

Profession
Professional
Professionalism

Professional socialization
Professionalization

How does one become a pharmacist? At first glance, the answer to this question appears simple and straightforward: a person attends pharmacy school, gains the requisite amount of education and training, passes a qualifying examination, obtains a license, and finds a job. Actually, that is how someone attains the qualifications to practice as a licensed pharmacist. To *become* a pharmacist, a man or women also must be socialized.[1] Robert Merton defined socialization as "the process by which people selectively acquire the values and attitudes, the interests, skills and knowledge —in short, the culture—current in the groups of which they are, or seek to become, a member. It refers to the learning of social roles."[2] All functioning members of a society undergo a process of primary socialization whereby individuals learn their major identifying roles within a culture, such as gender, ethnicity, and religious beliefs. These identities are inculcated primarily within the family. Secondary socialization occurs when people join a group after their identities have been formed through earlier primary socialization. When someone takes a new job, he or she quickly learns the mores of the new work culture and how to function in this adult role.

In the case of most pharmacists today who practice in the community setting, their role is one that mixes two distinct identities, professional and commercial.[3] One hundred years ago, these two identities were compatible, but during the last 40 years they have diverged as pharmacy practice and the healthcare marketplace have evolved.[4] New pharmacists entering the workforce, especially in community settings, often discover an environment that contradicts the ideals of professional practice taught in pharmacy school, leading to disillusionment or "realistic disenchantment."[3,5] Moreover, the hopes of educators and leaders that lengthened education (PharmD degree) and innovative practice models (pharmaceutical care) would expand the societal role of pharmacists and elevate their stature have failed to be realized fully, though progress is evident. As a result, the subject of professional socialization (professionalization) in pharmacy has attracted increased attention in recent years. Scholars continue to explore definitions and frameworks as well as interventions to develop and assess professionalism. However, academic pharmacy still struggles to develop consensus on definitions and disseminate strategies that are proven to reach a desired end. This topic will continue to garner attention in the foreseeable future as the Center for the Advancement of Pharmaceutical Education (CAPE) identified professionalism as an educational outcome under the domain of personal and professional development.[6] With the Accreditation Council for Pharmacy Education adopting the CAPE 2013 Educational Outcomes in the 2016 Accreditation Standards and Guidelines for the Doctor of Pharmacy Program, a structure and process for developing and assessing student professionalism is expected for all Doctor of Pharmacy programs.[7]

This chapter explores this topic from the historical roots of its development to present day strategies and challenges in developing and assessing professionalism.

THE HISTORY OF PHARMACY'S PROFESSIONAL EVOLUTION

Merton's definition of socialization is generally accepted, but the same cannot be said about the meaning of the word *profession*. The *Oxford English Dictionary* retains a traditional view of the term: "The occupation which one professes to be skilled in and to follow a vocation in which a professed knowledge of some department of learning or science is used in its application to the affairs of others or in the practice of an art founded upon it. This applies specifically to the three learned professions of divinity, law, and medicine; also to the military profession."[8] Historically, an individual made a claim or "profession" to have the requisite abilities to fulfill a socially accepted and understood role such as *pharmacist*. Fully established in American society by the middle of the 1800s, pharmacists were retailers of medicines, spices, oils, flavorings, sponges, cosmetics, and sundry other "drugstore items." Their professional claim rested on their specialized skill in preparing drugs and compounding medicines upon a physician's prescription order. In the late 1800s the American public began to value paper credentials (school diplomas and governmental licenses) as indicators of professional competency as much as personal reputation. Pharmacy, with its dual cultures, however, has clung to both individualistic (drugstore proprietor) and collective (licensed graduate) approaches to pursuing societal recognition.[9]

Definitions of *profession* and *professionalism* abound, and scholars have struggled to find ones that fit pharmacy well.[10] Throughout the 20th century, authors did not include pharmacists as full professionals, classifying them as semiprofessionals or "incomplete professionals."[11-13] They observed that most pharmacists spent their days selling packaged goods in a commercialized retail setting. Moreover, even in their "professional" practice—filling prescriptions—pharmacists lacked autonomy; they were just following the orders of physicians.[11-14] For this reason, Supreme Court Justice Warren Burger deemed pharmacists no more professional than store clerks selling law books.[15]

Pharmacy historian Glenn Sonnedecker, building on Carr-Saunders and Thorner, put forward a useful set of "essentials" or traits that result in an occupation attaining professional status:

> *A relatively specific, socially necessary function upon the regular performance of which the practitioner depends for his livelihood and social status; a special technique, competence in which is demanded, resting upon a body of knowledge embracing generalized principles, the mastery of which requires theoretic study; a traditional and generally accepted ethic subordinating its adherents' immediate private interests to the most effective performance of the function; and a formal association fostering the ethic and improvement of performance.*[16]

For pharmacy in the count-and-pour era of the 1950s, Sonnedecker's traits were an ambitious target. The "socially necessary function" of the pharmacists in 1960 was to dispense medications according to a physician's order. Compounding, the crux of community pharmacy's professional claim from the 1870s through the 1940s, had all but disappeared. Mass manufacturers made almost all end dosage forms. Laws prohibited generic substitution and limited refills. Pharmacists were not allowed to discuss the content or actions of drugs with their patients. In fact, to protect patients, pharmacists did not put the name of the medicine on the prescription container. Pharmacists were often called "the most over-educated professionals" because they possessed a large "body of knowledge" in the chemical sciences but their "special technique" was little demanded.

The pharmacy profession, represented by the American Pharmaceutical Association (APhA), did possess a "generally accepted ethic," put forward in the APhA Code of Ethics. This code, like those of other occupations, was "a detailed, explicit, operational blue-print of norms of professional conduct, a public recital of desirable and undesirable actions having an impact upon the character of a professional and its functional reliability"[17](pp39–40). The APhA had revised its code periodically since the founding of the organization in 1852. A few excerpts from the 1952 version illustrate the restricted role of the pharmacists in the count-and-pour era:

> The primary obligation of pharmacy is the service it can render to the public in safeguarding the preparation, compounding, and dispensing of drugs and the storage and handling of drugs and medical supplies...

> The pharmacist holds the health and safety of his patrons to be of first consideration; he makes no attempt to prescribe for or treat disease or to offer for sale any drugs or medical device merely for profit...

> The pharmacist willingly makes available his expert knowledge of drugs to the other health professionals...

> The pharmacist does not discuss the therapeutic effect of composition of a prescription with a patient. When such questions are asked, he suggests that the qualified practitioner [i.e., the physician] is the proper person with whom such matters should be discussed[17] (pp155–6).

Despite the high-sounding tone of the code, readers should remember that in the early 1950s the vast majority of pharmacists worked in small, independent shops that prospered by the sale of over-the-counter medicines, tobacco products, candy, magazines, greeting cards, and other similar merchandise. Prescription sales brought in less than 25% of the average community pharmacy's income.[18] Most of the young men who entered pharmacy aspired to be drugstore owners, and to achieve this goal they first had to become pharmacists. Generally, they had experience as stock boys, soda jerks, or store clerks, and had already been socialized in the "drug business," not unlike the apprentice apothecaries of the late 1800s.

CLINICAL PHARMACY

In the middle of the 1960s, a major paradigm shift in the profession occurred with the rise of the *clinical pharmacy* movement. Innovative pharmacists, mainly in hospital settings, actively sought to expand their practice roles through the staffing of drug information centers, adoption of unit dose distribution methods, and other ideas that pushed daily practice beyond mundane counting and pouring, licking, and sticking. In the late 1960s and early 1970s, pharmacy educators embraced the new model of pharmacists as drug information specialists and medication counselors. Biology, psychology, and therapeutics courses were added to the chemistry and physical pharmacy subjects that dominated curricula in the 1950s and early 1960s. Rotations in hospitals and clinics exposed pharmacy students to collaborative practices. In turn, pharmacy students were encouraged to look forward to careers as clinical pharmacists.[19] Graduates in the 1970s often sought placement in hospital settings with prospects for advanced practice, but soon discovered that most open positions were to be found in community pharmacies. There the opportunities for clinical pharmacy were few and far between. Most pharmacists continued to spend their days dispensing prescriptions without providing additional services. The result was frustration and disappointment among young practitioners.

A number of pharmacy scholars in the mid-1970s noticed this trend among beginning pharmacists, which educator Robert Buerki had earlier called "realistic disenchantment."[5] Henri Manasse, in his dissertation and a series of articles that followed it, explored this phenomenon with an eye toward the important role of socialization.[20] In a classic article published in 1975, Manasse, Stewart, and Hall argued that the underlying cause was a pattern of "inconsistent socialization," that is, "the process by which the individual develops or acquires incompatible or conflicting behaviors, beliefs and values from formal or informal sources due to the absence of uniformity or agreement within the idealized group model into which he is being socialized"[21] (p. 658). In the case of pharmacy, the environment in which a student completed his or her practical experience was key. If that environment contradicted the ideals inculcated within the classroom, "role conflict" resulted[21] (p. 658).

During the clinical pharmacy era (1965–1990), pharmacy educators attempted to rectify the inconsistent-socialization problem through lengthening and altering the experiential learning portions of the curriculum. Studies done on the professionalism of students as they progressed through school, clerkships, and early work experiences, however, revealed no improvement or even a decline in their social and occupational attitudes.[22-24] Cynicism and anxiety increased.[25] Negative experiences with supervisors or physicians tended to push students into passivity and discouragement.[26] And those graduates who worked in community pharmacy found an environment as commercialized and professionally discouraging as in the 1950s.[27,28]

PHARMACEUTICAL CARE

The *pharmaceutical* care concept introduced by Helper and Strand in the late 1980s seemed to offer pharmacy something it had lacked for full growth as a profession: a set of universal shared values within the occupation. In addition to their traditional roles of filling prescriptions with due diligence, pharmacists were to accept full responsibility for drug therapy outcomes. They would actively care for patients and be their therapeutic advocates. When Douglas Hepler spoke at the Pharmacy in the 21st Century Conference in 1989, the gathered group of American pharmacy leaders endorsed pharmaceutical care as the future of the profession's direction.[29] During this same time period, the American Council on Pharmaceutical Education announced its intent to accredit after 2001 only those programs that led to the doctor of pharmacy degree. The Omnibus Budget Reconciliation Act of 1990 (OBRA'90) included provisions calling for pharmacists to utilize their expertise to promote rational drug out-comes.[30] The scene was set for major professional advancement through dual paradigm shifts in education and in the practice model.[31]

The 1990s, initially heralded as the "pharmaceutical care era," witnessed huge growth in the prescription drug sector of health care, with subsequent efforts to control exploding costs through a group of methods euphemistically called "managed care." Caught between a burgeoning number of prescriptions to fill and time spent wrangling with pharmacy benefits managers over coverage issues, most community pharmacists had no real time to "care." When the first generation of students educated within the pharmaceutical care paradigm entered the hectic and restrictive realm of community pharmacy, they expressed disappointment and disillusionment, just like their predecessors a generation before.

In 1995, a special American Association of Colleges of Pharmacy (AACP) committee looked at the situation and made this stark observation:

> *It has been argued that students are presented the ideal, patient-oriented perspective by pharmacy educators, only to have those levels of expectations unsupported and unmet as they progress through the curriculum, gain experience in the real world, and enter practice. If students are unclear about what should be expected of them, as a result of mixed, inconsistent messages during socialization, they might experience role ambiguity where they are unsure exactly what their role should be. Their behaviors could be significantly swayed by the opinions of powerful others (e.g., employers, physicians, patients). The difference in role expectations (by some pharmacists) in current practice may not be consistent with the role expectations of recent graduates (they are trained at a higher level to pursue expanded roles) culminating in role stress/strain and a dissatisfaction with practice[3] (p. 85).*

The committee recommended "continuing efforts within AACP to encourage faculty to give comparable attention to professional socialization as to optimizing the traditional academic components. These two educational (professional socialization and academic learning) processes should be planned as mutually dependent and mutually reinforcing contributions to student growth in achieving the overall educational goals adopted by the faculty"[3] (p. 87).

PRESENT DAY CONCEPTS AND PRINCIPLES

Since the mid-1990s, a large number of studies, task force reports, and white papers have been generated on the subject of pharmacy student professionalism and professionalization. Of special value is the "White Paper on Pharmacy Student Professionalism," the product of a joint task force of members from the American Pharmaceutical Association's Academy of Students of Pharmacy and the AACP Council of Deans.[32] It returned to first principles, providing valuable contemporary definitions of key concepts:

Profession: An occupation whose members share ten common characteristics:

1. Prolonged specialized training in a body of abstract knowledge
2. A service orientation
3. An ideology based on the original faith professed by members
4. An ethic that is binding on the practitioners
5. A body of knowledge unique to the members

6. A guild of those entitled to practice the profession

7. A set of skills that form the technique pf the profession

8. Authority granted by society in the form of licensure or certification

9. A recognized setting where the profession is practiced

10. A theory of societal benefits from the ideology

Professional: A member of a profession who displayed the following ten traits:

1. Knowledge and skills of a profession

2. Commitment to self-improvement of skills and knowledge

3. Service orientation

4. Pride in profession

5. Covenantal relationship with the client

6. Creativity and innovation

7. Conscience and trustworthiness

8. Accountability for his/her work

9. Ethically sound decision making

10. Leadership

Professionalism: The active demonstration of the traits of a professional.

Professional socialization (professionalization): The process of inculcating a profession's attitudes, values, and behaviors in a professional. The goal of professional socialization is to develop professionalism, as defines by the ten character traits above.[32]

While authors have suggested additional tenets, concepts, frameworks and taxonomies for professionalism since the task force's work, the definitions and recommendations of the task force continue to resonate today. First of all, the task force contended that "students have a significant role in advancing the process of professional socialization" and that the concepts of professionalism should be introduced to students on their first day in school. Students should take on two parallel tasks from that day: learning how to assume more responsibility for patient care and more responsibility for their own professional development. Second, the task force recommended that schools of pharmacy create structured programs to facilitate "the development of professional attitudes, behaviors, and identity." The task force gave advice concerning recruitment, admissions, educational programs, and experiential learning. Finally, the task force recognized that practicing pharmacists had a "critical role in professional socialization." It insisted that practitioners avoid situations that reinforce inconsistent socialization. Instead, they were to serve "as professional mentors and role models to recent pharmacy graduates and pharmacy students."[32] These recommendations have been realized in the works of many scholars, shaping of accreditation standards and guidelines, and definition of educational outcomes. The CAPE 2013 educational outcomes defines professionalism as "Exhibit(ing) behaviors and values that are consistent with the trust given to the profession by patients, other healthcare providers, and society."[6]

PRESENT DAY INITIATIVES AND STRATEGIES TO DEVELOP PROFESSIONALISM

Hammer applied professional socialization literature to academic pharmacy by citing the need to recognize and consider; the attitudes and behaviors students possess at entry to a professional pharmacy program, the modeling of professionalism by faculty and practitioners, and the culture of environments where students develop.[33] As one group of authors puts it, "Schools of pharmacy exist to develop professionally mature pharmacy practitioners who can render pharmaceutical care."[10] This is a far cry from the educational *raison d'être* of the Philadelphia College of Pharmacy in 1821, which was to provide a night finishing school for those learning pharmacy (and being socialized) during the day through apprenticeship in a shop, wholesaler, or factory. Hammer encouraged schools to;

- infuse elements of professionalism in their mission statements and develop their codes of ethics or statements of professionalism,
- orient student services and advising to professional development,
- highlight professionalism in recruitment materials,
- assess professionalism as a component of admissions criteria,
- orient students to professional life,
- implement didactic programming,
- support extracurricular activities, and
- foster professionalism in experiential education.[33]

As a result, students today are encouraged to take consider themselves student pharmacists and take on a persona of what they imagine a professional pharmacist might be.

In 2011, an AACP Professionalism Task Force focused on the status of the development of professionalism in schools and colleges of pharmacy. Per their report, the Task Force identified continuing barriers and challenges to professionalism within the Academy. Common barriers included:

- lack of effective instruments to assess student professionalism at the time of admissions and throughout the curriculum;
- behaviors of faculty members, preceptors, and practicing pharmacists that sometimes fail to model excellent professional behaviors and skills;
- decreased faculty morale in some institutions;
- ineffective advising and a lack of career development opportunities; and
- difficulty in identifying the true cause of antiprofessionalism culture within professional education."[34]

Duncan-Hewitt summarized a potential need for more profound student and mentor cognitive and moral development. Citing the work of Latif and Berger as well as unpublished admissions assessments, students were reported as entering pharmacy school at a lower than anticipated level of cognitive and moral maturity leading to difficulty with accountability and responsibility. Therefore, education must be developmentally congruent to these needs in both focus and strategies.[35]

Strategies across the lifespan of pharmacy education have been summarized in the literature, though most of these strategies seem focused on the beginning and end of pharmacy education as opposed to a more longitudinal focus. Colleagues at Samford described the use of a required reading of professionalism essays rooted in the humanities prior to students attending orientation. The readings and related orientation discussions were deemed an effective approach to nurturing and encouraging professionalism. Students were engaged in the discussions and reported an increased awareness of the importance of professionalism.[36] Interprofesisonal colleagues at the University of Cincinnati coordinated an interprofessional student orientation focused on health care and professionalism, including a field experience. Surveys of students showed an increase in awareness of the importance of professionalism in the patient care setting and their individual profession's contributions to health care.[37] Kelley and colleagues compared undergraduate first-year experience (FYE) programming to pharmacy education programing for developing professional attitudes and behaviors. While similar experiences were pursued, FYE included more reflective writing activities, peer mentoring and diversity activities than the compared professional pharmacy programs.[38]

Hammer described strategies to improve professionalism during experiential education including stating explicit expectations, setting high standards, treating students respectfully, giving frequent, timely and specific feedback to students, evaluating students' professional behavior, and soliciting student feedback for the site and preceptors.[39] Boyle and colleagues described a process for stating expectations and evaluating student professional behavior. All experiential courses required 100% acceptable professionalism ratings to pass a rotation. While the vast majority of students met the criteria, nine students did not and were required to remediate and engage in further professional development.[40]

ASSESSMENT OF PROFESSIONALISM

Many have commented on the difficulty of measuring professionalism, yet they feel they know when it is being displayed. Some literature has described assessment strategies for professionalization in pharmacy education. A learning activity on addiction pharmacy requiring students to work in teams to influence decision makers for the pharmacist societal role in managing drug addiction was observed to allow professionalization to occur and be assessed via the quantity and quality of online activity, grading via rubrics and student report via survey.[41]

Chisholm and colleagues developed and validated an instrument named the Pharmacy Professionalism Instrument at the University of Georgia. The instrument included 18 items that measured, with satisfactory reliability, six tenets of professionalism including excellence, respect for others, altruism, duty, accountability, and honor/integrity.[42] Kelley and colleagues described an additional validated tool named the Professionalism Assessment Tool (PAT) implemented across seven schools. The PAT utilized 33-items across five domains of professionalism including: 1) reliability, responsibility and accountability; 2) lifelong learning and adaptability; 3) relationships with others; 4) upholding principles of integrity and respect; and 5) citizenship and professional engagement.[43] Bradford and colleagues, through administration of the student self-assessed Behavioral Professionalism Assessment, showed a significant positive correlation between self-reported professionalism and involvement in student organization activities.[44]

ONGOING CHALLENGES

After years of philosophizing about professional socialization in pharmacy, faculty members have pursued interventions and suggested some concrete assessments of professionalism to facilitate evaluation of student advancement. Is there a professionalism crisis in a 21st century pharmaceutical education? A number of pharmacy educators advocating for "more professionalism" have lamented the "erosion of values and civility" and a general "demoralization of society."[39,40] An analysis of student experiences in training demonstrated that the perceived importance of learning a science core limited professional socialization. Students shared that they did not focus on professional identity until after this core was achieved; their education began with a heavy emphasis on scientific knowledge; the abundance of material fostered rote memorization; and social pharmacy was valued, but not viewed as essential to developing a professional identity.[45] Faculty members may be contributing as much to the problem as they are the solution. The profession continues to struggle with consensus on definitions, a relative lack of shared strategies, and a lack of solidified assessment tools. The continuing presence of different perceptions may result in the problem worsening as inconsistency leads to a lack of trust between a school and students for any initiative related to professionalization.

Despite the importance of pharmacy schools in the development of the pharmacists, we should remember what Manasse, Kabat, and Wertheimer observed in 1976:

> *The focus of the professional socialization process is on how*
> *professional aspirants exchange their lay views and imagery*
> *of a profession for those the profession ascribes to itself. In this*
> *layman-to-professional exchange, students acquire a self-image*
> *within the context of their professional role and, at the same*
> *time, begin to adjust to professional demands and uncertain-*
> *ties. The major feature of professional socialization is that the*
> *process occurs under strictly defines conditions and is admin-*
> *istered by the "gate-keeping" professional group. What cannot*
> *be controlled in professional socialization are those behaviors of*
> *the "socialize" which are exhibited outside the sphere of profes-*
> *sional practice.[46]*

SUMMARY

From the colonial period up to the start of the 20th century, American pharmacy was an apprenticeship-based trade whose leadership sought to transform it into a modern, credentialed profession. Despite the development of much more rigorous educational requirements from the 1920s to the 1990s—from two-year PhG courses to six-year PharmD programs—pharmacy continues to struggle for full professional recognition. Socialization, once simply regarded as the means through which a newcomer adopted the culture of the pharmacy workplace, has recently gained the attention of educators and leaders hoping to utilize this process consciously to inculcate values of caring and professionalism in pharmacy students.

In 1996, William Zellmer put forward a simple mission for American pharmacists: "Let's dedicate ourselves to remaking this occupation of ours into a profession that gives people what they want and need. This is not an agenda that we can assign to someone else. Each of us must take personal responsibility for making this happen."[47] Rather than laying the responsibility for change upon pharmacy students and graduates, let us work to understand more fully the subculture that is pharmacy and accept the strengths of its dual identity. Rather than forcing abstract (and unreachable) ideals of *professionalism* upon the young, it might be better for all pharmacists to rededicate themselves to the traditional values of *pharmacy*: expertise, accuracy, diligence, and integrity.

REFERENCES

1. Schwirian, P.M. & Fachinetti, N.J. (1975). Professional socialization and disillusionment: The case of pharmacy. *Am J Pharm Educ* 39:18.

2. Merton, R.K., Reader, G.G., & Kendall, P.L. (1957). *The student-physician.* Cambridge, MA: Harvard University Press, 40–41. For further discussion of the cultural concept in pharmacy, see Zellmer, W.A. (1992). The culture and subcultures of pharmacy. *Am J Hosp Pharm* 49:841

3. Chalmers, R.K., Adler, D.S., Haddad, A.M., et al. (1995). The essential linkage of professional socialization and pharmaceutical care. *Am J Pharm Educ* 59:85–90.

4. For two differing opinions on this divergence, see Parks, L.M. (1961). What price professionalism. *Am J Pharm Educ* 25:527–34 and Franckem, D.E. (1969).Let's separate pharmacies and drug stores. *Am J Pharm* 141:161–76.

5. The term realistic disenchantment was coined by Robert Buerki in the mid-1960s; see Buerki, R.A. (1977). Pharmacist Smyth and druggist Smith—a study in professional aspirations. *Am J Pharm Educ* 41:28–33.

6. Medina, M.S., Plaza, C.M., Stowe, C.D., et.al. (2013). Center for the advancement of pharmacy education 2013 educational outcomes. *Am J Pharm Educ* 77(8), Article 162.

7. Accreditation Council for Pharmacy Education. (2016). Accreditation standards and key elements for the professional program in pharmacy leading to the doctor of pharmacy degree. https://www.acpe-accredit.org/pdf/Standards2016FINAL.pdf. Accessed February 7, 2016.

8. Oxford English Dictionary. (1933). *Profession*. Oxford, England: Oxford University Press, 6:1427

9. Higby, G.J. (1986). Professionalism and the nineteenth-century American pharmacist. *Pharm History* 28:155–24.

10. Hammer, D.P., Berger, B.A., Beardsley, R.S., & Easton, M.R. (2003). Student professionalism. *Am J Pharm Educ* 67:96.

11. Flexner, J.A. (1931). A vanishing profession. *Atlantic Monthly* 98:16–25.

12. McCormack, T.H. (1956). The druggists' dilemma: problems of a marginal occupation. *Am J Sociol* 61:308–15.

13. Wilensky, H.L. (1964). The professionalization of everyone? *Am J Sociol* 60:141.

14. Denzin, N.K. & Mettlin, C.J. (1968). Incomplete professionalization: The case of pharmacy. *Social Forces* 46:375–81.

15. Flannery, M.A., Buerki, R.A., & Higby, G. (2007). 150 years of American pharmacy as reflected in its trade press. 151(May):58; The professionalism issue. (1976). *Drug Topics* 120(June):10.

16. Sonnedecker, G.A. (1961). To be or not to be—professional. *Am J Pharm* 133:243–54.

17. Buerki, R.A., & Vottero, L.D. (1994). *Ethical responsibility in pharmacy practice*. Madison: American Institute of the History of Pharmacy, 39–40.

18. Jackson, R.A., Worthen, D.B., & Garner, D.D. (2003). Total income for pharmacy owners at record highs. *America's Pharmacist* 125:29–31.

19. Parascandola, J., Brodie, D.C., Benson, R.A., Francke, D.E., Whitney, H.A., & Rodowskas, C.A. (1976). Clinical pharmacy in historical perspective. *Drug Intell Clin Pharm* 10:505–28.

20. Manasse, H.R. (1974). *The states and process of socialization in the profession of pharmacy* [PhD dissertation]. University of Minnesota.

21. Manasse, H.R., Stewart, J.E., & Hall, R.H. (1975). Inconsistent socialization in pharmacy—a pattern in need of change. *J Am Pharm Assoc* 15:616–21, 658.

22. Manasse, H.R., Kabat, H.F., & Wertheimer, A.I. (1977). Professional socialization in pharmacy: A cross-sectional analysis of dominant value characteristics of agents and objects of socialization. *Soc Sci Med* 11:653–9.

23. Speranza, K.A. & McCook, W.M. (1978). The effects of an institutional clinic experience on pharmacy student professional status perceptions. *Am J Pharm Educ* 42:11–4.

24. Hatoum, H.T. & Smith, M.C. (1987). Identifying patterns of professional socialization for pharmacists during pharmacy schooling and after one year practice. *Am J Pharm Educ* 51:7–17.

25. Hatoum, H., Smith, M.C., & Sharpe, T.R. (1982). Attitudes of pharmacy students towards psychological factors in health care. *Soc Sci Med* 16:1240–1.

26. Broadhead, R. & Facchinetti, N. J. (1985). Clinical clerkship in professional education: a study in pharmacy and other ancillary professions. *Soc Sci Med* 20:231–40.

27. Anderson, Rd. (1977). The peril of deprofessionalization. *Am J Hosp Pharm* 34:133–9.

28. Speedie, M. (2006).Introductory experiential education: a means for introducing concepts of healthcare improvement. *Am J Pharm Educ* 70:145.

29. Conference on Pharmacy in the 21st Century, October 11–14, 1989, Williamsburg, VA. *Am J Pharm Educ* 1989;53(suppl):1S–78S.

30. Brushwood, D.B., Catizone, C.A., & Coster, J.M. (1992). OBRA 90: What it means to your practice. *US Pharmacist* 17:64–72.

31. Higby, G.J. (1997). American pharmacy in that twentieth century. *Am J Health-System Pharm* 54:1814.

32. APhA-AACP task Force on Professionalism. (2000). White paper on pharmacy student professionalism. *J Am Pharm Assoc* 40:96–102.

33. Hammer, D.P. (2000).*Professional Attitudes and Behaviors*: The "A's and B's" of professionalism. *Am J Pharm Educ* 64:455–64.

34. Popovich, N.G., Hammer, D.P., Hansen, D.J., et al. (2011). Report of the AACP professionalism task force, May 2011. *Am J Pharm Educ* 75:Article S4.

35. Duncan-Hewitt, W. (2005). The development of a professional: Reinterpretation of the Professionalization problem from the perspective of cognitive/moral development. *Am J Pharm Educ* 69:Article 6.

36. Bumgarner, G.W., Spies, A.R., Asbill, C.S., et. al. (2007). Using the humanities to strengthen the concept of professionalism among first-professional year pharmacy students. *Am J Pharm Educ* 71:Article 28.

37. Brehm, B., Breen, P., Brown, B., et. al. (2006). An interdisciplinary approach to introducing professionalism. *Am J Pharm Educ* 70:Article 81.

38. Kelley, K.A., DeBisschop, M., Donaldson, A.R. et. al. (2009). Professional socialization of pharmacy students: Do we have the right ingredients and the right formula for success? *Curr Pharm Teach Learn* 1:103–9.

39. Hammer, D. (2006). Improving student professionalism during experiential learning. *Am J Pharm Educ* 70:59.

40. Boyle, C.J., Beardsley, R.S., Morgan, J.A., & de Bittner, M.R. (2007). Professionalism: A determining factor in experiential learning. *Am J Pharm Educ* 71:31.

41. Roche, C. (2014). "Addiction pharmacy" and the professionalization process: Technology-enhanced assessment of reflective practice and teamwork. *Pharmacy* 2:175–194.

42. Chisholm, M.A., Cobb, H., Duke, L., et. al. (2006). Development of an instrument to measure professionalism. *Am J Pharm Educ* 70:Article 85.

43. Kelley, K.A., Stanke, L.D., Rab, S.M., et. al. Cross-validation of an instrument for measuring professionalism behaviors. (2011). *Am J Pharm Educ* 75:Article179.

44. Bradford, D., Watmore, P., Hammer, D., et. al. (2011). The relationship between self-reported professionalism and student involvement in pharmacy organizations at one college of pharmacy: an exploratory analysis. *Curr Pharm Teach Learn* 3:283–9.

45. Taylor, K.M. & Harding, G. (2007). The pharmacy degree: The student experience of professional training. *Pharm Educ* 7:83–8.

46. Manasse, H.R., Kabat, H.F., & Wertheimer, A.I. (1976). Professional socialization in pharmacy I: a cross-sectional analysis of personality characteristics of agents and objects of socialization. *Drugs Health Care* 3(3):4.

47. Zellmer, W.A. (1996). Searching for the soul of pharmacy. *Am J Health Syst Pharm* 53:1911–6.

CHAPTER 7

ORGANIZATIONAL CHANGE

Salisa C. Westrick, PhD, Benjamin S. Teeter, MS

LEARNING OBJECTIVES:

1. Discuss external factors outside the organization that encourage organization changes.
2. Compare and contrast Lewin's Change Model and Kotter's Eight Stage Model.
3. Utilize Force Field Analysis to identify forces for and against a given change.
4. Outline factors influencing program sustainability.
5. Recognize and overcome common hidden traps in decision-making.

KEY TERMS

Champion

Decision making

Force Field Analysis

Kotter's Eight-Stage Model for
 Leading Change

Lewin's Change Model

Program evaluation

Sustainability

QUEST FOR CHANGE:
VALUE-DRIVEN HEALTHCARE

Between 1980 and 2010 the cost of healthcare spending per person in the United States increased from $1,110 to $8,402 annually.[1] A variety of factors play a role in the rising cost of healthcare in the United States, some of which can be addressed by pharmacists in their daily practice. For example, avoidable healthcare costs associated with medication non-adherence have been estimated to be between $100 billion and $300 billion annually in the United States.[2] Additionally, a June 2013 publication estimated that preventable adverse drug events caused by medication errors and mismanaged polypharmacy in elderly patients accounted for $15.9 billion to $29.7 billion of avoidable healthcare costs annually.[3] As a result of rising healthcare costs, third-party payers put forth efforts to control costs of healthcare while improving health outcomes.

Several strategies are implemented to control costs of healthcare. For example, payers may increase restrictions on access to costly drugs by utilizing preferred drug lists and prior authorization.[4] Another strategy may involve increasing patients' cost-sharing, resulting in greater financial burden to plan beneficiaries.[5,6] Health care providers are also affected by payers' cost control strategies. For example, health care providers are pressured to engage in generic substitution and therapeutic interchange of less costly drugs.[7] In addition, pharmacy benefits managers have been aggressive in establishing the deepest discounts in reimbursement formulas for drugs.[8] Because of the discounts, profit margins for pharmaceuticals are decreased.[9] Hence, pharmacies may have to increase their volume in order to maintain the same level of profits and obtain different venue to earn their revenues.

In addition to controlling healthcare costs, payers' attentions have been given to provide quality care and improve patient outcomes.[10–13] Improving the quality of care provided is one of the major goals of the Patient Protection and Affordable Care Act that was signed into law in 2010. As part of this law, many health plans are being evaluated and given star ratings based on quality metrics. Beneficiaries can then compare plans based on these ratings and select the plan that best fits their needs. This leads to an increase in competition between plans trying to attract new beneficiaries and because of this, plans are searching for ways to improve the quality of care provided by the providers with whom they contract, including pharmacists and pharmacies. Patient outcomes are commonly used as indicators of plan quality or pharmacy performance. Health promotion and disease prevention activities have been implemented by many health plans as one of the effective ways to improve patient outcomes. For instance, Medication Therapy Management Services (MTMs) can be implemented by pharmacists to improve health outcomes and be able to receive reimbursement for the services. Additionally, to facilitate pharmacy participation in patient care services, some health plans are offering bonus payments to pharmacies that effectively manage their patients' medications and encourage medication adherence.

In summary, as a result of rising health care costs and the movement towards value-driven health care, payers have implemented various strategies to control costs and improve health outcomes. These strategies have left pharmacists with both threats and opportunities. The threats relate to decreasing profit margins for pharmaceuticals and the opportunities to provide patient care services and improve quality of care call for change from a traditional product focus to a patient focus.

MECHANISMS TO CHANGE PHARMACY PRACTICE

Optimizing patient outcomes is a goal of pharmacy practice.[14] To achieve this goal, the practice of pharmacy needs to shift its focus from traditional dispensing activities to patient care activities and from the focus on processes to patient outcomes. One approach is to change the attitudes, skills, and behaviors of individual pharmacists to deliver innovative patient care services. Using the individual approach, numerous studies have shown that during the intervention period, patient outcomes and pharmacists' satisfactions improved.[15-18] However, these innovative services were not sustained beyond the intervention period.[19,20] Some have suggested that it may be because the individual approach does not consider the complexity of organizations.[19,21,22]

An alternative approach to facilitate pharmacy practice change is to target the change at the organizational level. This organization-level approach recognizes that: (a) individuals have limited capabilities to make independent decisions regarding adoption and implementation of patient care services and (b) individuals' values and behaviors are influenced by the organization and the environment.[22] A better understanding of change at the organizational level may help organizational leaders and pharmacists effectively initiate, manage, and sustain change in their organizations for today's practice environment.

ORGANIZATIONAL CHANGE IN PHARMACY PRACTICE

Change at the organization-level can be unplanned or planned. Unplanned change generally happens over a period of time. An unplanned change typically is not planned by leaders in the organization, but rather is influenced by the external environment. Examples of unplanned change include a growth in part-time pharmacists, an increase in the number of female pharmacists in the workforce, and new federal and state law and regulations. Even though this type of change is not planned by leaders in the organization, it shapes the way work is scheduled, organized, and managed. In contrast, a planned change occurs as leaders recognize the need for the organization to change and carefully design a plan to accomplish the change. This planned change can be used to improve organizational performance or solve problems within the organization. Typically, in the planned-change situations, members of the organization are conscious and aware of the change. In this chapter, organizational change is referred to as a planned change within an organization such as a plan to implement a medication therapy management service. Two change models are introduced as they can be used to guide pharmacists when planning a change in their organizations.

Most organizational change theories originated from Lewin's change model.[23] Lewin's change model suggests that organizational behavior is the results of two sets of forces: driving forces and restraining forces (see Figure 7-1). Driving forces include forces or factors that initiate and push for change. On the other hand, restraining forces can be thought of as barriers to change. These forces resist a change and seek to maintain the status quo (i.e., current state of affairs). At the status quo, both sets of force are about equal. Therefore, at the status quo, the state of organizational behavior is maintained and stable. To shift from the status quo to the desired state, the driving forces must exceed the restraining forces. To ensure that driving forces exceed the restraining forces, the following options can be implemented: increasing the strength of the existing driving forces, adding new driving forces, reducing the strength of the existing restraining forces, and a combination of these options. For instance, the number of prescriptions dispensed in a pharmacy is stable because group norms maintaining the status quo are equivalent to the manager's pressures for change to a higher dispensing rate. This level can be increased to the manager's desired level by increasing manager's pressures to dispense prescriptions at a higher rate, by modifying the group norms to support higher levels of efficiency, or by using a combination of both strategies.[24] It is important to note that addressing driving forces without modifying restraining forces may increase the strength of the restraining forces. Therefore, it is recommended that restraining forces must be modified during the change process. Organizations can choose to modify restraining forces alone or in conjunction with driving forces.

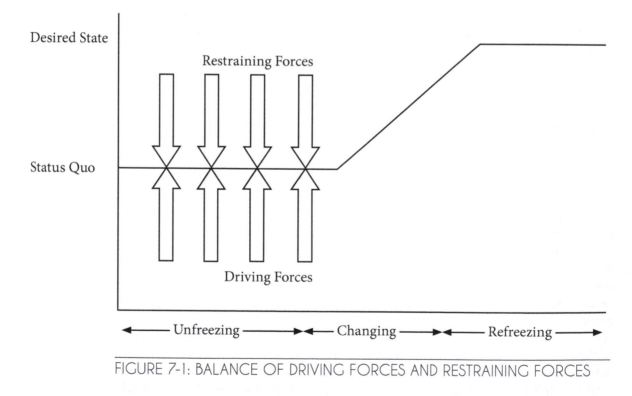

FIGURE 7-1: BALANCE OF DRIVING FORCES AND RESTRAINING FORCES

Lewin developed a three-stage model of planned change that explained how to initiate, manage, and stabilize the change process. The three stages are unfreezing, changing, and refreezing.[23]

1. *Unfreezing*

Unfreezing is the stage where change is initiated. As previously stated, the current level of organizational behavior is stabilized because of the balance between restraining forces and driving forces. Hence, in order to make any organizational change, the balance of these forces needs to be modified. At this stage, various strategies can be implemented to ensure that the driving forces exceed the restraining forces. Leaders can begin the unfreezing process by introducing information that shows discrepancies between behaviors desired by leaders' and employees' current behaviors. For example, to get pharmacy staff interested in improving patient adherence, organizational leaders should compare the pharmacy's current patient adherence rate with the adherence rates among the competitors. By doing so, the discrepancies will disconfirm the usefulness or appropriateness of pharmacy staff's present behaviors or attitudes and, hence, create the motivation to change. The leaders and pharmacists may also introduce rewards to strengthening the driving forces at this stage. Rewards are used to motivate pharmacy staff to move towards the change direction.

2. *Changing*

The changing stage happens when the existing behavior shifts to the desired level. During this stage, employees learn new concepts and new ways of doing things. They develop new behaviors, values, and attitudes. In order to be successful in shifting to the desired level, it is important that employees are provided with information, assistance, and encouragement during the change process. It is highly recommended that organizational leaders communicate clearly and openly with employees on the benefits of changing their behaviors and how the change will affect them and the organization as a whole. Furthermore, leaders must pay attention to problems that arise during this change process. Once problems are discovered, leaders must deal with them immediately.

3. *Refreezing*

Organizational leaders stabilize change during the refreezing stage by helping employees integrate the changed behavior or attitude into their normal way of doing things. This is accomplished by using positive reinforcement, such as rewards, to encourage the desired behavior. Further, organizational leaders can establish feedback systems as a way to reinforce desired behaviors and prevent employees from relapsing back to the previous behavior. Additional coaching and modeling also are used at this point to reinforce the stability of the change.

CASE EXAMPLE 1

Dr. Smith is the new owner of Auburn Pharmacy, an independently-owned community pharmacy in Alabama. After working as a staff pharmacist at Auburn Pharmacy for 10 years, the previous owner decided to retire and sold the pharmacy to Dr. Smith. There are three other pharmacists employed at the pharmacy, five technicians, and eight other employees whose jobs range from medication inventory management to store clerk. The majority of Auburn Pharmacy's revenue comes from dispensing medications. Due to reduced reimbursements for prescription medications, Dr. Smith believes some change needs to be made to provide patient care and become more patient-focused while delivering value driven healthcare to the patients of Auburn Pharmacy. In the past he has considered the following options: 1) increasing automation to give pharmacists more time to counsel patients, 2) updating the computer system to identify patients who have not picked up their prescriptions or who are prescribed to high-risk medications, 3) offering influenza, pneumococcal, and herpes zoster vaccinations, and 4) medication synchronization for patients with multiple medications. Implementing any of these options would require a change in the focus of the organization and, of course, money. Dr. Smith knows the process of implementing change will be difficult because many of his employees are happy with the way things are done currently at the pharmacy, but he feels that a change in the focus of the organization is necessary.

1. Following Lewin's Change Model, what activities should Dr. Smith engage in during the unfreezing stage?

2. In the changing stage of Lewin's Change Model, what can Dr. Smith do to help his employees develop new attitudes toward patient care activities and value driven healthcare?

3. Once Dr. Smith has implemented the desired changes, how can he ensure the change will be permanent?

As explained above, Lewin's model provides a framework to explain the change processes within an organization. Since the model is rather broad in nature, it may not identify specific actions for any particular plans. In order to determine specific actions to accomplish a desired goal, a Force Field Analysis can be utilized.

Force Field Analysis is a method for listing, discussing, and evaluating the various forces for and against a proposed change. Force Field Analysis derives from Lewin's three-step model of change discussed earlier. The basis of Force Field Analysis is that there are two types of factors affecting organizational change: restraining forces and driving forces. Force Field Analysis helps leaders look at the big picture by analyzing all of the forces impacting the change and weighing the strength of restraining forces and driving forces. Once the strength of restraining forces and driving forces is identified, strategies to reduce the impact of the opposing forces and strengthen the supporting forces can be developed.

To conduct a Force Field Analysis, it must start with describing the current situation and determining a goal or change to be implemented. Second, a list of all restraining forces that hinder the change and driving forces that promote the change is compiled and recorded into two different columns. Examples of driving forces are pressure from leaders, monetary and nonmonetary rewards, and new mandates. Examples of restraining forces include investment cost of new automated technology, limited space and resources, and fear of automated processes. A list of restraining forces and driving forces can be collected through various methods such as questionnaires, interviews, observations, and records.[24] Once all driving forces and restraining forces are identified, the next step is to assign a score to each force impacting change in terms of its strength from 1 (weak) to 5 (strong). Strength of each force is based on personal belief and input from organizational members.[24] After each force is rated, a total score for each of the two columns is calculated. The total score for restrainin g force reflects the strength of forces that act against change. Likewise, the total score for driving forces reflects the strength of forces that promote change. After the total scores for driving forces and restraining forces are calculated, leaders must decide whether the goal or change is still feasible. If so, the next step is to develop a manageable course of action to strengthen the existing driving forces, create new driving forces, weaken existing restraining forces, or a combination of these actions.

Figures 7-2a and 7-2b illustrates how a Force Field Analysis can be used to determine a course of action related to the adoption of a new automated dispensing machine in a community pharmacy. In Figure 7-2a, a list of restraining forces and driving forces is compiled and recorded into two different columns. After the strength of each force is determined, the total scores for driving forces and restraining forces are calculated. The current situation shows that the total score for the driving forces is lower than the total score for the restraining forces. Thus, at the current situation, the goal may not be accomplished. Figure 7-2b shows how an action plan is determined using the results of the force field analysis. As previously stated, to make effective change, the total score for the driving forces must be greater than the restraining forces. This can be accomplished by taking appropriate actions. For example, the community pharmacy could implement the following actions such as a communication plan to address concerns about resistance to change and a training session on the new automated dispensing machine to allow employees to familiarize themselves and to reduce the fear. After possible actions are developed, the next step is to determine the new scores assuming that these actions successfully take place. Please note that, in this example, only the restraining forces are modified. It is possible to develop other action plans to increase the strength of the driving forces and/or add new driving forces. Figure 7-2b illustrates that after the action plans are implemented, a change to an automated dispensing process is possible as the total score for the driving forces is higher than the total score for the restraining forces.

DRIVING FORCES (STRENGTH)	Goal: Adoption of a new automated dispensing machine	RESTRAINING FORCES (STRENGTH)
Free up pharmacists' time to develop and implement patient care services (4)		Staff frightened of new technology (4)
Reduce dispensing errors (3)		Cost of a new technology (3)
Improve efficiency of dispensing service (2)		Staff resistance to change to automated processes (3)
Increase number of prescriptions dispensed (2)		Loss of staff overtime (2)
		Disruption of workflow during change (2)
Total Score = 11		Total Score = 14

FIGURE 7-2A: FORCE FIELD ANALYSIS FOR THE ADOPTION OF AN AUTOMATED DISPENSING MACHINE: ASSESSING THE POSSIBILITY OF CHANGE

DRIVING FORCES (STRENGTH)	Goal: Adoption of a new automated dispensing machine	RESTRAINING FORCES (STRENGTH)

DRIVING FORCES (STRENGTH)

Free up pharmacists' time to develop and implement patient care services (4)

Reduce dispensing errors (3)

Improve efficiency of dispensing service (2)

Increase number of prescriptions dispensed (2)

Total Score = 11

Goal: Adoption of a new automated dispensing machine

RESTRAINING FORCES (STRENGTH)

Staff frightened of new technology (1) Training plan

Cost of a new technology (3)

Staff resistance to change to automated processes (1)

Loss of staff overtime (2)

Disruption of workflow during change (2)

Communication plan

Total Score = 9

FIGURE 7-2B: FORCE FIELD ANALYSIS FOR THE ADOPTION OF AN AUTOMATED DISPENSING MACHINE: AFTER THE IMPLEMENTATION OF ACTION PLANS

In summary, a Force Field Analysis allows organizational leaders and pharmacists to look at a planned change in terms of forces for and against the change and proactively design actions to effectively manage the change.

CASE EXAMPLE 2

Consider the Auburn Pharmacy scenario in Case Example 1. Dr. Smith is attempting to change the organization from a dispensing pharmacy to a more patient-centered, value-driven pharmacy. Using Figures 7-2a and 7-2b for guidance, conduct a Force Field Analysis for one of the four options Dr. Smith is considering. Are there more driving forces or restraining forces? What strategies can be used to reduce to restraining forces?

KOTTER'S EIGHT-STAGE MODEL FOR LEADING CHANGE

Building on Lewin's Change Model, Kotter[25] studied over 100 organizations to identify the errors that organizations make that lead to unsuccessful change. Kotter determined that there were eight common errors that occur during the change process and, from these eight errors, his Eight-Stage Model was created. Figure 7-3 lists and defines the stages in Kotter's model. As can be seen, the first 4 stages coincide with Lewin's "unfreezing" stage, stages 5 through 7 coincide with the "changing" stage, and stage 8 with the "refreezing" stage. In order to lead a successful change, all eight steps must be worked through completely. Additionally, failing to reinforce the early stages will result in an unsuccessful change. For example, if a sense of urgency is not reinforced throughout the change process, the crisis the change will help to avert or the opportunity the change will allow the organization to capitalize on will be forgotten. The inevitable result is an unsuccessful change.

UNFREEZING

1. **Establishing a sensen of urgency**
   - Examine competition and market
   - Identify and discuss crises, potential crises, or major opportunities

2. **Forming a powerful guiding coalition**
   - Assemble a group that can help lead the change
   - Get the group to work together as a team

3. **Creating a vision**
   - Create a vision to help direct the change effort
   - Develop strategies for achieving that vision

4. **Communicating the vision**
   - Use every vehicle possible to constantly communicate the new vision and strategies
   - Lead by example with coalition to teach new behaviors

↓

CHANGING

5. **Empowering others to act on the vision**
   - Getting rid of obstacles to change
   - Changing systems of structures that seriously undermine the vision
   - Encouraging non-traditional ideas, activities and actions

6. **Planning for and creating short term wins**
   - Planning for visible performance improvements
   - Creating those improvements
   - Recognizing and rewarding employees involved in the improvements

7. **Consolidating improvements and creating still more change**
   - Using increased visibility to change systems, structures and policies that don't fit the vision
   - Hiring, promoting, and developing employees who can implement the vision
   - Reinvigorating the process with new projects, initiatives, and change agents

↓

REFREEZING

8. **Institutionalizing new approaches**
   - Articulating the connection between the new behaviors and success of the business
   - Developing the means to ensure leadership development and succession

FIGURE 7-3: RELATIONSHIPS BETWEEN KOTTER'S EIGHT-STEP MODEL (1995) AND LEWIN'S CHANGE MODEL (1951)

Dr. Smith of Auburn Pharmacy is familiar with both Lewin's Change Model and Kotter's Eight-Stage Model. Because of the structure of the Eight-Stage Model, he believes it will be the best choice to ensure a successful change to Auburn Pharmacy. He is attempting to change the organization from a dispensing-focused pharmacy to a patient-centered, value-driven pharmacy.

1. What can Dr. Smith do to establish a sense of urgency?
2. Which employees do you think should be included in the guiding coalition? Why?
3. What strategies should be used to communicate the change vision?
4. How can Dr. Smith generate short term wins?

Organizational leaders of pharmacy and pharmacists are encouraged to use Lewin's change model and Kotter's Eight-Stage Model as guidance when developing a plan to implement patient care services. Once patient care services are implemented, leaders of the organization and pharmacists must ensure that effective patient care services are sustained in the practice. This step has been highlighted in both Lewin's and Kotter's Models.

SUSTAINABILITY OF PATIENT-CARE SERVICES

Patient care services, like other innovations, have their life cycle.[26-29] Generally, new services proceed through a series of overlapping stages.[26,27,29] The first stage, initiation, occurs when an organization senses demands of the current system, searches for possible alternatives, and evaluates these alternatives.[29] The second stage, development and adoption, happens when the service is put to the test in a real context.[29] At this stage, to be successful, the service should be reinvented or modified to accommodate the organization's needs and structure.[27] Next, the service proceeds to the third stage, implementation, when the program is put into full practice.[29] At this stage, the adopting organization needs to allocate its resources to ensure the success of the implementation phase.[27,29] The next stage, sustainability, occurs when organizational members no longer think of the service as a new idea and the service becomes part of the organization.[27] Lastly, dissemination stage involves the diffusion of the service to other practice sites.[29]

After a new service is implemented, discontinuation of the program can occur at any stage.[27] Premature termination of effective services can be costly to the organization as substantial time and resources have been invested in the services, to pharmacy staff as discontinuation of services may affect pharmacy staff emotionally and/or financially, and to customers as they may count on the continuation of the services.[30] Hence, organizational leaders of the organization and pharmacists should not undermine the topic of sustainability of patient-care services. The following section will give guidance into how to build sustainable patient-care services. Specifically, the importance and the definition of sustainability are discussed and factors influencing greater sustainability are identified. Leaders and pharmacists should take these factors in consideration during the planning phase.[30,31]

SUSTAINABILITY

Many pharmacies are conducting patient care services that are new to their organizations. Some of these new services will enjoy long-term survival, and some will be terminated after an initial operating period.[32] In this chapter, sustainability is defined as "a service's ability to continue delivering intended services to their targeted audience over the long term and to keep with their goals and objectives for their service."[33] Using this definition, patient care services that cannot achieve the set goals and objectives, after proper implementation, should not endure for a long period of time.[34]

After developing and initially implementing a new patient care service, leaders of the pharmacy and pharmacists make a decision whether to continue or reject the service.[27] The decision to continue the program delivery increases the sustainability of the service. In contrast, the pharmacy may make a decision to reject the service. There are two types of rejection: replacement and disenchantment.[27] Replacement happens when the pharmacy rejects one type of patient care service in order to adopt a better service that supersedes the previous one. Disenchantment refers to when the pharmacy rejects the service as a result of dissatisfaction with its performance and does not replace it with any other patient care services.[27] Dissatisfaction can be caused by many reasons. For example, the pharmacy may decide, after proper implementation and careful evaluation, that the service did not meet set goals and objectives and, as such, the service is terminated. In this case, the service is well implemented but did not bring desired benefits to the pharmacy; hence, it is logical to discontinue the service. In other situations, however, dissatisfaction can be the result of poor planning or an improper implementation. In these cases, rejection as a result of dissatisfaction should have been prevented had the service been better planned and implemented.

Research shows that failure to sustain services is often caused by not incorporating a focus on sustainability during the planning phase.[35-37] Goodman and Steckler observed that sustainability is often a latent concern in many health promotion programs.[30] That is, organizations hope to see the services continue, however, in the absence of early and active planning, the conditions that would enhance the degree of sustainability are not created and, as a result, sustainability does not occur.[30] Hence, in order to heighten the program sustainability, organizational leaders must move from a passive approach to sustainability to an active use of programmatic approaches that maximize long-term sustainability. As such, organizational leaders of organizations and pharmacists needs to have a clear understanding of factors influencing greater sustainability.[31] The following section discusses five factors that were consistently supported as important factors influencing the extent of sustainability.[29]

1. *Champion*

Program champions are influential individuals within the implementing organization acting as program advocates.[31] Champions make decisive contributions to the service by actively and enthusiastically promoting the service.[32,38] As such, effective champions must overcome indifference or resistance that the new idea may provoke in an organization.[27] Service sustainability is greatly facilitated when the champion has three specific attributes: (a) a mid to upper-level administrative position within the organization; (b) an acute sense of the types of trade-offs that are necessary to influence others to support the service; and (c) negotiating skills that facilitate the formation of coalitions among those individuals who are favorably disposed toward the service.[32]

Literature has shown strong evidence of the effect of champions on increasing the success of innovations[27,38,39] and service sustainability.[26,29,32] That is, the presence of a champion who strongly advocates the continuation of the service increases the service's sustainability. In fact, sustainability is almost guaranteed if there is a champion.[26] For example, results of a study of discontinuation of the fluoride mouth rinse program in public school districts showed that an internal champion played a key role in initial adoption of the service and in preventing it from discontinuation.[28] Accordingly, to ensure the success of patient care services, leaders of the organization should consider developing a champion to advocate for the sustainability of the services.

> Example to illustrate roles of champion in pharmacy (adapted from Stecker and Goodman),[32] John Howard is a Medication Therapy Management Service coordinator for a large chain pharmacy. Pharmacist Howard successfully facilitates the sustainability of MTM services among participating pharmacies. Before the implementation of MTM services, he first has to understand how managers and staff pharmacists at the participating pharmacies perceive the MTM services. By appreciating the perceptions that members of the pharmacies hold in relation to the service, Pharmacist Howard is in a position to negotiate with each member to foster a favorable impression of the service. Once favorable perceptions begin to emerge, he establishes links among individuals who jointly advocate for the service. Because each member may have different interests in supporting a particular service, a coalition is formed among different individuals. By forming a coalition to support the implementation of MTM services, individual interests become mutual interests. During the implementation phase, Pharmacist Howard frequently visits the participating pharmacies to ensure that they have the necessary resources to carry out the MTM services. Furthermore, he continues to influence upper-level management to support the continuation of MTM services.

2. *Modifiability of patient care services*

As previously discussed, sustainability is an ability of patient care services to continuously deliver intended services to clients over time. This suggests important notions in continuation without limiting itself to any particular form.[31] That is, a service must adjust or adapt to new needs and circumstances if it is to continue.[29] Research studies consistently show that services that were modifiable were more likely to be sustained.[26,31,34,40] O'Loughlin and colleagues found that programs that underwent modification during implementation were almost three times more likely to be sustained than those that remained in their original format.[35]

In pharmacy practice, in order to have patient care services with high level of sustainability, patient care services should be modifiable to fit with the organizational operations. This is especially true if the services have been developed elsewhere (e.g., by professional organizations, academia, or other practice sites). Since these services may not fit well with the new context, leaders of the organization and pharmacists must engage in thoughtful modifications of components of the service to fit the new organizational context. On the other hand, if the service is developed internally, it is suggested that a service should be designed in a way that it can be subdivided into different parts, can be delivered in a variety of sequences or formats, or has alternative content and educational materials.[35]

3. *Fit within the host organization*

To increase sustainability of the service, the fit between service and organization is necessary.[26,32,35,41,42] Organizational fit refers to a service's compatibility with the organization's mission, values, norms, and core operations.[32] Results from various research studies consistently suggest that services that fit well with the organization were likely to remain more viable than those that required adjustment within the organization to accommodate the intervention.[26,32,35,41] This could be because services that could be sold as contributing to the organization's goals were more likely to receive internal support and resources that allowed them to be sustained.[29] Furthermore, activities that could readily fit into existing tasks and procedures were more likely to have the support of operating staff members.[29]

To illustrate the importance of a service-organization fit, the case of a health promotion program in a community mental health center is used.[32] The mental health center's mission was oriented to clinical services in mental health and substance abuse. The health promotion program was a newer concept and ancillary to this mission. Due to the poor fit between the organization's mission and the promotion program, the program became isolated from the center's core functions. Because the program was not a principal concern of the organization, the health promotion program was underfunded, had high staff turnover, lacked consistent implementation, and was eventually rejected.

Similar scenarios could happen in a pharmacy if leaders fail to determine the fit between their organization and patient care services. For example, if a pharmacy is oriented to dispensing, a patient care service that requires intensive scheduled sessions with patients may not be sustainable and eventually may be terminated. Hence, to prevent this type of scenario from occurring, leaders and pharmacists should examine how closely the service aligns with the organizational mission, values, and core operations.

4. *Integration with existing operations*

The fourth factor is related to integration between patient care services and core operations. Research has consistently shown that stand-alone services are less likely to be sustained than services that are well integrated with existing operations.[34,40,43] This may be because stand-alone services tend to create jealousy and are less likely to attract funding from the central pool.[43] As such, leaders and pharmacists should plan to incorporate a new service as an integral part of core functions rather than a stand-alone activity.[40]

An example of integrated and non-integrated patient care services in pharmacy practice is illustrated by two types of pharmacy-based vaccination services. Generally, a pharmacist or a pharmacy can be involved in vaccination services through two different mechanisms: (a) contracting with outside providers, generally nurses, to administer vaccines in community pharmacies and (b) using staff pharmacists to administer vaccines at their practice site.[44,45] The first mechanism is referred to as an "outsourced vaccination service" and the second is referred to as an "in-house vaccination service." Generally, in-house vaccination service providers offer walk-in services and/or by appointment,[44] which requires a greater degree of integration with existing workflow and scheduling. Since an outsourced vaccination service is normally offered as a stand-alone service and offered for fewer than four days a year,[44] it is easier to be terminated when compared to an in-house vaccination service that requires a greater degree of integration with existing organizational operations. Therefore, to foster greater sustainability among vaccination services, organizational leaders and pharmacists should incorporate vaccination services into an existing workflow by offering in-house vaccination services rather than outsourced services.

5. Program Assessments and Evaluations

In order to ensure that the service meets the set objectives and the service is correctly implemented, the organization needs to conduct continuous assessments and evaluations.[31,34,35,46] The use of assessment and evaluations allows organizations to continuously monitor and revise both objectives and processes to improve the delivery of the service. Information obtained from the assessments and evaluations can be used to inform the decision makers whether any improvements need to be made to the service. The importance of evaluation was supported by Evashwick and Ory; they interviewed 20 organizations that implemented successful sustainable innovation health services.[40] Their study suggested that outcomes and process evaluations were vital to the service's success.[40]

In pharmacy practice, after a patient care service is implemented, it is strongly recommended that the leaders and pharmacists conduct routine assessments of process and outcomes of the service. The following example illustrates how assessment approaches can be utilized in a pharmacy-based diabetic management service. The success in patient recruitment should be assessed by reviewing the number of new patients who successfully enrolled in the service and by reviewing the number of diabetic patients who could have been recruited. Furthermore, patient outcomes such as A1C and adherence should also be assessed. Data obtained from the routine assessments can be used to inform the decision makers, the champions, and pharmacists who are involved in the diabetic management service if modifications are necessary and to convince the decision makers to continue the support for the diabetic management service.

Dr. Smith from Auburn Pharmacy knows the five factors that are important to sustainability and that a solid plan for sustainability should be established prior to implementing any service or innovation. As listed in Case Example 1, Dr. Smith is considering the following options for Auburn Pharmacy: 1) increasing automation to give pharmacists more time to counsel patients, 2) updating the computer system to identify patients who have not picked up their prescriptions or who are prescribed to high-risk medications, 3) offering influenza, pneumococcal, and herpes zoster vaccinations, and 4) medication synchronization for patients with multiple medications. If Dr. Smith elects to offer immunization services, give examples of three strategies that can be implemented so that the immunization services are sustained over time and suggest how Dr. Smith should approach these strategies.

Organizational leaders and pharmacists play critical roles in making decisions related to how to initiate, manage, and sustain patient care services. In some instances, decision makers are not able to make the most rational decision as they are susceptible to cognitive biases and/or use mental shortcuts to simplify or oversimplify decisions.[47] The following section discusses these cognitive biases and mental shortcuts that can prevent decision makers from making effective decisions.

HIDDEN TRAPS IN DECISION-MAKING

Making decisions is the most important job of organizational leaders.[48] Every day, decisions are being made.[49] Decisions in pharmacy practice can range from a small decision such as when to place an order for a cold medication to a big decision such as whether to implement a Medication Therapy Management service. A number of factors can affect how organizational leaders make decisions. Due to the complexity inherent in decision-making, decisions cannot be made completely objectively and rationally.[50] Rather, decision makers usually bring cognitive biases from their beliefs and experiences into the situation[51] or use mental shortcuts to help make decisions.[51,52] Mental shortcuts are used to explain how people make decisions, typically when facing complex problems or incomplete information. These shortcuts are simple and usually effective, but sometimes they can mislead the decision makers to think differently or choose a different outcome than they might otherwise.[53] Hence, decision makers must be cautious about decision traps affecting how they make decisions. The following section describes three common decision traps and how to overcome them.

STATUS QUO TRAP

In a decision-making context, the status quo refers to the existing state of affairs.[54] In business settings, it refers to existing goals or objectives and the existing plans, strategies, and tactics for attaining those goals.[54] Research has consistently shown that decision makers prefer to continue with existing goals and plans instead of other, better alternatives.[54-58] As a result, organizations avoid making changes or breaking with the status quo despite the opportunity to put those resources to more effective use.[48,54]

March and Simon provided an explanation for why organizations prefer maintaining their status quo over choosing other alternatives.[50] They suggested that the retention of the status quo is likely when a current stage is satisfactory.[50] That is, as long as the status quo stage produces positive outcomes, it is unlikely for decision makers to search for superior alternatives. Additionally, even if decision makers are presented with information about superior alternatives, they may, in fact, refuse to invest further time on exploring the better alternatives.[54] Furthermore, research shows that, in some cases, despite negative outcomes produced by the status quo, decision makers discount the negative information, change organizational goals to fit the situation, or retain hope in the eventual success of the status quo.[54]

Similar to other organizations, decision-making in pharmacy may be affected by the status quo trap. Hence, decision makers need to recognize and overcome the status quo tendency. For example, decision makers should be vigilant in examining alternatives by regularly reviewing how organizational goals are achieved by the status quo when compared to other alternatives.[52,54] It is important that decision makers objectively and rationally explore and evaluate all alternatives, including the status quo alternative.[59] To reduce potential status quo tendency, it may be helpful to have an outside, independent, or separate review of the status quo.[54] Selection of one best alternative should only come after the complete evaluations of all possible alternatives.

SUNK COST TRAP

Sunk costs are defined as costs that have already been incurred and cannot be recovered to any significant degree.[60] Decision makers have a tendency to continue an endeavor once an investment in time, money, or effort has been made at an earlier time, even though the endeavor may no longer produce satisfactory outcomes.[48,61] In other words, decision makers affected by the sunk cost trap are described as if they have too much invested to quit.[62] When they are affected by the sunk cost trap, decision makers have a tendency to continue to invest more money and personnel into a poor performance plan with the hopes of an improvement in the outcomes.

Sunk costs are taken in consideration in the decision-making process because decision makers perceive sunk costs as losses, and hence, results in risk seeking behaviors such as continuing the same endeavor to avoid these losses.[60] Therefore, it is crucial that organizational leaders be aware of the influence of past decisions and past investments and do not allow the effect of sunk cost to cloud judgment. The following two scenarios, adapted from Arkes and Blumer,[60] illustrate the sunk cost effect in pharmacy practice.

Scenario 1: As the owner of an independent pharmacy, you have invested $40,000 of the pharmacy's money into remodeling a patient consultation room, purchasing computer software and hardware, and training staff pharmacists in order to provide state-of-the-art MTM services. Your pharmacy's goal is to secure a contract with a large self-insured employer to provide MTM services for their employees. When the project is 80% completed, another pharmacy begins to market their MTM services to the self-insured employer that your pharmacy is targeting. It is apparent that the competitor's services are much better and more attractive to the target employer than the services that your pharmacy is developing. Since this employer is the only possible target group, the question is: should you invest the last $10,000 to finish your plan for the MTM services, yes or no?

Scenario 2: As the owner of an independent pharmacy, you have received a suggestion from one of your staff pharmacists. The suggestion is to use $10,000 of the pharmacy's money to invest in remodeling a patient consultation room, purchasing necessary computer software and hardware, and training staff pharmacists in order to provide state-of-the-art MTM services. These actions will help the pharmacy to secure a contract with a large self-insured employer to provide MTM services for their employees. However, another pharmacy recently begins to develop their MTM services to the self-insured employer that your pharmacy is targeting. It is apparent that the competitor's services are much better and more attractive to the target employer than the services that your pharmacy could develop. Since this employer is the only possible target group, the question is: should you invest $10,000 to develop the MTM services, yes or no?

What was your answer to each of the scenarios? A higher proportion of people would choose to continue to invest in the MTM services in the first scenario and would opt out in the second scenario. As previously stated, this phenomenon is referred to as the sunk cost effect. Decision makers have a greater tendency to continue an endeavor once an investment in time, money, or effort has been made. In this first scenario, $40,000 has already been invested in developing MTM services; therefore, decision makers are likely to continue to invest resources into the MTM service endeavor.

Sunk cost traps can be avoided if decision makers seek out and listen to people who were not involved in the previous decision-making and/or past investments. This is because people who are not attached to the previous investment and decisions are in a more neutral position to make decisions when sunk costs are present. Furthermore, in order to prevent employees from perpetuating mistakes and justifying their past actions, decision makers must develop a nonpunitive culture.[52] In this way, organizations do not tie negative consequences to the outcome of decisions, especially when the individual has little control over the outcomes.[54]

CONFIRMING-EVIDENCE TRAP

The confirming-evidence trap is a bias that leads decision makers to seek out information to support their existing beliefs and points of view, while avoiding any contradictory information.[48,63,64] Research has shown that, once a single idea is chosen, decision makers typically spend little time exploring other alternatives.[65] This trap not only affects how decision makers seek information but also affects how they interpret evidence.[48] When decision makers are affected by the confirming evidence trap, they put too much weight on supporting information and too little to those that are conflicting[48] or to unintentionally select or distort facts to suit their preferences.[47] This confirming-evidence trap happens because naturally, people are drawn to information that supports their subconscious beliefs, thoughts, and opinions.

In order to avoid this trap, a key is to avoid a limited search for alternative solutions.[59] Generally, when decision makers promote a single idea, the limited-search trap is set to the single idea rather than expanding the search for other alternatives.[59,66] Hence, decision makers should seek advice from others who are objective in their decision-making and/or are not emotionally attached to a particular idea. In this way, others can help uncover options that would otherwise be undiscovered.[59] It is crucial for decision makers to gather all evidence from multiple perspectives, examine it with equal rigor and avoid the tendency to accept the confirming evidence without questioning it thoroughly.[63] Furthermore, decision makers may find it helpful to build counterarguments themselves by asking reasons for choosing different options or asking someone to argue against the option decision makers are contemplating.[48]

Status quo trap, sunk cost trap and confirming-evidence trap are common psychological traps that can mislead decision makers when they make decisions. Decision makers should keep in mind that these traps work in concert with each other. Typically, the effect of traps is more prominent when a decision is made quickly, under uncertainty, and/or based on gut instincts. Hence, organizational leaders and pharmacists should avoid these traps in order to make effective decisions.

CASE EXAMPLE 5

Dr. Smith decides to meet with his staff pharmacists to discuss the changes that he believes need to occur in Auburn Pharmacy. He explains the four options that he has been considering and described why he believes moving toward offering patient care services and providing value-driven health care is important. At the end of the meeting, Dr. Smith gives the other pharmacists the opportunity to give their opinions about his proposed changes. The following are their responses:

> Pharmacist Murray: We have already put so much money into finally getting the pharmacy situated so that we can dispense medications quickly and correctly. I say we just continue to make changes to our layout so that we can dispense more medications and if we need to hire another technician that would be better than investing in some robot.

> Pharmacist Rockefeller: I have a friend who is a pharmacist at Alabama Pharmacy and she just simply hates it. She said they started offering vaccinations and there is just never enough time to keep up with everything. With our heavy workload here dispensing medications, I don't want to end up hating my job like her.

> Pharmacist Miller: I think all this talk about the need to change to a patient-centered pharmacy is just a fad. The way we do things is how we have always done them and it works. We've been open here for 20 years and have always been successful. Believe me, this fad will pass.

1. What kind of trap is Pharmacist Murray falling into?
2. What kind of trap is Pharmacist Rockefeller falling into?
3. What kind of trap is Pharmacist Miller falling into?
4. Dr. Smith is aware of the decision traps the above three pharmacists are fallen in. What can Dr. Smith do to overcome this problem?

SUMMARY

In today's practice environment, quality of care and optimizing patient outcomes are important. To achieve this goal, the practice of pharmacy needs to shift its focus from traditional dispensing activities to patient care activities and from process-oriented to outcome-oriented practice. Organizational leaders and pharmacists are encouraged to use an organization-level approach to initiate, manage, and sustain change in their organizations. Lewin's change model, Force Field Analysis, and Kotter's Eight Stages Model can be used as guidance to develop a course of action to accomplish changes within the organization. It is important that organizational leaders incorporate five factors contributing to sustainability of patient care services into the plan at an early stage of the planning process. Organizational leaders must ensure that a patient care service that will be implemented: (a) has a champion, (b) fits well within the organization, (c) can be modifiable, (d) can be integrated with existing operations, and (e) is regularly assessed and evaluated. Further, organizational leaders and pharmacists must be cautious about decision traps affecting their decisions. Common traps discussed in this chapter are status quo trap, sunk cost trap, and confirming evidence trap. Strategies to overcome these traps are also discussed in this chapter.

REFERENCES

1. Kaiser Family Foundation. (2012). Costs. *JAMA* 308(12):1197–1197.

2. Iuga, A.O. & McGuire, M.J. (2014). Adherence and health care costs. *Risk Manag Healthc Policy* 7:35–44.

3. IMS Institute for Healthcare Informatics. (2013). *Avoidable costs in U.S. healthcare: The $200 billion opportunity from using medicines more responsibly.*
   Parsippany, NJ: IMS Institute for Healthcare Informatics.

4. Soumeral, S. (2004). Benefits and risks of increasing restrictions on access to costly drugs in Medicaid. *Health Aff. (Millwood)* 23(1):135–146.

5. Wright, B.J., Carlson, M.I., Edlund, T., Devoe, J., Gallia, C., & Smith, J. (2005). The impact of increased cost sharing on Medicaid enrollees. *Health Aff. (Millwood)* 24(4):1106–1116.

6. Artiga, S., Rousseau, D., Lyons, B., Smith, S., & Gaylin, D. (2006). Can states stretch the Medicaid dollar without passing the buck? Lessons from Utah. *Health Aff. (Millwood)* 25(2):532–540.

7. Wallack, S.S., Weinberg, D.B., & Thomas, C. P. (2004). Health plans' strategies to control prescription drug spending. *Health Aff. (Millwood)*. 23(6):141–148.

8. Lipton, H., Kreling, D.H., Collins, T., & Hertz, K. (1999). Pharmacy benefit management companies. *Annu. Rev. Public Health* 20:361–401.

9. Garis, R.I. & Clark B.E. (2004). The spread: pilot study of an undocumented source of pharmacy benefit manager revenue. *J. Am. Pharm. Assoc.* 44(1):15–21.

10. Fireman, B., Bartlett, J., & Selby, J. (2004). Can disease management reduce health care costs by improving quality? *Health Aff. (Millwood)* 23(6):63–75.

11. Galvin, R. (2006). Pay-for-performance: too much of a good thing? A conversation with Martin Roland. *Health Aff. (Millwood).* 2006 Web Exclusives;25:pw412–w419.

12. Health care quality. (2005). *Health Aff. (Millwood)* 24(5):1367.

13. Buffington, D.E. (2007). Future of medication therapy management services in delivering patient-centered care. *Am. J. Health. Syst. Pharm.* 64(15):S10–S12.

14. Hepler, C. & Strand, L. (1990). Opportunities and responsibilities in pharmaceutical care. *Am. J. Hosp. Pharm.* 43(533–543).

15. Huyghebaert, T., Farris, K.B., & Volume, C.I. (1999). Implementing pharmaceutical care: insights from Alberta community pharmacists. *Can. Pharm. J.* 132:41–45.

16. Herborg, H., Soendergaard, B., Frokjaer, B., Fonnesbaek, L., & Hepler, C. (1996). Pharmaceutical care value proved. *International Pharmacy Journal* 10:167–168.

17. Shibley, M.C. & Pugh, C.B. (1997). Implementation o f pharmaceutical care services for patients with hyperlipidemias by independent community pharmacy practitioners. *Ann. Pharmacother.* 31(6):713–719.

18. Barner, J.C., Brown, C.M., Shepherd, M.D., Chou, J.Y., & Yang, M. (2002). Provision of pharmacy services in community health centers and migrant health centers. *J. Am. Pharm. Assoc.* 42(5):713–722.

19. Farris, K.B. & Schopflocher, D.P. (1999). Between intention and behavior: an application of community pharmacists' assessment of pharmaceutical care. *Social Science and Medicine* 49:55–66.

20. Odedina, F.L., Segal, R., Hepler, C.D., Lipowski, E., & Kimberlin, C. (1996). Changing pharmacists' practice pattern: pharmacists' implementation of pharmaceutical care factors. *Journal of Social and Administrative Pharmacy.* 13(2):74–88.

21. Baldridge, J.V. & Burnham, R.A. (1975). Organization innovation: individual, organizational, and environmental impacts. *Adm. Sci. Q.* 20(2):165–176.

22. Scott, W.R. (2003). *Organizations: Rational, natural, and open system.* 5 ed. Upper Saddle River, New Jersey: Prentice Hall.

23. Lewin, K. (1951). *Field Theory in Social Science.* New York: Harper and Row.

24. Cummings, T.G. & Worley, C.G. (1993). *Organization development and change*. 5 ed. St. Paul, MN: West Publishing Company.

25. Kotter, J.P. (1995). Leading change: Why transformation efforts fail. *Harvard business review*. 73(2):59–67.

26. Goodman, R.M. & Steckler, A.B. (1989). A model for the institutionalization of health promotion programs. *Fam. Community Health* 11(4):63–78.

27. Rogers, E.M. (2003). *Diffusion of Innovation* (5th ed.). New York: Free Press.

28. Scheirer, M.A. (1990). The life cycle of an innovation: adoption versus discontinuation of the fluoride mouth rinse program in schools. *J. Health Soc. Behav.* 31(2):203–215.

29. Scheirer, M.A. (2005). Is sustainability possible? A review and commentary on empirical studies of program sustainability. *American Journal of Evaluation*. 26(3):320–348.

30. Goodman, R.M. & Steckler, A.B. (1987–88). The life and death of a health promotion program: an institutionalization case study. *Int. Q. Community. Health. Educ.* 8(1):5–21.

31. Shediac-Rizkallah, M.C. & Bone, L.R. (1998). Planning for the sustainability of community-based health programs: conceptual frameworks and future directions for research, practice and policy. *Health Educ. Res.* 13(1):87–108.

32. Steckler, A.B. & Goodman, R.M. (1989). How to institutionalize health promotion programs. *Am. J. Health Promot.* 3(4):34–44.

33. Bamberger, M. & Cheema, S. (1990). *Case studies of project sustainability: implications for policy and opeations from asian experience*. Washington, DC: The World Bank.

34. Glaser, E.M. (1981). Durability of innovations in human service organizations: A case study analysis. *Knowledge: Creation, Diffusion, Utilization*. 3:167–185.

35. O'Loughlin, J., Renaud, L., Richard, L., Gomez, L.S., & Paradis, G. (1998). Correlates of the sustainability of community-based heart health promotion interventions. *Prev. Med.* 27:702–712.

36. Yin, R.K. (1979). *Changing urban bureaucracies: how new practices become routinized*. Lexington, MA: Lexington Books.

37. Shediac, M.C. & Bone, L. R. (1998). Planning for the sustainability of community-based health programs: conceptual frameworks and future directions for research, practice and policy. *Health Educ. Res.* 13(1):87–108.

38. Achilladelis, B., Jervis, P., & Robertson, A. (1971). A *study of success and failure in industrial innovation*. Sussex, England: University of Sussex Press.

39. Howell, J.M. & Higgins, C.A. (1990). Champions of technological innovation. *Adm. Sci. Q.* 35:317–341.

40. Evashwick, C. & Ory, M. (2003). Organizational characteristics of success-ful innovative health care programs sustained over time. *Fam. Community Health.* 26(3):177–193.

41. Gladwin, J., Dixon, R.A., & Wilson, T.D. (2002). Rejection of an innovation: health information management training materials in east Africa. *Health Policy Plan.* 17(4):354–361.

42. Westrick, S.C. & Breland, M.L. (2009). Sustainability of pharmacy-based innovations: The case of in-house immunization services. *J Am Pharm Assoc* (2003) 49(4):500–508.

43. Bossert, T.J. (1990). Can they get along without us? Sustainability of donor-supported health projects in Central America and Africa. *Social Science and Medicine* 30(1015–1023).

44. Chamnanmoh, S. (2004). *Adoption of Immunization Services in Pharmacies.* Madison: Social and Administrative Sciences in Pharmacy, University of Wisconsin-Madison.

45. Savino, L.B. (1998). Your pharmacy and immunizations. *America's Pharma-cist* 120(7):49–53.

46. Stange, K.C., Goodwin, M.A., Zyzanzki, S.J., & Dietrich, A.K. (2003).Sustain-ability of a practice-individualized preventive service delivery intervention. *Am. J. Prev. Med.* 25(296–300).

47. Teach, E. Avoiding decision traps. *CFO.* Vol 202004:97–99.

48. Hammond, J.S., Keeney, R.L., & Raiffa, H. The hidden traps in decision mak-ing. *Harvard Business Review.* Vol 842006:118–126.

49. Anonymous. (1999). Discussing desirability of decisions. *New Zealand Man-agement* 46(8).

50. March, J.G. & Simon, H. A. (1957). *Organizations.* New York: Free Press.

51. Kahneman, D. & Tversky, A. (1979). Prospect theory: An analysis of decision under risk. *Econometrica* 47(2):263–292.

52. Anderson, K. Making all of the right decisions. *Food Manufacture.* Vol 741999:2–4.

53. Tversky, A. & Kahneman D. (1974). Judgment under uncertainty: heuristics and biases. *Science.* 185(4157):1124–1131.

54. Silver, W.S. & Mitchell, T.R. (1990). The status quo tendency in decision mak-ing. *Organizational Dynamics* 18(4):34–46.

55. Hambrick, D.C., Geletkanycz, M.A., & Fredrickson, J. W. (1993). Top execu-tive commitment to the status quo: some tests of its determinants. *Stategic Management Journal* 14(6):401–418.

56. Geletkanycz, M.A. (1995). The salience of culture's consequences: the effects of cultural values on top executive commitment to the status quo. *Stategic Management Journal* 18(8):615–634.

57. Samuelson, W. & Zeckhauser, R. (1998). Status quo bias in decision making. *Journal of Risk and Uncertainty* 1:7–59.

58. Schweitzer, M. (1995). Multiple reference points, framing, and the status quo bias in health care financing decisions. *Organizational Behavior & Human Decision Processes* 63(1):69–72.

59. Nutt, P.C. (2004). Expanding the search for alternatives during strategic decision-making. *Academy of Management Executive* 18(4):13–28.

60. Arkes, H. & Blumer, C. (1985). The Psychology of Sunk Cost. *Organ. Behav. Hum. Decis. Process.* 35:124–140.

61. Zeelenberg, M. & van Dijk, E. (1997). A reverse sunk cost effect in risky decision making: Sometimes we have too much invested to gamble. *Journal of Economic Psychology* 18:677–691.

62. Teger, A.L. (1980). *Too much invested to quit.* New York: Pergamon Press.

63. Anderson, K. Decision-making traps. *Broadcast Engineering.* Vol 411999:106.

64. Anderson, K. Decisions. *Food Manufacture.* Vol 741999:2–4.

65. Nutt, P.C. (2002). *Why decisions fail.* San Francisco, CA: Berrett-Koehler.

66. Nutt, P.C. (2004). Averting decision debacles. *Technological Forecasting and Social Change* 71:239–265.

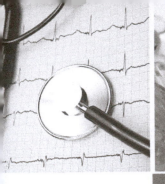
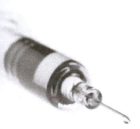
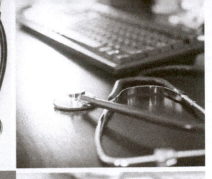
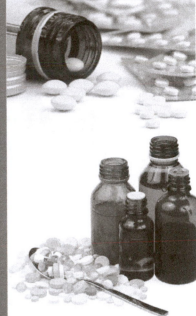
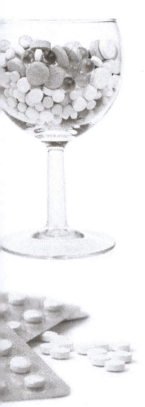
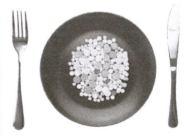
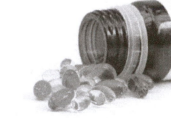
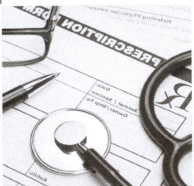

TREATMENT PLANNING AND PARTICIPATION

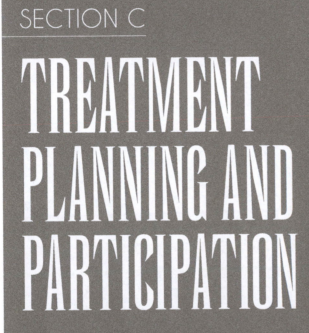
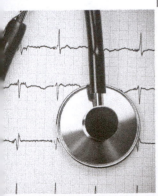
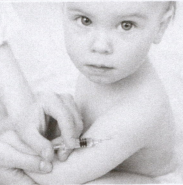
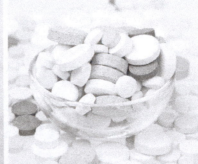

CHAPTER 8

PRESCRIBING BEHAVIOR

Kent E. M. Groves, MSc, PhD, CChem, Neil J. MacKinnon, M.Sc. (Pharm), Ph.D., FCSHP, Ingrid Sketris, PharmD., MPA (HSA), John-Michael Gamble, BScPharm, PhD

LEARNING OBJECTIVES:

1. Describe the various influences on prescribing behavior.
2. Compare and contrast the differences between direct to physician marketing and direct to consumer advertising.
3. Evaluate which physician practice characteristics have the largest impact on prescribing behavior.
4. Distinguish which physician profile characteristics have the largest impact on prescribing behavior.
5. Outline the emerging role of social media on prescribing.

KEY TERMS

Channel propensity

Direct to consumer advertising

Direct to physician marketing

Innovation diffusion

Physician profiles

Prescribing

Prescribing behavior

Contributed by Neil J. MacKinnon, Kent E. Groves, Ingrid Sketris, & John-Michael Gamble.

INTRODUCTION

"The factors that influence a physician's decision to prescribe a particular drug, order a diagnostic test, or follow another course of action are numerous and complex."[1]

The factors influencing physicians' prescribing[i] behavior and the context or system in which they work, including medical, non-medical, physician and non-physician variables, have been extensively studied by various disciplines.[2-19]

This chapter discusses the various influences on physician prescribing behavior. It discusses the strategies used by pharmaceutical industry marketers to provide physicians and, in some countries, patients with new information about their products. It also discusses the ways in which managers and clinical leaders in the health care system provide information on optimal approaches to prescribing in the health system. This chapter also discusses theories, models and frameworks that review how physicians acquire, and incorporate prescribing practices into their clinical practice.

One of the system factors that has resulted in increased complexity in the prescribing environment is the increasing number and type of non-physician prescribers.[20] For example, in the United States, there are over 95,000 certified physician assistants and 180,000 nurse practitioners.[21] In many countries, pharmacists have received prescribing privileges.[22] In addition, their regulatory frameworks, the degree of independence or level of physician supervision, and the drug types they can prescribe varies across jurisdictions.[22-29]

Challenges to influencing prescribing behavior in this environment include the different prescribing training requirements and roles, professional communities of practice, sources of drug information, reimbursement, and organizational infrastructures. In addition, multiple prescribers can lead to increased adverse drug events.[30] Providing optimal prescribing in the face of multiple prescribers includes enabling integrated patient-centered collaborative care models and using such tools as common electronic health records and team communication mechanisms.[27,28,31-33] Pharmaceutical manufacturers influence not only physicians, but also non-physician prescribers.

While there remain gaps in the literature, specifically in the areas relating to the interdependency between marketing activities and physician specific characteristics, our goal in this chapter is to bring the insights from the existing body of literature together into one place.

We have identified the primary models, theories, and frameworks that provide insight into our understanding of the variables that influence prescribing behavior. Additionally, we will present models used by the pharmaceutical industry in their development of marketing strategy to increase sales of prescription pharmaceuticals.

The traditional marketing approach, followed by the pharmaceutical industry globally, was to target its efforts toward the physician (Figure 8-1).[34] This model still exists,

---

[i] While there are many prescribers in the health professions, physicians account for the majority of prescriptions written.

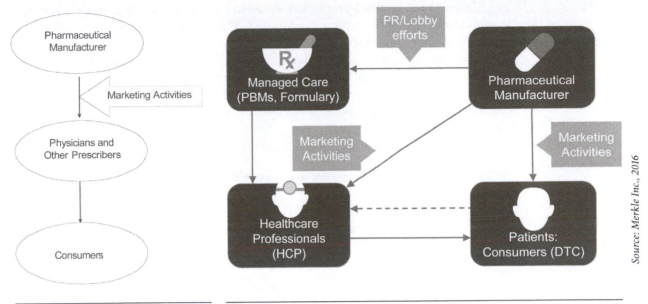

Source: Merkle Inc., 2016

FIGURE 8-1: HISTORICAL
PHARMACEUTICAL INDUSTRY
MARKETING STRATEGY

FIGURE 8-2: PHARMACEUTICAL INDUSTRY
MARKETING STRATEGY

especially in markets in which direct-to-consumer advertising (DTCA) is not permitted. Even in markets in which DTCA is not permitted, DTCA within the United States has a spillover or halo effect in many western cultures through print, broadcast and electronic and social media.

DTCA (in the United States) over the last 15 years has resulted in a two-pronged marketing approach. This strategy consists of a continued focus on the physician, while targeting a complementary (and concurrent) message toward the consumer[ii] (Figure 8-2), with the objective of educating and informing the end user, and peripherally, influencing (reinforcing) the physician's interpretation of the message.[35] In markets like the United States, the two channels are acknowledged and pursued. In other Western markets, DTCA is more restricted,[iii] with the exception of New Zealand.[36,37]

In the European Union, brands cannot be promoted by advertising that tries to stimulate consumer-physician interaction, although providing education is permitted. A push to weaken this ban was defeated in 2004. A proposal to reform DTCA has been proposed in the past.[38] In the absence of a "DTCA friendly regulatory environment," traditional marketing efforts may be complemented through the efforts of voluntary health agencies and patient disease advocacy groups who may lobby to have particular drugs added to a jurisdictional formulary.

[ii] In this chapter, we will use the term *consumer* exclusively as consumers are the end target of a marketing message, thus, consumers may be health professionals as well as patients.

[iii] In Canada, drugs may be advertised to consumers, but either the name of the drug appears with no medical condition mentioned, or the medical condition appears with no drug named.[210]

In addition to the targeted promotion we see in Figures 8-1 and 8-2, there is another level of consideration, as outlined in Figure 8-3. In this scenario, primary influences typically include physician-specific factors, and secondary influences include non-physician characteristics, such as those individuals or groups that may influence the physician's decision. Additionally, as we have witnessed the rapid adoption of social media over the past five years, channel (or medium) is also assuming a key role in reach, impact, and likelihood to prescribe.

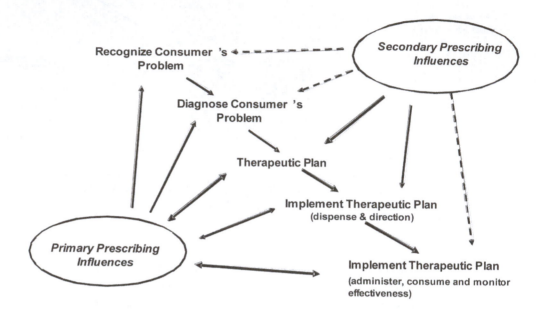

FIGURE 8-3: FLOW OF INFLUENCE WITHIN THE MEDICATION USE SYSTEM (PRESCRIBERS DECISION PROCESS)

adapted from Hepler (155)

Understanding the extent to which primary and secondary factors influence prescribing activity is critical, as these factors, to a greater or lesser extent, predicate the defined market size for a specific product. That is, the professional identification and diagnosis of a condition, association of that condition with a specific intervention, developing a list of possible therapeutic options, and the subsequent selection of one intervention over another will be a direct artifact of the activities and nature of the physician population. And, more importantly, this will be a direct artifact of the success of the pharmaceutical company in reaching and influencing that group of prescribers.

Ultimately, the complexity of prescribing behavior is a function of the relationship between physician variables, consumer variables, and the environment.

While there are numerous factors that may influence a physician's prescribing behavior, the factors that influence a consumer's decision process (Figure 8-4) regarding their request for use of a pharmaceutical intervention for an identified condition must also be recognized and considered. Within the context of health care consumers, we can see that the decision process involves recognition of a problem, which may lead to either evaluation of alternatives prior to visiting a physician, followed by a conscious decision to accept the physician's recommendation. This decision process is subsequently influenced by external stimuli as well as their own characteristics.[39,40] In 2016, market "noise" and market stimuli is assuming a greater influence on the consumer, through a broader range of media and channels, that historically had limited influence (Figure 8-5).

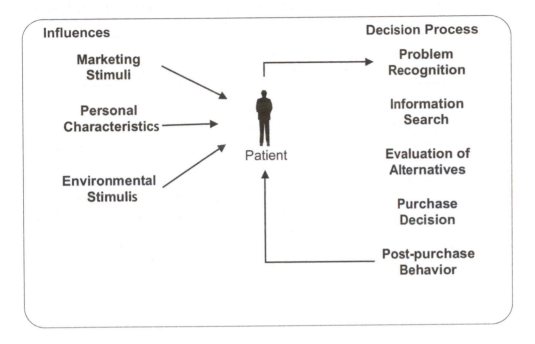

FIGURE 8-4: CONSUMER DECISION MAKING PROCESS

adapted from Kotler et al, 2005 (ref)

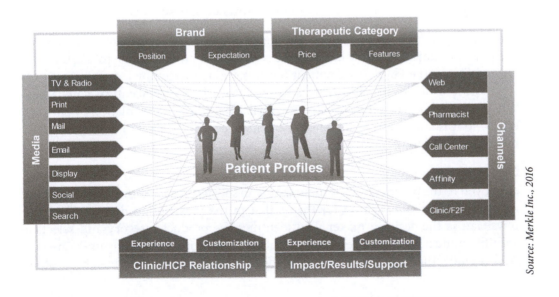

FIGURE 8-5: MARKETING STIMULI: CONSUMER/PATIENT INFLUENCE MODEL—CIRCA 2015

The consumer's role in influencing the physician is recognized, and one approach is to consider employing the traditional business to consumer marketing approach. While the model in Figure 8-4 is a construct based on the consumer decision-making literature,[41-45] this direction of strategic evaluation involves another entire body of literature, one that is not directly related to the focus of this chapter. That is, combining an appropriate marketing mix within the context of the existing external stimuli to ultimately influence the consumer's decision process.

THE PHYSICIAN AS A CONSUMER

We typically think of consumers as one of two types; those who buy for their own consumption, or those who buy for someone else. Marketers tend to position their messages to target one of these two types of consumers. Physicians, however, are unique in their "consumer/consumption" role. They are unique in that they are neither the consumer nor the purchaser. Although they may recommend (prescribe) a product, they are not necessarily concerned or influenced by the price of the product. Their reward for the "purchase" may be vicariously provided through seeing improvements in the health of a patient (in this case, the ultimate consumer) or, in some situations, through incentives from the manufacturer or purchaser. Of course, many other factors influence this as well. These may include:

- Other reward systems such as pay-for-performance in some US healthcare settings
- Budget incentives[46]
- Third party survey and patient-reported outcomes
- Managed care initiatives around reward for post-treatment response and re-engagement
- Key opinion-leader (KOL) status and associated speaker engagements

Providing payments to physicians for their various roles in promoting drugs for the pharmaceutical industry has become regulated to protect public interest. In the United States, the Physician Payment Sunshine Act, enacted by Congress in 2010, regulates the disclosure of payments to physicians by pharmaceutical companies. The payments began to be reported in April 2013 when the regulations went into effect, so it is still too early to determine impact on patient-physician relationships, prescribing and health care costs.[47-49]

Given the unique nature of the physician as a consumer, the marketing strategies employed in the pharmaceutical industry are in sharp contrast to those used in other markets. The primary reason for this is that in the prescription drug market, the physician is the decision maker who identifies the product category and selects a specific product from the alternatives within that category on the consumer's behalf. Additionally, there is typically more freedom to create and deliver insight in other industries, pharmaceutical advertising is heavily regulated, with a significant portion of all messaging allocated for fair balance messaging.[50]

The most appropriate comparison between the physician as consumer and other markets is with that of an agency relationship, in which, in this case, the physician is the agent[34,51-53] or advocate for the consumer.[54] While it is the physician who makes the decision in collaboration with the consumer, it is still the consumer who uses the product and ultimately takes responsibility for payment of the product.

In consideration of their role as intermediaries and key decision makers in the prescribing process, it is to be expected that physicians would become the target of the marketing activities associated with prescription drugs. For years, a variety of means available to the pharmaceutical industry to communicate their message to physicians has been employed.[55-57] The metric against which the industry measures the success of their marketing effort is the volume of drugs sold, or more specifically, the number of prescriptions written by the physician. The actual writing of a prescription is thus indicative of a physician's recognition that a product is the best alternative to address the consumer's condition, and it is also the primary metric that measures prescribing behavior. This being said, while a prescription written is a measure of marketing success, the actual dispensing of the product, and adherence to the medication may be subject to a greater variety of variables over which there is less control.[31]

While it is not within the scope of this chapter to discuss government or specific jurisdictional policy relative to prescribing, it needs to be recognized as an influencing variable on prescribing behavior. The primary issues of policy relate to the eligibility of patients for benefits, comprehensiveness of prescription drug coverage (formulary listings, cost-sharing mechanisms, etc.), and the pricing of prescription drugs. Indeed, prescribers must be responsive to costs of medications especially given that up to 5–10% of medication non-adherence related to costs.[58,59]

INFLUENCES ON PRESCRIBING BEHAVIOR

"It is important to understand what influences physician decision-making, to ensure that resources and tools are made available to help physicians make appropriate and cost-effective choices that lead to the best possible care."[1]

Given the most intuitive measure of prescribing behavior is prescribing (a treatment decision), we need to consider this action at its basic level, namely, the adoption of a new innovation by the physician. The drivers that can have a dramatic influence on changes in prescribing behavior are represented graphically in Figure 8-6. Given this, our next step, then, is to discuss the concepts of innovation diffusion and adoption, as it provides insight into the nature of the metric associated with prescribing behavior, specifically, prescribing. The next four areas of consideration relative to prescribing behavior include pharmaceutical marketing activity (direct to consumer and direct to professional), practice characteristics or the clinical profile, and the physician profile or related demographics and channel propensity, namely, an individual's affinity for a particular channel (e.g.; web via hand-held device, e-detailing, direct mail response, pharmaceutical representative, key opinion leader video on a notepad, etc.).

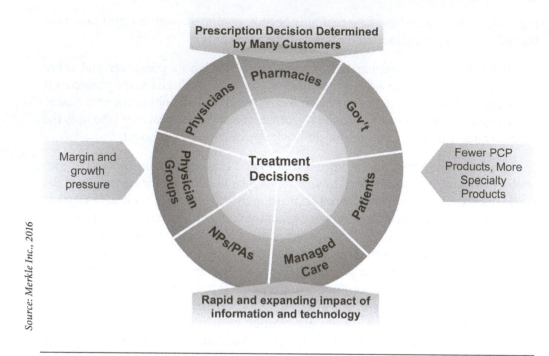

FIGURE 8-6: DRIVERS INFLUENCING PRESCRIBING BEHAVIOR

Source: Merkle Inc., 2016

INNOVATION DIFFUSION AND ADOPTION

Given that, in the end, the question is really "to prescribe or not to prescribe," it is important to gain insight into the current thought on diffusion and adoption, and its role in understanding the issues related to influencing prescribing behavior. This portion of the chapter thus focuses on the adoption of new technologies in general, not specifically innovations associated with health care.

Extensive literature reviews on the theories, models and frameworks to implement new innovations in health care have been conducted.[33,60-63] Improving prescribing (increasing appropriate use and decreasing inappropriate and misuse) in a complex clinical environment with busy prescribers can be difficult. Theories, models and frameworks can assist in designing and evaluating strategies for prescribing behavior change at the individual prescriber, organization and health care system levels. These frameworks may also aid in determining mechanisms for success or failure in different contexts, in other words, what strategies work for whom and how.[61,63]

At the organizational level, a key classic theory, and one of the most highly cited is Everett M Rogers "Diffusion of Innovations" which is the theory detailed in our chapter.[64,65] Other theories at the organization level include human factors/systems engineering, organizational learning, complexity science etc.[61,63] Some theories relate to understanding context and social interactions between individuals within and across organizations.[63,66]

At the individual level, theories from such disciplines as psychology, sociology, and education have examined such factors as attitude, motivation, and cognition.[61,62] Other paradigms relate to understanding the development of prescribing habits or clinical mindlines (tacit guidelines influenced by both literature evidence and inter-actions with peers, opinion leaders, patients and others).[33]

A recent framework, the Theoretical Domains Framework, relevant to the individual and the organization examined over 30 behavior change theories and developed 14 theoretical domains (84 component constructs) about such factors as an individuals' knowledge, skills, beliefs about capabilities and consequences, and intentions as well as the environment and resources. This framework can be used to understand barri-ers and enablers prior to implementing a prescribing change strategy.[62]

We focus on Rogers' diffusion of innovations theory and provide information more specific to the adoption of prescription drugs. A review of the adoption of technology provides insight into key variables that may be directly involved in physician adop-tion, or more specifically, the variables likely to influence prescribing behavior.

Diffusion is the process by which an *innovation* is *communicated* through certain *channels* over *time* among the members of a *social system*.[64] Whereas, the innovation is an idea, practice or object that is perceived as new by an individual or other unit of adoption. Time is an important element in diffusion, as it is involved in the process by which an individual passes from first knowledge to adoption or rejection, as well as the innovativeness or speed by which an innovation is adopted relative to the other members of the social system.

Initially, adoption was studied by various research traditions. By the late 1970s, they had effectively merged. Several disciplines became integral to studying prescribing behavior, namely; Marketing, Public Health and Medical Sociology. A study commis-sioned by the Charles Pfizer Company established our fundamental understanding of the diffusion and adoption of new drugs by physicians.[67] While some elements of this diffusion model have been questioned,[68] much of the initial research conducted by Coleman and colleagues, remains relevant. The success of marketing managers in launching a new product is often measured by rate of adoption and retention among a target audience.

Physicians are not passive recipients of innovations. They seek them out; they experi-ment with them and evaluate them; they worry about them; they collaborate with peers and seek reinforcement; they modify them and attempt to adapt them to their specific circumstances; they challenge them; and may even become emotionally attached to them. Physicians may do this in isolation, or with other members of their social system.

Within the context of prescribing behavior, we need to recognize that the adopter is an actor who interacts purposefully and creatively with a complex innovation[60] and plays a critical role in the diffusion of innovations, both within health service orga-nizations, and the medical community at large.

Probably two of the more important considerations for adoption, as proposed by Peay and Peay, are preparedness to prescribe the new drug, and presentation of par-ticular circumstances which are appropriate for its use.[69] An individual's prepared-ness to prescribe a "new" drug is an independent variable, which may be predicted, depending on the physician, consumer, and environmental information available.

TABLE 8-1: STEPS IN THE INNOVATION-DECISION PROCESS

1. KNOWLEDGE—CHARACTERISTICS OF THE DECISION MAKING[v]
a. Socio-economic characteristics
b. Personality variables
c. Communication behavior
2. PERSUASION – PERCEIVED CHARACTERISTICS OF THE INNOVATION
a. Relative advantage
b. Compatibility
c. Complexity
d. Trialability
e. Observability
3. DECISION
a. Adoption
b. Rejection
4. IMPLEMENTATION
5. CONFIRMATION
a. Adoption—continued
b. Adoption—discontinuance
c. Rejection—continued
d. Rejection— later adoption

[v] *In this case, the decision making unit is typically the physician, but may also be considered the combination of the physician and the consumer.*

To appreciate the variables that may influence physician adoption, one must revisit the innovation-decision process.[64] Prior conditions required to create an environment that will lead to the physician innovation-decision process taking place include previous practice, felt needs/problems, innovativeness, norms of the social system, and presence of circumstances appropriate for trial. If these conditions are met, it is more likely that an individual or group will seek out knowledge, be open to persuasion, decide to initiate trial, implement and evaluate, as described in Table 8-1.

When considering the traditional approach to adoption, one might determine that the characteristics of the adopter and the adoption environment are stable over time. Waarts et al., however, suggest that the driving factors in adopting innovations will change as the diffusion of the innovation within the market progresses.[70] That is, while it is well-known that different groups of adopters have different characteristics concerning the rate of innovation adoption,[64] the factors explaining the adoption of innovations will not be stable over the diffusion process, but will change as larger numbers of individuals adopt the innovation. Waarts suggests that in the first stages of adoption of innovation by organizations, the most important stimulating factors are a combination of internal drivers (personal characteristics), whereas subsequent adopters are more influenced by a mix of stimulating factors focusing on the practical issues.[70] This insight is supported by the marketing mix used by industry, in which combinations of direct to consumer, journal and physician detailing changes with the nature and "perceived innovativeness" of the drug.[71] Within the actual "communication mix" utilized by industry to reach physicians, channels (e-mail, e-detail, peer to peer, sales rep), frequency are mix are all adjusted based on the profile of the target physician audience.

Another consideration in the adoption process relates to individual versus team decisions. Contrary to the traditional five steps associated with individual trial and adoption proposed by Rogers,[64] Wozniak suggests that adoption and technical acquisition decisions are made jointly by team members, and that the influences of the determinants of that decision differ with the timing of adoption and the channels of information dissemination.[72] The traditional steps may not occur successively, but different stages may need to occur concurrently to achieve maximum response. His work also concurs with earlier research with respect to differences between the individuals at various stages of adoption. He indicates that early adopters find information more useful in the early stages of adoption decision process than in the later stages.

Olshavsky questions the individual's approach to innovation evaluation.[73] The traditional marketing assumption has been that individuals faced with a new stimulus engage in some type of attribute by attribute evaluation, in which the interpretation of the innovation is a function of the elements or attributes of the stimulus. Olshavsky suggests that people may be more inclined to establish evaluative criteria by placing the new stimulus into an existing category, thus simply giving the innovation the same evaluation that it gives other category members. This suggests that all innovations are not adopted using an attribute approach as suggested in Rogers' step 2, "persuasion—perceived characteristics of the innovation" (Table 8-1). Olshavsky suggests that there are four other processes influencing evaluation: forming evaluative criteria, forming expectation about the innovation concept, assessing satisfaction with an old product, and comparing the new and the old products.

An intuitive consideration in adoption is that "'early' adopters are more likely to adopt," and consequently, "prescribers are more likely to prescribe." Health research in this area has been limited.[74] Shih and Venkatesh found that adopters with higher use-diffusion levels (that is, they use a newly adopted product more often and in a greater variety of ways), are not only more satisfied with the current innovation, but are more interested in adopting future innovations.[75] Marinova determined that innovation effort takes shape over time under two opposing forces: market knowledge diffusion (how will I use this product in the future?) which propels innovation and satisfaction with past performance (I am content and am not interested in new applications or innovations?), which hinders innovation.[76] This, in turn, may impact adoption of "perceived similar" products within a product category.

If behavior predicts behavior, preparedness to prescribe a new drug as proposed by Peay and Peay thus becomes a critical step in the process toward actually prescribing.[69] Considering behavior, McDonald proposed that there may be a number of behavioral variables that influence the likelihood of prescribing. These may include, among others, individual prescribing habits, size of the practice, location of the practice, and the nature of their social groups. The role of collective behavior on individual adoption[77] as well as the role of social networks on diffusion and adoption[78] are recognized.

Often it is the multiple interactions that arise in various settings that determine the success or failure of an innovation and its subsequent dissemination. Different product markets may exhibit different adoption characteristics, thus impacting the extrapolation of insights between products and markets.

PHARMACEUTICAL MARKETING ACTIVITY

Manufacturers must determine how to strategically present "new" drugs to the target audiences. New product success is dependent on many variables, some that they can control (promotion, price, channels of distribution, etc.) and some that they cannot control (regulation, scientific evaluation leading to publication, independent third party reviews, formulary status and patient insurer coverage, etc.). Additionally, success of the new drug depends on the nature of the physicians (primary influences), and whether they will perceive the new product as a radically differentiated offering (discontinuous innovation) or as a minor variation of existing functionalities (dynamically continuous innovation).[73,79,80] These primary influences are identified within the context of the environment in which the physician practices, or may relate to the characteristics of the physicians themselves.

DIRECT TO PHYSICIAN MARKETING

It seems intuitive to suggest that the probability of prescribing a drug is a function of the marketing effort expended on that particular product. This marketing effort may be more specifically defined as corporate or academic detailing (a core of individuals who visit physician's offices) and the associated drug "trial samples," and other commercial sources of information to promote a particular drug. The use and expense associated with free drug samples is a long-standing industry practice[81,82] and has been demonstrated to be an excellent way to introduce new products or dislodge a market leader.[83] These two categories—detailing and product sampling—are complimentary, and together they typically account for over 65% of the total drug promotional expenditures.[71,84,85] A physician who was interviewed as part of a study looking at how the pharmaceutical industry influences prescribing through the use of samples said "when [pharmaceutical companies] provide samples, [doctors] usually, instead of following guidelines, they usually end up writing a prescription they were provided a sample, and once they give the patient a sample and the medication works, then they tend to continue prescribing the same medication. So whatever is available from some pharmaceutical company with free drugs, that's what they would use."[86]

While there is some disagreement on the impact that drug promotion has on adoption (some physicians go so far as to suggest that they are not influenced by pharmaceutical marketing, but they believe that their colleagues are influenced),[87] if a particular promotional tactic does not work, the pharmaceutical industry would most likely discontinue its use. Hawkins and Hoch suggested that low involvement processing leads to poorer memory, but greater belief.[88] That is, the less time an individual spends thinking about a given point or observation, the more likely they are to consider it true; conversely, they may be less likely to remember it. This work is supported in part by Prosser et al. who defined general practitioners as largely reactive recipients, rather than active searchers of new drug information, and in many instances relied heavily on the pharmaceutical industry as the major information source.[89]

Given the pharmaceutical industry's approach to its market (brief, frequent visits), we now start to gain insight as to why physicians feel that they do not believe that they are influenced by the marketing activities of industry, even though research would tell us otherwise.[90,91] Watkins et al. have even gone on to say that general practitioners who receive information and visits from the pharmaceutical industry are responsible for higher prescribing costs and prescribe in a less rational manner than their peers who function without direct pharmaceutical industry influence.[92] Additionally, Muijrers et al. found a negative relationship between prescribing according to evidence-based general practical guidelines and the frequency of visits by pharmaceutical sales representatives.[93]

An extension of the physician's "perceived resilience or imperviousness" to advertising is the consensus among both high and low prescribing populations of physicians that they like to prescribe drugs with which they are familiar, which means that there may be some reluctance to prescribe new medications.[94] When considering the definition and application of the word "familiar," we know that brand names have greater impact on choice in situations where minimal quality information is available on product alternatives.[95] That is, when choosing between two similar products, the familiar brand name is often considered when less qualitative information is available for the comparator. This, in turn, can have a significant impact on usage (prescription) when that brand name is associated with pioneer or a "first-to-market" in-category product.[96] Leffler suggested that brand loyalty may result from the high costs of acquiring new information or of learning by experience, and subsequently may generate persistence in prescribing patterns, thus influencing physician responsiveness to promotional efforts.[97]

There is support for the relationship between physician satisfaction with their pharmaceutical sales representatives and their prescribing behavior,[98] and for the influence of drug company representatives through product information dissemination.[99] Work by Watkins et al. suggested that frequent contact with a drug representative was significantly associated with a greater willingness to prescribe new drugs and to agree to consumers' requests for drugs that may not be clinically indicated.[100] Additionally, promotional impact should not be limited to the perception that a manufacturer is simply communicating their message. While publication of new evidence may be associated with modest changes in individual practice, industry led promotional activity appears to have a greater influence on the adoption of this new evidence.[101]

Changes in prescribing behavior are not simply a function of the marketing or advertising dollars spent, but more a function of the message and the target audience. Kerr et al. noted that the increase in cyclooxygenase-2 (COX-2) inhibitor prescribing in Australia coincided with a period of energetic marketing to the medical profession, which promoted the message that the new COX-2 inhibitors were "safer" than traditional non-steroidal anti-inflammatory drugs (NSAIDs).[102] Additionally, retrospective work by Van den Bulte on the original study done by Coleman with respect to the medical community's understanding of tetracycline, suggests that it was through aggressive marketing efforts targeted at the physician population, and not social contagion, that this product gained in popularity and application.[68]

With the exception of recent work by Mizik et al., limited academic literature documents the efficiency of marketing directly to physicians through detailing. Mizik quantified the impact of detailing, and determined that detailing and free drug samples have a modest influence on the number of new prescriptions issued by a physician.[103] Interestingly, this impact is only significant when one considers the lagged effect (future response resulting from a current action). That is, immediate impact is less significant that future impact. Mizik demonstrated the residual impact of marketing activity six months after the fact, but other studies have demonstrated a persistent effect on product sales for more than 12 months.[104]

Gonul, interpreting feedback from a panel of physicians, found that a certain level of detailing positively influences prescribing, but excessive detailing becomes counter-productive.[105] Gonul's work is supported by the work of Manchanda and Chintagunta, who demonstrated that there are optimal levels of marketing, after which incremental increases are negatively elastic.[106] That is, the percentage increase in prescribing declines relative to a similar percentage increase in marketing expenditure.

When pursued by governments, hospitals and health management organizations, detailing is referred to as academic detailing. While this form of detailing has been shown to be a very effective technique to encourage adoption of clinical practice guidelines,[107–111] its widespread adoption is less likely as it is expensive,[112] and, as noted by Mizik and others,[103,113,114] physicians are not always receptive to this approach.

While a positive impact of product detailing, of free drug samples and journal advertising on prescribing of drugs has been found, it is often difficult to quantify, as their activities are not mutually exclusive. Jones et al. found no clear relationship between the extent of drug advertising and the amount of prescribing by GPs[115] and suggested that while advertising in journals is only one of many factors which influence general practitioners to prescribe, it is probably not a major influence. Interestingly, there is very little work discussing the impact of drug samples, independent of the pharmaceutical representative. Schumock made an attempt to quantify this, and his results suggested that free samples influenced prescribing decisions, but the information disseminated by pharmaceutical sales representatives had no significant impact. It would seem that it is difficult to separate one from the other,[116] and the covariance, or relationship between the two cannot be discounted.

Although it may be difficult to separate journal advertising from the marketing mix, and relate it back to response, it is an element of pharmaceutical industry's approach to market, and probably needs to be evaluated concurrently with the total marketing spending vs sales (prescriptions). Majumdar suggested that new evidence published in peer-reviewed journals is associated with modest changes in clinical practice, but more active promotional strategies are required to accelerate the adoption of new evidence in routine clinical practice.[101] The use of active promotional strategies was supported in earlier work by Hurwitz et al., who demonstrated that promotion outlays by market entrants contribute to expanding their market share, but price discounts have only a weak short-run effect on entrants' market share.[117]

Additionally, the predictable decline in promotional expenditure that is linked to an impending loss of patent status has been associated with a decline in prescriptions.[118] While the focus here has been on the influence of personal promotion, namely pharmaceutical sales representative details and office visits, the range of channels and media that are used today to reach physicians is much broader, and, depending on the therapeutic area, specialty and stage of the product's lifecycle all may have a greater or lesser contribution to prescribing behavior (Figure 8-7). In general, all pharmaceutical marketing activities have been documented to have some effect on prescribing behavior, but detailing is particularly effective.

DIRECT TO CONSUMER ADVERTISING (DTCA)

DTCA has been permitted in the United States since the 1990s with FDA guidance in 1997 providing information requirements related to broadcast media.[119] The FDA DTCA guidance continues to evolve with guidance on social media published in 2014[119] and draft guidance for risk communication recommending the use of non-technical language, and supporting "Drug Facts" type consumer summaries in 2015.[120,121] The regulation and monitoring of direct to consumer marketing in its various print, broadcast and online media platforms remains challenging.[119]

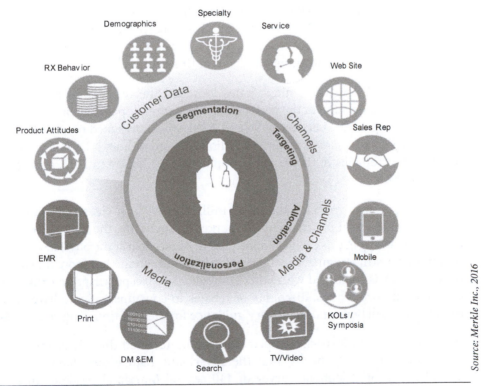

Source: Merkle Inc., 2016

FIGURE 8-7: HEALTH CARE PRACTITONER PRESCRIBING INFLUENCE MODEL

In most industrialized countries, other than the United States and New Zealand, DTCA of prescription pharmaceuticals is not permitted. In Canada, in 2000, Health Canada published a policy paper that allowed "reminder advertisements" for prescription drugs for the public. While DTCA may be perceived as being a US phenomenon, the print and broadcast media images generated may be accessed by patients outside the United States (even though many note they are designated for US consumers) and may influence physician prescribing in many countries.[119] Indeed, DTCA crosses international borders via pharmaceutical industry product websites, paid ads for online search engines, podcasts, mobile apps and social media. About 30% of Canadian consumers are exposed to US direct to consumer ads.[122-124] The DTCA share of all marketing expenditures is significant and has increased since the 1990s but is still considerably less than promotional activities to health care professionals. The amount spent on DTCA via online platforms is increasing due to cost efficiency and increased ability to target specific market segments.[119] In 2011, $ 4 billion was spent on DTCA.[121]

One key study that determined the impact of US DTCA outside of the United States found that in Vancouver, British Columbia, Canada, 87.4% of consumers in the study had actually seen prescription drug advertisements.[125]

Physicians often state that they are not influenced by any form of targeted marketing activity,[90,126] be that pharmaceutical representative, journal advertisement, or the consumer themselves. Despite this, there has been much written about the marketing efficiency of DTCA, and its subsequent impact on prescribing behavior through the medium of the consumer, who makes a direct brand or product category request to their physician.[127] Even prior to the advent of DTCA, physicians indicated that one of the most common reasons for the use of many medications was consumer demand.[128] In a qualitative study of 25 physicians and how pharmaceutical companies try and influence their prescribing of NSAIDs, one physician said "direct consumer advertising is the bane of every working physician in this country."[86]

In 1997, the FDA in the United States loosened the regulations associated with DTCA. In consideration of the period post-1997, annual spending on DTCA for prescription drugs tripled between 1996 and 2000, when it reached nearly $2.5 billion.[84] By 2004, this figure had exceeded $4 billion,129 and although DTCA spending has fluctuated, it remains in this range, dropping to $3.8 billion in 2013, and up to $4.5 billion in 2014.[130]

Despite the increase from less than $500 million in 1995, DTCA still accounts for less than 15% of the total pharmaceutical marketing spending, the majority of pharmaceutical spending in this category continues to be targeted at the physician, indicating that industry still recognizes that physician targeted activity has more impact. Sometimes, DTCA is combined with other strategies, such as prescription drug coupons, that market cost-savings, discounts or rebates to consumers. Some have called for increased regulations and regulatory guidance for prescription drug coupon use.[82]

Initially, it was unclear what impact advertising targeted directly at the consumer would have. In 1998, shortly after the advertising regulations changed, Peyrot et al. did a random telephone survey of 440 central Maryland residents in an effort to determine prescription drug knowledge and drug requesting behavior.[131] Their study suggested that while DTCA had an effect on drug requesting, it was unclear whether requesting led to changes in prescribing behavior. This work was supported in part by Mehta and Purvis, who determined that a broad range of individuals value DTCA, but they also determined that there was some variance among demographics (age, education, gender) with respect to comprehension, agreement with the message, and the expected impact of the message on the individual's anticipated exchange with their physician.[132]

Zachry et al. took the approach of using a time series design on specific products advertised from January 1992 to December 1997.[133] Their results suggested that the DTCA expenditure was associated with physician diagnosing and physician prescribing only for certain drugs and drug classes. However, even when a statistically significant association was found, DTCA was deemed to account for only a modest amount of the variance associated with diagnosing and prescribing.

Vogel et al. assessed the effects of DTCA on the pharmaceutical industry's approach to market in the United States using economic models.[134] While their models suggest that DTCA affects the price and quantity demanded of pharmaceutical products indirectly via its effect on changes in consumer demand, they gained little insight into the impact the pharmaceutical industry's approach to marketing has on prescribing trends.

Rosenthal et al. (for the Kaiser Family Foundation)[35] measured the impact of DTCA on market share within a therapeutic class, as well as on an entire therapeutic class, which is effectively a multi-stage budgeting structure. They examined monthly data from August 1996 to December 1999 for five therapeutic classes, including on all the drugs in each class. Their results suggest an average advertising elasticity of 0.1, in which one would realize a 1% increase in sales following a 10% increase in DTCA spending with variation between drug classes.

Mintzes et al. linked DTCA to increased prescribing.[125] They surveyed a split population of physicians and their consumers, with one study taking place in Vancouver, Canada, and the other in Sacramento, California. While consumers in both markets reported seeing DTCA, Sacramento consumers reported more advertising exposure and requested more advertised drugs than consumers in Vancouver, but in both settings, consumers with higher exposure to advertising requested more advertised drugs. Consumers with higher self-reported exposure to advertising, had conditions that were potentially treatable by advertised drugs, and/or had greater reliance on advertising and subsequently requested more advertised medicines. The results of this study suggest that more advertising leads to more requests for advertised medicines, and ultimately more prescriptions. This study corroborates the work by Donohue et al. whose research on the effects of DTCA suggested that not only was DTCA of antidepressants associated with an increase in the number of people diagnosed with depression, but it was also associated with an increase in the number who initiated medication therapy.[135]

Conversely, in a study of 34 drugs in three therapeutic categories, Ruiz-Conde and colleagues found that DTCA does not affect the rates of physicians trying new medications. Instead, they argue that "during the first 12 months after the introduction of a new drug, [pharmaceutical company marketing] managers should concentrate their efforts mainly on direct-to-physician activities."[136]

Monson and Fink co-authored a commentary on DTCA, where they argue that the two major areas of concern are: 1. The increase in prescribing of newly approved and heavily advertised medications, which may place patients at an increased risk of experiencing an adverse drug reaction, and 2. increased healthcare costs associated with "medicalizing" uncommon, cosmetic, and natural conditions. They also note that drugs targeted for DTCA often include expensive "me too" drugs that have little benefit over existing medications.[137] A study of DTCA exposure and the prescribing of statins did conclude that DTCA may promote overtreatment of statins and over-diagnosis of high cholesterol.[138]

In summary, the weight of evidence in the United States suggests that DTCA has a primary impact on the consumer, followed by a secondary influence on the physician and their prescribing behavior.

PRACTICE CHARACTERISTICS (CLINICAL PROFILE)

This section considers those elements of a physician's practice that relate to consumer demographics, the physical location of the practice, and the nature of the practice (sole practitioner or multiple person clinic), and their subsequent influence on their prescribing behavior. While it is intuitive to consider that physician practice characteristics have a synergistic influence, Table 8-2 illustrates the predictive power (likelihood to prescribe) of given elements in the early stage of a product lifecycle.

CONSUMER PROFILE AND DEMOGRAPHICS

"Taking a patient's desires, beliefs, and capabilities into account is an important element of patient-centred care. As a result, family physicians may select one treatment over another because it is more popular with their patients."[1]

The issues that are addressed in this section refer to identifying the types of consumers that are influenced by DTCA, and the consumer demographics that lead to influence on physician prescribing behavior.

Stevenson et al. indicated that in interviews with 21 general practitioners (GPs) in the Birmingham Health Authority, 100% of the respondents believed that they had experienced pressure for a prescription from consumers, and they all indicated that they had prescribed when they would not have otherwise done so.[139]

TABLE 8-2: VARIABLE INFLUENCE (SIGNIFICANCE) IN LIKELIHOOD TO RESPOND TO A BRANDED MESSAGE FOR A WIDELY WRITTEN ANTI-HYPERTENSIVE

MODEL VARIABLE	SIG LEVEL	BUSINESS INTERPRETATION
Metropolitan	***	PCPs in metropolitan areas are less likely to respond
Pre 12 Months: ARx Samples	***	PCPs who received more ARx* samples in the last 12 months are more likely to respond
Low Group Practice Size	***	PCPs who practice alone OR belong to small group practice (1 to 3 PCPs) are more likely to respond
Pre 6 Months: BRx Details	***	PCPs who received more BRx* details in the last 6 months are more likely to respond
Pre 12 Month BRx Portfolio NRx Share	**	PCPs with larger BRx* share are more likely to respond

*** Significant at 99% level
** Significant at 95% level
*A & B are both brands from a single corporation's cardiovascular franchise

Britten et al. considered the variables that influence consumers with respect to their attitudes toward medicines and their expectations for a prescription.[140] The study took place in South London, England and surveyed 544 consumers waiting in GP offices. Since they were in England, the influence of DTCA was likely limited. The primary factors influencing consumers' expectations for a prescription were determined to be:

1. Demographic variables that included gender, age, marital status, period of time at the same address, age leaving school, ethnic group, employment status, and prescription status (extent of coverage).
2. Organizational variables which included day of the week and appointment status.
3. Illness variables including symptoms, reason for the visit and self-medication.
4. Attitudes toward medicine, as measured by individuals' level of agreement with a variety of statements about medicines and their role in health and wellness.

Unlike Britten, Mamdani suggested that demographics, particularly age and household income, did not play a role in consumer expectations, but did appear to influence physician prescribing.[141] This study determined that physicians in the province of Ontario, Canada, practicing in low income neighborhoods, were more likely to prescribe lower priced generic drugs for their elderly consumers, regardless of the consumers' drug coverage. This work is consistent with research by Soumerai and Avorn on the impact of copayments among lower income populations,[142] and by Tamblyn et al. on the impact of cost sharing among elderly persons and welfare recipients.[143] In both studies, a demonstrated decrease in the use of essential drugs was established.

Stewart et al. in the Netherlands assessed the effects of GP and consumer characteristics on prescribing behavior.[144] He measured adherence to the global WHO pharmacotherapeutic guidelines[145] in combination with Barber's good prescribing guidelines.[40] The study of 251 GPs from 190 practices suggested adherence to prescribing guidelines (effectively, factors influencing prescribing behavior) were influenced by two sets of variables, practice characteristics, and consumer characteristics. Consumer characteristics were either directly related to the consumer, or were aggregated to a categorized consumer level. Directly related variables of age and gender were shown to influence adherence to prescribing guidelines, while the aggregated variables mean costs, mean volume, and different WHO anatomic therapeutic chemical classifications of drugs (effectively variance in drug selection for given conditions) were shown to influence prescribing.

Bradley suggested that consumer factors, such as age, ethnicity, social class, and education influence prescribing; however, factors that were equally important were the physician's prior knowledge of the consumer, the physician's feeling towards the consumer, communication problems, and the doctor's desire to try to preserve the doctor-consumer relationship.[146] Additional work by Bradley,[16] and McKinlay,[147] while recognizing the many considerations (including medical, social, and logistic) that influence the decision to prescribe in general practice, note that prescribing depends on the complex interaction of many disparate influences.

Bennett focused on the variables that might influence the likelihood of switching a consumer from one drug to another.[148] Her work focused on switching consumers from non-selective (NS)-NSAIDs to COX-2s. A surprisingly low percentage (17%) of incumbent NS-NSAID users were switched to COX-2s. Older, female consumers were more likely to be switched from NS-NSAIDs to COX-2s, but one of the reasons may be that physicians believe females are more prone to gastrointestinal toxicity.

Tamblyn et al. suggested that a high proportion of elderly in a practice was associated with a greater likelihood of prescribing any new drug, but at the same time, there was a lower rate of new drug utilization among members of this cohort with multiple prescriptions.[149] Again, while it may seem intuitive that consumer's age might influence prescribing, this influence may simply be a function of their current drug regimen, and subsequently it is just as likely to influence more prescribing, as it is to influence less prescribing.

Another demographic variable, education, may have some influence on prescribing, but this hasn't been tested. Mehta did, however, determine that individuals with advanced education are more acceptable to new approaches to health care, and most likely have insight and interest in new drugs,[132] but it is unknown as to whether this converted into a change in prescribing.

Sears and colleagues identified gaps in communication about medications between patients with chronic illness and their Primary Care Physicians (PCPs) across multiple countries and they recommended that "healthcare providers need to be trained to recognize how cultural differences, socio-economic factors, and personal values and beliefs can impact, both positively and negatively, effective communication."[150]

In summary, while there is a large volume of research which supports the impact of consumer demographics on physician prescribing, the results are inconsistent, and seem to reinforce the requirement that individual jurisdictional variables be taken into consideration. That is, extrapolations between similar populations in different geographic areas may be less representative than previously thought, and the inconsistency in influence simply reinforces the need for geographic (and geodemographic) specific analysis.

LOCATION OF PRACTICE

Following consumer demographics, the second practice consideration has to do with how the population influences the practice. One example of population influences that has been studied is whether they are in a rural or urban setting. This location, in turn, may have an impact on a variety of factors ranging from the characteristics of the physicians and the consumers, relative access to new information, continuing medical education and possibly extent of their contact with industry representatives. Another issue with respect to rural practitioners is their individual profiles, and those of their practices. Rural physicians tend to be older and more likely to be male than their urban counterparts.[19,151,152] Additionally, the consumer profile of the rural practice tends to be more elderly than that of the urban practice. These variances may in turn have an effect on prescribing given the influence of consumer age and physician gender as an influence on prescribing.

Tamblyn's research indicated that new drug utilization was lower among generalists and specialists practicing in rural Quebec, and suggested that this may be a function of the characteristics of physicians who elect to practice in rural areas, their isolation from the influence of peers and colleagues, or possibly the reduced frequency of visits from pharmaceutical marketing representatives.[149] One deficiency with this observation, however, relates to what is defined as rural and urban. Tamblyn indicated that Quebec uses "tarification" territories, which are classified as remote, rural, and urban, to establish levels of physician remuneration. Unfortunately, these territories are not further defined by population density.

Stewart defined rural practices as physicians operating in an area with a population density of less than 1500 addresses per square kilometer, and urban as those with more than 1500 addresses per square kilometer.[144] While his work suggested that the location of the practice was significant with respect to adherence with prescribing best practices, he did not indicate the extent to which physicians in a rural or urban practices were likely to prescribe.

Rural practitioners in Australia (obtained from a defined database of the rural workforce agency) felt that their remoteness and the remoteness of their consumers had an influence on their prescribing activities.[151] Cutts and Tett's work further suggested that of the 142 responding doctors practicing in rural Queensland (55% survey response rate), their propensity to prescribe a new drug was inversely proportional to the amount of monitoring required of the consumer following prescription. In general, rural physicians in this study had prescribed fewer new medicines than their urban counterparts, but again we have a similar problem with the definition of rural. In another paper, Cutts and Tett suggested that the prescribing of recently marketed drugs was more likely by doctors practicing in less remote rural areas.[153]

NATURE OF PRACTICE

There are many considerations related to the nature of practice. These include organizational factors (whether the practice is solo or group, access to other health professionals (e.g. nurse practitioners, types of information technology available, and types of patients in the practice including number and types of diseases, socioeconomic status, etc). The latter relates to the opportunity the physician has to interact with other practitioners, and also addresses the influence of knowledge opinion leaders on prescribing behavior. This is not to say that sole practitioners do not interact with their peers, but merely suggests that there is a greater opportunity for informal interaction among individuals working in the same clinic.

PRACTICE SIZE (NUMBER OF PATIENTS)

While it may seem intuitive, the frequency of opportunities available to prescribe a new drug influences whether it can be adopted into practice and used. As Peay and Peay suggest, in order for the drug to be prescribed, the doctor must be prepared to use it, and the treatment situation must be appropriate for its use.[69] Effectively, the presence of more patients likely to benefit from a specific drug in physician's practice increases the likelihood of drug trial.

The increase in the number of situations available in which to prescribe a given drug influences the likelihood of trial. However, as the number of drugs introduced into a given patient's regimen increases, the likelihood of prescribing a new drug into the patient's mix decreases. Tamblyn suggests that one explanation may be a function of the physician's lack of confidence and understanding of co-morbidity and contraindications between multiple interventions.[149] Interestingly, Redelmeier et al. suggested that there is an inverse correlation between the presence of a chronic disease and the likelihood of treatment of an unrelated disorder.[154] Howlett et al. suggested that while effective medical treatment is not likely withheld, depending on physician specialty, there may be varying degrees of adoption of new interventions for specific conditions (in this case congestive heart failure).[155]

The presence in a physician's patient population of health conditions for which a given drug is recommended is likely to have an influence on trial of that drug. The experience from this initial trial will have a significant effect on continued use (adoption), or conversely, discontinued use (relinquishment), of a drug. This was supported by Buban, who suggested that, in the case of new agents to treat cancer, one of the most significant influences on the adoption of paclitaxel was physician experience with paclitaxel to treat late-stage breast cancer.[156] Buban also suggested that perceptions of the relative advantages of a new drug are formed through individual experience with the drug, and through their interactions with other practitioners.

PRACTICE SIZE (NUMBER OF PHYSICIANS)

Physicians often rely on conversations with fellow physicians to help direct their decision-making. While this may be convenient, especially within a group practice, the advice received may not be evidence-based.[1]

While adoption of a new drug as a consequence of interacting with colleagues within the same practice was supported through early research by Coleman et al.,[157] as mentioned previously, the implications of this study were subsequently questioned by Van Den Bulte et al., who suggested that the social influence was overstated, and it was more than likely simply aggressive marketing which led to the rapid adoption of tetracycline.[68] Despite this work by Van den Bulte, the fact that people act in accordance with a frame of reference produced by the groups to which they belong is a long-accepted premise, and is supported throughout the literature.[158] Peers and individuals from the physician's normative social group have influence as supported by Ajzen's work on planned behavior.[159] While improving prescribing requires physician education, the type of educational interventions and continuing professional development that is most effective is still being determined.[160,161]

Steffensen et al., determined that, while physicians in single-handed practices and those in partnerships both adopted new drugs, the median time for adoption (as defined by their first prescription) in partnership practices was 10 days (mean = 41) while in single handed practices it was 52 days (mean = 119).[162] With partnership practices adopting new drugs faster, Steffensen and his team concluded that the continuous professional stimulation and other social factors are responsible for the accelerated adoption. These findings were supported by Dybdahl who reduced the number of independent variables, and also found that larger practice size had a positive influence on adoption time, with partnership practices demonstrating the most rapid rate of new product adoption.[74]

The rate of relinquishment or adoption, if initial observations are less than favorable may also be influenced. Cranney et al. surveyed 76 physicians in an attempt to determine why GPs do not implement evidence-based guidelines.[163] While their work suggested that single-handed GPs were enthusiastic about peer-based continuing medical education, as it provided them with the peer interaction they lacked, this study was qualitative, lacked sample size, and was not really representative. Interestingly, Peay and Peay suggested earlier that the inclination to innovate is not related to the number of other doctors with whom the doctor practices, but is more likely to be influenced by commercial advertising.[69] Prosser et al. supported both the work of Peay et al. and Cranney et al., and demonstrated that prescribing of new drugs is related to the mode of exposure to pharmacological information, the social influences on decision making, risk perception, frequency of pharmaceutical representative visits, and individual experience with the drug.[89,164]

In Finland, a government sponsored program aimed at changing clinical practice to enhance rational prescribing has proven to be effective when using GPs as facilitators of their continuing medical education programs, and results at the local level have suggested that critical thinking and willingness to consider change of practice(s) has been achieved.[165] This approach has been subsequently supported through research by Maue et al. suggesting that implementation strategies that utilize well-respected physician champions (key opinion leaders, educational influencers) in the practice sites may improve guideline compliance,[166] and by Cutts et al. who identified factors such as access to continuing medical education and specialists as having an influence on prescribing.[153]

There is a greater possibility of seeing or hearing about new products if there is more than one individual in an office or peer group, or, if the physician regularly interacts with peers and opinion leaders through other associations. This interaction is also an opportunity for professional development, as suggested by Pearson et al. in their study of interns, by which every prescription charted is an opportunity for learning,[167] and subsequently influencing their development as effective practitioners. This notion of practical application and trial to establish prescribing and therapeutic insight is supported by the steps in adoption, and was supported by Jones et al. who found that the progression from first use to regular use is an important step in the drug innovation process.[99]

Previous experience with a drug that has resulted in a positive or favorable outcome, may lead to a less than thorough investigation of the consumer's condition and evaluation of other options available to treat a consumer prior to prescribing. Denig's in-depth interview with 61 GPs determined that fully 40% made recommendations out of habit, without undertaking any specific contemplation of the consumer's condition.[168] Schwartz et al. also observed that prescribers asserted that their own clinical experience indicated that these drugs were actually the therapies of choice in the conditions presented, despite contrary research evidence.[128] Physicians may remain with their previous prescribing patterns as defined by habit and experience in spite of new literature suggesting other alternatives.

Allery et al. considered physician characteristics from the perspective of changing their practice. In a study of 50 GPs, they found that organizational factors, education, and contact with professionals was influential in changing their clinical practices.[169] The weakness of this study is that the aforementioned variables account for less than 50% of the changes in clinical behavior. Additionally, the small sample size and the large number of independent variables make it difficult to confidently measure the influence of professional contact.

Landon et al. suggested that physicians in solo and two person practices appear to have a more aggressive treatment style than those physicians in group practices.[170] While the definition of aggressive is associated with the propensity to request clinical tests, there is no indication that this activity is causal to prescribing. Additionally, this study is limited by the use of physician-reported behavior based on vignettes rather than measures of actual clinical decisions. A similar observation was made by O'Neill and Kuder who noted that being in a solo practice had a greater association with the propensity of a physician to ordering a service (tests),[171] but as with Landon, it was not indicated if this was associated with actual prescribing.

Ashworth et al. considered physician motivation to change within the context of GPs who had joined a general practice covering a geographic locality in south London, UK.[172] Within the context of the UK's Primary Care Commissioning Group structure, it appears that one of the lead motivators for change was related to a collectivist (team) perspective amongst GPs who are prepared to consider the prescribing implications for their fellow GPs. Contrary to Ashworth, however, Simon et al.[110] demonstrated that both group and individual academic detailing improved antihypertensive prescribing over and above usual care, while Watkins et al. suggested that the effects of interventions in larger practices appear to be less significant given the logistics of getting all the physicians together at one time.[113]

While it seems logical that GPs that have access to an informal peer network may be more likely to prescribe (new interventions), the opposite of this may also be true. That is, informal feedback from peers may result in a tendency to decrease their levels of prescribing. While the literature supports the latter, research by Watkins has suggested that there may be a greater tendency to prescribe among sole practitioners practicing in markets of individuals with low income, with minimal academic detailing.[92] This insight was supported in part by Peay and Peay who determined that the number of other doctors with whom the doctor practices was not a significant predictor of innovativeness.[69]

Carthy et al., suggested some physicians didn't consult with their colleagues because they were either confident in their own decisions or they didn't want to subject themselves to potential criticism.[173]

Outside of the influence of colleagues in a practice environment is the issue of the influence of individuals in peer groups, colleagues operating in different clinics, markets or environments, as well as opinion leaders whose experience and insight is respected and deemed relevant. Soumerai et al., suggests that working with opinion leaders and providing performance feedback can accelerate the adoption of some alternative acute myocardial infarction (AMI) therapies.[174] This recommendation suggests that local physicians have the potential to be influenced by local peer/opinion leaders. The weakness of this study, however, was the inability to control a variety of other factors that may have led to the adoption of the alternative AMI therapies. Soumerai's proposal on the influence of local opinion leaders was supported by Sbarbaro.[5] While he suggested that the endorsement of national professional guidelines by local opinion leaders may have a positive influence on the impact of professional guidelines, it may also be effective to provide performance feedback comparing the physician's results to peers. While these observations were more of a commentary, again there may be intuitive value here.

Hepler reinforced the value of the opinion leader among health professionals by suggesting that physicians tend to value autonomy and be socially powerful. To this end, institutional pharmacists are well advised to seek out opinion leaders who have power and know how to use it. Having the support of such an individual can increase the ability to influence appropriate drug use (prescribing behavior) within a physician population.[9]

PHYSICIAN PROFILE

The final consideration within the context of practice characteristics relates to a number of physician dependent factors. This area has always been recognized as playing a role in the likelihood of a physician prescribing a particular product, given a specific condition. An extensive review of physician influences by Hemminki categorized influencing variables into education, advertising, colleagues, regulations and control measures, societal and consumer demands and doctor characteristics.[175] While there are a number of areas of influence, considered in this review are the areas of gender, age, training and background, and experience.

GENDER

While there is very little in the literature that considers the influence of gender on prescribing, there are also relatively few studies that have been conducted in the area of consumer behavior on gender differences.[176] Most research in this area tends to focus on the female (or collective) consumer because of their significant purchasing power, and in the case of some of the benchmark studies on consumer styles index and decision making, the influence of gender on the consumer decision making process is not weighted.[177,178] To this end, the research in this area is inconclusive, and often contradictory. Thus, while the challenge is to determine the influence of gender on prescribing, when considering the physician as a consumer, we must recognize that males and females want different products and they are likely to have different ways of thinking about obtaining them.

A review of the consumer behavior literature[179–181] identifies men as more independent, confident, competitive, externally motivated, and more willing to take risks. A recent study of 358 male and female shoppers between the ages of 18 and 44 further suggests that men use more information and communication technology products than women and show a greater interest in these products.[176] Even though age profile is not truly reflective of the physician population in this study, this observation suggest that we may anticipate a greater propensity among male physicians to have an interest in new technology (new medications) and subsequently, the prescribing of new drugs.

Tamblyn et al. found that male general practitioners had higher rates of new drug use than females, but this trend was not significant after adjusting for other physician and practice characteristics such as year of graduation and the profile of the consumers in their practice.[149] This pattern, while not significant, relates to the work by Mitchell and Walsh that suggests that male physicians are more confident than female physicians in initiating new medical treatments,[176] and to work by Groves indicating a greater propensity among males to prescribe COX-2s relative to their female counterparts.[19]

Work by Steffensen et al. concurs with Tamblyn's research, and suggests that there is an association between late adoption and the independent variables of female gender, smaller practice, low diagnostic activity per consumer, and a general restrictive attitude toward pharmacotherapy.[162] While this study was qualitative, and as such did not have the ability to test for these variables independently, it does suggest that the characteristics of the "light" prescriber[iv] tend to fit into the conservative physician typology.

Inman et al. divided a sample of physicians involved in the UK's prescription event monitoring scheme into six segments, defined by the relative values of prescriptions of new drugs issued per consumer over a seven year period, commencing in 1984.[182]

[iv] Issues fewer prescriptions per patient visit than the general physician population.

From an initial sample of over 28,000 physicians, they selected representative subsets from each segment. Their results suggest that female gender was strongly associated with the likelihood of not prescribing, or prescribing less than their male colleagues. While this is significant, given the low relative prescribing ratios, the logic here suggested that females may have more part-time practices, and spend more time with their consumers. Subsequently, they have less propensity to test new drugs, and have less time to do so. The propensity to not prescribe was also supported through research by Duetz et al. who found that female physicians were more inclined to discontinue antihypertensive drug therapy than their male counterparts.[183]

Thus, while we seem to have a trend, none of the studies have conclusively developed a relationship between gender and prescribing. Additionally, the research in this area did not appear to identify gender as a primary focus, but as an artifact that was identified following testing against some previously defined primary hypotheses.

AGE

In consideration of the influence of age, sociologists, psychologists, and marketers have done much to document the resistance to change common among the elderly.[184] The combined observations from the literature are best summarized with the recognition that the older the consumer, the more negative the view toward technology, and the lower the use of various technologies (including new prescription drugs).

While Peay and Peay's work demonstrates a level of agreement with the consumer literature, and suggests that age was significant in predicting innovativeness in high risk therapy, it also suggested that the results were not stable when controlling for specialty or a specific drug.[69] Despite this, they did suggest that older doctors are less innovative than younger ones. Hemminki summarized the influence of age with the suggestion that more appropriate prescribers were younger, more cosmopolitan and modern,[175] albeit the definition of appropriate is subjective, and isn't necessarily reflective of the degree of adoption. This observation is supported by the work of Lacy et al. who determined that older physicians prescribed proton pump inhibitors more often than younger physicians for mild or intermittent gastroesophageal reflux disease, without really giving consideration to non-prescription solutions.[185]

Steffensen et al.'s work supported the commonly held belief that rate of adoption is a function of physician characteristics, but also suggested that the rate of adoption may be influenced by the drug characteristics as well. Within this context, they identified several physician variables that may influence prescribing (gender was mentioned earlier) including age. In this case, physicians greater than 50 years old were more likely to be categorized as late prescribers (although the validity of these results may be questionable due to the small sample size). Freiman's work supported this proposal by demonstrating that the likelihood of prescribing a new drug decreases as the physician ages.[186]

While Tamblyn didn't specifically measure for age, she did consider year of graduation from medical school (which may be considered as a relative age variable).[149] Given this, her results suggested that year of graduation had no influence on rates of adoption among GPs. Using a similar approach to Tamblyn, Helin-Salmivaara et al.'s work on the adoption of COX-2s, demonstrated that clinical experience of the physician, measured as the number of years since graduation, had no significant effect on adoption.[187] In a different study of early prescribers of COX-2s, early, high volume prescribers were more likely to be older and more experienced (and male and operating in a rural practice).[188] While age may play a role in prescribing behavior, research has been unable to consistently establish the extent of its influence.

TRAINING, BACKGROUND AND EXPERIENCE

Hemminki's review of the literature on the influence of education on drug prescribing led her to conclude that education positively influences the quality of prescribing.[175] Quality of prescribing, however, is subjective with respect to the level of prescribing, and as a result means little in our attempt to measure educational influence on prescribing. Work by Landon et al. suggested that there is no evidence of a consistent practice style across GPs when presented with representative clinical scenarios.[170] This was supported through research by Tamayo-Sarver et al. with emergency physicians and the study of their prescribing practices for opioids, which noted that while some physicians tended to interpret information provided in similar ways across conditions, they couldn't find any physician or practice characteristics that were significantly associated with physician responses.[189]

In effect, Hemminki's review of the literature of the day (pre-1975) simply suggested that there was no significant difference in prescribing among doctors graduating from different medical schools. This observation is supported in part by Tamblyn, whose physician sample was representative of four medical schools in Quebec.[149] Her results demonstrated no variance between the traditional schools. However, the school which uses a problem-oriented medical curriculum has demonstrated higher relative prescribing rates of new drugs versus the traditional curriculum format. Conversely, it has been argued that the "lessons learned in medical school and clinical residency may have the great influence on a physician's decision-making."[1]

While Tamblyn has suggested that the type of educational format offered by the medical school may influence prescribing, she also demonstrated that specialists had higher relative rates of drug utilization then GPs. Helin-Salmivaara et al. suggested this early adoption and more frequent utilization of drugs may relate to the concept that prescribing a new drug may enhance reputation better than prescribing an older drug.[187] Garjon and colleagues found that specialists adopted new drugs faster than PCPs in seven out of eight drugs included in their study.[190]

The dynamics of a physician's practice may be correlated to physician age and experience, and, as such, may be interchangeable. As their practice becomes more stable/predictable, and the physicians become more familiar with their consumers and their specific conditions, the physicians may become more risk averse, and less inclined to try new drugs or interventions that they do not have a regimen of experience with. Contrary to this logic, however, is the acknowledgment that familiarity may lead to the desire to try alternative products among that portion of a physician's consumer population that has not responded to traditional treatments. Work by Armstrong et al.[191] suggested that behavior change follows a dramatic or conflictual clinical event (a product doesn't work), while Bennett et al.[148] suggested that physicians with consumer history (experience and knowledge of the consumer's health and drug regimen over time) are more likely to switch consumers to new drugs, particularly if they have the personal experience or insight into the results associated with previously prescribed interventions.

This latter body of research ties in with the notion that when physicians know what works for them, they are less likely to actively consider all possible alternatives, and are likely to go with the familiar, given that the effect on consumer's health outcomes is likely to be similar.[173,192,193] Conversely, when an intervention isn't working through their own trials, they are more likely to seek out new alternatives.

In a study of prescribing among GPs in Ireland, Bourke and Roper found that the physicians who have a track record of early adoption tend to continue to be the early adopters of new drugs as they enter the marketplace.[194]

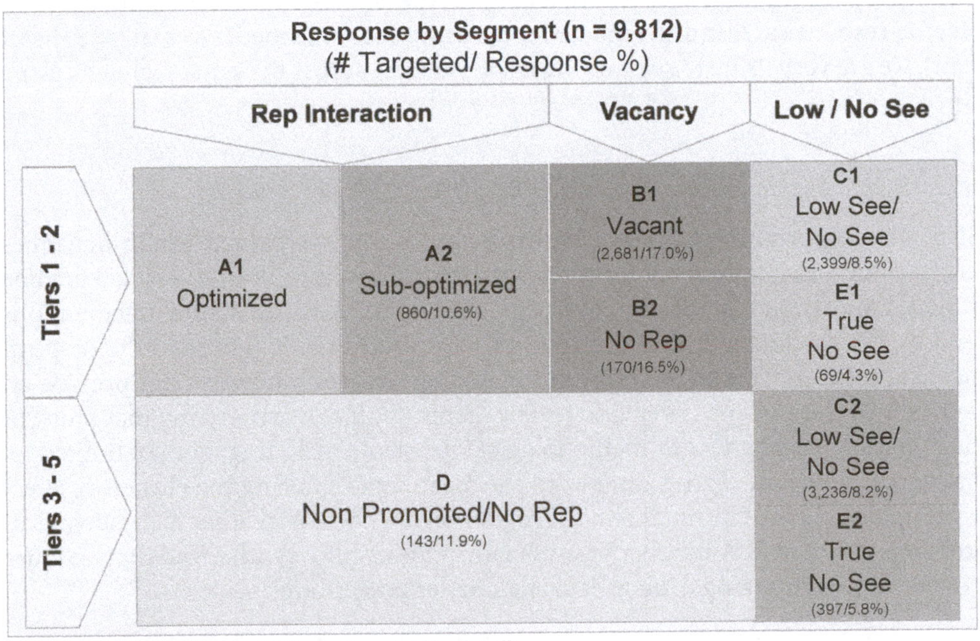

•Optimized: received >80% of planned Rx details
•Sub-Optimized: received 30to 80% of planned Rx details
•Low See/No See: received <30% of planned Rx details
•True No See/Non-Promoted: received no Rx details

FIGURE 8-8: CAMPAIGN RESPONSE TO RX MESSAGING

SOCIAL MEDIA, CHANNEL PROPENSITY, AND SEGMENTATION

We have demonstrated in this chapter that there are a number of variables that influence physician prescribing behavior. While individually they all have some level of influence, collectively they can have a synergistic, or potentially an antagonistic effect. In Figure 8-8, you can see the influence of a number of variables that ultimately had an impact on the level of engagement between PCPs and a brand. Starting with target segmentation that considers whether or not the PCPs are receiving an optimal number of details from the sales force, through to their perceived value to the brand (defined by their categorical writing and represented by a tier ranking). This audience was messaged uniformly using a combination of direct mail and e-mail messages sent out six times, over a period of four months. While the overall response rate in this example was 10.8%, it ranged from a low of 5.8% to a high of 17.0%. The variance in response rates (click through on e-mail and/or returning a reply card from the direct mail piece) across the entire target population demonstrates the influence of unique profile variables on message response and engagement.

If we look beyond the profile of the PCP, it is important to consider message uptake, namely, did they see/read/comprehend the message. While this, in itself, plays a key role in prescribing as we move beyond 2016, an even greater consideration becomes "channel propensity". That is, which media (e.g.; e-mail, direct mail, pharma sales rep details, social media such as Sermo or Medscape) are the PCPs you are trying to reach most comfortable. Said another way, while gender, practice size and training may influence prescribing, the way in which you try to reach your target audience with your message may be just as important. Just as we saw in Figure 8-8 with varying response across different audiences using the same media (e-mail and direct mail), we are very likely to see varying response rates across the same segments using different media.

HEALTHCARE ORGANIZATIONS' INTERVENTIONS TO IMPROVE PRESCRIBING

Given the importance of optimizing drug use to improve patient health outcomes and provide value for money from pharmaceuticals, a large body of evidence, some of which has been discussed above (e.g., opinion leaders), exists for interventions used by health care organizations to improve prescribing. It is beyond the scope of this chapter to review these intervention studies in detail; however, we provide an overview of the current systematic review literature. It is worth noting that much of the literature is fraught with methodological problems including, but not limited to, inadequate controls, regression toward the mean, and ignoring the clustering effect of group practices. Majumdar and colleagues review these and other methodological problems in detail.[195] A number of systematic reviews have synthesized the literature surrounding optimizing drug use through better prescribing.

Irwin et al.[196] conducted a review of systematic reviews that evaluated practice-level quality improvement interventions in the context of primary care. They concluded that point-of-care reminders, computerized advice, and educational outreach visits (i.e., academic detailing) had the largest effect on prescribing behavior. Shojania et al.[197] meta-analyzed 21 randomized or quasi-randomized trials testing computerized reminders targeting prescribing behavior and found a 3.3% (Interquartile range [IQR] 0.5% to 10.6%) and 6.2% (IQR 3.0 % to 28.0%) absolute improvement when pooling the median and maximum outcome from included studies, respectively. Similarly, Gillaizeau et al.[198] synthesized the evidence for computerized advice on drug dosage and concluded there were benefits over routine care but the evidence was fraught with studies with a high risk of bias. O'Brien et al.[199] reviewed intervention trials assessing the impact of educational outreach visits on prescribing behavior and found a consistent effect across 17 trials with an absolute improvement of 4.8% (IQR 3.0% to 6.3%). Irwin et al. also found that multifaceted interventions generally being more effective than single interventions, although this was not consistent across all studies. These findings are consistent with the broader literature on changing healthcare provider behavior that suggests reliable effective strategies include educational outreach, reminder systems, and interactive workshops.[200]

Other interventions have variably consistent evidence. For example, Ivers et al.[201] assessed 39 randomized controlled trials evaluating audit and feedback interventions targeting suboptimal prescribing. Upon meta-analyzing trials with an unclear or low risk of bias, they calculated a weighted mean adjusted risk difference of 13% (IQR 3% to 17%). Larger effects were observed when the baseline performance was low, when the information came from a trusted source (e.g., a senior colleague or supervisor), when repeated feedback was provided, when written and verbal feedback was provided, and when explicit targets and action plans were integrated into the intervention. Other interventions with variably effective strategies for modifying the behavior of healthcare professionals include local opinion leaders, local consensus, patient mediated interventions. Moreover, the use of champions, facilitators, formal leadership, and marketing and mass media strategies may enhance interventions targeting behavior change.[200]

To keep up-to-date with the literature on behavior change in the healthcare, one may consult specialized repositories including the Cochrane Effective Practice and Organization of Care (EPOC) Group Specialized Register or the Canadian Agency for Drugs and Technologies in Health (CADTH) Rx For Change database—a searchable database of interventional research regarding behavior change in healthcare including prescribing behavior (www.cadth.ca/rx-change). The Rx For Change database classifies studies according to the intervention scheme of the EPOC group which includes over 50 types of interventions under five overarching categories of professional, financial, organizational, structural, and regulatory interventions. Provider and patient oriented interventions are embedded within these categories.

The implementation of effective interventions in a sustainable manner for the health system remains a challenge. Several countries have coordinated national hubs (e.g., The National Prescribing Centre, UK; The National Prescribing Service, Australia; The Best Practice Advocacy Centre, New Zealand) to combat the under, over, and misuse of medications. Interestingly, the National Prescribing Service has developed a single competency framework for all prescribers in the UK.[202] This goal of this framework is to aid all type of prescribers to safe and effective prescribing for all types of prescribers including physicians, dentists, and non-traditional prescribers (e.g., pharmacists, nurses, optometrists, among others). Although the magnitude of success of these national initiatives aimed at improving prescribing is unknown, these large scale organizational interventions provide guidance towards best practices for optimization of medication use. Furthermore, gaps in the evidence base remain even within understanding the effectiveness and cost-effectiveness of interventions aimed at suboptimal prescribing. A scoping review by Faria and colleagues identified evidence gaps in areas such as prescribing low-cost generics, cost-effectiveness, and documentation, and suggest that decision modelling will help in prioritizing future research and implementation of effective policies in the health system.[203] Other challenges include the heterogeneity of interventions and the reporting of the interventions tested and the health systems in which they were delivered. Even the most effective strategies targeting an improvement in prescribing appear to be modestly effective at best. With the rise in prevalence of more sophisticated electronic medical systems integrated with computerized physician order entry, e-prescribing, chronic disease management pathways, among other point of care patient management tools, further research is required to test the most cost-effective delivery of single and multifaceted interventions aimed to optimize prescribing behavior.

SUMMARY

As stated in the introduction to this chapter, physician prescribing behavior is complex. It is a function of the relationship between physician factors, consumer factors, and the environment. The body of literature in this field has grown substantially in recent years, from the early work of Hemminki in the 1970s to Segal and Hepler in the 1980s to a critical mass of researchers such as Denig, Tamblyn, and others over the past 30 years. With this growth has come greater understanding of the role of these various factors and their influence on prescribing behavior. While more knowledge about physician decision-making is beneficial it its own right, there are at least three critical caveats about prescribing behavior.

First, one of the challenges associated with the isolation of physician and patient characteristics is the fact that these variables do not function in isolation of each other, and tend to exhibit varying degrees of covariance. Additionally, influence may further be a function of non-measured variables such as practice geography, jurisdiction, beliefs and value, or even sampling bias. Thus, it is obvious from the literature that there are physician characteristics that influence prescribing, but the challenge is determining which have the greatest influence and their weight of influence relative to the presence of other variables, and given sets of circumstances or prescribing situations. For example, Jones et al. made the observation that practice variables only explain a small proportion of the variance in prescribing, and that prescribing decisions are complex and idiosyncratic and will not be fully explained by easily identifiable general practitioner characteristics.[204] McKinlay et al. suggested that variability in decision making is not entirely accounted for by strictly rational Bayesian inference.[147] In addition, "like other clinical decisions, prescribing decisions are influenced by a number of complex factors, some of which may be out of the hands of the family physician. For example, a specialist may write the initial prescription but the family doctor provides the follow-up, prescription renewals, and monitoring of the medication use,"[1]

Second, patient involvement in the prescribing decision-making process has increased as there has been movement away from the paternalistic medical model, however, there is still much work to be done to determine the optimal role for the patient in this process. Indeed, shared-decision making is integral to patient-centered care. Legare et al.[205,206] showed a substantive improvement in antibiotic prescribing for acute respiratory infections when patients were engaged in the treatment decision-making process. Nonetheless, as per discussion in this chapter, there are times when the patient can influence prescribing for the worst, for example, when asking the physician for a medication they saw on television or that a friend is taking that may not be appropriate for them. Still, patients that are knowledgeable about their disease and medications and who demonstrate intelligent adherence can greatly increase the probability of an optimal outcome from a prescription. A study by Gardner and colleagues highlighted the difference between physician and patient preferences in the choice of drugs.[207] Patients and family physicians were surveyed about their perceived importance of 12 differentiating factors when selecting an antidepressant. Overall, there was moderate disagreement between the patients and physicians, including considerable disagreement on the importance of uncommon serious side effects, cost and dosing schedule.

Third, the evolution of social media and access to information immediately will continue to influence the physician/patient/prescribing relationship. Patients and physicians regularly use tablets and mobile devices to access information real-time, and also receive promotional messages, offers, formulary status, coverage, and co-pay data during a visit. As physician access continues to decline, peer to peer networks, e-detailing, and digital access and downloads will continue to play a greater role in the pharma-physician relationship.

Fourth, while influencing prescribing can result in improved patient outcomes, prescribing is only one part of the medication-use system. Other essential elements of this system include: (1) timely recognition of drug indications and other signs and symptoms relevant to drug use, (2) safe, accessible, and cost-effective medicines, (3) distribution, dispensing, and administration of drug products with appropriate patient advice, (4) intelligent adherence, (5) monitoring, (6) documentation and communication, and (7) performance measurement.[208] Even a prescription that is entirely appropriate and evidence-based does not necessitate an optimal outcome. As Segal and Wang argue, "the medical literature supports the assertions that prescribing 'the drug of choice' does not guarantee a good patient outcome and that poor outcomes probably have more to do with what happens after a drug is prescribed."[3]

Acknowledgements: The authors would like to acknowledge Jonathan Penm who assisted with the literature search and with Melanie Fulton who provided administrative support.

REFERENCES

1. Health Council of Canada. (2010). *Decisions, decisions: Family doctors as gatekeepers to prescription drugs and diagnostic imaging in Canada.* Toronto, ON: Health Council of Canada.

2. Groves, K.E., Flanagan, P.S., & MacKinnon, N.J. (2002). Why physicians start or stop prescribing a drug: literature review and formulary implications. *Formulary* 37(4):186–94.

3. Segal, R. & Wang, F. (1999). Influencing physician prescribing. *Pharm Pract Manag Q* 19(3):30–50.

4. Gill, P., Mäkelä, M., Vermeulen, K., et al. (1999). Changing doctor prescribing behaviour. *Pharm World Sci* 21(4):158–67.

5. Sbarbaro, J.A. (2001). Can we influence prescribing patterns? *Clin Infect Dis* 33(Suppl 3):S240–4.

6. Parrino, T.A. (2005). Controlled trials to improve antibiotic utilization: a systematic review of experience, 1984–2004. *Pharmacotherapy* 25(2):289–98.

7. Pippalla, R., Riley, D., & Chinburapa, V. (1995). Influencing the prescribing behaviour of physicians: a metaevaluation. *J Clin Pharm Ther* 20(4):189–98.

8. Wilson, A. L. (1994). Influencing prescribers. *Top Hosp Pharm Manage* 14(3):40–6.

9. Hepler, C.D., Segal, R., & Freeman, R.A. (1981). How physicians choose the drugs they prescribe. *Top Hosp Pharm Manage* 1(3):23–44.

10. Raisch, D.W. (1990). A model of methods for influencing prescribing: Part I. A review of prescribing models, persuasion theories, and administrative and educational methods. *DICP* 24(4):417–21.

11. Raisch, D.W. (1990). A model of methods for influencing prescribing: Part II. A review of educational methods, theories of human inference, and delineation of the model. *DICP* 24(5):537–42.

12. Grol, R. & Grimshaw, J. (2003). From best evidence to best practice: effective implementation of change in patients' care. *Lancet* 362(9391):1225–30.

13. Anderson, G.M. & Lexchin, J. (1996). Strategies for improving prescribing practice. *CMAJ* 154(7):1013–7.

14. Carter, A.O., Strachan, D., & Appiah, Y. (1996). Physician prescribing practices: What do we know? Where do we go? How do we get there? *CMAJ* 154(11):1649–53.

15. Vuckovic, N. & Nichter, M. (1997). Changing patterns of pharmaceutical practice in the United States. *Soc Sci Med* 44(9):1285–302.

16. Bradley, C.P. (1992). Uncomfortable prescribing decisions: a critical incident study. *BMJ* 304(6822):294–6.

17. Weiss, M.C., Fitzpatrick, R., Scott, D.K., & Goldacre, M.J. (1996). Pressures on the general practitioner and decisions to prescribe. *Fam Pract* 13(5):432–8.

18. Einarson, T.R. (2005). The Authority/pharmacotherapy Care Model: An explanatory model of the drug use process in primary care. *Res Social Adm Pharm* 1(1):101–17.

19. Groves, K.E. (2006). *The influence of pharmaceutical marketing activity, practice characteristics and physician profile on physician prescribing behaviour* [PhD thesis]. NS, Canada: Dalhousie University.

20. Tranmer, J.E., Colley, L., Edge, D.S., Sears, K., VanDenKerkhof, E., & Levesque. L. (2015). Trends in nurse practitioners' prescribing to older adults in Ontario, 2000–2010: A retrospective cohort study. *CMAJ open* 3(3):E299–304.

21. Loxterkamp, D. (2014). What a doctor is good for. *BMJ* 349(g6894).

22. Mossialos, E., Courtin, E., Naci, H., et al. (2015). From "retailers" to health care providers: transforming the role of community pharmacists in chronic disease management. *Health Policy* 119(5):628–39.

23. Maier, C.B. (2015). The role of governance in implementing task-shifting from physicians to nurses in advanced roles in Europe, US, Canada, New Zealand and Australia. *Health Policy* 119(12):1627–35.

24. Law, M.R., Ma, T., Fisher, J., & Sketris, I.S. (2012). Independent pharmacist prescribing in Canada. *Can Pharm J (Ott)* 145(1):17–23.e1.

25. Freund, T., Everett, C., Griffiths, P., Hudon, C., Naccarella, L., & Laurant, M. (2015). Skill mix, roles and remuneration in the primary care workforce: Who are the healthcare professionals in the primary care teams across the world? *Int J Nurs Stud* 52(3):727–43.

26. Gadbois, E.A., Miller, E.A., & Tyler, D., & Intrator, O. (2015). Trends in state regulation of nurse practitioners and physician assistants, 2001 to 2010. *Med Care Res Rev* 72(2):200–19.

27. Creedon, R., Byrne, S., Kennedy, J., & McCarthy, S. (2015). The impact of nurse prescribing on the clinical setting. *Br J Nurs* 24(17):878–85.

28. Nelson, S., Turnbull, J., Bainbridge, L., et al. (2014). *Optimizing scopes of practice: New models of care for a new health care system.* Ottawa, ON: Canadian Academy of Health Sciences.

29. Smith, A., Latter, S., & Blenkinsopp, A. (2014). Safety and quality of nurse independent prescribing: a national study of experiences of education, continuing professional development clinical governance. *J Adv Nurs* 70(11):2506–17.

30. Tamblyn, R.M., McLeod, P.J., Abrahamowicz, M., & Laprise, R. (1996). Do too many cooks spoil the broth? Multiple physician involvement in medical management of elderly patients and potentially inappropriate drug combinations. *CMAJ* 154(8):1177–84.

31. Weiss, M.C., Platt, J., Riley, R., et al. (2015). Medication decision making and patient outcomes in GP, nurse and pharmacist prescriber consultations. *Prim Health Care Res Dev* 16(05):513–27.

32. Greenhalgh, T., Howick, J., & Maskrey, N. Evidence based medicine: a movement in crisis? *BMJ* 348:g3725.

33. Wieringa, S. & Greenhalgh, T. (2015). 10 years of mindlines: A systematic review and commentary. *Implement Sci* 10(45).

34. Gönül, F.F., Carter, F., Petrova, E., & Srinivasan, K. (2001). Promotion of prescription drugs and its impact on physicians' choice behavior. *J Market* 65(3):79–90.

35. Rosenthal, M.B., Berndt, E.R., Donohue, J.M., Epstein, A.M., & Frank, R.G. (2003). *Demand effects of recent changes in prescription drug promotion.* Menlo Park, CA: Henry J. Kaiser Family Foundation.

36. Semin S, Aras Ş, & Guldal, D. (2007). Direct-to-consumer advertising of pharmaceuticals: developed countries experiences and Turkey. *Health Expectations* 10(1):4–15.

37. Mintzes, B. (2006). *What are the public health implications? Direct-to-consumer advertising of prescription drugs in Canada.* Ottawa, ON: Health Council of Canada.

38. Health Action International. *Direct to consumer advertising revisited by European commission, "Deja-vu all over again?"* (Accessed Feb, 8, 2016, at http://haieurope.org/wp-content/uploads/2012/01/4-Oct-2006-HAI-Europe-Press-Release-DTCA-by-EU-Commission-Deja-vu-all-over-again.pdf).

39. Jenkings, K.N., & Barber, N. (2004). What constitutes evidence in hospital new drug decision making? *Soc Sci Med* 58(9):1757–66.

40. Barber, N. (1995). What constitutes good prescribing? *BMJ* 310(6984):923–5.

41. Horton, R.L. (1979). Some relationships between personality and consumer decision making. *J Market Res* 16(2):233–46.

42. Turley, L.W. & LeBlanc, R.P. (1995). Evoked sets: a dynamic process model. *J Mark Theory Pract* 3(2):28–36.

43. Kotler, P., Armstrong, G., & Cunningham, P.H. (2005). *Principles of Marketing* 6th ed (Canadian). Toronto, ON: Pearson Education Canada.

44. Solomon, M., Zaichkowsky, J., & Polegato, R. (2005). *Consumer behaviour: Buying, having, and behaving* 6th ed. Toronto, ON: Prentice Hall.

45. Olshavsky, R.W. & Granbois, D.H. (1979). Consumer decision making-fact or fiction? *J Consum Res* 6(2):93–100.

46. Landon, B.E. (2006). Is pay-for-performance moving north? P4P prospects in the Canadian healthcare system. *Healthc Pap* 6(4):28–33.

47. Alkhaled, L., Kahale, L., Nass, H., et al. (2014). Legislative, educational, policy and other interventions targeting physicians' interaction with pharmaceutical companies: a systematic review. *BMJ Open* 4(7):e004880.

48. Sismondo, S. (2013). Key opinion leaders and the corruption of medical knowledge: what the Sunshine Act will and won't cast light on. *J Law Med Ethics* 41(3):635–43.

49. Frishman, W.H. (2016). Reflections on the physicians payment sunshine act. *Am J Med* 129(1):3–4.

50. Peters, B. & Ferrence, H.D. *Compliance in pharmaceutical advertising, fair balance and the role of contact centers.* (Accessed Feb, 8, 2016, at http://www. pharmacompliancemonitor.com/compliance-in-pharmaceutical-advertising-fair-balance-and-the-role-of-contact-centers/5217/).

51. Rochaix, L. (1998). The physician as perfect agent: a comment. *Soc Sci Med* 47(3):355–6.

52. Mooney, G. & Ryan, M. (1993). Agency in health care: getting beyond first principles. *J Health Econ* 12(2):125–35.

53. Mott, D.A., Schommer, J.C., Doucette, W.R., & Kreling, D.H. (1998). Agency theory, drug formularies, and drug product selection: implications for public policy. *J Public Policy Mark* 17(2):287–95.

54. MacLeod, S.M. (1996). Improving physician prescribing practices: bridge over troubled waters. *CMAJ* 154(5):675–7.

55. McTavish, J.R. (1999). What did Bayer do before aspirin? Early pharmaceutical marketing practices in America. *Pharm Hist* 41(1):3–15.

56. Angus, D.E. & Karpetz, H.M. (1998). Pharmaceutical policies in Canada. *Pharmacoeconomics* 14(1):81–96.

57. Lublóy, Á. (2014). Factors affecting the uptake of new medicines: a systematic literature review. *BMC Health Serv Res* 14(469).

58. Law, M.R., Cheng, L., Dhalla, I.A., Heard, D., & Morgan, S.G. (2012). The effect of cost on adherence to prescription medications in Canada. *CMAJ* 184(3):297–302.

59. Aitken, M. & Valkova, S. (2013). *Avoidable costs in U.S. healthcare: The $200 billion opportunity from using medicines more responsibly.* Parsippany, NJ: IMS Institute for Healthcare Informatics.

60. Greenhalgh, T., Robert, G., Macfarlane, F., Bate, P., & Kyriakidou, O. (2004). Diffusion of innovations in service organizations: systematic review and recommendations. *Milbank Q* 82(4):581–629.

61. Nilsen, P. (2015). Making sense of implementation theories, models and frameworks. *Implement Sci* 10(53).

62. Cane, J., O'Connor, D., & Michie, S. (2012). Validation of the theoretical domains framework for use in behaviour change and implementation research. *Implement Sci* 7(37).

63. Davey, P. (2015). The 2015 Garrod Lecture: Why is improvement difficult? *J Antimicrob Chemother* 70(11):2931–44.

64. Rogers, E.M. (1995). *Diffusion of innovations* 4th ed. New York, NY: Free Press.

65. Estabrooks, C.A., Derksen, L., Winther, C., et al. (2008). The intellectual structure and substance of the knowledge utilization field: A longitudinal author co-citation analysis, 1945 to 2004. *Implement Sci* 3(49).

66. Bate, P. (2014). Context is everything. In: Riddell Bamber, J. (Ed.), Perspectives on context. *A selection of essays considering the role of context in successful quality improvement.* London: Health Foundation, 1–30.

67. Coleman, J.S., Katz, E., & Menzel, H. (1966). *Medical innovation: A diffusion study.* Indianapolis: The Bobbs-Merrill Company.

68. Van den Bulte, C. & Lilien, G.L. (2001). Medical innovation revisited: Social contagion versus marketing effort. *Am J Sociol* 106(5):1409–35.

69. Peay, M.Y. & Peay, E.R. (1994). Innovation in high risk drug therapy. *Soc Sci Med* 39(1):39–52.

70. Waarts, E., Everdingen, Y.M., & Hillegersberg, J. (2002). The dynamics of factors affecting the adoption of innovations. *J Prod Innovation Manage* 19(6):412–23.

71. Ma, J., Stafford, R.S., Cockburn, I.M., & Finkelstein, S.N. (2003). A statistical analysis of the magnitude and composition of drug promotion in the United States in 1998. *Clin Ther* 25(5):1503–17.

72. Wozniak, G.D. (1993). Joint information acquisition and new technology adoption: Late versus early adoption. *Rev Econ Stat* 75(3):438–45.

73. Olshavsky, R.W. & Spreng, R. A. (1996). An exploratory study of the innovation evaluation process. *J Prod Innovation Manage* 13(6):512–29.

74. Dybdahl, T., Andersen, M., Søndergaard, J., Kragstrup, J., & Kristiansen, I.S. (2004). Does the early adopter of drugs exist? A population-based study of general practitioners' prescribing of new drugs. *Eur J Clin Pharmacol* 60(9):667–72.

75. Shih, C. & Venkatesh, A. (2004). Beyond adoption: Development and application of a use-diffusion model. *J Market* 68(1):59–72.

76. Marinova, D. (2004). Actualizing innovation effort: the impact of market knowledge diffusion in a dynamic system of competition. *J Market* 68(3):1–20.

77. Granovetter, M. (1978). Threshold models of collective behavior. *Am J Sociol* 83(6):1420–43.

78. Valente, T.W.(1996). Social network thresholds in the diffusion of innovations. *Social Networks* 18(1):69–89.

79. Carpenter, G.S. & Nakamoto, K. (1989). Consumer preference formation and pioneering advantage. *J Market Res* 26(3):285–98.

80. Boulding, W. & Christen, M. (2003). Sustainable pioneering advantage? Profit implications of market entry order. *Marketing Science* 22(3):371–92.

81. Groves, K., Sketris, I., & Tett, S. (2003). Prescription drug samples–does this marketing strategy counteract policies for quality use of medicines? *J Clin Pharm Ther* 28(4):259–71.

82. Mackey, T.K., Yagi, N., Liang, B.A. (2014). Prescription drug coupons: evolution and need for regulation in direct-to-consumer advertising. *Res Social Adm Pharm* 10(3):588–94.

83. Marks, L.J. & Kamins, M.A. (1988). The use of product sampling and advertising: Effects of sequence of exposure and degree of advertising claim exaggeration on consumers' belief strength, belief confidence, and attitudes. *J Market Res* 25(3):266–81.

84. Rosenthal, M,B., Berndt, E.R., Donohue, J.M., Frank, R.G., & Epstein, A.M. (2002). Promotion of prescription drugs to consumers. *N Engl J Med* 346(7):498–505.

85. Mack J. (2013). Pharma promotional spending in 2013. *Pharma Marketing News* 13(5):1–6.

86. Naik, A.D., Woofter, A.L., Skinner, J.M., & Abraham, N.S. (2009). Pharmaceutical company influence on nonsteroidal anti-inflammatory drug prescribing behaviors. *Am J Manag Care* 15(4):e9–15.

87. Kondro, W. (2007). Academic drug detailing: an evidence-based alternative. *CMAJ* 176(4):429–31.

88. Hawkins, S.A.& Hoch, S.J. (1992). Low-involvement learning: Memory without evaluation. *J Consum Res* 19(2):212–25.

89. Prosser, H., Almond, S., & Walley, T. (2003). Influences on GPs' decision to prescribe new drugs-the importance of who says what. *Fam Pract* 20(1):61–8.

90. Avorn, J., Chen, M., & Hartley, R. (1982). Scientific versus commercial sources of influence on the prescribing behavior of physicians. *Am J Med* 73(1):4–8.

91. Guldal, D. & Semin, S. (2000). The influences of drug companies' advertising programs on physicians. *Int J Health Serv* 30(3):585–95.

92. Watkins, C., Harvey, I., Carthy, P., Moore, L., Robinson, E., & Brawn, R. (2003). Attitudes and behaviour of general practitioners and their prescribing costs: a national cross sectional survey. *Qual Saf Health Care* 12(1):29–34.

93. Muijrers, P.E., Grol, R.P., Sijbrandij, J., Janknegt. R., & Knottnerus, J.A. (2005). Differences in prescribing between GPs: impact of the cooperation with pharmacists and impact of visits from pharmaceutical industry representatives. *Fam Pract* 22(6):624–30.

94. Jacoby, A., Smith, M., & Eccles, M. (2003). A qualitative study to explore influences on general practitioners' decisions to prescribe new drugs. *Br J Gen Pract* 53(487):120–5.

95. Jiang, P. (2004). The role of brand name in customization decisions: A search vs experience perspective. *J Prod Brand Manag* 13(2):73–83.

96. Gorecki, P.K. (1986). The importance of being first: The case of prescription drugs in Canada. *Int J Ind Organ* 4(4):371–95.

97. Leffler, K.B. (1981). Persuasion or information? The economics of prescription drug advertising. *J Law Econ.* 24 (1):45–74.

98. Scharitzer, D. & Kollarits, H.C. (2000). Satisfied customers: Profitable customer relationships: Pharmaceutical marketing: How pharmaceutical sales representatives can achieve economic success through relationship management with settled general practitioners—An empirical study. *Total Qual Manage* 11(7):955–65.

99. Jones, M.I., Greenfield, S.M., & Bradley, C.P. (2001). Prescribing new drugs: qualitative study of influences on consultants and general practitioners. *BMJ* 323(7309):378–81.

100. Watkins, C., Moore, L., Harvey, I., Carthy, P., Robinson, E., & Brawn, R. (2003). Characteristics of general practitioners who frequently see drug industry representatives: National cross sectional study. *BMJ* 326(7400):1178–9.

101. Majumdar, S.R., McAlister, F.A., & Soumerai, S.B. (2003). Synergy between publication and promotion: comparing adoption of new evidence in Canada and the United States. *Am J Med* 115(6):467–72.

102. Kerr, S.J., Mant, A., Horn, F.E., McGeechan, K., & Sayer, G.P. (2003). Lessons from early large-scale adoption of celecoxib and rofecoxib by Australian general practitioners. *Med J Aust* 179(8):403–7.

103. Mizik, N. & Jacobson, R. (2004). Are physicians "easy marks"? Quantifying the effects of detailing and sampling on new prescriptions. *Manag Sci* 50(12):1704–15.

104. Dekimpe, M.G. & Hanssens, D.M. (1995). The persistence of marketing effects on sales. *Market Sci* 14(1):1–21.

105. Gönül, F.F., Carter, F., & Wind, J. (2000). What kind of patients and physicians value direct-to-consumer advertising of prescription drugs. *Health Care Manag Sci* 3(3):215–26.

106. Manchanda, P. & Chintagunta, P.K. (2004). Responsiveness of physician prescription behavior to salesforce effort: An individual level analysis. *Mark Lett* 15(2-3):129–45.

107. Coenen, S., Van Royen, P., Michiels, B., & Denekens, J. (2004). Optimizing antibiotic prescribing for acute cough in general practice: a cluster-randomized controlled trial. *J Antimicrob Chemother* 54(3):661–72.

108. Solomon, D.H., Van Houten, L., Glynn, R.J., et al. (2001). Academic detailing to improve use of broad-spectrum antibiotics at an academic medical center. *Arch Intern Med* 161(15):1897–902.

109. Zwar, N., Wolk, J., Gordon, J., Sanson-Fisher, R., & Kehoe, L. (1999). Influencing antibiotic prescribing in general practice: a trial of prescriber feedback and management guidelines. *Fam Pract* 16(5):495–500.

110. Simon, S.R., Majumdar, S.R., Prosser, L.A., et al. (2005). Group versus individual academic detailing to improve the use of antihypertensive medications in primary care: a cluster-randomized controlled trial. *Am J Med* 118(5):521–8.

111. Schuster, R.J., Terwoord, N.A., & Tasosa, J. (2006). Changing physician practice behavior to measure and improve clinical outcomes. *Am J Med Qual* 21(6):394–400.

112. Fretheim, A., Oxman, A.D., Håvelsrud, K., Treweek, S., Kristoffersen, D.T., & Bjørnda, A. (2006). Rational prescribing in primary care (RaPP): a cluster randomized trial of a tailored intervention. *PLoS Med* 3(6):e134.

113. Watkins, C., Timm, A., Gooberman-Hill, R., Harvey, I., Haines, A., & Donovan, J. (2004). Factors affecting feasibility and acceptability of a practice-based educational intervention to support evidence-based prescribing: a qualitative study. *Fam Pract* 21(6):661–9.

114. Polinski, J.M., Brookhart, M.A., Katz, J.N., et al. (2005). Educational outreach (academic detailing) regarding osteoporosis in primary care. *Pharmacoepidemiol Drug Saf* 14(12):843–50.

115. Jones, M., Greenfield, S., Bradley, C. (1999). A survey of the advertising of nine new drugs in the general practice literature. *J Clin Pharm Ther* 24(6):451–60.

116. Schumock, G.T., Walton, S. M., Park, H.Y., et al. (2004). Factors that influence prescribing decisions. *Ann Pharmacother* 38(4):557–62.

117. Hurwitz, M.A .& Caves, R.E. (1988). Persuasion or information? Promotion and the shares of brand name and generic pharmaceuticals. *J Law Econ* 31(2):299–320.

118. Stafford, R.S., Furberg, C.D., Finkelstein, S,N., Cockburn, I.M., Alehegn, T., & Ma, J. (2004). Impact of clinical trial results on national trends in α-blocker prescribing, 1996-2002. *JAMA* 291(1):54–62.

119. Kim, H. (2015). Trouble spots in online direct-to-consumer prescription drug promotion: a content analysis of FDA warning letters. *Int J Health Policy Manag* 4(12):813.

120. Robertson, C.T. (2015). New DTCA Guidance—Enough to Empower Consumers? *N Engl J Med* 373(12):1085–7.

121. Schwartz, L.M. & Woloshin, S. (2013). The Drug Facts Box: Improving the communication of prescription drug information. *Proc Natl Acad Sci U S A*; 110 (Suppl 3):14069–74.

122. Mintzes, B., Morgan, S., Wright, J.M. (200900. Twelve years' experience with direct-to-consumer advertising of prescription drugs in Canada: A cautionary tale. *PLoS One* 4(5):e5699.

123. Mintzes, B. (2012). Advertising of prescription-only medicines to the public: Does evidence of benefit counterbalance harm? *Public Health* 33(1):259.

124. Lexchin, J. & Mintzes B. (2014). A compromise too far: A review of Canadian cases of direct-to-consumer advertising regulation. *Int J Risk Saf Med* 26(4):213–25.

125. Mintzes, B., Barer, M.L., Kravitz, R.L., et al. (2003). How does direct-to-consumer advertising (DTCA) affect prescribing? A survey in primary care environments with and without legal DTCA. *CMAJ* 169(5):405–12.

126. Scott, I.A. (2006). On the need for probity when physicians interact with industry. *Intern Med J* 36(4):265–9.

127. Roth, M.S. (2003). Media and message effects on DTC prescription drug print advertising awareness. *J Advert Res* 43(02):180–93.

128. Schwartz, R.K., Soumerai, S.B., & Avorn J. (1989). Physician motivations for nonscientific drug prescribing. *Soc Sci Med* 28(6):577–82.

129. Donohue, J.M. (2006). Direct-to-consumer advertising of prescription drugs: Does it add to the overuse and inappropriate use of prescription drugs or alleviate underuse? *Int J Pharm Med* 20(1):17–24.

130. Dobrow, L. (2014). Pharma DTC spending jumps almost 21% in 2014. Accessed Feb, 8, 2016, at http://www.mmm-online.com/agency/pharma-dtc-spending-jumps-almost-21-in-2014/article/404922/.

131. Peyrot, M., Alperstein, N.M., Van Doren, D., & Poli, L.G. (1998). Direct-to-consumer ads can influence behavior. *Mark Health Serv* 18(2):26.

132. Mehta, A. & Purvis, S.C. (2003). Consumer response to print prescription drug advertising. *St* 43(2):194–206.

133. Zachry, W.M., Shepherd, M.D., Hinich, M.J., Wilson, J.P., Brown, C.M., & Lawson K.A. (2002). Relationship between direct-to-consumer advertising and physician diagnosing and prescribing. *Am J Health Syst Pharm* 59(1):42–9.

134. Vogel, R.J., Ramachandran, S., & Zachry, W.M. (2003). A 3-stage model for assessing the probable economic effects of direct-to-consumer advertising of pharmaceuticals. *Clin Ther* 25(1):309-29.

135. Donohue, J.M., Berndt, E.R., Rosenthal, M., Epstein, A.M., & Frank, R.G. (2004). Effects of pharmaceutical promotion on adherence to the treatment guidelines for depression. *Med Care* 42(12):1176–85.

136. Ruiz-Conde, E., Wieringa, J.E., & Leeflang, P.S. (2014). Competitive diffusion of new prescription drugs: The role of pharmaceutical marketing investment. *Technol Forecast Soc Change* 88:49–63.

137. Monson, K.E. & Fink, J.L. 3rd. (2014). Direct-to-consumer advertising: Implications for the pharmacist and other health professionals. *Ann Pharmacother* 48(7):916–8.

138. Niederdeppe, J., Byrne, S., Avery, R.J., & Cantor, J. (2013). Direct-to-consumer television advertising exposure, diagnosis with high cholesterol, and statin use. *J Gen Intern Med* 28(7):886–93.

139. Stevenson, F.A., Greenfield, S.M., Jones, M., Nayak, A., & Bradley, C.P. (1999). GPs' perceptions of patient influence on prescribing. *Fam Pract* 16(3):255–61.

140. Britten, N., Ukoumunne, O.C., & Boulton, M.G. (2002). Patients' attitudes to medicines and expectations for prescriptions. *Health Expect* 5(3):256–69.

141. Mamdani, M.M., Tu, K., Austin, P.C., & Alter, D.A. (2002). Influence of socioeconomic status on drug selection for the elderly in Canada. *Ann Pharmacother* 36(5):804–8.

142. Soumerai, S.B., Avorn, J., Ross-Degnan, D., & Gortmaker S. (1987). Payment restrictions for prescription drugs under Medicaid. *N Engl J Med* 317(9):550–6.

143. Tamblyn, R., Laprise, R., Hanley, J.A., et al. (2001). Adverse events associated with prescription drug cost-sharing among poor and elderly persons. *JAMA* 285(4):421–9.

144. Stewart, R.E., Vroegop, S., Kamps, G.B., Van Der Werf, Ger, Th., & Meyboom-de Jong, B. (2003). Factors influencing adherence to guidelines in general practice. *Int J Technol Assess Health Care* 19(3):546–54.

145. World Health Organization. (1987). *The rational use of drugs*. Geneva, CH: WHO Press.

146. Bradley, C.P. (1992). Factors which influence the decision whether or not to prescribe: the dilemma facing general practitioners. *Br J Gen Pract* 42(364):454–8.

147. McKinlay, J.B., Potter, D.A., & Feldman, H.A. (1996). Non-medical influences on medical decision-making. *Soc Sci Med* 42(5):769–76.

148. Bennett, K., Teeling, M., & Feely, J. (2003). "Selective" switching from non-selective to selective non-steroidal anti-inflammatory drugs. *Eur J Clin Pharmacol* 59(8-9):645–9.

149. Tamblyn, R., McLeod, P., Hanley, J.A., Girard, N., & Hurley, J. (2003). Physician and practice characteristics associated with the early utilization of new prescription drugs. *Med Care* 41(8):895–908.

150. Sears K, Bishop A, MacKinnon NJ. Do you hear what I hear? (2014). Communication practices about medications between physicians and clients with chronic illness in Canada. *J Participat Med* 15(6):e2.

151. Cutts, C. & Tett, S.E. (2003). Doctors perceptions of the influences on their prescribing: a comparison of general practitioners based in rural and urban Australia. *Eur J Clin Pharmacol* 58(11):761–6.

152. Baldwin, L., Rosenblatt, R.A., Schneeweiss, R., Lishner, D.M., & Hart, L.G. (1999). Rural and urban physicians: Does the content of their practices differ? *J Rural Health* 15(2):240–51.

153. Cutts, C. & Tett, S.E. (2003). Influences on doctors' prescribing: Is geographical remoteness a factor? *Aust J Rural Health* 11(3):124–30.

154. Redelmeier, D.A., Tan, S.H., & Booth, G.L. (1998). The treatment of unrelated disorders in patients with chronic medical diseases. *N Engl J Med* 338(21):1516–20.

155. Howlett, J.G., Cox, J.L., Haddad, H., Stanley, J., McDonald, M., & Johnstone, D.E. (2003). Physician specialty and quality of care for CHF: different patients or different patterns of practice? *Can J Cardiol* 19(4):371–7.

156. Buban, G.M., Link, B.K., & Doucette W.R. (2001). Influences on oncologists' adoption of new agents in adjuvant chemotherapy of breast cancer. *J Clin Oncol* 19(4):954–9.

157. Coleman, J., Menzel, H., & Katz, E. (1959). Social processes in physicians' adoption of a new drug. *J Chronic Dis* 9(1):1–19.

158. Bearden, W.O. & Etzel, M.J. (1982). Reference group influence on product and brand purchase decisions. *J Consum Res* 9(2):183–94.

159. Ajzen, I. (1991). The theory of planned behavior. *Organ Behav Hum Decis Process* 50(2):179–211.

160. Rosenstein, A.H. & Shulkin, D. (1991). Changing physician behavior is tool to reduce health care costs. *Health Care Strateg Manage* 9(9):14–6.

161. Grimshaw, J., Eccles, M., & Tetroe. J. (2004). Implementing clinical guidelines: current evidence and future implications. *J Contin Educ Health Prof* 24(S1):S31–7.

162. Steffensen, F.H., Sorensen, H.T., & Olesen, F. (1999.) Diffusion of new drugs in Danish general practice. *Fam Pract* 16(4):407–13.

163. Cranney, M., Warren, E., Barton, S., Gardner, K., & Walley, T. (2001). Why do GPs not implement evidence-based guidelines? A descriptive study. *Fam Pract* 18(4):359–63.

164. Prosser, H. & Walley, T. (2003). New drug uptake: qualitative comparison of high and low prescribing GPs' attitudes and approach. *Fam Pract* 20(5):583–91.

165. Helin-Salmivaara, A., Huupponen, R., Klaukka, T., & Hoppu, K. (2003). Focusing on changing clinical practice to enhance rational prescribing—collaboration and networking enable comprehensive approaches. *Health Policy* 66(1):1–10.

166. Maue, S.K., Segal, R., Kimberlin, C.L., & Lipowski, E.E. (2004). Predicting physician guideline compliance: an assessment of motivators and perceived barriers. *Am J Manag Care* 10(6):383–91.

167. Pearson, S., Rolfe, I., & Smith, T. (2002). Factors influencing prescribing: An intern's perspective. *Med Educ* 36(8):781–7.

168. Denig, P., Haaijer-Ruskamp, F., Wesseling, H., & Versluis, A. (1991). Impact of clinical trials on the adoption of new drugs within a university hospital. *Eur J Clin Pharmacol* 41(4):325–8.

169. Allery, L.A., Owen, P.A., Robling, M.R. (1997). Why general practitioners and consultants change their clinical practice: a critical incident study. *BMJ* 314(7084):870–4.

170. Landon, B.E., Reschovsky, J., Reed, M., & Blumenthal, D. (2001). Personal, organizational, and market level influences on physicians' practice patterns: results of a national survey of primary care physicians. *Med Care* 39(8):889–905.

171. O'Neill, L. & Kuder, J. (2005). Explaining variation in physician practice patterns and their propensities to recommend services. *Med Care Res Rev* 62(3):339–57.

172. Ashworth, M., Armstrong, D., Colwill, S., Cohen, A., & Balazs, J. (2000). Motivating general practitioners to change their prescribing: the incentive of working together. *J Clin Pharm Ther* 25(2):119–24.

173. Carthy, P., Harvey, I., Brawn, R., & Watkins, C. (2000). A study of factors associated with cost and variation in prescribing among GPs. *Fam Pract* 17(1):36–41.

174. Soumerai, S.B., McLaughlin, T.J., Gurwitz, J.H., et al. (1998). Effect of local medical opinion leaders on quality of care for acute myocardial infarction: a randomized controlled trial. *JAMA* 279(17):1358–63.

175. Hemminki, E. (1975). Review of literature on the factors affecting drug prescribing. *Soc Sci Med* 9(2):111–5.

176. Mitchell, V. & Walsh, G. (2004). Gender differences in German consumer decision-making styles. *J Consum Behav* 3(4):331–46.

177. Sproles, G.B. & Kendall, E.L. (1986). A methodology for profiling consumers' decision-making styles. *J Consumer Aff* 20(2):267–79.

178. Sproles, E.K. & Sproles, G.B. (1990). Consumer decision-making styles as a function of individual learning styles. *J Consum Aff* 24(1):134–47.

179. Chang, J. & Samuel, N. (2004). Internet shopper demographics and buying behaviour in Australia. *J Am Acad Bus* 5(1/2):171–6.

180. Roy Dholakia, R. (1999). Going shopping: key determinants of shopping behaviors and motivations. *Int J Retail & Distribution Manag* 27(4):154–65.

181. Fischer, E. & Arnold, S.J. (1994). Sex, gender identity, gender role attitudes, and consumer behavior. *Psychol Market* 11(2):163–82.

182. Inman, W. & Pearce, G. (1993). Prescriber profile and post-marketing surveillance. *Lancet* 342(8872):658–61.

183. Duetz, M.S., Schneeweiss, S., Maclure, M., Abel, T., Glynn, R.J., & Soumerai, S.B. (2003). Physician gender and changes in drug prescribing after the implementation of reference pricing in British Columbia. *Clin Ther* 25(1):273–84.

184. Gilly, M.C. & Zeithaml, V.A. (1985). The elderly consumer and adoption of technologies. *J Consum Res* 12(3):353–7.

185. 1Lacy, B.E., Crowell, M.D., Riesett, R.P., & Mitchell, A. (2005). Age, specialty, and practice setting predict gastroesophageal reflux disease prescribing behavior. *J Clin Gastroenterol* 39(6):489–94.

186. Freiman, M.P. (1985). The rate of adoption of new procedures among physicians: the impact of specialty and practice characteristics. *Med Care* 23(8):939–45.

187. Helin-Salmivaara, A., Huupponen, R., Virtanen, A., & Klaukka, T. (2005). Adoption of celecoxib and rofecoxib: A nationwide database study. *J Clin Pharm Ther* 30(2):145–52.

188. Groves, K.E., Schellinck, T., Sketris, I., & MacKinnon, N.J. (2010). Identifying early prescribers of cycloxygenase-2 inhibitors (COX-2s) in Nova Scotia, Canada: Considerations for targeted academic detailing. *Res Social Adm Pharm* 6(3):257–67.

189. Tamayo-Sarver, J.H., Dawson, N.V., Cydulka, R.K., Wigton, R.S., & Baker, D.W. (2004). Variability in emergency physician decision making about prescribing opioid analgesics. *Ann Emerg Med* 43(4):483–93.

190. Garjón, F.J., Azparren, A., Vergara, I., Azaola, B., & Loayssa, J.R. (2012). Adoption of new drugs by physicians: a survival analysis. *BMC Health Serv Res* 12(56).

191. Armstrong, D., Reyburn, H., & Jones, R. (1996). A study of general practitioners' reasons for changing their prescribing behaviour. *BMJ* 312(7036):949–52.

192. Denig, P., Witteman, C.L., & Schouten, H.W. (2002). Scope and nature of prescribing decisions made by general practitioners. *Qual Saf Health Care* 11(2):137–43.

193. Nazareth, I., Freemantle, N., Duggan, C., Mason, J., & Haines, A. (2002). Evaluation of a complex intervention for changing professional behaviour: the Evidence Based Out Reach (EBOR) Trial. *J Health Serv Res Policy* 7(4):230–8.

194. Bourke, J. & Roper, S. (2012). In with the new: the determinants of prescribing innovation by general practitioners in Ireland. *Eur J Health Econ* 13(4):393–407.

195. Majumdar, S.R., Lipton, H.L., & Soumerai, S.B. (2012). Chapter 25. Evaluating and improving physician prescribing. In Strom, B.L., Kimmel, S.E., & Hennessy, S. (Eds.), *Pharmacoepidemiology* 5th ed. Chichester, UK: Wiley-Blackwell, 402–422.

196. Irwin, R., Stokes, T., & Marshall, T. (2015). Practice-level quality improvement interventions in primary care: a review of systematic reviews. *Prim Health Care Res Dev* 16(6):556–77.

197. Shojania, K.G., Jennings, A., Mayhew, A., Ramsay, C.R., Eccles, M.P., & Grimshaw. J. (2009). The effects of on-screen, point of care computer reminders on processes and outcomes of care. *Cochrane Database Syst Rev* 3.

198. Gillaizeau, F., Chan, E., Trinquart, L., et al. (2013). Computerized advice on drug dosage to improve prescribing practice. *Cochrane Database Syst Rev* 11.

199. O'Brien, M.A., Rogers, S., Jamtvedt, G., et al. (2007). Educational outreach visits: effects on professional practice and health care outcomes. *Cochrane Database Syst Rev* 4.

200. Canadian Institutes for Health Research. *Moving into action: We know what practices we want to change, now what? An implementation guide for health care practitioners.* (Accessed Feb, 8, 2016, at http://www.cihr-irsc.gc.ca/e/45669.html).

201. Ivers, N., Jamtvedt, G., Flottorp, S., et al. (2012). Audit and feedback: effects on professional practice and health care outcomes. *Cochrane Database Syst Rev* 6.

202. National Prescribing Centre. (2012). *A single competency framework for all prescribers.* (Accessed Feb, 8, 2016, at http://www.webarchive.org.uk/wayback/archive/20140627112901/http://www.npc.nhs.uk/improving_safety/improving_quality/resources/single_comp_framework_v2.pdf).

203. Faria, R., Barbieri, M., Light, K., Elliott, R.A., & Sculpher, M. (2014). The economics of medicines optimization: policy developments, remaining challenges and research priorities. *Br Med Bull* 111(1):45–61.

204. Jones, M.I., Greenfield, S.M., Jowett, S., Bradley, C.P., & Seal, R. (2001). Proton pump inhibitors: A study of GPs' prescribing. *Fam Pract* 18(3):333–8.

205. Legare, F., Labrecque, M., Cauchon, M., Castel, J., Turcotte, S., & Grimshaw, J. (2012). Training family physicians in shared decision-making to reduce the overuse of antibiotics in acute respiratory infections: a cluster randomized trial. *CMAJ* 184(13):E726–34.

206. Stiggelbout, A.M., Van der Weijden, T., De Wit, M., et al. (2012). Shared decision making: really putting patients at the centre of healthcare. *BMJ* 344(e256).

207. Gardner, D.M., MacKinnon, N., Langille, D.B., & Andreou, P. (2007). A comparison of factors used by physicians and patients in the selection of antidepressant agents. *Psychiatr Serv* 58(1):34–40.

208. MacKinnon, N.J. (2007). *Safe and effective: The eight essential elements of an optimal medication-use system*. Ottawa, ON: Canadian Pharmacists Association.

209. Hepler, C.D. & Grainger-Rousseau, T.J. (1995). Pharmaceutical care versus traditional drug treatment. Is there a difference? *Drugs* 49(1):1–10.

210. Health Canada. (2003). *Legislative renewal—issue paper; direct to consumer advertising (DTCA) of prescription drugs*. Ottawa, ON: Government of Canada.

CHAPTER 9

ENGAGING PATIENTS IN HEALTHCARE AND DECISION-MAKING: UNDERSTANDING AND FACILITATING THE PROCESS

Michael R. Gionfriddo and Anthony W. Olson

LEARNING OBJECTIVES:

1. Summarize the contemporary understanding of the decision making process and behavior change.
2. Describe factors that influence patients when making decisions in the face of illness.
3. Examine the role of the pharmacist in facilitating and engaging in the decision making process with patients.
4. Identify tools, technologies, approaches, and resources that can be applied in activating patients in their treatment decisions as it relates to medication use both inside and outside of clinical encounters.
5. Evaluate the importance and relevance of decision making for patients and healthcare professionals as it pertains to health outcomes.

KEY TERMS

Bias

Choice architecture

Conformity pressure

Heuristic

Information environment

Informed decision making

Paternalistic decision making

Shared decision making

Threat of disease

INTRODUCTION

In Chapter 3, different theoretical models of health behavior were presented to provide a helpful framework for understanding how patients respond to illness. This chapter will explore in more detail how patients make decisions in the face of illness. Some of these decisions, like the day-to-day taking of medications, are made without consulting a healthcare provider. However, pharmacists are increasingly in a position to partner and guide decisions with patients such as optimizing their medication treatment (i.e. medication therapy management) to best fit their needs, beliefs, and lifestyle. Grasping how patients experience, respond to, and are impacted by illness helps facilitate meaningful communication, partnership, and individualized person-centered care by pharmacists. By the end of the chapter, readers will understand the factors influencing patient decision making and how to engage patients in this process.

INTRODUCTION TO DECISION MAKING

People make decisions every day, from deciding whether to pick up their medications from their community pharmacy (i.e. often a conscious decision) to choosing the route that brings them there (i.e. often a subconscious decision). Some characteristics of decision making are universal to the human race, while others are more specific to an individual's unique qualities, background, and role (i.e. patient vs. practitioner, mother vs. daughter). Contemporary understanding of the mental processes by which individuals make decisions are best represented by two distinct, but interfacing operating systems colloquially known as "System 1" and "System 2."[1]

System 1 represents the effortless, automatic, and innate mental programming that produces and expresses "impressions, intuitions, intentions, and feelings" stimulated by internal and external cues. In contrast, System 2 represents the mental activities that are more effortful, time-consuming, and self-conscious with a primary function to evaluate the constant suggestions delivered by System 1. If suggestions put forth by System 1 are approved by System 2, impulses from System 1 become beliefs and voluntary actions.[1]

TABLE 9-1: TWO COGNITIVE SYSTEMS USED IN DECISION MAKING.[2]

SYSTEM 1	SYSTEM 2
Associative Linking/Pattern Recognition	Deductive
Automatic	Controlled
Effortless	Effortful
Rapid	Slow
Reduced Vigilance/Intuition	Heightened Awareness/Critical Thinking
Subconscious	Conscious
Programmable Skills	Rule-following

Consider a patient recently diagnosed with diabetes type 1. Initially, they will struggle through the multi-step process to appropriately prepare, administer, and dispose of their insulin. This is because the unfamiliar task requires conscious and effortful decisions by System 2 at each step of the process, which cumulatively depletes cognitive resources and capacity. However, over time, the knowledge and skills necessary to complete these tasks transfers to System 1, which explains how a patient that has adequately managed their diabetes with insulin for years can complete the same tasks appropriately and automatically without any cognitive effort.[2]

It may be helpful to conceptualize your brain as a computer with System 1 representing pre-programmed applications that take environmental cues to quickly yield an output. Many refer to this as their "intuition" or "gut-feeling." In contrast, System 2 is the limited amount of working memory (i.e. moment-to-moment cognitive capacity) at any given time to activate, revise, replace, or write the programming in System 1 to better reflect the demands and information in the external environment. In other words, it is your conscious thought.

System 2 fully engages only when System 1 encounters a question or situation for which it can't generate an adequate suggestion. Otherwise, System 2 operates at a fraction of its capacity in order to conserve energy and cognitive resources. In one sense, System 2 acts as a filter for System 1, overriding impulses that conflict with other values, beliefs, or ideas. For example, although many people are distressed by the idea or act of inserting a needle into their skin, they still consciously allow it to happen to deliver a vaccination or another medication that they believe will help them. Not surprisingly, the entire experience can be stress-inducing and exhausting.

For all intents and purposes, there is simply not enough time and cognitive capacity available in most of us to deliberately analyze everything with System 2. Fortunately, System 1 provides mental shortcuts, known as "heuristics," that are extraordinarily useful and necessary in successfully navigating everyday life. Unfortunately, heuristics can also lead to errors, otherwise known as biases.[2]

There have been many studies on biases and heuristics resulting in terms such as "anchoring bias," availability bias," and "representative bias." In essence, each type refers to a situation where the associations, beliefs, and skills programmed into System 1 don't adequately represent the situation that judgements and decisions are being applied to. For example, a "50% chance of avoiding a heart attack within 10 years by taking a statin" is evaluated differently from a "50% chance of having a heart attack within 10 year while taking a statin." The framing of this identical information in terms of gains or losses to lead to different results because System 1 relies heavily on causal thinking (i.e. x happened before y, therefore x causes y) where order and other presentational factors can heavily influence the interpretation and evaluation of the same information.[1] In contrast, although a statistical approach to thinking would lead to a more logical conclusion, this type of thinking is not innately programmed into System 1. This does not mean that statistical thinking cannot be "reprogrammed" into System 1, but that it would require sustained effort and training via System 2 to make it so. An awareness of the processes and influences that lead to biases such as these is particularly important in health care given the monetary, safety, and quality of life related costs derived from suboptimal decisions.

DECISION MAKING IN HEALTHCARE

Many daily decisions directly impact health. One of the goals of pharmacy is to partner and guide decisions with patients such as optimizing their medication treatment (i.e. medication therapy management) to best fit their needs, beliefs, and lifestyle. To do so requires a grasp of how patients experience, respond to, and are impacted by illness. This is necessary to facilitate meaningful communication, partnership, and individualized person-centered care by pharmacists.

DECISION MAKING AND THE EXPERIENCE OF ILLNESS

Disease is the presence of a physiologic abnormality, while illness is how that disease is experienced by an individual.[3] How a person experiences illness is shaped by a many factors (e.g. cultural, societal, experiential, etc.) that are often either tacit or unspoken unless intentionally elicited. Just as the newly diagnosed patient with diabetes type 1 utilizes System 2 to consciously program skills of delivering insulin, the patient and partnering clinician must deliberately explore how to comprehensively understand and work through how patients experience illness. Failure to do so may result in non-adherence, dissatisfaction with care, and worse quality of care.[3]

The patient's understanding and behavioral response to illness is dependent upon his or her own experiences as well as information from the experiences of others. The sum of these components creates a perceived "threat of disease," which is the combination of the person's perceived susceptibility to the disease as well as the perceived severity to a disease. This threat is influenced by physical factors, sociocultural factors, and personal factors. According to the Health Belief Model described in Chapter 3, one's perceived threat of disease affects how a person responds to the disease.

For example, if a person does not perceive a disease as a threat, they might not seek treatment. Issues can arise when there are disagreements between the medical model of disease and the person's view of disease.

In the case of a physical perceived threat of disease, or a disruption of one's body, consider conditions such as mild hypertension and hypercholesterolemia. In the absence of a diagnosis, patients may not experience any illness as there is nothing to experience given the asymptomatic nature of these diseases. Once diagnosed however, patients may experience illness as a result of anxiety, worry, or other manifestations of being labeled as sick.[4] It is also possible that when diagnosed, patients may not view these conditions as a threat and may not adhere to therapy as a result.[5] Studies utilizing the Beliefs about Medicines Questionnaire have found that those patients who do not view their medicines as a necessity are often less adherent than those who view them as a necessity.[6] Working with patients to understand their medication-related beliefs may improve adherence either from better understandings by the patient, or treatment plans more aligned with the patient's beliefs.

This situation may also occur in diseases like asthma where symptoms come and go. Studies of people with asthma find that people hold a variety of beliefs related to asthma and asthma medicine with a subset believing that no symptoms means that they no longer have asthma.[7] This belief has a direct consequence on health, as failure to take preventer medication such as inhaled corticosteroids puts them at a higher risk of exacerbation.[8]

The perceived threat of disease extends beyond the symptoms (i.e. physical) and can also be influenced by an individual's culture or society. Cultural differences can lead to different interpretations of the causes and appropriate treatment of illness. Consider for example, the case of a young Chinese man who Western clinicians determined was likely suffering from depression. The stigma associated with mental illness led the patient to treat his ailment as a physical illness caused by an imbalance of humors. The man's ethnic community discouraged the use of Western medicine and encouraged self-treatment with traditional Chinese medicine aimed at curing the physical illness (i.e. the imbalance of humors). When he did present to the hospital, he initially declined psychotherapy but eventually accepted both psychotherapy and antidepressants, which resolved his depression, but he continued to deny that his illness was not physical in nature. Each culture has a logic which may seem irrational to others, but by striving to understand an individual's culture and establishing a common ground, clinicians can communicate in a culturally sensitive manner and develop culturally sensitive treatment plans.[3]

Finally, the threat of illness can also disrupt one's sense of self.[9,10] The degree to which a person integrates an illness into their identity affects their response to and treatment decisions for that illness.[11] For instance, an individual may not accept the illness as part of their identity, and it is not perceived as threat (except perhaps as a threat to their current identity), and therefore the illness is not treated appropriately. The integration of an illness into a person's identity is dependent on many factors including prior experience with the illness, either first hand (self/family/friends with illness) or second hand (how society/culture views the illness e.g. stigma; remember how cultural stigma influenced denial of a diagnosis of depression above, or what the individual has heard or read about the illness; and the perceived impact on current identity, which includes how someone understands themselves as valuable with or without illness and how they see illness affecting how they live their life and the various roles they play.

Regardless of whether the illness itself is accepted, the treatment also has effects on identity. For example, in a study on patients with asthma participants felt that when they were on medication they were not themselves.[12] In a separate study, adolescents with asthma commented about how taking the asthma medicine acted as a reminder that they were sick or not normal and this reminder was unwelcome and in some cases contributed to non-adherence.[13]

Knowledge, whether gained through direct or secondhand experience, affects how individuals make decisions in response to illness. Arthur Kleinman offers an illustrative example.[3] He describes the case of an elderly woman who was recovering from pulmonary edema associated with congestive heart failure. From the time of her admission she had greatly improved and was asymptomatic but was acting rather strange. The woman induced vomiting and frequently urinated in bed and became agitated when asked to stop. Upon questioning the patient, it was uncovered that she came from a family of plumbers and understood anatomy as a system of pipes and the chest had two pipes one to the mouth and one to the urethra. Additionally, she understood that her condition caused water to build up in the lungs. Her attempts at vomiting and urination were attempts to remove this water, much like the water pill she was taking. After discussing with the patient that the body's plumbing was more complex and that her behavior would not help, the patient acknowledged her misconceptions and stopped her "strange" behavior. As clinicians it is important that we explore patients' prior knowledge of an illness or treatment as this may expose potential misconceptions or misunderstandings, which once addressed may facilitate communication as well as adherence.

All of the factors described thus far help to shape a person's values. Values can loosely be defined as a set of beliefs or principles that define what is important and therefore inform action.[14] While some values may be informed by personal experience, others may be informed by things like culture, family, or society. Values inform decision making and are used in the construction of preferences, which are made in response to specific situations an individual faces. Preferences can include things like preferring oral over injectable medications, preferring generic vs. brand name medication, or preferring quality over quantity of life. Understanding what an individual values, what shapes that value, and how that value informs a preference can facilitate and inform communication and decision-making between clinician and patient and potentially improve adherence and avoid misunderstandings like those described throughout this section.

CONTEXTUAL FACTORS INFLUENCING DECISION MAKING

Contextual factors that influence decision making can be defined as conditions that elicit a motivation to act for an outcome separate from the act in and of itself. These can be partitioned into two general categories: (1) Accessible Resources and (2) Social Influences.

Accessible resources refer to the available means and assets that create and limit the reasonable choices available to each patient. Depending on the individual, System 1 has an inventory of resources related to areas that are frequently used. These include things like cost, transportation, time, language, safety, storage, and lifestyle. In general, individuals have an automatic response to whether they can pay for a medication, how to get from location to another to access the medication, how much time they can devote to obtaining the medication, how to communicate with others, and so on. When utilization of these resources deviates or extends from the norm, System 2 springs into action to find a potential solution. If a patient's insurance will not cover medical care and they do not have enough income to support an out-of-pocket purchase, they may seek out alternatives or experts that know of alternatives (i.e. pharmacists and other healthcare professionals) such as charity care, which provides free or discounted services to patients with low-income.

Much like how society affects the personal experience of illness, social influences also affect how patient's make decisions. Social influences can be split into two pieces: the (1) information environment and (2) conformity pressures.

The information environment refers to the contextual cues from the actions and beliefs others that are then perceived by the patient to be optimal for themselves. Similar but slightly distinct, conformity pressure refers to a concern or interest by the patient about what others may think of them that drives them to follow the crowd to evade scrutiny or obtain praise. These inter-related concepts have been applied in research to show that things like teenage pregnancy and obesity are contagious (i.e. if the close friend of an individual gains weight, it increases that individual's risk to do the same) when controlling for other associated risk factors.[2]

In essence, status quo of the information environment and conformity pressures are programmed into System 1. They automatically indoctrinate the suggestions sent to System 2 for conscious and effortful deliberation. The origin and content of these suggestions may range from memorable advice from a healthcare professional, cultural norms, or even direct-to-consumer advertising (DTCA) from a drug company. In fact, patients who either use DCTA as an information source and/or have a relevant disease condition are more likely to request their physicians for advertised medications. Even in countries besides the United States and New Zealand where DTCA is not officially permitted, patients' expectations and decisions for medications can be influenced on the Internet.[15]

Interestingly, these effects are not isolated to patients alone as physician prescribing and treatment decisions have been shown to be influenced by patient expectations. In a study of general practice in Australia, patients who expected medication were nearly three times as likely to receive it; when the general practitioner thought that the patient expected medication, they were 10 times more likely to write a prescription.[16]

As these examples show, both patients and clinicians bring varying contextual resources, information, and pressures to any interaction between them. The preceding section also shows there are a number of intrinsic factors also relevant to this exchange. For all intents and purposes, each party brings content that is necessary and relevant to making an optimal health decision.

A MEETING OF EXPERTS: DECISION MAKING BETWEEN CLINICIANS AND PATIENTS

As highlighted above, patients make decisions about their healthcare on a daily basis, often without directly interacting with a clinician. These decisions are driven by their personal experience with disease, their ingrained understanding of the disease and treatment, and various contextual issues. When patients interact with the healthcare system, they bring with them this experience, knowledge, and understanding of their own unique circumstances. They are the experts in their values, context, and experience with disease.[17,18] Clinicians, while occasionally seen as gatekeepers to treatment, can also be conceptualized as partners in health as they bring additional professional expertise to the interaction. Clinicians are experts in the general course of the disease and the general effectiveness of different treatments. By working together towards a common goal the two experts can help craft a plan of care that best fits with the best available evidence as well as the patient's values, context, and goals.[19] In order to understand this process and its implications, we will review the historical and current context of the patient pharmacist relationship, how patients and pharmacists can work together to make decisions, and how this process can be facilitated and implemented in routine pharmacy practice.

HISTORICAL CONTEXT OF THE PHARMACIST-PATIENT RELATIONSHIP

For most of the 20th century, pharmacists did not focus on providing direct patient care. In fact, the American Pharmacists Association (APhA) Code of Ethics in 1952 stated the "pharmacist does not discuss the therapeutic effects or composition of a prescription with a patient."[20] Instead, pharmacists were the professionals that compounded the prescriptions written by the physician, consulted with patients regarding non-prescription remedies, and provided the neighborhood kids with a free beverage from the soda fountain now and again. These services were primarily offered in small neighborhood pharmacies that operated at slower paces relative to today. It was not uncommon for families to be serviced by only a single pharmacist or pharmacy for several years, which provided an ideal context for the development of personalized relationships.

The ubiquity of this pharmacy practice and delivery model had drastically changed by the 1980s when incorporated chain pharmacies utilized large scale manufacturing of drug products that economically out-competed more traditional pharmacies. These large chain pharmacies maximized customer convenience and transactional efficiency with a business model dependent on high product volumes delivered to a large population by minimal staff. Around the same time, pharmacists began to carve out roles as clinicians due to changes in education, technology, and clinical practice. The focus of pharmacy began shifting from the drugs patients take to the people that take them.[20,21] These shifts led to significant changes in the nature and extent of the pharmacist-patient relationship.

PHARMACIST-PATIENT RELATIONSHIPS

Pharmacists today are providing a variety of clinical services to populations growing in number and complexity under tighter and tighter time constraints. The consequently higher workloads have led to larger turnover rates as well as more part-time and "float" pharmacists. These demands have led to a more efficient and convenient delivery system ill-suited for cultivating and maintaining more personalized relationships familiar to many middle-age or older patients. At the same time, the value and ability of pharmacists to serve clinical roles have risen given their unique medication expertise and accessibility relative to other healthcare practitioners. In other words, although pharmacists are more clinically prepared than ever, many have lost the practice contexts conducive to developing personalized relationships. This is important because although the patient's perceived clinical competence and expertise in the pharmacist is very important to the quality of the pharmacist-patient relationship, so is the perception of the pharmacist's trustworthiness, caring nature, and availability for frequent contact.[22-24] It is these latter characteristics that are more ideally formed over time. It could therefore be argued that the space separating the pharmacist's knowledge, skills, and experience from the patient's health views, preferences, and background is potentially greater and more important than ever before.

These conditions call for new approaches to either replace or reclaim the value and support lost from the adjusted pharmacist-patient relationship dynamic operating in a time-limited environment. New tools accounting for new conditions are needed to bridge the space between patients and pharmacists. It means moving beyond structural vestiges currently guiding typical patient-pharmacist interactions by intentionally reflecting on how to optimally organize decision making contexts. Taking responsibility for organizing the decision making context is known as "choice architecture." A core tenet of this concept is that arbitrary characteristics in design can subtly influence how decisions are made.[2] Think back to the example from earlier in the chapter that showed how different framing of the impact on statins regarding the chances of having heart attack in 10 years influenced different interpretations and evaluation of the same information.[1] Diligent reflection upon and intentional construction of the decision-making context is important because of its influence in what decisions are made. From this lens, the development and implementation of pharmaceutical care attempts to do this.

Pharmaceutical care is defined by the relationship between pharmacist and patient.[25] In the classic definition, the patient grants authority to the pharmacist who, in turn, gives competence and commitment to the patient. The concept was transformative for pharmacy practice and sparked a dialogue on the ways pharmacists can interact with patients, ranging from relationships based on authority and deference to mutual respect and collaboration. Although there are many ways that patients and clinicians can make decisions together, the following will focus on three approaches: (1) paternalistic, (2) informed, and (3) shared.

Historically, most decisions in medicine have been made paternalistically, with minimal patient input.[26] The clinician makes decisions guided by their own beliefs about what is best for the patient. The patient's role throughout the process is passive and there is no explicit consideration of their values or goals. This approach is most appropriate in urgent situations or situations when there is a "technical" decision to be made. Technical decisions can be thought of as decisions where there is only one reasonable course of action (e.g. which drug or procedure to use to stop active bleeding).

An informed approach to decision making swings the balance of power away from the clinician and towards the patient. Both the clinician and patients are active and treated as experts in the decision making process. However, the clinician serves primarily as a source of medical information for the patient who utilizes the information to make the decision. This approach may be appropriate in some situations concerning over the counter medications (e.g. choosing among a variety of antiseptic preparations).

Both of these approaches may be appropriate in certain situations, but each has limitations. A paternalistic approach fails to consider the patient's situation and fails to acknowledge their input or expertise. While an informed approach considers these things, it undervalues the importance of communication and the relationship between clinician and patient.

In shared decision making, the patient and clinician engage in a dialogue that leads to a mutual understanding of the patient's situation values, and goals that leads to deliberation over the available evidence and options and culminates in a decision.[26,27] It requires a relationship built on mutual respect and trust, support, good communication, and conscious acknowledgment of issues that need to be addressed. The process and outcomes may appear different in each situation given its patient specific nature. Decision making done this way has the potential to improve patient outcomes,[28] and is considered both an ethical imperative,[29,30] and the pinnacle of patient-centered care.[31]

FACILITATING SHARED DECISION MAKING IN PHARMACY PRACTICE

In order to facilitate the translation of shared decision making into practice several tools and training programs have been developed.[28,32,33] While the majority of these have been developed for use by physicians, there is emerging research applying them in pharmacy practice

Decision aids, a broad category of tools that utilize choice architecture to organize and optimize the context in which patients make decisions, can be used to facilitate shared decision making.[34] They have been shown to improve communication, patient knowledge and risk perception, reduce decisional conflict, and stimulate patients to take a more active role in decision making.[28] The majority of these tools have been developed to help patients prepare for a shared decision making conversation with their clinicians and typically provide patients with information about the available options, with some also providing values clarification exercises. Some tools however, have been developed for use within the clinical encounter. These tools recognize the expertise in the encounter and thus generally contain less information and act as starting point for meaningful conversations. These tools are potentially more relevant to pharmacy practice as they do not require identification of or contact with the patients ahead of time.

Tools used within the encounter can broadly be broken down into three categories: (1) Issues-based (2) Risk-based and (3) Template-based.

Issue-based tools utilize salient issues around a given decision to help the patient and clinician have meaningful conversations around the situation facing the patient. Examples of these types of tools include Option Grids[®35] (www.optiongrid.org) and the Diabetes Medication Choice decision aid.[36,37] In the Diabetes Medication Choice tool Figure 9-1 (which is available both in paper and electronic format: https://diabetesdecisionaid.mayoclinic.org/) several salient issues pertinent to choosing medicines for diabetes are presented. Patients can then choose which of those issues is most pertinent to their situation. A discussion then occurs around that issue and why it is important. As they explore the patient's situation, other cards may be chosen by either the patient or clinician to help expand upon or better understand the situation. This is important as issues may interact with one another (for example a patient may consider weight loss the most important issue, but when cost is considered, the option that causes the most weight loss may not be preferred). After a process of deliberation, the clinician and patient together decide which course of action best fits with the patient's preferences and context.

Considerations

Metformin
In the first few weeks after starting Metformin, patients may have some nausea, indigestion or diarrhea.

Insulin
There are no other side effects associated with Insulin.

Pioglitazone
Over time, 10 in 100 people may have fluid retention (edema) while taking the drug. For some it may be as little as ankle swelling. For others, fluid may build up in the lungs making it difficult to breathe. This may resolve after you stop taking the drug. 10 in 100 people at risk of bone fractures who use this drug will have a bone fracture in the next 10 years. There appears to be a slight increase in the risk of bladder cancer with this drug.

Liraglutide/Exenatide
Some patients may have nausea or diarrhea. In some cases, the nausea may be severe enough that a patient has to stop taking the drug. There are reports of pain in the abdomen that may be caused by inflammation of the pancreas with these agents.

Sulfonylureas
Glipizide, Glimepiride, Glyburide
Some patients get nausea, rash and/or diarrhea when they first start taking Sulfonylureas. This type of reaction may force them to stop taking the drug.

Gliptins
A few patients may get nose and sinus congestion, headaches, and perhaps be at risk of problems with their pancreas.

SGLT2 Inhibitors
Urinary tract infections and yeast infections are more common among patients taking this medication.

Daily Routine
Metformin · Insulin · Pioglitazone · Liraglutide / Exenatide · Sulfonylureas (Glipizide, Glimepiride, Glyburide) · Gliptins · SGLT2 Inhibitors

Weight Change

Medication	Weight Change
Metformin	None
Insulin	4 to 6 lb. gain
Pioglitazone	More than 2 to 6 lb. gain
Liraglutide/Exenatide	3 to 6 lb. loss
Sulfonylureas (Glipizide, Glimepiride, Glyburide)	2 to 3 lb. gain
Gliptins	None
SGLT2 Inhibitors	3 to 4 lb. loss

Cost

These figures are estimates and are for comparative reference only. Actual out-of-pocket costs vary over time, by pharmacy, insurance plan coverage, prescription and dosage. Under some plans, name brands may be comparable in cost to generics.

Medication	Per day	Per 3 months
Metformin (Generic available)	$0.10 per day	$10 / 3 months
Insulin (No generic available – price varies by dose)		
Lantus: Vial, per 100 units $10; Pen, per 100 units $43		
NPH: Vial, per 100 units $6; Pen, per 100 units $30		
Short acting analog insulin: Vial, per 100 units $10; Pen, per 100 units $43		
Pioglitazone (Generic available)	$10.00 per day	$900 / 3 months
Liraglutide/Exenatide (No generic available)	$11.00 per day	$1,000 / 3 months
Sulfonylureas Glipizide, Glimepiride, Glyburide (Generic available)	$0.10 per day	$10 / 3 months
Gliptins (No generic available)	$7.00 per day	$620 / 3 months
SGLT2 Inhibitors (No generic available)	$8.00 per day	$750 / 3 months

Blood Sugar (A1c Reduction)

Medication	A1c Reduction
Metformin	1 – 2%
Insulin	Unlimited %
Pioglitazone	1%
Liraglutide/Exenatide	0.5 – 1%
Sulfonylureas (Glipizide, Glimepiride, Glyburide)	1 – 2%
Gliptins	0.5 – 1%
SGLT2 Inhibitors	0.5 – 1%

Low Blood Sugar (Hypoglycemia)

Medication	Severe	Minor
Metformin	No Severe Risk	0 – 1%
Insulin	1 – 3%	30 – 40%
Pioglitazone	No Severe Risk	1 – 2%
Liraglutide/Exenatide	No Severe Risk	0 – 1%
Sulfonylureas (Glipizide, Glimepiride, Glyburide)	Less than 1%	21%
Gliptins	No Severe Risk	1%
SGLT2 Inhibitors	No Severe Risk	3 – 4%

Daily Sugar Testing (Monitoring)

Medication	Monitoring
Metformin	No monitoring necessary.
Insulin	Monitor once or twice daily, less often once stable.
Pioglitazone	No monitoring necessary.
Liraglutide/Exenatide	Monitor twice daily after meals when used with Sulfonylureas. Otherwise not needed.
Sulfonylureas (Glipizide, Glimepiride, Glyburide)	Monitor 2 - 5 times weekly, less often once stable.
Gliptins	No monitoring necessary.
SGLT2 Inhibitors	No monitoring necessary.

FIGURE 9-1. THE DIABETES MEDICATION CHOICE TOOL

The use of the Diabetes Medication Choice tool could be used during medication therapy management consultations and may be most useful if a collaborative practice agreement to manage patients with diabetes is in place. A feasibility study examining the use of the tool in pharmacy encounters was conducted at the Mayo Clinic and use of the tool was found to be feasible and acceptable to both pharmacists and patients (Morgan Jones PharmD, written communication, November 2015).

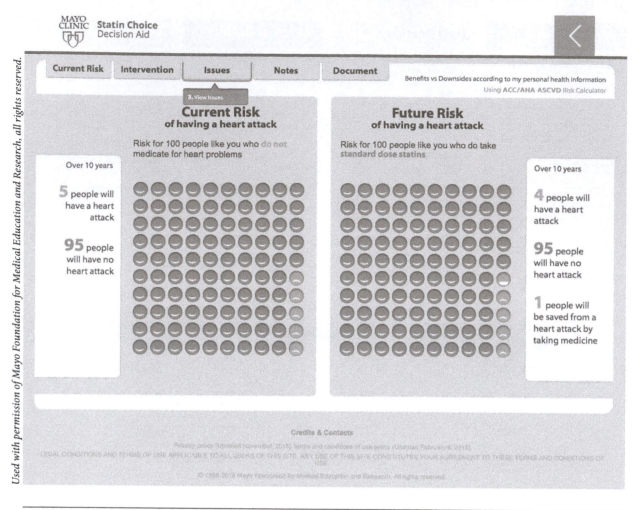

FIGURE 9-2. THE STATIN CHOICE TOOL

The second category of decision aids are risk based tools. An example of a risk based tool is the Statin Choice tool.[38,39]

This tool calculates the risk of a heart attack, given the patient's risk factors, with and without a statin. It presents the risk as an icon array (separating out as natural frequencies the number that will have a heart attack, the number that will not, and the number that will benefit from a statin), as well as highlighting the risk in words and numbers in colors that correspond to the icon array. In addition, the tool has a section that highlights some pertinent issues regarding statin therapy, but when tested in a randomized trial, the majority of the decision-making process occurred around the issue of risk (Victor Montori MD, oral communication, November 2015). This tool could also be used in medication therapy management encounters to discuss with patients the pros and cons of using a statin medication given their risk.

Finally, decision aids could be template-based. These templates may or may not be decision specific. The templates could either prompt patients to engage in the decision making or prompt clinicians to cover the essential components of shared decision making. A feasibility study using a template-based tool for shared decision making was conducted in medication therapy management encounters focused on mental health and was found to be feasible and acceptable by both patients and pharmacists.

A variety of training programs have been developed to facilitate the adoption of these tools and the general principles of shared decision making. For example, AHRQ has begun holding "train the trainer" workshops for its SHARE approach, a 5-step process for shared decision making: (1) Seek your patient's participating, (2) help your patient explore and compare treatment options, (3) assess your patient's values and preferences, (4) reach a decision with your patient, and (5) evaluate your patient's decision.[40] As of November 2015, only 3.3.% of participants in this program were pharmacists (Michelle Treager PhD, written communication, November 2015), however the hope is that these pharmacists will be training pharmacists at their home institutions in shared decision making.[40] The SHARE approach was developed by AHRQ to support the implementation of shared decision making. In theory, training clinicians would improve the use of shared decision making however, the heterogeneous nature of existing training programs precludes a generalizable conclusion on the effectiveness of training programs.[33]

ENGAGING PATIENTS OUTSIDE THE CLINICAL ENCOUNTER

Shared decision making engages patients in the process of making decisions within the context of a clinical encounter. However, many of the decisions that patients make occur outside of this context, particularly via the Internet and mobile technology. It is estimated that the number of health-related mobile apps is greater than 40,000 varying in target audience (e.g. healthcare professionals, patients, etc.) and functions like clinical decision tools, communication, EHR access, drug information, and more.[41] A Pew Research Center report released in April 2015 reports that 64% of American adults own a smart phone and that 62% of this group use their phone for health-related information.[42] Applications provide the ability for patients and healthcare providers to record, access, store, and share health information in real-time on platforms such as Microsoft's Health Vault. The application and use of choice architecture principles in these mobile health apps are still being explored, but there is little doubt they are and will be relevant in health behaviors and decisions.

BARRIERS TO ENGAGING PATIENTS

While engaging patients in their healthcare is generally seen as a good thing and a step towards more patient-centered care, there are several barriers which make engaging patients in their healthcare challenging.[43] Understanding these barriers and what can be done to overcome them will further facilitate patient engagement.

One the most commonly cited barriers to engaging patients is time. Whether it's a busy clinical practice or a busy community pharmacy, clinicians are pressed for time.[21] However, it is possible that engaging patients may not take additional time and in some cases may even save time. Shared decision making has not been consistently found to take additional time.[28,44] Additionally, research indicates that in primary care consultations a wide variety of topics are covered and not always in a way that is well organized.[45] Tools to facilitate patient engagement and shared decision making may help to better organize the conversation, creating time for more meaningful conversations or may create time to discuss additional topics.

While the barrier of time is universal, what is partially unique to pharmacists is that patients and other professionals may not see a role for pharmacists in engaging patients in their healthcare. Surveys of both patients and physicians have shown mixed support for clinical pharmacy services.[21,46,47] Multiple surveys have shown that the majority of patients supported expanded pharmacy services beyond dispensing.[46,47] A survey out of Canada however found that more people consider themselves customers at the pharmacy rather than patients (65% vs. 15%).[48] Even if patients feel comfortable with pharmacists in roles beyond dispensing they may be too embarrassed to ask the pharmacist a question or feel that it is inappropriate to do so.[49] These feelings are less likely to be present if the patient has a good relationship with the pharmacist.[24]

The physical environment of many community pharmacies does not facilitate engaging patients in meaningful discussions regarding their health and healthcare. Having a calm quiet area to be able to discuss the patient medication-related and other health-related concerns will facilitate pharmacist-patient communication and collaboration.

In addition to the barriers listed above, pharmacists themselves may be uncomfortable engaging patients. Training pharmacists and pharmacy student in communication and how to engage patients and collaborate with them in the management of their health is necessary. In addition, tools to help facilitate pharmacist-patient interactions like those mentioned in this chapter may help to overcome this barrier.

SUMMARY

This chapter began with a general introduction to decision making and then went on to discuss how patients make decisions in response to illness. After covering how different facets of the illness experience affect decision making, contextual factors were briefly covered. Patients carry these experiential and contextual factors with them in the clinical encounter and eliciting, understanding, respecting, and integrating them into the decision making process is a part of person-centered care. Tools to facilitate this process both within and outside the clinical encounter were then presented and common barriers reviewed. The reader should now understand how the patient experience of illness and their context shapes decision making. Further, the reader should be able identify ways to facilitate meaningful conversations around the patient's experience in order to inform decision making and encourage patient engagement in healthcare.

Acknowledgements: The authors gratefully acknowledge Nathaniel Rickles PharmD, PhD, Nicky Britten PhD, Janine Morgall-Traulsen PhD, and Paul Bissell, PhD for their insights on this chapter. Portions of this chapter are based on their work "Patient Decision-Making: Responses to Illness and Treatment" in *Social and Behavioral Aspects of Pharmaceutical Care*, Second Edition, 2010.

REFERENCES

1. Kahneman, D. (2011). *Thinking, fast and slow.* New York: Farrar, Straus, and Giroux. http://www.amazon.com/Thinking-Fast-Slow-Daniel-Kahneman/dp/0374533555. Accessed November 14, 2015.

2. Thaler, R.H. & Sunstein, C.R. (2009). *Nudge: Improving decisions about health, wealth, and happiness.* 2nd ed. New York City: Penguin Group. http://www.amazon.com/Nudge-Improving-Decisions-Health-Happiness/dp/014311526X. Accessed November 14, 2015.

3. Kleinman, A., Eisenberg, L., & Good, B.(1978). Culture, illness, and care: clinical lessons from anthropologic and cross-cultural research. *Ann Intern Med.* 88(2):251–258. http://www.ncbi.nlm.nih.gov/pubmed/626456. Accessed November 11, 2015.

4. Pickering, T.G. (2006). Now we are sick: Labeling and hypertension. *J Clin Hypertens.* 8(1):57–60. doi:10.1111/j.1524-6175.2005.05121.x

5. DiMatteo, M.R., Haskard, K.B., & Williams, S.L. (2007). Health beliefs, disease severity, and patient adherence: a meta-analysis. *Med Care.* 45(6):521–528. doi:10.1097/MLR.0b013e318032937e

6. Horne, R., Chapman, S.C.E., Parham, R., Freemantle, N., Forbes, A., & Cooper, V. (2013). Understanding patients' adherence-related beliefs about medicines prescribed for long-term conditions: a meta-analytic review of the Necessity-Concerns Framework. *PLoS One* 8(12):e80633. doi:10.1371/journal.pone.0080633

7. Halm, E.A., Mora, P., & Leventhal, H. (2006). No symptoms, no asthma: The acute episodic disease belief is associated with poor self-management among inner-city adults with persistent asthma. *Chest* 129(3):573-580. doi:10.1378/chest.129.3.573

8. Bårnes, C.B. & Ulrik, C.S. (2015). Asthma and adherence to inhaled cortico-steroids: current status and future perspectives. *Respir Care* 60(3):455–468. doi:10.4187/respcare.03200

9. Kelly, M.P. & Field, D. (1996). Medical sociology, chronic illness and the body. *Sociol Heal Illn.* 18(2):241–257. doi:10.1111/1467-9566.ep10934993

10. Conrad, P. & Barker, K.K. (2010). The social construction of illness: key insights and policy implications. *J Health Soc Behav.* 51 Suppl(1_suppl):S67–S79. doi:10.1177/0022146510383495

11. Adams, S., Pill, R., & Jones, A. (1997). Medication, chronic illness and identity: The perspective of people with asthma. *Soc Sci Med.* 45(2):189–201. http://www.ncbi.nlm.nih.gov/pubmed/9225407. Accessed November 14, 2015.

12. Hansson Scherman, M. & Löwhagen, O. (2004). Drug compliance and identity: reasons for non-compliance. Experiences of medication from persons with asthma/allergy. *Patient Educ Couns.* 54(1):3–9. doi:10.1016/S0738-3991(03)00199-X

13. Kintner, E. (1997). Adolescent process of coming to accept asthma: a phenomenological study. *J Asthma* 34(6):547–561. http://www.ncbi.nlm.nih.gov/pubmed/9428301. Accessed November 14, 2015.

14. Epstein, R.M. & Peters, E. (2009). Beyond information: exploring patients' preferences. *JAMA* 302(2):195–197. doi:10.1001/jama.2009.984

15. Mintzes, B., Barer, M.L., Kravitz, R.L., et al. (2003). How does direct-to-consumer advertising (DTCA) affect prescribing? A survey in primary care environments with and without legal DTCA. *CMAJ* 169(5):40–412. http://www.pubmedcentral.nih.gov/articlerender.fcgi?artid=183290&tool=pmcentrez&rendertype=abstract. Accessed November 14, 2015.

16. Cockburn, J. & Pit, S.(1997). Prescribing behaviour in clinical practice: patients' expectations and doctors' perceptions of patients' expectations—a questionnaire study. Br *Med J.* 315(30 August):520–523. http://go.galegroup.com/ps/retrieve.do?sort=RELEVANCE&docType=Article&tabID=T002&prodId=EAIM&searchId=R1&resultListType=RESULT_LIST&searchType=AdvancedSearchForm&contentSegment=&currentPosition=1&searchResultsType=SingleTab&inPS=true&userGroupName=umn_wil. Accessed November 14, 2015.

17. Mieg, H. (2006). Social and sociological factors in the development of expertise. In: Ericsson, K. et al. (Eds.), *The Cambridge handbook of expertise and expert performance.* Cambridge, MA: Cambridge University Press.

18. Tuckett, D., Boulton, M., Olson, C., & Williams, A. (1985). *Meeting between experts: An approach to sharing ideas in medical consultations.* London: Tavistock. doi:10.1111/1467-9566.ep11346994

19. Hoffmann, T.C., Montori, V.M., & Del Mar, C. (2014). The connection between evidence-based medicine and shared decision making. *JAMA* 312(13):1295. doi:10.1001/jama.2014.10186

20. Higby, G.J. (2002). The continuing evolution of american pharmacy practice, 1952–2002. *J Am Pharm Assoc.* 42(1):12. doi:10.1331/108658002763538017

21. Schommer, J.C. & Gaither, C.A. (2014). A segmentation analysis for pharmacists' and patients' views of pharmacists' roles. *Res Social Adm Pharm.* 10(3):508–528. doi:10.1016/j.sapharm.2013.10.004

22. Berger, B.A. (1993). Building an effective therapeutic alliance: competence, trustworthiness, and caring. *Am J Hosp Pharm.* 50(11):2399–2403. http://www.ncbi.nlm.nih.gov/pubmed/7818615. Accessed November 14, 2015.

23. Worley, M.M. & Schommer, J.C. (1999). Pharmacist-patient relationships: factors influencing quality and commitment. *J Soc Adm Pharm.* 16(3/4):157–173.

24. Hermansen, C.J. & Wiederholt, J.B. (2001). Pharmacist-patient relationship development in an ambulatory clinic setting. *Health Commun.* 13(3):307–325. doi:10.1207/S15327027HC1303_5

25. Hepler, C.D. & Strand, L.M. (1990). Opportunities and responsibilities in pharmaceutical care. *Am J Hosptial Pharm.* 47:533–534.

26. Charles, C., Gafni, A., & Whelan, T. (1999). Decision-making in the physician-patient encounter: revisiting the shared treatment decision-making model. *Soc Sci Med.* 49(5):651–661. http://www.ncbi.nlm.nih.gov/pubmed/10452420. Accessed November 14, 2015.

27. Elwyn, G., Lloyd, A., May, C., et al.(2014). Collaborative deliberation: a model for patient care. *Patient Educ Couns.* 97(2):158–164. doi:10.1016/j.pec.2014.07.027

28. Stacey, D., Légaré, F., Col, N.F., et al. (2014). Decision aids for people facing health treatment or screening decisions. *Cochrane database Syst Rev.* 1:CD001431. doi:10.1002/14651858.CD001431.pub4

29. Drake, R.E. & Deegan, P.E. (2009). Shared decision making is an ethical imperative. *Psychiatr Serv.* 60(8):1007. doi:10.1176/appi.ps.60.8.1007

30. Elwyn, G., Tilburt, J., & Montori, V. (2013). The ethical imperative for shared decision-making. *Eur J Pers Centered Healthc.* 1(1):129. doi:10.5750/ejpch.v1i1.645

31. Barry, M.J. & Edgman-Levitan, S. (2012). Shared decision making—pinnacle of patient-centered care. *N Engl J Med.* 366(9):780–781. doi:10.1056/NEJMp1109283

32. Légaré, F., Stacey, D., Turcotte, S., et al. (2014). Interventions for improving the adoption of shared decision making by healthcare professionals. *Cochrane database Syst Rev.* 9:CD006732. doi:10.1002/14651858.CD006732.pub3

33. Légaré, F., Politi, M.C., Drolet, R., Desroches, S., Stacey, D., & Bekker, H. (2012). Training health professionals in shared decision-making: an international environmental scan. *Patient Educ Couns.* 88(2):159–169. doi:10.1016/j.pec.2012.01.002

34. Johnson, E.J., Shu, S.B., Dellaert, B.G.C., et al. (2012). Beyond nudges: Tools of a choice architecture. *Mark Lett.* 23(2):487–504. doi:10.1007/s11002-012-9186-1

35. Dartmouth Institute for Health Policy and Clinical Practice. (2015). *Option Grid.* http://optiongrid.org/. Accessed November 14, 2015.

36. Mullan, R.J., Montori, V.M., Shah, N.D., et al. (2009). The diabetes mellitus medication choice decision aid: a randomized trial. *Arch Intern Med.* 169(17):1560–1568. doi:10.1001/archinternmed.2009.293

37. Branda, M.E., LeBlanc, A., Shah, N.D., et al. (2013). Shared decision making for patients with type 2 diabetes: a randomized trial in primary care. *BMC Health Serv Res.* 13(1):301. doi:10.1186/1472-6963-13-301

38. Mann, D.M., Ponieman, D., Montori, V.M., Arciniega, J., & McGinn, T. (2010). The Statin Choice decision aid in primary care: A randomized trial. *Patient Educ Couns.* 80(1):138–140. doi:10.1016/j.pec.2009.10.008

39. Weymiller, A.J., Montori, V.M., Jones, L.A., et al. (2007). Helping patients with type 2 diabetes mellitus make treatment decisions: statin choice randomized trial. *Arch Intern Med.* 2007;167(10):1076–1082. doi:10.1001/archinte.167.10.1076

40. Agency for Healthcare Research and Quality. (2015). SHARE Approach Workshop. *Share Approach Work.* http://www.ahrq.gov/professionals/education/curriculum-tools/shareddecisionmaking/workshop/index.html. Accessed November 10, 2015.

41. Boulos, M.N.K., Brewer, A.C., Karimkhani, C., Buller, D.B., & Dellavalle, R.P.(2014). Mobile medical and health apps: state of the art, concerns, regulatory control and certification. *Online J Public Health Inform.* 5(3):229. doi:10.5210/ojphi.v5i3.4814

42. Pew Research Center. (2015). The smartphone difference. *Pewinternet.org.* http://www.pewinternet.org/files/2015/03/PI_Smartphones_0401151.pdf. Accessed November 14, 2015.

43. Légaré, F., Ratté, S., Gravel, K., & Graham, I.D. (2008). Barriers and facilitators to implementing shared decision-making in clinical practice: update of a systematic review of health professionals' perceptions. *Patient Educ Couns.* 73(3):526–535. doi:10.1016/j.pec.2008.07.018

44. Légaré, F. & Thompson-Leduc, P. (2014). Twelve myths about shared decision making. *Patient Educ Couns.* 96(3):281–286. doi:10.1016/j.pec.2014.06.014

45. Tai-Seale, M., McGuire, T.G., & Zhang, W. (2007). Time allocation in primary care office visits. *Health Serv Res.* 42(5):1871–1894. doi:10.1111/j.1475-6773.2006.00689.x

46. Kelly, D.V., Young, S., Phillips, L., & Clark, D. (2014). Patient attitudes regarding the role of the pharmacist and interest in expanded pharmacist services. *Can Pharm J (Ott).* 147(4):239–247. doi:10.1177/1715163514535731

47. American Pharmacists Association. (2014). How are you perceived by patients and the general public? *pharmacist.com.* http://www.pharmacist.com/how-are-you-perceived-patients-and-general-public. Accessed November 14, 2015.

48. Perepelkin, J. (2011). Public opinion of pharmacists and pharmacist prescribing. *Can Pharm J Rev des Pharm du Canada* 144(2):86–93. http://cph.sagepub.com/content/144/2/86.full.pdf. Accessed November 14, 2015.

49. Chewning, B. & Schommer, J.C. (1996). Increasing clients' knowledge of community pharmacists' roles. *Pharm Res.* 13(9):1299–1304. doi:10.1023/A:1016001428511

INTERPERSONAL COMMUNICATION FOR PATIENT CARE

Lourdes G. Planas and Carol J. Hermansen-Kobulnicky

LEARNING OBJECTIVES:

1. Describe how the functions of interpersonal communication relate to patient care delivery.
2. Discuss the importance of developing rapport with patients and identify strategies a pharmacist can take to build rapport.
3. Identify various reasons for information exchange during the patient care process.
4. Discuss the extent and content of interpersonal communication for patient care services that researchers have measured, such as counseling and drug therapy assessment.
5. Distinguish among individual, interpersonal, and environmental factors associated with patient-pharmacist communication.

KEY TERMS

Consumer medication information

Drug therapy problems

Drug-related needs

Environmental factors

Individual factors

Information exchange

Interpersonal communication

Interpersonal perceptions

Medication therapy management

Open-ended questions

Patient care process

Rapport

Therapeutic relationship

INTRODUCTION

Understanding pharmacist-patient communication is critical for pharmacists to help patients optimize their drug therapy outcomes. The type and extent of communication that can take place between a patient and pharmacist depend on many individual, interpersonal, and environmental factors. For example, what attitudes about patient counseling does the pharmacist possess? What kind of communication does the patient expect from the pharmacist? How does the pharmacist's work setting facilitate or hinder communication?

This chapter introduces key issues pertaining to interpersonal communication for patient care. Specific issues examined are:

- the nature and significance of interpersonal communication for patient care;
- the extent of interpersonal communication for patient care; and
- factors that influence interpersonal communication for patient care.

It is important to be aware of these issues because interpersonal communication is a fundamental social and behavioral aspect of patient care.

NATURE OF PHARMACIST-PATIENT INTERPERSONAL COMMUNICATION FOR PATIENT CARE

Effective interpersonal communication is vital for patient care. It is essential in pharmacist-patient interactions to (1) establish rapport, (2) build therapeutic relationships, (3) promote dialogue for accurate information exchange, and (4) implement a patient care process by engaging patients in collaborative problem solving to identify, resolve, and prevent drug therapy problems (DTPs). Figure 10-1 depicts the interplay of these four behaviors at the intersections of interpersonal communication, patient-centeredness, problem solving, and patient care. In this figure and chapter, patient care, and specifically pharmacist-provided patient care is defined

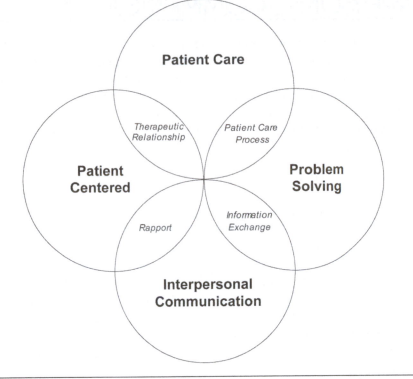

Patient Care

Therapeutic Relationship

Patient Care Process

Patient Centered

Problem Solving

Rapport

Information Exchange

Interpersonal Communication

FIGURE 10-1. NATURE OF INTERPERSONAL COMMUNICATION IN PATIENT CARE

using pharmaceutical care practice as a framework. Pharmaceutical care practice is "a practice in which the practitioner takes responsibility for a patient's drug-related needs, and is held accountable for this commitment."[1]

Interpersonal communication in patient care serves two basic functions: (1) establish rapport and (2) promote information exchange (see the bottom of Figure 10-1). Moving up the left side of the figure, we see that establishing rapport with patients using a patient-centered approach is instrumental to building a therapeutic relationship. A therapeutic relationship is a collaborative alliance between a patient and a provider for the purpose of optimizing the patient's medication experience and outcomes.[1] Moving up the right side of Figure 10-1, we see that information exchange between a patient and pharmacist for the purpose of problem solving is instrumental to implement the patient care process, in which a pharmacist (in collaboration with a patient and other health care professionals) collects and assesses patient information, develops and implements an individualized patient-centered plan, and monitors, evaluates, and modifies the plan as needed.[2] Building a therapeutic relationship with patients and implementing the patient care process are the primary provider roles in patient care practice (see the top of Figure 10-1).[1]

In the next three sections of the chapter, we will further examine elements appearing in Figure 10-1. All of these elements contribute to the social and behavioral nature and significance of interpersonal communication for patient care.

INTERPERSONAL COMMUNICATION

Interpersonal communication involves interaction between two people. A basic model used to understand communication is presented in Figure 10-2.[3,4] The model includes five elements: sender, receiver, message, feedback, and barriers. In the process, a sender encodes and transmits a message to a receiver, who then decodes and receives the message. For effective communication to occur, the receiver must assign the same meaning as the sender intended. The receiver assigns meaning based on his or her experiences, definitions, and knowledge.

The message is the element that is transmitted from the sender to the receiver. In pharmacy, for example, this may be information directed to a patient (receiver) about how to use a medication (from the pharmacist as sender) or it could be a question asked by a patient (sender) to a pharmacist (receiver). Messages are transmitted verbally using words via spoken or written language and nonverbally (without words). Nonverbal communication includes eye contact, facial expressions, gestures, posture, proximity (distance between two people), and paralanguage (tone, volume, inflection). The majority of messages that people send are nonverbal in nature, ranging from approximately 55% to 93%.[5,6] Nonverbal communication is not always done consciously, for example, body language is typically a reflection of a person's emotions or emotional state.[7] What we mean to communicate is not always what is ultimately conveyed, in part, due to incongruity of verbal and nonverbal messages. If the words do not match the tone or behavior, typically it is the tone or behavior (the nonverbal components) that are believed.[7] An example of an incongruent message would be stating you agree ("Yes, that will work") while looking down and shaking your head from side to side (indicating "No, it won't work").

Feedback is the process by which the receiver transmits his or her understanding of the message back to the sender. During feedback, the receiver and sender switch

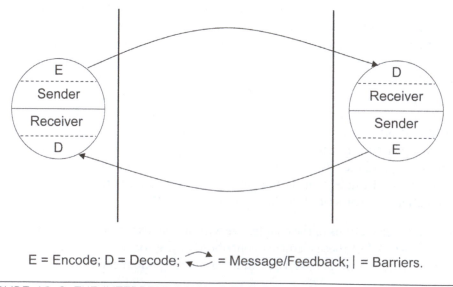

E = Encode; D = Decode; 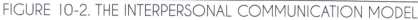 = Message/Feedback; | = Barriers.

FIGURE 10-2. THE INTERPERSONAL COMMUNICATION MODEL

roles. Feedback can range from a simple head nod to repeating back a set of medication instructions. Feedback is crucial for effective communication and mutual understanding because it permits the sender and receiver to confirm the accuracy of the message.

An example of feedback important to patient safety is "Check-Back," a tool used to close the communication loop among professionals, including pharmacists.[8] The key to using Check-Back successfully is to ensure the sender of the message verifies from the receiver that the message was not only received, but also accepted, understood, and/or confirmed. Without this verification, some say communication does not truly take place, as one does not know if the intended message was received. Although seemingly simple, it is a critical tool to use in healthcare. A common usage for pharmacists is when receiving a verbal prescription order. In this example, the pharmacist systematically uses Check-Back to verify each part of the order.

Barriers in the communication process can distort messages and cause misunderstandings. There are two major categories of barriers: personal and environmental. Each category consists of many types of barriers (Table 10-1). Some barriers are obvious (e.g., loud background noise), while others are not (e.g., the patient having a previous unpleasant encounter with another pharmacist). Likewise, some barriers are easier than others to minimize or overcome. For example, a pharmacist may feel rushed and speak in a hurried tone. Although not intentional, a patient might interpret the pharmacist's tone as disinterest in the patient. Overcoming this type of barrier may require a reworking of the environment or work flow processes, or it may simply require the pharmacist to stop and take a breath before speaking.

TABLE 10-1 COMMON INTERPERSONAL COMMUNICATION BARRIERS IN PHARMACIST-PATIENT INTERACTIONS

CATEGORY	TYPE	EXAMPLE
PERSONAL	PSYCHOLOGICAL	EMOTIONAL STATE (E.G., RUSHED)
	Internal noise	Competing thoughts
	Social	Lack of prior relationship
	Historical	Previous unpleasant encounter
	Cultural	Differences in use of eye contact
	Semantic	Not understanding words (e.g., medical terms)
ENVIRONMENTAL	PHYSICAL	HIGH PRESCRIPTION COUNTER
	Setting	Lack of private area
	External noise	Phones ringing

Adapted from Mehrabian A. Silent messages. *Belmont, CA: Wadsworth, 1971.*

The model presented in Figure 10-2 emphasizes the dynamic and transactional nature of interpersonal communication by acknowledging that messages and feedback are sent simultaneously between sender and receiver. When acting as a sender, pharmacists should send messages in their clearest form and ask for feedback to determine if the message was received as intended. This could include verifying the patient can hear the pharmacist or read the font size of the written materials. Likewise, when acting as a receiver, pharmacists should offer feedback to check if they understood the message as intended from the sender. An example of this would be paraphrasing what the patient has said when explaining the culturally-related conflict the patient has with fasting while taking the medication. These activities make communication a two-way process intended to establish shared meaning. It is important to anticipate potential barriers and develop strategies to minimize them so that effective communication can occur. One way to overcome communication barriers is to develop rapport with patients.

RAPPORT FOR BUILDING THERAPEUTIC RELATIONSHIPS

Rapport is an interpersonal communication component that, through a patient-centered approach, is instrumental to building a therapeutic relationship (see left portion of Figure 10-1, moving upward). The American Heritage Dictionary defines rapport as "a relationship, especially one of mutual trust or emotional affinity."[9] Rapport is synonymous with "understanding." A pharmacist who establishes rapport with a patient, therefore, attempts to relate to a patient's needs and experiences while developing trust and a positive emotional bond.

LISTENING AND EMPATHY

Two major interpersonal communication behaviors for developing rapport with patients are listening and empathic responding. Listening is less well-developed communication skill for most, yet it is the most frequently needed communication skill. Of our time spent communicating, approximately half is spent listening, while the remaining time is divided between talking, reading, and writing.[10,11] Effective listening is not listening with the intent to reply, but rather listening with the intent to understand.[12]

Effective listening can be passive or active. In passive listening, we remain silent using nonverbal communication and minimal words such as "yes" or "okay." Active listening involves paraphrasing or summarizing our understanding of the sender's message and reflecting it back for verification. This verification or feedback process enhances our ability to decode the sender's message in a way that is intended to be congruent with what was said. Also, our reflection to the sender of what they conveyed can help the sender feel understood. Feeling understood by a health care provider can lessen patients' negative emotions that accompany illness and health care experiences. This is evidenced by the positive relationship between patient-centered communication and patient satisfaction in the medical literature.[13]

Empathic responding is another interpersonal communication behavior that helps develop rapport. Patients communicate how they feel, whether verbal or nonverbal, in the messages they send. Expressing empathy is acknowledging the feelings, attitudes, and thoughts of another. It involves taking the other person's perspective by imagining yourself in their situation.[14] Empathic responses are free from judgment and advice. The main characteristic that distinguishes empathy from active listening is that an empathic response acknowledges emotion and content (e.g., the reason for the emotion), while active listening primarily paraphrases or summarizes content without including emotion. An example of an empathic response is a pharmacist saying, "You're discouraged [emotion] because your doctor prescribed more medications for you [reason for the emotion]."

OTHER WAYS TO DEVELOP RAPPORT WITH PATIENTS

In addition to listening and expressing empathy, there are other ways to develop rapport with patients and to therefore, create an atmosphere conducive to developing an understanding of their needs and preferences. These include, but are not limited to, using the patient's name and clarifying expectations for the patient encounter.[15] Also, rapport can be built by validating the thoughts and opinions of the other person. To achieve this in a patient care context, the pharmacist can foster a dialogue by not interrupting, by inviting questions and concerns from the patient, and by being sensitive to cultural differences and any other patient needs that may be influenced by how and what the pharmacist communicates. Nonverbal behaviors are also critical components of communication that should not be overlooked when attempting to build rapport. For example, while conversing with a patient face-to-face, it is important to use eye contact about 50% or 70% percent of the time, respectively, depending on whether speaking or listening, respectively. It is also important to note that cultural groups use eye contact differently from each other. Having an open stance by leaning in towards the patient and being careful not to fold one's arms across the chest can help to show you are open to, and not disinterested in, what is being said.

Active listening and empathy along with other easily incorporated strategies to build rapport with patients can help patients feel understood and able to trust a pharmacist as someone who genuinely cares about them. Rapport between a patient and a pharmacist is necessary for patient-centered care. The dimensions of patient-centered care have been identified as: understanding a patient's illness experience, perceiving each patient as unique, fostering an egalitarian relationship with a patient, building a therapeutic alliance with a patient, and developing self-awareness of one's personal effects on patients.[16] Consistent with these dimensions, a central tenet of patient-centered care is involving patients in the decision-making process to meet therapeutic goals that they and their healthcare providers endorse. It has even been suggested that rapport building may be just as valuable, if not more, than the discussion of options when involving patients in the decision-making process.[17] Similarly, asking open-ended questions and having personal dialogue with patients establishes patient loyalty.[18] Establishing rapport is a foundation for building a therapeutic relationship.

THERAPEUTIC RELATIONSHIP

In their influential work, Hepler and Strand defined a therapeutic relationship as "a mutually beneficial exchange in which the patient grants authority to the provider and the provider gives competence and commitment (accepts responsibility) to the patient."[19] They characterized this relationship as a covenant, or a solemn and binding agreement between patient and provider.[20] One of the most important outcomes of a therapeutic relationship between a patient and a provider is shared decision-making towards goals of therapy. This is accomplished with greater patient involvement through trust, dialogue, and collaboration. Thus, pharmacists who build therapeutic relationships with patients are able to elicit more information necessary to help patients with their medications.[1]

INFORMATION EXCHANGE FOR PATIENT CARE PROCESS

The right side of Figure 10-1 portrays information exchange as an interpersonal communication component which, when conducted for the purpose of problem solving, is instrumental to the patient care process. Information exchange denotes a back-and-forth pattern of communication between patient and provider. In the context of performing the patient care process, information exchange is used to: (1) collect patient-specific information, (2) assess drug-related needs in order to identify DTPs; (3) develop and (4) implement a care plan that includes goals of therapy and interventions to prevent or resolve DTPs; and (5) perform a follow-up to compare patient outcomes to goals of therapy, evaluate interventions, and assess the patient for any new DTPs.[1,2]

INDIAN HEALTH SERVICE MODEL OF PHARMACIST-PATIENT CONSULTATION

The most widely-used model for counseling patients about their medications is an example of information exchange in action. These techniques developed by the Indian Health Service (IHS) are widely known in pharmacy.[21-23] The IHS patient counseling approach consists of three steps: (1) assess the patient's knowledge about medication, (2) provide information to supplement patient's knowledge, and (3) verify the patient's recall and understanding. The ultimate goals are to ensure patients understand how to use and what to expect from their medications. Expanding on this, the questions can be used to improve the quality of information exchanged to help prepare patients to make appropriate decisions regarding their drug therapy. In this section of the chapter, we will describe how this approach has been traditionally used as well as how an expanded application can enhance the patient care process.

Using the IHS patient counseling approach, pharmacists ask a series of prime questions to ascertain what patients know about their medication: What did your doctor tell you the medication is for? How did your doctor tell you to take/use the medication? What did your doctor tell you to expect from the medication? These questions are among those listed in the first column of Table 10-2. Based on a patient's answer to each prime question and any necessary follow-up questions, the pharmacist provides information to assure adequate patient knowledge (second column of Table 10-2). At the conclusion of the prime question-answer-information sequences, the pharmacist asks the patient to repeat the most pertinent information. This last step in the IHS patient counseling approach is a form of feedback that enables the pharmacist to check that the patient recalls what has been discussed. The IHS refers to it as the "Final Verification;"[21-23] however, others refer to this same idea of verifying recall and understanding as "Teach-back."[24]

TABLE 10-2: INFORMATION EXCHANGE TO ASSESS PATIENT KNOWLEDGE, PROVIDE DRUG INFORMATION, AND IDENTIFY DRUG THERAPY PROBLEMS

EXAMPLE QUESTIONS TO ASSESS PATIENT KNOWLEDGE OF NEW DRUG THERAPY	DRUG INFORMATION TO PROVIDE TO SUPPLEMENT PATIENT KNOWLEDGE AND NEEDS[2,3]	DRUG-RELATED NEED[1]	POTENTIAL DRUG THERAPY PROBLEM[1]	ASSESS DRUG THERAPY PROBLEMS AFTER PATIENT HAS INITIATED DRUG THERAPY[1,26]
What did your doctor tell you the medication is for?[21] What will you take the medication for?	Purpose of medication	Appropriate	1. Unnecessary drug therapy 2. Additional drug therapy needed	Assess whether every medication has an appropriate indication; if any therapeutic duplications exist; and if the patient has an untreated indication that would benefit from new pharmacological therapy, or a treated indication that would benefit from adjunct therapy.
What did your doctor tell you to expect?[21] How will you know the medication is working?	Techniques and specific criteria for self-monitoring of response Benefits of medication (short-term, long-term)	Effective	3. Ineffective drug 4. Dosage too low	Assess patient perceptions of effectiveness (including long-term benefits and/or risk minimization); how condition is being monitored by patient and/or physician, and results of monitoring from each; whether the medication is the most effective for the patient; and whether the dose, frequency, or duration of drug therapy is too low to produce the desired response or outcome.
What did your doctor tell you to expect?[21] What possible side effects will you watch for? What should you do if you experience a specific side effect?	Common or potentially dangerous side effects; symptoms, frequency, duration, and severity What to do to avoid or manage side effects, when to contact physician or pharmacist Precautions for use	Safe	5. Adverse drug reaction 6. Dosage too high	Assess signs and symptoms of adverse effects and toxicity, and what the patient has been doing to avoid or manage these; and whether the dose, frequency, or duration of drug therapy is too high and producing undesirable toxic effects.
How did your doctor tell you to take/use the medication?[21] Tell me in your own words how you will take/use this medicine.	Dosage (e.g., 1 tablet, 2 capsules) Dosage schedule that fits patient routine How to take What to do if a dose is missed Duration of use Proper preparation and storage	Adherence	7. Nonadherence	Assess how patient is taking/using each medication (e.g., times of day; number of doses missed in a typical week and reasons for missed doses; frequency of use and maximum doses in fixed interval of "as needed" medications; patient demonstration of use of drug delivery devices such as inhalers).

DRUG-RELATED NEEDS AND DRUG THERAPY PROBLEMS

The three IHS prime questions encompass four drug-related needs that patients have (i.e., drug therapy is *appropriate, effective, safe,* and the patient is able and willing to *adhere* to the regimen; third column of Table 10-2).[1] The IHS prime questions regarding purpose of the medication and how to take/use the medication correspond to appropriateness and adherence, respectively. The question regarding what to expect addresses the two remaining needs, effectiveness and safety. Each of these four drug-related needs, if not appropriately fulfilled, can result in a drug therapy problem (DTP) (fourth column of Table 10-2).[1,25]

The final column of the table lists important factors about which to inquire when assessing for DTPs *after* a patient has initiated drug therapy.[1,26] For example, informing a patient about what to expect from his medication in terms of effectiveness, instructing him how to monitor his response, and helping him to set goals for his therapy can empower him to know whether the medication is working as intended. Through monitoring parameters of effectiveness (e.g., blood pressure), a patient can detect a lack of medication effectiveness that may be due to a DTP associated with a suboptimal dosage (e.g., dosage too low) or because the medication is not the most effective one for this patient (e.g., ineffective drug). Unless a patient understands how to monitor his response to treatment, he may not be able to assist with the detection of this type of DTP. Additionally, educating a patient about how to take his medication, including how to best fit a prescribed regimen into his daily routine, instructing him about what to do when he misses a dose, and discussing the duration of use (e.g., chronic) may encourage adherence. Through monitoring how a patient is taking his medication, such as by assessing the number of, and reasons, for missed doses, a pharmacist can identify and address a DTP of nonadherence. In essence, the information exchange that occurs during the IHS patient counseling approach during an initial or subsequent dispensing can foster problem solving to identify potential DTPs and prevent or reduce their occurrence.

PATIENT CARE PROCESS

The patient care process is comprised of five steps: (1) collect information, (2) assess information, (3) develop care plan, (4) implement care plan, and (5) follow-up evaluation. It is a comprehensive and systematic problem solving process.[1,2] The purposes of this process are to attain the most appropriate, effective, safe, and convenient drug therapy for the patient; to identify, resolve, and prevent any DTPs that could interfere with this attainment; and to ensure positive patient outcomes.

During the collection and assessment steps of the patient care process, a pharmacist explores a patient's drug-related needs.[1] This includes asking questions to ascertain what the patient wants, does not want, and knows about his drug therapy. A comprehensive assessment for the DTPs listed in Table 10-2 is also performed, which can include modifications of the IHS prime questions. To assess drug therapy appropriateness, a pharmacist can ask for what purpose each medication is being taken. This questioning helps not only to identify gaps in the patient's knowledge; it also can complement the pharmacist's own understanding of the patient's medication use to identify unnecessary drug therapy, such as therapeutic duplications. A modification of the prime question pertaining to medication use can be used to assess how the patient is *actually* taking his medication (e.g., "How do you take the medication?"). The prime question regarding what to expect can be divided into two separate questions addressing safety and effectiveness. Patients can be questioned about the incidence and severity of adverse effects. Additionally, they can be asked about their response to treatment, especially with regard to achieving therapeutic goals. Examples of question adaptations include: "What problems have you had with the medication?" and "How do you know if the medication is working?"

The third and fourth steps of the patient care process involve the care plan.[1] During these steps, a patient and pharmacist collaborate to establish a list of possible actions to address all drug-related needs and DTPs. Based on a patient's preferences and guided by a pharmacist's expertise, clinical guidelines, and other evidence in the literature, the most appropriate interventions are selected. Additionally, therapeutic goals are set in conjunction with a patient's needs and values. The planned resolution of DTPs in a care plan is important because these problems can interfere with patients achieving desired therapeutic goals. Care plans should also prevent potential DTPs that can minimize the probability of the patient attaining therapeutic goals.

The final step of the patient care process is the follow-up evaluation during which the pharmacist assumes responsibility for a patient's drug therapy outcomes. The follow-up evaluation is conducted to determine the extent of intervention success, if therapeutic goals were met, and if any new DTPs have developed.[1] A pharmacist's involvement in the follow-up evaluation is proactive. In re-assessing for DTPs, the process begins again. Thus, the patient care process is a continuous collaborative communication process with the follow-up evaluation providing important feedback.

SUMMARY

At its most basic level, information exchange is a dialogue: a series of questions and answers between two individuals. Such information exchange can occur during more formalized appointments between pharmacists and patients or more informally while a patient is receiving a refill medication. In the context of problem solving, it becomes a means to assess a patient's drug-related needs and ensure he understands how to use his medication. In the previously discussed context of patient care (right side of Figure 10-1), the patient care process is a comprehensive and systematic problem solving process that relies heavily on effective information exchange between a pharmacist and patient.

Feedback is crucial in many aspects of interpersonal communication for patient care and is necessary for mutual understanding in the interpersonal communication process. Listening and empathy are forms of feedback to help patients feel understood and to enhance rapport. Verifying that a patient understands aspects of his drug therapy and effectively adapting one's communication to a patient's needs are accomplished by eliciting feedback from the patient. Lastly, the patient care process becomes a continuous process when follow-up evaluations are conducted to receive feedback on the success of interventions and the achievement of therapeutic goals.

THE PAST AND CURRENT STATE OF PHARMACIST-PATIENT COMMUNICATION

The pharmacy profession has undergone a major evolution since the latter part of the 20th century, most notably the clinical pharmacy and pharmaceutical care eras.[19,27] While the social, ethical, and professional roles of pharmacists have changed, so has the extent of interpersonal communication, specifically pharmacist-patient communication. The more that pharmacists accept responsibility for patients' drug-related needs and are held accountable for this commitment,[1] the greater the extent of and importance of interpersonal communication that is required between the pharmacist and patient.

PATIENT COUNSELING

HISTORICAL CONTEXT

In 1952, the Pharmacist Code of Ethics stated, "The pharmacist does not discuss the therapeutic effect or composition of a prescription with a patient."[28] More than 20 years later, change was occurring. The student group of the American Pharmacists Association (APhA), now the Academy of Student Pharmacists (ASP), adopted a resolution stating "APhA-ASP embraces an active role in further educating the public about the professional health care role of the pharmacist and in informing the patient how to effectively analyze and understand the information on prescription and nonprescription drugs."[29] This is one of the earliest policy statements acknowledging the importance of pharmacists communicating with patients. A few years later in 1977, APhA adopted policy statements that explicitly state the professional obligation of pharmacists to educate patients face-to-face about their prescription medications to optimize drug therapy.[30]

More than a decade later, an important event for pharmacy was the implementation of the Omnibus Budget Reconciliation Act of 1990 (OBRA '90). A stipulation in this act requires pharmacists to offer to counsel Medicaid recipients about their new prescriptions and to conduct prospective drug utilization reviews.[31] Since its implementation in 1993, most states have expanded state regulations to include all patients receiving new prescriptions.

EXTENT OF PATIENT COUNSELING

Before 1974, pharmacist-patient communication was not well documented or studied. Between 1974 and 1993, in the decades following the profession's acknowledgement of this important role, researchers sought to quantify the percentage of patients receiving counseling and information from pharmacists, focusing on community pharmacy practice. Using direct observation, mock patients (secret shoppers posing as patients), and mail surveys, studies reported 20–40% of patients who received a prescription also received oral (spoken) counseling from a pharmacist.[32-37]

There appears to have been an upward trend in the occurrence of patient counseling in community pharmacies since the implementation of OBRA '90, however, variations exist. Studies published between 1995 and 2006 using patient surveys, mock patients, and direct observation of interactions have reported counseling occurring in approximately 57–70% of pharmacist-patient encounters.[38–43] In more recent secret shopper studies involving new prescription dispensing, counseling was reported in only 42–43% of observed pharmacist-patient encounters.[44,45] However, in a 2014 observational study, pharmacy personnel offered to counsel 100% during the over 2000 pharmacist-patient encounters involving both new and refilled prescriptions, with 89% of patients having accepted the offer to be counseled.[43] The differences in these numbers (42% versus 89%) are notable and may have been influenced by both state regulations and the research methods used.

CONTENT OF PATIENT COUNSELING

In addition to studying the occurrence of patient counseling, some studies have observed the content of communication between pharmacists and patients. The most common types of information relayed to patients are directions for medication use[36,46] and side effects,[36] as well as the purpose of the medication, and solicitation of feedback and administrative (also referred to as "technical") elements such as generic substitutions or price.[46] Research into what types of information patients desire when receiving a new prescription reveal the top three being side effects, directions for use, and information about interactions.[47,48] A discrepancy is found when comparing these two lists; information about interactions, although desired by patients, is not commonly provided by pharmacists.

By asking questions, a patient can receive additional information not volunteered by the pharmacist. Indeed, research into patients' question-asking behaviors show that when patients ask community pharmacists questions, compared to when they do not, patients are more likely to receive information about contraindications, how the medication works, what it replaces ("continuity of therapy"), generic substitution availability, price, and refill renewals ("administrative elements").[46] Because few of these topics are traditionally included during a consultation, when a patient asks a question, it can clearly make the encounter more patient-centered. Thus, inviting questions from patients is likely to alter the content of the information exchange.

Another important way to influence information exchange and build rapport is to evoke the patient's perspective by asking questions of patients. Doing so elicits patient input and ideas, and improves the likelihood of providing patient-centered care. A study of community pharmacies in New Mexico observed pharmacists asking patients questions in 36% of encounters,[40] with more than one drug therapy question being asked in only 6% of these encounters. Open-ended questions were asked in only 7% of observed encounters. This is notable when one considers the need for questions to assess the major types of DTPs.

Open-ended questions convey a willingness to listen and increase patient participation, and thus provide a more patient-centered approach. In contrast, closed-ended questions reduce a patient's degree of openness and increase passivity.[49] For example, asking, "Do you have any questions?" is a closed-ended question that is more easily answered as "no" while asking an open-ended question such as "What questions do you have?" offers an opportunity for the patient to voice their questions or concerns.

WRITTEN PRESCRIPTION INFORMATION

Written prescription information, also known as Consumer Medication Information (CMI), is an important component of communicating with patients. Growing numbers of CMI are required to be Medication Guides (MedGuides) to more adequately address the higher risks of certain drug products.[50] Written prescription information is intended to supplement and/or complement, not replace, oral patient counseling. Over the past three decades, the percentage of patients who receive written prescription information has increased from 15% to 59% in 1982 and 1994,[38] respectively, to about 89% between 1999 and 2001.[51–53] In two secret shopper studies, 94–100% of shoppers received CMI when dispensed a new prescription drug.[44,54]

Pharmacists would do well to use CMI and MedGuides, where applicable, to start important conversations about benefits and risks (e.g., side effects) of prescription medication use. To date, little has been done to test the best approach to use written information during an oral consultation. Future research is needed to ascertain the most effective means to share this information with patients and to improve patient engagement in the exchange, and the knowledge gained and used by patients.

Providing patient counseling and written information can help to ensure patients understand important aspects of their medications for informed treatment decision-making and problem-solving. Most patient counseling encounters focus on providing information for the immediately prescribed medication. What happens when the patient begins taking the medication? How effective is it? What problems are experienced? How well is the patient able to adhere to the regimen? These questions are answered when pharmacists take the time to speak with patients to identify, resolve, and prevent DTPs that interfere with achieving therapeutic goals. Patient counseling and written prescription information are useful communication tools. They alone, however, do not comprise all necessary pharmacist-patient communication to deliver patient care intended to help patients optimize their medication use and outcomes.

EXPANDING BEYOND PATIENT COUNSELING

The extent of pharmacist-provided patient care, including medication therapy management (MTM) services, is summarized in this section. MTM services provide direct patient care opportunities requiring pharmacist-patient communication. The Medicare Modernization Act of 2003 specifies that pharmacists or other qualified healthcare practitioners provide MTM services for eligible patients enrolled in the Medicare prescription drug benefit.[55] MTM is a strategy that incorporates the philosophy of pharmaceutical care and the patient care process into pharmacy practice for a defined patient population.[2,56] The core elements of an MTM service are designed to, among other things, improve care and enhance communication among patients and pharmacists in community pharmacies.[57] Under Medicare Part D, these services require an interactive one-on-one discussion with the patient to complete an annual Comprehensive Medication Review with quarterly Targeted Medication Reviews, with subsequent person-to-person follow-up preferred.[58]

In this section we first describe pharmacists' self-reports of performing specific patient care activities. Measures of patient care activities vary, but generally include screening patient profiles, patient counseling, patient-oriented DTP identification and solving, and documentation. Second, we examine DTPs identified in studies that specifically sought to implement and evaluate patient care practices. Because the patient care process is a comprehensive problem solving process, investigating the extent of DTP identification in intervention studies is also a marker of patient care provision. Examining the types of DTPs that are commonly identified and comparing this to the types of DTPs that require more direct pharmacist-patient communication offer insight into the extent of interpersonal communication that occurs in patient care practices.

PHARMACIST-PROVIDED PATIENT CARE

The extent of patient care provided by pharmacists primarily has been studied using surveys and claims analyses. Several of these studies are summarized next.

Research looking at the impact of MTM services on pharmacist-patient communication reveals a positive impact. Studies show patients are very satisfied with the MTM-based interactions they have with pharmacists[59-61] and that patients believe a benefit of MTM is improved communication with their pharmacists.[61] Future observational research is needed to examine the quality of pharmacist-patient communication during a Comprehensive Medication Review interview, for example, or during Targeted Medication Review follow-up discussions with patients. With the lack of reimbursement being a notable barrier to providing services such as MTM, it is important to recognize that the potential for pharmacists to bill for these types of services is greater now than at any other time in the profession's history.[62]

During the years after implementation of OBRA '90 and before the Medicare Modernization Act, community pharmacist activities in assessment, monitoring, and documentation were generally low. Researchers in Florida surveyed community pharmacists about their implementation of pharmaceutical care services.[63] Respondents reported moderate levels of patient record screening, patient consultation, and verification of patient understanding. They reported very low levels of patient assessment, implementation of therapeutic objectives and monitoring plans, and documentation. The extent of pharmaceutical care provision in West Virginia rural community practices was determined by surveying pharmacy owners and managers.[64] Activities that respondents indicated performing most frequently pertained to patient communication, reviewing patients' medication profiles, and obtaining and maintaining patient information. Drug therapy monitoring, which included medication adherence, therapeutic effect, and adverse effects, was the least frequently reported activity. Although 30% of North Carolina pharmacists responding to a mail survey indicated they provided pharmaceutical care services, only 20% indicated ensuring appropriate pharmacotherapy, ensuring patients' understanding of and adherence to their treatment, and monitoring and reporting outcomes.[65]

Based on analyses of MTM services provided by community pharmacists in 47 states between 2000 and 2006, interventions have evolved from patient education regarding medications for acute illnesses to consultation-type services with prescribers regarding chronic medications, as well as a higher proportion of older patients.[66] Since 2007, the APhA has conducted annual national surveys of pharmacists involved in patient care services. Between 63% and 79% of pharmacists have reported providing MTM services, with an upward trend when year-to-year percentages are compared.[67-73] In 2013, a majority of these pharmacists indicated they often or always conduct a comprehensive medication review, create a personal medication record/list, develop a patient medication-related action plan, provide interventions/recommendations to providers, and maintain documentation.[74] These increases from previous years in assessment, monitoring, and documentation activities are notable; however, the pharmacists who responded to the APhA surveys are not representative of all pharmacists.

As these studies demonstrate, patient care implementation by community pharmacists has increased since the latter part of the 20th century. Previously, activities that were distinct to patient care and MTM services were performed less frequently than those that are more in line with OBRA '90 (i.e., screening patients' medication records and counseling them about their medications).[31] Much of this increase is likely due to MTM's focus on monitoring activities to identify and resolve DTPs.

AMOUNTS AND TYPES OF DRUG THERAPY PROBLEMS

In addition to pharmacists' self-reports, the extent of pharmaceutical care provision in studies in which pharmaceutical care services are implemented can be measured by the number of DTPs. In many instances, DTP identification, resolution, and follow-up evaluation rely on pharmacist-patient communication (e.g., medication history, assessing patient's response to treatment).

For example, screening patients' medication records for drug-drug interactions or therapeutic duplications requires very little pharmacist-patient communication. In contrast, interviewing patients about their response to treatment or presence of symptoms requires more information exchange and direct patient contact (e.g., suboptimal response due to a low dosage, needing an additional medication prescribed for an untreated indication, or nonadherence).

Pharmaceutical care intervention studies that have measured the numbers of identified and resolved DTPs report an average of about two to three DTPs per patient per year.[75-84] With regard to types of DTPs, under-treatment appears to be a prevalent problem. Consistently, the three most common types of DTPs identified tend to be needing additional drug therapy, low dosage, and nonadherence (Table 10-3). For example, a patient with hypertension whose blood pressure is not at goal may require an additional medication to be added to his regimen (i.e., additional drug therapy) or a dosage increase of a medication he is currently taking (i.e., low dosage). Additionally, a patient may have a suboptimal response due to not taking a medication as prescribed (i.e., nonadherence).

TABLE 10-3 TYPE AND PERCENTAGE OF DRUG THERAPY PROBLEMS IDENTIFIED IN PATIENT CARE STUDIES

APPROPRIATE	ISETTS ET AL.[80] (2008)	HARRIS ET AL.[81] (2009)	CONNOR ET AL.[82] (2009)	WITRY ET AL.[83] (2011)	ISETTS ET AL.[84] (2012)
Unnecessary drug therapy	6.0	2.0	8.0	14.2	5.0
Need additional drug therapy	33.9	49.6	22.9	30.1	21.2
EFFECTIVE					
Ineffective drug	11.6	4.4	0	8.4	7.3
Dosage too low	19.9	13.2	6.9	6.7	30.2
SAFE					
Adverse drug reaction	14.4	8.0	3.7	19.2	8.3
Dosage too high	4.9	5.2	1.6	3.7	8.0
ADHERENCE					
Nonadherence	9.6	17.6	55.3	17.6	20.0
TOTAL NUMBER OF DRUG THERAPY PROBLEMS PER PATIENT PER YEAR	2.2	3.0	1.7	1.5	3.8

The identification of these most common types of DTPs typically requires direct pharmacist-patient communication. These DTPs cannot be identified by merely screening a patient's medication profile, which requires little, if any, pharmacist-patient communication. Furthermore, monitoring of the resolution of these types of DTPs usually requires asking patients about their treatment response and medication adherence. In most community pharmacies, these are best accomplished by talking with patients. Medication refill dates in a patient's profile can provide an estimate of adherence. Late refill dates have been shown to predict pharmacist self-report of initiating discussion with patients about adherence;[85] however, speaking with a patient can uncover issues such as reasons for nonadherence and preferred solutions. Such communication could be initiated by the pharmacist when dispensing a refill using any discussion of "technical" topics such as cost or manufacturer changes.[86] This approach seems feasible with estimates of two-thirds of patients receiving refills wanting some type of information from the pharmacist,[48] and yet it would likely need to be implemented proactively and systematically due to the routine nature of refill dispensing.[86]

The last half-century has seen an evolution of pharmacist-patient communication, especially in the contexts of patient counseling and pharmaceutical care. The need for effective interpersonal communication between pharmacists and patients is expected to increase as more pharmacists move toward patient-centered care. Understanding factors associated with interpersonal communication for patient care can help improve its expansion. Such factors are discussed in the following section.

FACTORS ASSOCIATED WITH INTERPERSONAL COMMUNICATION FOR PATIENT CARE

Many factors influence pharmacist-patient communication. These factors can be divided into three types: individual, interpersonal, and environmental.

INDIVIDUAL FACTORS

PHARMACISTS

Factors that influence interpersonal communication for pharmacist-provided patient care include attitudes, self-efficacy beliefs, perceived behavioral control, and perceived responsibility of individual pharmacists. The word "perceived" appears in some of these terms because the influencing factor is an individual's report of his or her *perception*, which can vary among individuals in spite of similar circumstances.

An attitude is "a learned predisposition to respond in a consistently favorable or unfavorable manner with respect to a given object."[87] Attitudes can be measured as the sum of beliefs about the consequences of performing a behavior in which each belief is weighed by one's evaluations of these consequences.[87] As an example, a pharmacist may believe that patient counseling is helpful for patients, is important for pharmacists to do, takes a lot of time, and warrants reimbursement. Each of these beliefs is then weighted by its relative importance to the pharmacist. If a pharmacist believes helping patients is important regardless of the time needed, that pharmacist will set patient counseling as a priority and choose to provide it, regardless of perceived time limitations. Attitudes are determinants of peoples' intentions to perform behaviors, which are precursors to actual behavior.[87] Pharmacists' decisions to counsel patients and provide pharmaceutical care are influenced by their attitudes toward the pharmacist's role as a counselor ("Counselor Role Orientation")[34,88,89] and attitudes toward pharmaceutical care,[90,91] respectively. Likewise, pharmacists' attitudes about medication monitoring predict their behavioral intention to ask medication monitoring questions of a patient receiving a refill medication[85] and attitudes toward medication therapy management services predict intention to provide such services.[92] Pharmacists' concerns over liability due to malpractice suits and disciplinary actions by their state board of pharmacy may influence them to adhere to regulations that require making offers to counsel patients. A study of Texas pharmacists found their reports of these concerns to be positively related to reports of advising patients about taking contraindicated medications.[93]

Self-efficacy beliefs are "people's judgments of their capabilities to organize and execute courses of action required to attain designated types of performances."[94] Two important elements of self-efficacy beliefs are (1) an individual's confidence in his ability to perform certain tasks and (2) expectations that performing a task will lead to a particular outcome. Researchers investigating self-efficacy beliefs have asked pharmacists to indicate their level of confidence that they can successfully perform patient care behaviors.[63,64,90,95,96] Pharmacists' confidence in their patient counseling and referral services significantly predict self-report of patient care provision.[64] Self-efficacy beliefs have either directly predicted pharmacists' self-reports of pharmaceutical care provision[95] or influenced it indirectly through past behavior recency.[90] In the case of the latter, the more recently pharmacists had provided patient care, the greater their self-efficacy beliefs were (i.e., confidence by doing). Overcoming personal interactions, such as motivating patients who are not interested in receiving MTM and soliciting patient participation despite rejection, are relevant factors in self-efficacy to provide MTM.[96]

Perceived behavioral control is another factor that influences pharmacists. This factor relates to the pharmacist's sense of how much control she has over her performance of behaviors. Some studies have asked pharmacists to report their perceived ease or difficulty of providing pharmaceutical care.[63,90,95] These pharmacists have reported low perceived behavioral control for providing pharmaceutical care, which may be due to viewing little control over one's work environment. Other findings related to perceived behavioral control look at its relation to care delivery. For example, one study found that perceived behavioral control directly influenced both intention to provide pharmaceutical care and self-reported pharmaceutical care delivery.[63] Another study showed pharmacists' perceived behavioral control for providing medication therapy management services predicted intent to provide these services.[92] However, another study reported that perceived behavioral control did not directly influence pharmaceutical care delivery; instead, it directly influenced pharmacists' self-efficacy beliefs, which in turn directly influenced self-reported pharmaceutical care delivery. For example, pharmacists who lack appropriate models and strategies to implement pharmaceutical care will likely feel a low sense of perceived behavioral control, which may influence their confidence.[95] Therefore, a pharmacist's perceived behavioral control can be an appraisal process that frames how she views her work environment, and the extent to which she sets boundaries for future behavior.

A key component of pharmaceutical care is a pharmacist accepting responsibility for drug therapy outcomes. This responsibility has been described from philosophical and legal perspectives.[1,97–101] Researchers have found pharmacist-perceived responsibility for patients' drug therapy outcomes to be associated with self-report of pharmaceutical care provision and, therefore, the pharmacist-patient communication necessary to deliver that level of care.[102]

PATIENTS

Patient demographic characteristics are inconsistently associated with pharmacist-patient communication.[46,48,85] Patient age and gender may serve as cues to pharmacists for engaging in certain types of information exchange; however, different study methods reveal different findings. In an observation study of pharmacist-patient communication, older patients and men (compared to younger patients and women) were more often asked by the dispensing pharmacist for feedback and more often provided with medication monitoring information.[46] Contrary findings, however, using refill medication dispensing vignettes reveal pharmacists were more likely to report the intention to ask women (compared to men) medication monitoring questions, with no difference by age.[85]

When pharmacy patrons were asked what information they would like from the pharmacist when receiving both a new and refill prescription, responses varied by age and education level but not by gender.[48] When receiving a new medication, younger and more highly educated individuals, on average, reported wanting information about side effects, interactions, and/or precautions compared to those who were older and those having completed a less than or equal to high school education. When receiving a refill medication, respondents who completed high school or less were more likely to desire a review of medication information given when initially dispensed when compared to those having completed more than a high school education. In lieu of these findings, pharmacists may find less educated patients more receptive to discussing refills and they may especially need to discuss side effects and other risk information with those who are less educated and older, as these individuals may be less likely to seek out this type of information.

The variation in findings across age, gender, and education is notable, yet not definitive. No demographic characteristic can truly predict communication. Rather, it is the prior experience, expectations, and preferences of both the patient and pharmacist that are proposed to influence communication between these two individuals.[103] How these experiences, expectations, and preferences are realized relates to the perceptions formed within the pharmacist-patient communication dyad.

INTERPERSONAL PERCEPTIONS

Pharmacists and patients rely on perceptions of one another to define their relationships. Role perceptions also shape expectations of one another, which can influence resulting interactions. Thus, pharmacist-patient communication takes place within the context of interpersonal perceptions.

Pharmacists have reported that patient demand for receiving counseling and patient care activities are major determinants in their decisions to offer these services.[93,104,105] In fact, pharmacists' perceptions of patient demand are as important as actual patient demand in influencing pharmacists' provision of patient-oriented services.[106] Yet, studies have revealed that pharmacists may not fully understand what patients would like from them.[106-108]

Patients who have not received patient care services may not fully understand what pharmacists are capable of providing.[47,109,110] This shapes patients' perceptions of pharmacists, what they expect from pharmacists, and how they interact with them. When Counselor Role Orientation was examined among 1278 patients and 1518 pharmacists using data gathered between 1995 and 2010, researchers concluded little had changed over that time and that a moderately large subset of respondents were experiencing what they termed the dysfunctional "Care and Respect Cycle."[110] When pharmacists perceive too little time to counsel patients and choose not to provide care to patients, patients respond by not seeking the services of pharmacists, choosing to rely on their physician. This lack of respect by the patient for the pharmacist's skills then reinforces the pharmacist not providing the care needed. The authors argue that pharmacists must provide the care patients need in order for patients to grow to respect the skills pharmacists can provide, and that unless this is done, the dysfunctional cycle will continue.

Another way to consider how interpersonal perceptions may influence pharmacist-patient communication is to look at patient-perceived barriers to asking questions of a community-based pharmacist. Studies have found that some of the top barriers include the patient perceiving the pharmacist as unapproachable, too busy, or lacking in credibility[47,48] In attempting to overcome some of these barriers, creating awareness that pharmacists can be asked questions and being given questions to ask them is not enough to change patient behavior.[111] Addressing patients' fear and embarrassment as well as the perceived unapproachability and lack of credibility of pharmacists should be a priority as well.

For effective interpersonal communication, it is vital for both parties to understand one another. Studies reveal that patients and pharmacists generally disagree with one another regarding their respective roles in the pharmacist-patient relationship and regarding the benefits of pharmaceutical care services.[74,112,113] They also misunderstand each other's perceptions.[74,112]

In a Florida study, pharmacists were instructed to respond based on how they thought patients would answer, and patients were instructed to respond based on how they thought pharmacists would answer. "[Both] groups misunderstood each other's perceptions about the benefits of explaining to patients how to use their medications, developing follow-up plans measuring progress toward goals for the medication, and telling patients about other drugs that may cause problems with their medications."[74] The only issue on which both groups understood each other was making sure that patients understand information that is given to them. Generally, pharmacists thought that patients would perceive pharmaceutical care services to be more beneficial than patients actually did, thus overestimating patients' perceptions.[74,112] Additionally, patients underestimated the extent to which pharmacists would perceive these services to be beneficial to patients.[74]

A nationwide study surveyed pharmacists and patients about roles in the pharmacist-patient relationships.[113] Pharmacists and patients agreed on the *pharmacist's* information sharing role, which included talking with patients about monitoring side effects and taking prescription medications with over-the-counter products. Pharmacists and patients did not agree on the patient's information sharing role. Pharmacists reported stronger agreement than did patients that patients should discuss any medication problems and side effects with the pharmacist and keep the pharmacist up-to-date regarding changes in their health conditions. This pattern is consistent with other studies that have found that pharmacists rely on patients to initiate communication by volunteering information or asking questions.[46,64,114]

Ideally, pharmacists should be more proactive in initiating communication to identify potential and actual DTPs. This may increase patient expectations and respect for pharmacists' skills related to assisting with DTPs, and may help patients see the benefits of pharmaceutical care and participating more actively. In this study, pharmacists and patients' views also were different regarding collaboration. Pharmacists reported stronger agreement than did patients that *pharmacists* should show an interest and desire to assist patients with their healthcare-related and medication-related needs.[113] Pharmacists also more strongly agreed that *patients* should work with the pharmacist to manage their medications and help them deal with their healthcare needs. These patterns may have emerged because patient respondents were unfamiliar with these services, and thus did not know what pharmacists are capable of providing. Patients' knowledge of pharmacists' roles could be increased by exposing them to written materials about pharmacists' ability to provide patient care and medication management.[47]

ENVIRONMENTAL FACTORS

The environment in which communication takes places is an important component of the interpersonal communication process between pharmacist and patient. Some environmental factors originate in a specific practice setting, such as work flow issues. Others are more external in nature, such as federal regulations.

EXTERNAL ENVIRONMENT

External environmental factors originate at systems levels rather than at a specific pharmacy. Dominant factors of this kind that influence interpersonal communication in pharmaceutical care include federal and state regulations, practice models, payment models, and pharmacy education and training.

Over the last two decades, changes regarding the types of patient-oriented services provided by pharmacists have been mandated in federal and state regulations. As previously described, the passage of OBRA '90 requires Medicaid enrollees to receive an offer of counseling.[31] Since its passage and implementation, most states have extended the counseling requirement to all patients for new prescriptions.[39-42] State regulations vary in terms of their intensity which includes scope, stringency, and duration.[115] Pharmacies in states with more intense regulations tend to provide patient counseling more often and to a greater extent, including greater numbers of medication information items (e.g., drug name, purpose, directions for use) and asking patient questions to assess their understanding.[42] A state's regulations are considered more intense if they specifically address counseling and cover all patients (scope), require face-to-face counseling by a pharmacist or pharmacy intern/extern for all patients and their agents who present a new prescription (stringency), and if current regulations were implemented before OBRA '90 (duration).[42]

Several advances in pharmacy practice have expanded the opportunities for pharmacist-patient communication. The Washington CARE Project was one of the first to demonstrate the value of pharmacists addressing DTPs (termed "cognitive services").[116] The Asheville Project®[117] and the Diabetes Ten City Challenge[118] are practice model pilot projects, in which pharmacists served as coaches to patients, helping them better manage their diabetes. Appointment-Based Medication Synchronization programs in community pharmacies coordinate patients' multiple medication refills so they can be dispensed on the same day. They simultaneously allow pharmacists to have more focused times to speak with patients for medication management to improve medication adherence and persistence.[119]

Other advances include pharmacists working with primary care providers. The Patient-Centered Medical Home (PCMH) is a primary care model that offers important opportunities for pharmacists to work collaboratively with physicians and other health professionals to provide medication management services.[120-122] The key functions and attributes of the PCMH are that it is comprehensive, coordinated, accessible, and patient-centered with an emphasis on quality and quality improvement.[123] Collaborative Practice Agreements (CPAs) between pharmacists and physicians allow pharmacists to expand their scope of practice under protocol.[124] While stipulations vary by state, CPAs provide pharmacists opportunities to more closely monitor medication use and its outcomes, requiring communications with patients and their providers.

With practice advances have come changes to the external environments that impact reimbursement to pharmacies and pharmacists. These changes include Accountable Care Organizations and provider status for pharmacists. Accountable Care Organizations (ACOs) provide a payment model for hospitals, physicians, and other providers who collaborate to provide high quality, coordinated health care in that they share in the financial savings secured for the Medicare program[125] or private insurer. About half of ACOs have formal relationships with a pharmacy, arrangements that provide greater access to the Electronic Health Record (EHR) for pharmacists and, therefore, influence pharmacist-patient communication content.[126] Provider status has the potential to strongly impact the future of pharmacist-patient communication. Pharmacists have gained provider status in the state of California as of January, 2014[127] and at the time of this writing, efforts continue on the federal level to pursue provider status for pharmacists.[128] Such status has the potential to improve pharmacists' ability to directly provide and bill for services beyond dispensing that require more intensive communication with patients. The potential for pharmacists to bill for these types of services is greater now than at any other time in the profession's history.[62]

Pharmacy education is an environmental factor that continually influences interpersonal communication between pharmacists and patients. Pharmacy schools and their accrediting organizations recognize the importance of developing effective communication skills among its student pharmacists in both didactic and experiential learning programs.[129-132] More than half of U.S. schools of pharmacy offer separate communications courses as part of their required curricula while the remainder integrate communications across the curricula.[133] Assessments of students' communication skills focus more on dispensing a new prescription to patients than monitoring a patient's ongoing therapy,[133] a trend that may change as practice models extend into medication management. Expansion of early experiential programs has increased opportunities for student pharmacists to develop their patient communication skills while in school.[132]

After graduation, pharmacy residencies offer opportunities for communication skill development and use. In addition to health-system-based pharmacy residencies, community pharmacy residency programs are available to pharmacists who want to have more direct contact with patients. In a survey regarding community pharmacy residencies, 94% of current residents indicated the top skills emphasized in their community pharmacy residency were communication skills.[134] In addition, when asked what residency attributes were sought by current residents, the top two were patient care services offered and opportunities to develop innovative services—all attributes that both require good pharmacist-patient communication skills.

PHARMACY PRACTICE ENVIRONMENT

Practice setting characteristics, such as physical layout, workflow, use of a drive-thru and busyness influence a pharmacist's activities.[108,135] Workflow, for example, can influence whether or not a pharmacist is the person who hands a prescription and offers counseling to a patient. Prescription transfer by the pharmacist predicts the occurrence of communication.[88] Workflow modifications and adequate numbers of trained staff are usually necessary for a pharmacist to be able to transfer completed prescriptions to patients. Such modifications have increased pharmacists' counseling offers to patients; however, these increases have not resulted in more patients receiving counseling.[136,137] Patient expectations regarding counseling are likely contributors to the lack of increase in counseling, despite more offers. In one study that examined patient use of drive-through windows at 22 community pharmacies, findings revealed that when compared to use of a "walk-up" (in-store) window, patients who used a drive-through window spent less time talking with a pharmacist and subsequently, received less information.[43] This same study found that pharmacists spent less time talking with patients at either window with higher levels of busyness.

Busyness is another factor that influences the extent of pharmacist-patient communication.[43,49,88,89,135] In a study of 306 community pharmacists in eight states using secret shoppers, pharmacies that were considered busier had a lower percentage of pharmacists talking with patients, providing any specific medication information, and asking any questions to assess patient understanding.[42] When surveyed, community pharmacy patrons reported a pharmacist seeming busy or unapproachable as a barrier to asking that pharmacist questions.[47,48] When busyness has been examined, however, it has not always been a factor in pharmacist-patient communication, so its influence is unclear.[36] Pharmacists who are very busy may perceive a lack of time to communicate with patients. Indeed, perceived lack of time is commonly cited as a barrier to counseling patients.[88,104,135]

Some workplace factors have less to do with the actual setting and are more related to contextual cues. Indeed, research has not found any difference between chain and independently owned pharmacies regarding occurrence and content of pharmacist-patient communication.[42] Workplace situational factors are part of the environment at a particular moment.[63] For example, pharmacists tend to counsel patients more for new prescriptions than for refill prescriptions, especially if the patient is unfamiliar with the medication.[46,138] The occurrence of pharmacist-patient communication is influenced by the perceived importance of information relayed during the encounter, particularly if pharmacists perceive potentially serious consequences to the patient.[88,138]

Studies evaluating factors that influence pharmacists' provision of pharmaceutical care generally place greater emphasis on individual factors, such as attitude toward providing pharmaceutical care, over reimbursement and practice setting characteristics.[63,64,91,139] The primary reason for this preference is because individual factors are within a pharmacist's control, whereas many environmental factors are not.[139] However, the practice environment is arguably important due to its influence on how pharmacists perceive control over their work surroundings. Building on ways to empower pharmacists within the workplace to build self-efficacy and perceived behavioral control will likely be an important need as the profession continues to advance its communication-dependent practice models.

SUMMARY

Interpersonal communication is a fundamental social and behavioral aspect of patient care practice. Effective interpersonal communication is necessary to establish rapport with patients by understanding their needs, concerns, and experiences. Rapport serves as a foundation for building a therapeutic relationship with patients and having them participate in decision-making processes to meet their therapeutic goals. Interpersonal communication is also important to promote dialogue between pharmacists and patients so that information can be exchanged. Information exchange is critical for conducting the patient care process to identify, resolve, and prevent DTPs that could interfere with patients' therapeutic goals. Common DTPs encountered in patient care practices require direct pharmacist-patient communication. As more pharmacists become patient care providers, they will need effective interpersonal communication skills to help patients optimize their drug therapy outcomes.

A variety of factors influence pharmacist-patient communication. Attempts to increase interpersonal communication in patient care practices should incorporate interventions that influence personal, interpersonal, and environmental factors. Both pharmacist and patient perceptions must be included.

This chapter describes the nature, extent, and influencing factors of interpersonal communication for patient care practice. Understanding these issues is crucial for pharmacists to help patients optimize their drug therapy outcomes.

REFERENCES

1. Cipolle, R.J., Strand, L.M., & Morley, P.C. (2014). *Pharmaceutical care practice: The patient-centered approach to medication management.* 3rd ed. New York: McGraw–Hill.

2. Joint Commission of Pharmacy Practitioners. Pharmacists' patient care process. (2014).

3. Shannon, C.E. & Weaver, W. (1949). *The mathematical theory of communication.* Urbana, IL: University of Illinois Press.

4. Schramm, W. (1954). How communication works. In Schramm, W. (Ed.). *The process and effects of mass communication.* Urbana, IL: University of Illinois Press, 3–26.

5. Mehrabian, A. (1971). *Silent messages.* Belmont, CA: Wadsworth.

6. Poytos, F. (1983). New perspectives in nonverbal communication. New York: Pergamon Press.

7. Pease, A. & Pease, B. (2004). *The definitive book of body language*. New York: Bantam Books.

8. TeamSTEPPS Fundamentals Course: Module 3. Communication. (2014). Rockville, MD: Agency for Healthcare and Research Quality.

9. Rapport. American Heritage dictionary. Random House. (Accessed August 30, 2015, at http://dictionary.reference.com/browse/rapport)

10. Burley-Allen, M. (1995). *Listening: the forgotten skill*. 2nd ed. Hoboken, NJ: John Wiley & Sons, Inc.

11. Adler, R.B., Rosenfeld, L.B., & Proctor, R.F. (2006). *Interplay: the process of interpersonal communication*. 10th ed. New York: Oxford University Press, Inc.

12. Covey, S.R. (1989). *The 7 habits of highly effective people: powerful lessons in personal change*. New York: Free Press.

13. King, A. & Hoppe, R.B. (2013). "Best practice" for patient-centered communication: a narrative review. *J Grad Med Educ*. 5(3):385–3.

14. Rogers, C.R. (1980). *A way of being*. Boston, MA: Houghton Mifflin.

15. Rantucci, M.J. (2007). *Pharmacists talking with patients: A guide to patient counseling*. Philadelphia: Lippincott, Williams & Wilkins.

16. Mead, N. & Bower, P. (2000). Patient-centredness: a conceptual framework and review of the empirical literature. *Soc Sci Med*. 51(7):1087–110.

17. Ruiz-Moral, R. (2009). *The role of physician–patient communication in promoting patient–participatory decision making. Health Expect* 13(1):33–44.

18. Antunes, L.P., Gomes, J.J., & Cavaco, A.M. (2015). How pharmacist-patient communication determines pharmacy loyalty? Modeling relevant factors. *Res Social Adm Pharm*. 11(4):560–70.

19. Hepler, C.D. & Strand, L.M. (1990). Opportunities and responsibilities in pharmaceutical care. *Am J Hosp Pharm*. 47(3):533–43.

20. May, W.F. (1975). Code, covenant, contract, or philanthropy. *Hastings Cent Rep*. 5(6):29–38.

21. Pfizer, I. (1990). *Pharmacist-patient consultation program-Unit I: An interactive approach to verify patient understanding*. New York: National Health Care Operations.

22. Pfizer, I. (1993). *Pharmacist-patient consultation program-Unit II: How to counsel patients in challenging situations*. New York: National Health Care Operations.

23. Pfizer, I. (1995). *Pharmacist-patient consultation program-Unit III: Counseling to enhance compliance.* New York: National Health Care Operations.

24. Brega, A.G., Barnard, J., Mabachi, N.M. et al. (2015). *AHRQ health literacy universal precautions toolkit.* Rockville, MD. AHRQ Publication No.15-0023-EF.

25. Strand, L.M., Morley, P.C., Cipolle, R.J., Ramsey, R., & Lamsam, G.D. (1990). Drug-related problems: Their structure and function. *DICP* 24(11):1093–7.

26. Planas, L.G. & Er, N.L. (2008). A systems approach to scaffold communication skills development. *Am J Pharm Educ* 72(2):35.

27. Higby, G.J. (1996). From compounding to caring: An abridged history of American pharmacy. In Knowlton, C.H., Penna, R.P. (Eds.), *Pharmaceutical care.* New York: Chapman and Hall, 18–45.

28. American Pharmaceutical Association. (1952). Code of ethics. *J Am Pharm Assoc* 13(10):721–3.

29. American Pharmacists Association-Academy of Students of Pharmacy. (2012). *APhA-ASP Adopted Resolutions 1973-2012.* Washington, DC.

30. American Pharmacists Association. *Pharmacist/patient communication. Patient/pharmacist relationships.* APhA Policy Manual. (Accessed August 30, 2015, at http://www.pharmacist.com/policy-manual)

31. Omnibus Budget Reconciliation Act of 1990. (1990). Washington, DC: U.S. Government Printing Office, 152–1.

32. Rowles, B., Keller, S.M., & Gavin, P.W. (1974). Pharmacist as compounder and consultant. *Drug Intell Clin Pharm.* 8(5):242–4.

33. Ross, S.R., White, S.J., Hogan, L.C., & Godwin, H.N. (1981). The effect of a mandatory patient counseling regulation on the counseling practices of pharmacy practitioners. *Contemp Pharm Pract.* 4(2):64–8.

34. Mason, H.L. & Svarstad, B.L. (1984). Medication counseling behaviors and attitudes of rural community pharmacists. *Drug Intell Clin Pharm.* 18(5):409–14.

35. Carroll, N.V. & Gagnon, J.P. (1984).Consumer demand for patient-oriented pharmacy services. *Am J Public Health* 74(6):609–11.

36. Berardo, D.H., Kimberlin, C.L., & Barnett, C.W. (1989). Observational research on patient education activities of community pharmacists. *J Soc Admin Pharm* 6(1):21–30.

37. Raisch, D.W. (1993). Patient counseling in community pharmacy and its relationship with prescription payment methods and practice settings. *Ann Pharmacother* 27(10):1173–9.

38. Morris, L.A., Tabak, E.R., & Gondek, K. (1997). Counseling patients about prescribed medication: 12-year trends. *Med Care* 35(10):996–1007.

39. Perri, M., Kotzan, J., Pritchard, L., Ozburn, W., & Francisco, G. (1995). OBRA '90: The impact on pharmacists and patients. *Am Pharm* NS35(2):24–8, 65.

40. Sleath, B. (1995). Pharmacist question-asking in New Mexico community pharmacies. *Am J Pharm Educ* 59(4):374–9.

41. Schatz, R., Belloto, R.J. Jr., White, D.B., & Bachmann, K. (2003). Provision of drug information to patients by pharmacists: the impact of the Omnibus Budget Reconciliation Act of 1990 a decade later. *Am J Ther* 10(2):93–103.

42. Svarstad, B.L., Bultman, D.C., & Mount, J.K. (2004). Patient counseling provided in community pharmacies: effects of state regulation, pharmacist age, and busyness. *J Am Pharm Assoc* 44(1):22–9.

43. Odukoya, O.K., Chui, M.A., & Pu, J. (2014). Factors influencing quality of patient interaction at community pharmacy drive-through and walk-in counselling areas. *Int J Pharm Pract* 22(4):246–56.

44. Flynn, E.A., Barker, K.N., Berger, B.A., Lloyd, K.B., & Brackett, P.D. (2009). Dispensing errors and counseling quality in 100 pharmacies. *J Am Pharm Assoc* 49(2):171–80.

45. Kimberlin, C.L., Jamison, A.N., Linden, S., & Winterstein, A.G. (2011). Patient counseling practices in US pharmacies: effects of having pharmacists hand the medication to the patient and state regulations on pharmacist counseling. *J Am Pharm Assoc* 51(4):527–34.

46. Schommer, J.C., & Wiederholt, J.B. (1997). The association of prescription status, patient age, patient gender, and patient question asking behavior with the content of pharmacist-patient communication. *Pharm Res* 14(2):145–51.

47. Chewning, B., & Schommer, J.C.(1996). Increasing clients' knowledge of community pharmacists' roles. *Pharm Res* 13(9):1299–304.

48. Krueger, J.L. & Hermansen-Kobulnicky, C.J. (2011). Patient perspective of medication information desired and barriers to asking pharmacists questions. *J Am Pharm Assoc* 51(4):510–9.

49. Sleath, B. (1996). Pharmacist-patient relationships: authoritarian, participatory, or default? *Patient Educ Couns* 28(3):253–63.

50. U.S. Food and Drug Administration. *Drug and safety availability. Medication guides.* (Accessed August 30, 2015, at http://www.fda.gov/Drugs/DrugSafety/ucm085729.htm)

51. Svarstad, B.L., Bultman, D.C., Mount, J.K., & Tabak, E.R.(2003). Evaluation of written prescription information provided in community pharmacies: a study in eight states. *J Am Pharm Assoc* 43(3):383–93.

52. Stergachis, A., Maine, L.L., & Brown, L. (2002). The 2001 National Pharmacy Consumer Survey. *J Am Pharm Assoc* 42(4):568–76.

53. Svarstad B.L., Mount, J.K., & Tabak, E.R. (2005). Expert and consumer evaluation of patient medication leaflets provided in U.S. pharmacies. *J Am Pharm Assoc* 45(4):443–51.

54. Winterstein, A.G., Linden, S., Lee, A.E., Fernandez, E.M., & Kimberlin, C.L. (2010). Evaluation of consumer medication information dispensed in retail pharmacies. *Arch Intern Med.* 170(15):1317–24.

55. Federal Register. (January 28, 2005). (42 CFR Parts 400, 403, 411, 417, and 423).

56. McGivney, M.S., Meyer, S.M., Duncan-Hewitt ,W., Hall, D.L., Goode, J.V., & Smith RB. (2007). Medication therapy management: Its relationship to patient counseling, disease management, and pharmaceutical care. *J Am Pharm Assoc* 47(5):620–8.

57. Medication therapy management in pharmacy practice: core elements of an MTM service model (version 2.0). (2008). *J Am Pharm Assoc* 48(3):341–53.

58. Centers for Medicare and Medicaid Services. (April 7, 2015). CY2016 Medication therapy management program guidance and submission instructions. (Accessed August 30, 2015, at https://www.cms.gov/Medicare/Prescription-Drug-Coverage/PrescriptionDrugCovContra/Downloads/Memo-Contract-Year-2016-Medication-Therapy-Management-MTM-Program-Submission-v-040715.pdf)

59. de Oliveira, D.R., Brummel, A.R., & Miller, D.B. (2010). Medication therapy management: 10 years of experience in a large integrated health care system. *J Manag Care Pharm* 16(3):185–95.

60. Lauffenburger, J.C., Vu, M.B., Burkhart, J.I., Weinberger, M., & Roth, M.T.(2012). Design of a medication therapy management program for Medicare beneficiaries: qualitative findings from patients and physicians. *Am J Geriatr Pharmacother* 10(2):129–38.

61. Truong, H.A., Layson-Wolf, C., de Bittner, M.R., Owen, J.A., & Haupt, S. (2009). Perceptions of patients on Medicare Part D medication therapy management services. *J Am Pharm Assoc* 49(3):392–8.

62. Isetts, B.J. & Buffington, D.E. (2007). CPT code-change proposal: national data on pharmacists' medication therapy management services. *Am J Health Syst Pharm* 64(15):1642–6.

63. Odedina, F.T., Hepler, C.D., Segal, R., & Miller, D. (1997). The pharmacists' implementation of pharmaceutical care (PIPC) model. *Pharm Res* 14(2):135–44.

64. Venkataraman, K., Madhavan, S., & Bone, P. (1997). Barriers and facilitators to pharmaceutical care in rural community practice. *J Soc Admin Pharm* 4(4):208–19.

65. McDermott, J.H. & Christensen, D.B. (2002). Provision of pharmaceutical care services in North Carolina: a 1999 survey. *J Am Pharm Assoc* 42(1):26–35.

66. Barnett, M.J., Frank, J., Wehring, H., et al. (2009). Analysis of pharmacist-provided medication therapy management (MTM) services in community pharmacies over 7 years. *J Manag Care Pharm* 15(1):18–31.

67. American Pharmacists Association. (2008). *Medication Therapy Management Digest: Perspectives on MTM service implementation*. Washington, DC.

68. American Pharmacists Association. (2009). *Medication Therapy Management Digest: Perspectives on the value of MTM services and their impact on health care*. Washington, DC.

69. American Pharmacists Association. (2010). *Medication Therapy Management Digest: Perspectives on 2009: A year of changing opportunities*. Washington, DC.

70. American Pharmacists Association. (2011). *Medication Therapy Management Digest: Tracking the expansion of MTM in 2010: exploring the consumer perspective*. Washington, DC.

71. American Pharmacists Association. (2013). *Medication Therapy Management Digest: Pharmacists emerging as interdisciplinary health care team members*. Washington, DC.

72. American Pharmacists Association. (2014). *Medication Therapy Management Digest: The pursuit of provider status to support the growth and expansion of pharmacists' patient care services*. Washington, DC.

73. American Pharmacists Association. (2015). *Pharmacists' Patient Care Services Digest: Pharmacists improving patient access to health care*. Washington, DC.

74. Assa-Eley, M. & Kimberlin, C.L. (2005). Using interpersonal perception to characterize pharmacists' and patients' perceptions of the benefits of pharmaceutical care. *Health Commun.* 17(1):41–56.

75. Kassam, R., Farris, K.B., Burback, L., Volume, C.I., Cox, C.E., & Cave, A. (2001). Pharmaceutical care research and education project: pharmacists' interventions. *J Am Pharm Assoc* 41(3):401–10.

76. McDonough, R.P. & Doucette, W.R. (2003). Drug therapy management: an empirical report of drug therapy problems, pharmacists' interventions, and results of pharmacists' actions. *J Am Pharm Assoc* 43(4):511–8.

77. Doucette, W.R., McDonough, R.P., Klepser, D., & McCarthy, R. (2005).Comprehensive medication therapy management: identifying and resolving drug-related issues in a community pharmacy. *Clin Ther* 27(7):1104–11.

78. Isetts, B.J. (2007). *Evaluating effectiveness of the Minnesota Medication Therapy Management Care Program: Final report.* St. Paul, MN: Minnesota Department of Human Services. (Report no. B00749).

79. Isetts, B.J., Brown, L,M,, & Schondelmeyer, S,W., & Lenarz, L.A. (2003). Quality assessment of a collaborative approach for decreasing drug-related morbidity and achieving therapeutic goals. *Arch Intern Med* 163(15):1813–20.

80. Isetts, B.J., Schondelmeyer, S.W., Artz, M.B., et al. (2008). Clinical and economic outcomes of medication therapy management services: the Minnesota experience. *J Am Pharm Assoc* 48(2):203–11.

81. Harris, I.M., Westberg, S.M., Frakes, M.J., & Van Vooren, J.S. (2009). Outcomes of medication therapy review in a family medicine clinic. *J Am Pharm Assoc* 49(5):623–7.

82. Connor, S.E., Snyder, M.E., Snyder, Z.J., & Pater Steinmetz, K. (2009). Provision of clinical pharmacy services in two safety net provider settings. *Pharm Pract* 7(2):94–9.

83. Witry, M.J., Doucette, W.R., & Gainer, K.L. (2011). Evaluation of the pharmaceutical case management program implemented in a private sector health plan. *J Am Pharm Assoc* 51(5):631–5.

84. Isetts, B.J., Brummel, A.R., de Oliveira, D.R., & Moen, D.W. (2012). Managing drug-related morbidity and mortality in the patient-centered medical home. *Med Care* 50(11):997–1001.

85. Witry, M.J. & Doucette, W.R. (2015). Factors influencing community pharmacists' likelihood to ask medication monitoring questions: A factorial survey. *Res Social Adm Pharm* 11(5):639–50.

86. Witry, M.J. & Doucette, W.R. (2014). Community pharmacists, medication monitoring, and the routine nature of refills: a qualitative study. *J Am Pharm Assoc* 54(6):594–603.

87. Fishbein, M. & Ajzen, I. (1975). *Belief, attitude, intention, and behavior: An introduction to theory and research.* Vol 1. Reading, MA: Addison-Wesley.

88. Schommer, J.C. & Wiederholt, J.B. (1995). A field investigation of participant and environment effects on pharmacist patient communication in community pharmacies. *Med Care* 33(6):567–84.

89. Kirking, D. (1984). Evaluation of an explanatory model of pharmacists' patient counseling activities. *J Soc Adm Pharm* 2:50–6.

90. Odedina, F.T., Segal, R., Hepler, C.D., Lipowski, E., & Kimberlin, C. (1996). Changing pharmacists' practice pattern: pharmacists' implementation of pharmaceutical care factors. *J Soc Adm Pharm* 13(2):74–88.

91. Farris, K.B. & Kirking, D.M. (1995). Predicting community pharmacists' intention to try to prevent and correct drug therapy problems. *J Soc Adm Pharm* 12(2):64–79.

92. Herbert, K.E., Urmie, J.M., Newland, B.A., & Farris, K.B. (2006). Prediction of pharmacist intention to provide Medicare medication therapy management services using the theory of planned behavior. *Res Social Adm Pharm* 2(3):299–314.

93. Sitkin, S.B. & Sutcliffe, K.M. (1991). Dispensing legitimacy: The influence of professional, organizational, and legal controls on pharmacist behavior. *Res Sociol Organ* 8:269–95.

94. Bandura, A. (1986). *Social foundations of thought and action: A social cognitive theory.* Englewood Cliffs, NJ: Prentice Hall.

95. Farris, K.B. & Schopflocher, D.P. (1999). Between intention and behavior: An application of community pharmacists' assessment of pharmaceutical care. *Soc Sci Med* 49(1):55–66.

96. Martin, B.A., Chui, M.A., Thorpe, J.M., Mott, D.A., & Kreling, D.H. (2010). Development of a scale to measure pharmacists' self-efficacy in performing medication therapy management services. *Res Social Adm Pharm* 6(2):155–61.

97. Brushwood, D.B. & Hepler, C.D. (1996). Redefining pharmacist professional responsibility. In Knowlton, C.H. & Penna, R.P. (Eds.), *Pharmaceutical care.* New York: Chapman & Hall, 195–214.

98. Hepler, C.D. (1996). Philosophical issues raised by pharmaceutical care. In Haddad, A.M. & Buerki, R.A. (Eds.), *Ethical dimensions of pharmaceutical care.* Binghamton, NY: Haworth Press, 19–47.

99. Brushwood, D.B. (1991). The duty to counsel: Reviewing a decade of litigation. *DICP* 25(2):195–204.

100. Brushwood, D.B. (1995). The pharmacist's expanding legal responsibility for patient care. *J Soc Adm Pharm* 12(2):53–62.

101. Lynn, N.J. & Ellis, J.M. (1998). Pharmacists' liability into the year 2000. *J Am Pharm Assoc* 38(6):747–52.

102. Planas, L.G., Kimberlin, C.L., Segal, R., Brushwood, D.B., Hepler, C.D., & Schlenker, B.R. (2005). A pharmacist model of perceived responsibility for drug therapy outcomes. *Soc Sci Med* 60(10):2393–403.

103. Shah, B. & Chewning, B. (2006). Conceptualizing and measuring pharmacist-patient communication: a review of published studies. *Res Social Adm Pharm* 2(2):153–85.

104. Schommer, J.C. & Wiederholt, J.B. (1994). Pharmacists' perceptions of patients' needs for counseling. *Am J Hosp Pharm* 51(4):478–85.

105. Latif, D.A. (1998). Situational factors as determinants of community pharmacists' clinical decision making behavior. *J Am Pharm Assoc* 38(4):446–50.

106. Carroll, N.V. & Gagnon, J.P. (1984). Pharmacists' perceptions of consumer demand for patient-oriented pharmacy services. *Drug Intell Clin Pharm* 18(7-8):640–4.

107. Hirsch, J.D., Gagnon, J.P., & Camp, R. (1990). Value of pharmacy services: perceptions of consumers, physicians, and third party prescription plan administrators. *Am Pharm* NS30(3):20–5.

108. Herrier, R. & Boyce, R. (1994). Why aren't more pharmacists counseling? *Am Pharm* NS34(11):22–3.

109. Doucette, W.R, Witry, M.J., Alkhateeb, F., Farris, K.B., & Urmie, J.M. (2007). Attitudes of Medicare beneficiaries toward pharmacist-provided medication therapy management activities as part of the Medicare Part D benefit. *J Am Pharm Assoc* 47(6):758–62.

110. Schommer, J.C. & Gaither, C.A. (2014). A segmentation analysis for pharmacists' and patients' views of pharmacists' roles. *Res Soc Admin Pharm* 10(3):508–28.

111. Airaksinen, M., Ahonen, R., & Enlund, H. (1998). The "Questions to Ask About Your Medicines" campaign: an evaluation of pharmacists and the public's response. *Med Care* 36(3):422–7.

112. Assa, M. & Shepherd, E.F. (2000). Interpersonal perception: a theory and method for studying pharmacists' and patients' views of pharmaceutical care. *J Am Pharm Assoc* 40(1):71–81.

113. Worley, M.M., Schommer, J.C., Brown, L.M., et al. (2007). Pharmacists' and patients' roles in the pharmacist-patient relationship: are pharmacists and patients reading from the same relationship script? *Res Social Adm Pharm* 3(1):47–69.

114. Kirking, D.M. (1982). Pharmacists' perceptions of their patient counseling activities. *Contemp Pharm Pract* 5(4):230–8.

115. Cook, K., Shortell, S.M., Conrad, D.A., & Morrisey, M.A. (1983). A theory of organizational response to regulation: the case of hospitals. *Acad Manage Rev* (2):193–205.

116. Smith, D.H., Fassett, W.E., & Christensen, D.B. (1999). Washington State CARE Project: downstream cost changes associated with the provision of cognitive services by pharmacists. *J Am Pharm Assoc* 39(5):650–7.

117. Cranor, C.W., Bunting, B.A., & Christensen, D.B. (2003).The Asheville Project: long-term clinical and economic outcomes of a community pharmacy diabetes care program. *J Am Pharm Assoc* 43(2):173–84.

118. Fera, T., Bluml, B.M., & Ellis, W.M. (2009). Diabetes ten city challenge: Final economic and clinical results. *J Am Pharm Assoc* 49(3):383–91.

119. Holdford, D.A. & Inocencio, T.J. (2013). Adherence and persistence associated with an appointment-based medication synchronization program. *J Am Pharm Assoc* 53(6):576–83.

120. Abrons, J.P. & Smith, M. (2011). Patient-centered medical homes: primer for pharmacists. *Pharm Today* 17(5):52–64.

121. Kucukarslan, S.N., Hagan, A.M., Shimp, L.A., Gaither, C.A., & Lewis, N.J. (2011). Integrating medication therapy management in the primary care medical home: a review of randomized controlled trials. *Am J Health Syst Pharm* 68(4):335–45.

122. Nigro, S.C., Garwood, C.L., Berlie, H., et al. (2014). Clinical pharmacists as key members of the patient-centered medical home: An opinion statement of the Ambulatory Care Practice and Research Network of the American College of Clinical Pharmacy. *Pharmacother* 34(1):96–108.

123. Patient Centered Medical Home Resource Center. Agency for Healthcare Research and Quality. (Accessed August 30, 2015, at https://pcmh.ahrq.gov/)

124. Centers for Disease Control and Prevention. (2013). *Collaborative practice agreements and pharmacists' patient care services: A resource for pharmacists.* Atlanta, GA: U.S. Department of Health and Human Services.

125. Centers for Medicare and Medicaid Services. *Accountable care organizations.* (Accessed August 30, 2015, at https://www.cms.gov/Medicare/Medicare-Fee-for-Service-Payment/ACO/index.html?redirect=/aco)

126. Colla, C.H., Lewis, V.A., Beaulieu-Jones, B.R., & Morden, N.E. (2015). Role of pharmacy services in accountable care organizations. *J Manag Care Spec Pharm* 21(4):338–44.

127. Pharmacist provider status. California SB 493; 2013.

128. American Pharmacists Association. *Pharmacists provide care.* (Accessed August 30, 2015, at http://www.pharmacistsprovidecare.com/)

129. Svarstad, B.L. (1994). Development of behavioral science curricula and faculty in pharmacy: some issues requiring attention. *Am J Pharm Educ* 58(2):177–83.

130. Beardsley, R.S. (2001). Communication skills development in colleges of pharmacy. *Am J Pharm Educ* 65(4):307–14.

131. Medina, M.S., Plaza, C.M., Stowe, C.D., et al. (2013). Center for the Advancement of Pharmacy Education 2013 educational outcomes. *Am J Pharm Educ* 77(8):162.

132. Accreditation Council for Pharmacy Education. *Accreditation standards and guidelines for the professional program in pharmacy leading to the Doctor of Pharmacy degree: "Standards 2016."* (Accessed August 30, 2015, at www.acpe-accredit.org/pdf/Standards2016FINAL.pdf)

133. Kimberlin, C.L. (2006). Communicating with patients: skills assessment in US colleges of pharmacy. *Am J Pharm Educ* 70(3):67.

134. Unterwagner, W.L., Zeolla, M.M., & Burns, A.L. (2003). Training experiences of current and former community pharmacy residents, 1986–2000. *J Am Pharm Assoc* 43(2):201–6.

135. Raisch, D.W. (1993). Barriers to providing cognitive services. *Am Pharm* NS33(12):54–8.

136. Angelo, L.B., Ferreri, S.P. (2005).Assessment of workflow redesign in community pharmacy. *J Am Pharm Assoc* 45(2):145–50.

137. Angelo, L.B., Christensen, D.B.,& Ferreri, S.P. (2005). Impact of community pharmacy automation on workflow, workload, and patient interaction. *J Am Pharm Assoc* 45(2):138–44.

138. Schommer, J.C. & Wiederholt, J.B. (1994). Pharmacists' views of patient counseling. *Am Pharm* NS34(7):46–53.

139. Campagna, K.D. & Newlin, M.H. (1997). Key factors influencing pharmacists' drug therapy decisions. *Am J Health Syst Pharm* 54(11):1307–13.

CHAPTER 11

PHARMACEUTICAL CARE: INCORPORATING THE NEEDS AND PERSPECTIVES OF FAMILY CARERS

Sally-Anne Francis and Felicity Smith

LEARNING OBJECTIVES:

1. Illustrate the dependence of health care systems and patients on unpaid family carers, throughout the world, and their increasing prominence in health policy.

2. Explain the place of medicines-related activities as integral to the caring role of family carers.

3. Describe the diversity of medicines-related activities commonly undertaken by family carers of older people, young people with long-term conditions, and those depended on complex therapies.

4. Identify the extent and range of problems and concerns experienced by family carers, when assisting with medicines, and their potential contribution to carer-burden.

5. Synthesize how health professionals including pharmacists can more effectively support family carers in their medicines-related activities and thus optimize pharmaceutical care for the patients they assist.

Autonomy

Caring

Family carers

Medicines management activities

Medicines-related assistance

Systematic support

Unilateral decisions

INTRODUCTION

Informal care-giving is believed to be a major component of health care in all parts of the world. Unpaid carers have been defined as "people looking after, or providing some regular help for a sick, handicapped or older person living in their own or another provate household."[1] Unpaid carers span all age groups and, while usually a family member, may be a friend or neighbor. For the purposes of this chapter, all unpaid carers will be referred to as "family carers."

This chapter focuses on the place of family carers (also termed care-givers) in the medication management process and the implications for pharmaceutical care. Pharmacists are unusual among health care professionals in that they can commonly have face-to-face contact with the representative or family carer of a patient without the patient being present. This leads to both opportunities and challenges in the provision of pharmaceutical care.

In terms of opportunities, as illustrated in this chapter, family carers play a major and often essential role in the management of medicines for the person for whom they care. Thus, the contact that pharmacists may regularly have with a family carer enables them to identify and respond to medicines-related issues that arise in the context of the caring relationship.

The challenges are apparent. Initially, the pharmacist is dependent on identifying the family carer, or the carer themselves self-identifying, in order to offer assistance. The pharmacist may have to rely on the family carer for information about the patient and may be unable to make a first-hand assessment of a patient's needs. In performing medicines-related activities, family carers have their own problems and perspectives, and require information and support in order to be effective. This leads to further professional challenges in terms of how best to support the family carer in the patient's best interests while considering issues of patient respect, autonomy, and confidentiality.

Family carers make an enormous contribution to the health care system and in developing services in pharmaceutical care, the perspectives of family carers must always be considered. This chapter will first provide a brief overview of the extent of care-giving, highlighting its importance in health and social care. It will then describe the roles of family carers in the management of medicines, examining, in particular, family carers of older people, family carers of younger people with long term conditions, the range of medication-related activities that family carers undertake, and ways in which family carers and care-recipients work together to manage their medicines. It will draw on the research that has been undertaken from the perspectives of family carers, on their roles in assisting in the use of medicines together with the problems experienced and their concerns. The specialist requirements of some long-term conditions and the impact of advancing technologies, and their influence on the caring role will also be discussed.

This chapter will conclude with a discussion of the unique challenges in effective medicines management when caring for a person with dementia, and the implications of supporting family carers in the design of future pharmaceutical care services.

OVERVIEW OF CARE-GIVING

According to the United Nations population division,[2] the number of older persons (60 years or more) worldwide is projected to more than double to two billion by 2050, 19% of whom will be aged 80 years or more. Europe's population is projected to be the most aged in the world, with 34% of the population expected to be aged 60 or more by 2050, followed by Northern America with 27%. Notably, rapid growth of older populations will also be experienced in Africa, Latin America and the Caribbean, and Asia.

Incidence rates for dementia are also rising. Currently in the UK there are an estimated 800,000 people with dementia, and by 2021 this is expected to increase to one million. Over two-thirds of people with dementia live in the community and are supported in their daily living by 670,000 family carers.[3] With these demographic changes and the rising prevalence of dementia, it is anticipated there will be a commensurate rise in the numbers of, and dependence on, family carers.

Family carers of older people will often be older themselves and have their own health needs with some consequent functional limitations. As older people age, disease may progress; the burden on the family carer may increase at the same time as their ability to care diminishes. Family carers have been reported to have a chronic condition at more than twice the rate of non-family carers.[4] UK Census data found that the general health of carers deteriorated incrementally with the increasing hours of care provided.[3]

In 2009, more than 61 million family caregivers in the United States provided care to an adult with limitations in daily activities, at some time during the year.[5] In Australia, there are 2.7 million family carers who, on average, spend approximately 40 hours per week providing care. Although, it has been estimated that carers of someone with a mental illness spend on average 104 hours per week in the caring role.[6,7] According to UK census data,[3] there are around six million people providing unpaid care for an ill, frail or disabled family member or friend in England; over a third of carers are providing care for 20 hours or more per week. Unpaid care was highest for both men and women aged 50–64 years, with females taking on a greater share of the unpaid care burden. However many family carers, especially those in older age groups and caring for a spouse, are male. Furthermore, UK census data illustrated that there were more than 166,000 young carers aged 5–17 years, the majority providing 1–19 hours of care a week.

Family carers aged 50–64 years are most likely to care for an elderly parent. Daughters/sons (including in-laws) provide significant help for older people. The assistance they provide has to be accommodated alongside other commitments in their own home and working lives: 59% of family carers who care for someone over the age of 18 years either work, or have worked, while providing care; 62% have had to make some adjustments to their work life, including switching from full-time to parttime employment and giving up work entirely.[8] Becoming an unpaid carer in your 50s increases your chances of leaving the labor market for good, is associated with health problems, and restricts your social and leisure activities.[3]

In the United States, the estimated economic value of the services provided by family carers has been reported to be approximately $450 billion.[5] In Australia the estimated annual replacement value for unpaid care was over $40.9 billion.[6,9] In the UK the annual contribution of family carers to health care alone has been valued at £57.4 million.[10] Consequently, care-giving is, and will remain, an important component of healthcare worldwide.

In the UK, the essential contribution of family carers to health care is gaining increasing prominence. The latest document published by the British Government is the Carers Strategy: Second National Action Plan for 2014–16, which focuses on four key areas for the development of services:[11]

- To support those with caring responsibilities to self-identify as carers at an early stage, recognising the value of their contribution and involving them in designing local care provision and in planning individual care packages
- To enable carers to fulfil their education and employment potential
- To personalise support both for carers and care-recipients, enabling them to have a family and community life
- To support carers to remain mentally and physically well

ROLES OF FAMILY CARERS IN THE MANAGEMENT OF MEDICINES

The use of medicines is commonly a major component of the management of any medical condition. Older people experience more morbidity for which medicines will be required. Children and young people who require the long-term use of medicines are most likely to be principally cared for, and assisted by, their parents. Each has its own challenges; whereas young people with a chronic condition may take progressively greater responsibility for the use of their medicines as they grow up, an older care-recipient may become more dependent.

Providing assistance with the use of medicines would be expected to be an important part of the caring role. Despite this, research into the medicines-related aspects of informal caring and its associated challenges has been limited.[12–25]

Studies that have been conducted have shown the broad range of medicines-related activities that family carers undertake. Research has also highlighted the huge variation between family carers in the level of involvement they have, which will, of course, depend on the needs and wishes of the care-recipient. Medicines-related activities have been shown to be integral to care-giving: and this may explain why there have been so few studies focussing specifically on this aspect. While recognising the varying roles of family carers in assisting in the use of medicines, in order to address pharmaceutical care issues, we will separately discuss patterns of caring for older and young people.

FAMILY CARERS WHO ASSIST AN OLDER PERSON

The vast majority of unpaid carers providing medicines-related assistance for an older person are close relatives. Older people are major consumers of medicines, and many receive vital assistance from family carers in their use. The range of medicines-related activities that carers can assume is wide,[16, 19, 26] ranging from occasional assistance (e.g. collecting prescriptions from a doctor's office or pharmacy) to regular attendance as necessitated by frequent dosing regimens, assisting in the administration of different dosage forms and/or advising on the need for, and use of, various medicines. It is known that all medicines-related activities can present problems for carers. Ensuring that a person has a continuous supply of their medicines can be a challenging task, for example, different storage sites in the home, pack sizes, formulations and variable need for medicines can all contribute to these difficulties. When dosing regimens are frequent or complex, it can increase the burden especially for carers who have competing demands such as work commitments or children to look after. Problems and concerns are associated with all aspects of carers' activities when assisting with medicines.[26, 20, 25, 27, 28] A UK Government policy document for service development for older people acknowledged that at least half of older people may not be taking their medicines as 6 intended and that older people and carers should be more involved in therapy decisions and receive more information on the risks and benefits.[29]

Supporting both older people and their carers can present dilemmas for health professionals. Often, there are not any formal channels for providing information to carers, due to the awareness of services to preserve the confidentiality and autonomy of patients. However, as disease progresses, the difficulties associated with on-going support for carers so they remain effective in their roles need to be addressed. The provision of care with respect to the needs of both family carers and the older person that they assist, and within the changing context of the partnership between them, will present challenges for health professionals.[22]

MEDICINES-RELATED ASSISTANCE PROVIDED BY FAMILY CARERS OF OLDER PEOPLE

The number of different medication-related tasks undertaken by family carers varies (see Table 11.1). For family carers who assist with only a small number of tasks, these are most likely to be picking up prescriptions, taking them to the pharmacy and collecting the medicines. To provide appropriate pharmaceutical assistance and advice, health professionals (commonly pharmacists) would need to be aware of the range of responsibilities assumed by individual family carers.

TABLE 11-1: MEDICATION-RELATED ASSISTANCE THAT FAMILY CARERS PROVIDE FOR OLDER PEOPLE[19]

ACTIVITY	% WHO PROVIDE THIS
Ordering OP's prescriptions from the doctor's office (n=182)	81
Collecting OP's prescriptions from the doctor's office (n=183)	81
Taking OP's prescriptions to the pharmacy (n=183)	89
Collecting OP's prescription medication from the pharmacy (n=183)	97
Buying non-prescription medication or other remedies for OP(n=167)	60
Giving or lending medication to OP (n=181)	10
Reminding OP when to take medication (n=181)	55
Opening medication' containers for OP (n=182)	51
Assisting OP with taking or using medication (n=175)	34
Deciding how much medication OP should take or how often (n=178)	25
Noticing and managing OP's side-effects to medication (n=127)	58
Giving OP any other information or help with medication (n=156)	44

Note: OP = older person

PROBLEMS EXPERIENCED BY FAMILY CARERS IN THE MEDICINES-RELATED ROLES

Because a high proportion of family carers of older people are older themselves, it is not surprising that they may also experience some difficulties in the use of medicines, similar to those of their older family member. One-third of family carers, providing some medicines-related assistance rated their own health as either fair or poor, suggesting that they may have their own health needs which may affect their ability to care. It was also notable that family carers whose medication-related responsibilities included providing assistance in the home with the administration of medicines and/or advising on their use, were significantly more likely to find their caring role stressful.[19]

For the purposes of identifying the problems experienced by family carers, medicines management activities can be categorised into four main groups:[20]

- Activities associated with maintaining supplies of medicines, which include monitoring use and quantities in the home, liaising with doctor's offices and pharmacies in the ordering and collecting of new prescriptions

- Assisting with administration and reminding when doses are due
- Advising on the use of medicines, including interpreting information and making judgements of the need for, and appropriate use of, different products
- Communicating with the older person and health professionals

Family carers have been found to experience problems with all of these activities. Examining the types of problems that arise in relation to each of these categories provides some insight into pharmaceutical care needs of family carers, as well as indications on how these might be addressed. The discussion below is taken from a UK multicentre study that examined medication-related problems from the perspective of family carers.[19, 20]

MAINTAINING SUPPLIES OF MEDICINES

Many family carers experience difficulties in making sure there are always sufficient supplies of medicines in the home and that new supplies are ordered so that they arrive in time. This can be more of a problem when the older person is taking a number of different products or formulations, each with its own regimen, such that new supplies are needed at different times. For the convenience of the older person, medication may also be stored in different parts of the home. This complicates the monitoring of supplies. Family carers find that careful organisation is required to ensure that medicines are always available. This is often a time-consuming task.

Opening times of doctor's offices and pharmacies for some family carers are inconvenient, especially for those working or with family commitments. At the doctor's office, the need for advance ordering, dealing with unexpected changes on prescriptions, spotting errors, delays in updating of computer systems with new prescription requirements, different pack sizes for different products, all lead to problems.

Difficulties in pharmacy services include frequent low stocks and non-availability products necessitating return visits to the pharmacy. Provision of medications from different manufacturers, means that new supplies look different; family carers and older people worry that the wrong product has been dispensed. Labelling also sometimes leads to uncertainty, e.g. inadequate dose directions or dose changes about which the family carer or older person has not been informed. These problems can increase the burden of caring, as the family carer has to take steps to obtainclarification or rectify errors.

ASSISTING WITH ADMINISTRATION

Many older people use a large number of medicines, and a number of different formulations. Family carers often devise systems, such as removing tablets from containers in advance and arranging them so that the person for whom they care knows exactly what has to be taken and when. Frequent dosing schedules can mean that family carers have to be available to assist throughout the day. This may be difficult for family carers with other commitments. Some family carers, especially older family carers, experience similar difficulties to the older people in terms of remembering when the medicines are due, opening containers and reading labels.

When reviewing medication for older people, the dose regimens and formulations should be discussed with family carers and whenever possible take into account their other commitments. Frequent and complex medication regimens can be very onerous for family carers significantly increasing both the burden and the stress of caring.

ADVISING ON USE OF MEDICINES

Family carers inevitably have their own views and beliefs regarding the use of medicines, which will be reflected in the advice they give and the decisions they make. This can result in the family carers often taking an active role in questioning the appropriateness of the older person's medication. They may have concerns regarding the quantity of different medicines, the suitability of particular medicines, doubts about appropriate doses and/ or anxieties about side-effects.

The concerns of family carers and their perceptions of their responsibilities to try and ensure that their family member receives appropriate medicines can lead them to make independent decisions about doses, in terms of the need for individual medicines and the timing of doses. This may be dependent on the perceived clinical needs of the older person, but can also be in relation to meal times and/or to fit in with the family carer's own availability.

COMMUNICATING WITH THE CARE-RECIPIENT AND HEALTH PROFESSIONALS

Despite providing wide-ranging assistance with medicines, family carers receive very limited systematic support. Although some health professionals may be aware that a family carer assists the care-recipient, the family carer is not necessarily involved in consultations. There is often very little routine help for family carers in interpreting written information, such as printed leaflets in medicine packages, especially in relation to recognising side-effects and assessing their importance. Family carers need to understand how each product should be used and be able to assess if it is being used effectively. They are also often in the sole position of having to answer the older person's questions about their medicines and to reassure them. Presently, support for family carers, from health professionals including pharmacists, is very limited.

Family carers and older people work together in different ways in managing medicines.[22] In many cases, they work as a team, sharing responsibilities, discussing needs and information. However, it may not always be possible for family carers to elicit the co-operation of the older person. They may feel a need to make unilateral decisions that they believe are in the best interests of the older person. For example, a family carer may withhold information in the belief that they are protecting the older person from knowledge that they may find upsetting or that it would have a negative effect on the older person's adherence to their medication regimen.

Differing views between family carers and the older person for whom they are caring commonly complicate the caring role and have implications for the clinical care of the older person. Dilemmas for family carers can arise. These may be struggles by either the family carer or the older person to maintain some level of control over the use of medicines. Family carers may wish to ensure that the older person for whom they are caring receives appropriate drug therapy while also enabling them to maintain a level of independence and exercise autonomy in matters relating to their health care and medicines. Older people may wish to retain some control over their use of medicines and exercise their own judgements. The ability of family carers to manage complex medication regimens, sometimes in the context of difficult partnerships, can be a source of great anxiety.

Health professionals often feel a duty to observe confidentiality, but also will wish a patient to receive the most appropriate care. Autonomy has been defined as a person's ability and opportunity to make decisions relating to his/her own wishes.[30] In caring for older people, a balance needs to be found which respects the autonomy of the older person and ensures an appropriate level of confidentiality, while making available optimal information to enable family carers to be effective in their roles.[22] Caring is also dynamic. Health professionals cannot make assumptions regarding the relative needs of family carers and older people for support and information in relation to their medicines, based on a previous consultation or situation. A sudden or gradual change in the health of either family carer or older person may trigger changes in patterns of partnership and responsibility for medicines. Family carers and older people also have concerns for the future. Many family carers may worry about a possible deterioration in their own or their family member's health such that they are no longer able to care. Health professionals require a range of strategies and approaches that may be implemented with family carers and older people as each new situation presents.

FAMILY CARERS OF CHILDREN AND YOUNG PEOPLE

Caring is diverse. For those family carers looking after a child or young person with a chronic condition, managing medicines can be an important part of caring. Parents may have additional roles in terms of co-ordinating medicines use outside the home, e.g. in schools, at friends' homes, school trips etc. As children grow up, it is generally assumed that children will take on more responsibilities for their care and medicines. However, there has been only limited research into how responsibilities are shared within the home, the roles of parents as family carers in managing medicines and how this changes over time.

A study of young people 8–15 years with either asthma or diabetes examined medicines management in the home from the point of view of the young people themselves and their parents (i.e. the family carers).[23] Tables 2 and 3 describe which medicines-related activities were undertaken by the young people, the parents and/or shared between them.

TABLE 11-2: CHILDREN AND YOUNG PEOPLE WITH ASTHMA: SHARING OF MEDICINES-RELATED ACTIVITIES AND THEIR PARENTS (N=43)[23]

ACTIVITY	PERFORMED BY PARENT	SHARED BETWEEN YOUNG PERSON AND PARENT	PERFORMED BY YOUNG PERSON	% WHO PROVIDE THIS
Monitoring supplies and ordering prescriptions	38	1	2	2*
Collecting prescriptions	43	0	0	0
Remembering/reminding to take medicines	40	0	3	0
Administration of medicines	1	0	42	0
Decisions about the need for medicines**	25	0	5	13***

*seasonal asthma, requiring only one prescription per year
**relates to medicines prescribed for use as required
***decisions reported as responsibility of health professionals

TABLE 11-3: CHILDREN AND YOUNG PEOPLE WITH DIABETES: SHARING OF MEDICINES-RELATED ACTIVITIES AND THEIR PARENTS (N=26)[23]

ACTIVITY	PERFORMED BY PARENT	SHARED BETWEEN YOUNG PERSON AND PARENT	PERFORMED BY YOUNG PERSON
Monitoring supplies and ordering prescriptions	23	1	2
Collecting prescriptions	25	1	0
Remembering/reminding to monitor blood glucose levels	15	3	8
Monitoring of blood glucose levels	2	4	20
Remembering/reminding to administer insulin	13	4	9
Administration of insulin	5	11	10

In the case of young people with asthma, the responsibilities for obtaining supplies of medicines: monitoring supplies in the home, collaborating with health professionals for further prescriptions and collecting medicines from a pharmacy were generally taken by parents. In contrast, the young people commonly took responsibility for the administration of their medicines as well as some of the decision-making regarding the need for medicines. Similarly, the parents (family carers) of young people with diabetes generally took responsibility for maintaining supplies, but the young person usually monitored their own blood glucose levels and administered insulin.

Another study, focussing on young people with cystic fibrosis,[21] found that parents experienced difficulties in fitting a complex medication regimen into daily life while maximising the opportunities for their child to participate as fully as possible in educational and social activities. Parents mentioned the tension between the potential stigma of chronic conditions and the need to ensure adherence to medication regimens and special requirements while enabling integration into normal life.

Cystic fibrosis care in the UK involves health professionals in both the non-specialist and specialist sectors. Many parents experienced limitations in the knowledge and experience of non-specialists when asking for advice and support, in particular, parents described disagreeing with recommendations and advice; these conflicts can be stressful. Also, an added problem when care is shared between specialist and non-specialist centers is that the recommendations may differ. Parents, as family carers in these situations, have the added role of acting as advocate for their child in persuading reluctant non-specialist staff to follow the advice of the specialist centre (in whom they usually have more confidence).

Many studies have highlighted the limited involvement that children and young people have in consultations with health professionals. As a result, health professionals may well be unaware of the contrasting situation in the home, where young people are actively involved in medicines-related activities and exercise some autonomy regarding the use of their medicines. Young people also have their own priorities and concerns that they bring to decisions regarding the use of their medicines. Thus in supporting parents, as family carers, the perspectives of the young person should be sought.

Some studies have also uncovered potential conflicts between parents and young people, perhaps wider struggles for autonomy within the parent-young person relationship, that are reflected in decision-making about, and control regarding, the use of medicines.[31] In the case of the need for medication to avert life-threatening situations, any conflict would lead to a high level of anxiety.

Again, the caring role is dynamic in that the patterns of responsibility for medicines may change on a day-to-day basis, Circumstances that lead parents to increase their involvement include worsening of the condition or unsettled periods in home life. Situations that promote the transfer of responsibility for medicines to the young person include social and educational events, e.g. progressing to high school, staying overnight with friends and schools trips.[23]

A central aim of health policy is to find ways to encourage and empower young people to take a more active role in managing their health (which includes medicines). Collecting prescriptions from a pharmacy is the medicines-related activity that a young person is least likely to assume, partly due to legal constraints regarding the supply of medicines to minors. However, pharmacists will often see young people in the pharmacy, and the young person's lack of participation in any discussion should not be regarded as a reflection of a lack of wider involvement in the administration of their medicines and decisions about their use. At an early age, and with parental consent, engaging with young people in a positive way to inform them of the potential source of advice and support that pharmacists can provide regarding medicines use is an important aspect of developing a future constructive relationship with the young person. Supporting young people in making informed decisions may empower them to assume greater responsibility and appropriate management of their condition in the context of their daily lives. Health professionals, including pharmacists, may also wish to consider how they can facilitate the longerterm transfer of responsibility for medicines from parents to young people. Support for the transfer of responsibility for medicines, has been identified by family carers as a major issue for which advice is not necessarily available.

CARERS AND HIGH TECHNOLOGY PHARMACEUTICAL CARE

Increasingly, in many countries, the delivery of high technology pharmaceutical care is becoming feasible in the home. In many countries because of the rising costs of institutional provision, governments are open to new and diverse ways of delivering care. With many people with chronic health problems preferring to remain in their own homes, this has implications for family carers and their families.

A small qualitative study of patients with chronic obstructive pulmonary disease (COPD) illustrated the expert assistance family carers provided with prescribed nebulizer therapy, and the specific problems they experienced.[25] Carers assumed responsibility for practical assistance specific to nebulizer use, such as cleaning and maintenance, organizational, and therapeutic management. The carers commented on the difficulties they experienced with regards to obtaining equipment, the associated costs, and the problems with getting equipment serviced when it was in constant use. Effective use of nebulizers is essential for good management of COPD and to prevent exacerbations, which often result in a hospital admission. Many of the difficulties reported by carers could be anticipated to have a negative impact on patient outcomes.

In a study of young people with cystic fibrosis,[21] parents described having to be familiar with complex pharmaceutical delivery equipment including intravenous lines, nebulizers, and inhalers. They also reported stress and anxiety in having to deal with the supply of incorrect products and equipment. Parents felt they had to become "experts" in overseeing and making judgements about their child's therapy. Parents monitored the use of pancreatic enzymes, antibiotics, and inhalers. While many parents felt confident in these activities, others preferred a health professional to be involved.

A further study examined the daily lives of children/young people with diabetes mellitus and their families, when they were switched from multiple daily injections to insulin pumps.[32] While administration of insulin via pumps rather than injections was generally preferred because of benefits to glycaemic control, general well-being, and enabling young people to live more normal lives, it was reported that initially, parents experienced particular difficulties with the introduction of the new medical technology. In this study, the parents reported experiencing challenges in relation to learning about mechanical and operational aspects of the pump, the increased frequency of monitoring of blood glucose (sometimes resulting in disturbed sleep), and the complex tasks of carbohydrate counting, basal adjustments, and changing infusion sets. This study also illustrated the highly specialized roles undertaken by some family carers and the additional impact of the introduction of novel medical technologies.

To achieve policy goals for effective home-based care for people with complex health needs, pharmaceutical care that addresses the needs of family carers as well as those of the patients is essential. As regimens and equipment become more complex, the burden and strain on family carers, and the compromises in family life will increase. It is important for health professionals to take a holistic approach to the provision of pharmaceutical care in the home to achieve the best possible outcomes in relation to clinical care, wider health-related quality of life of patients, and the quality of life and burden on family carers. Effective communication pathways between specialist and non-specialist pharmacy services may help to provide educational support to the community-based pharmacist, which in turn would provide a further avenue of local support for parents and young people on specialist technologies when dealing with these dilemmas.

CARING FOR FAMILY AND FRIENDS WITH DEMENTIA

Assisting a person with dementia presents unique issues that need to be taken into account when designing pharmaceutical support services. When caring for a person with dementia, medicines-related activities can become more complex. Family carers may progressively assume greater responsibilities for all aspects of medicines use. Thus, the burden associated with medicines-related activities will often increase. Assistance required from carers will evolve as a consequence of limited memory and understanding, and possible lack of insight. The difficulties and burden of caring can be further compounded by potential or actual challenging behaviours, and upset regarding the progression and effects of disease. These can relate specifically to added problems in the administration of medicines, as well as ensuring optimal outcomes. Recent studies have found that carers of people with dementia have distinct needs regarding medication management activities, which contribute to carerburden and stress, which are often unacknowledged by health professionals.[33, 34]

FAMILY CARERS AND HEALTH PROFESSIONALS

Family carers have been found to be more proactive in seeking resources and talking to health professionals once they have self-identified.[35] However, problems can be compounded when health professionals may be hesitant to divulge what they see as confidential patient information, even though it is to that person's carer, resulting in the carer feeling uninformed and unsupported.[36] In the delivery of effective pharmaceutical care it is important that pharmacists are aware that they only see the "tip of the iceberg" of family carers' involvement unless they take proactive steps to delve further. More attention must be paid to the ethical dilemmas associated with the way in which health services and professionals respond to family carers' needs and support them in their caring roles.

All caring situations differ, depending on the needs of the person being cared for, the ability of the family carer to provide help, and the context of the partnership between both parties governing the dynamics of the caring role. The challenge for pharmacists is the lack of guidance on appropriate ways to effectively consult with carers of people with dementia and which information may be shared.

IMPLICATIONS FOR PHARMACEUTICAL CARE

Effective pharmaceutical care for family carers is dependent upon the pharmacist identifying family carers and taking time to understand their medication-related roles and associated problems. Many family carers will not self-identify or even identify with the term "carer" as they are simply a family member/friend/neighbour helping another family member/friend/neighbour.

Studies among family carers have identified a number of areas that may be improved to decrease the burden and anxiety associated with their medicines-related activities. For example, family carers would value effective systems of communication between prescribers and pharmacists to enable supplies to be ordered and prepared in advance. More streamlined ordering and collecting systems would reduce the burden associated with maintaining continuous supplies. Family carers highlighted the benefits of a pharmacist who was familiar with "their case" and could be proactive in addressing potential problems such as clarifying prescription changes, providing reassurance and being available for discussion.

While the administering of medicines occurs in the home, the descriptions by family carers of their roles and problems indicate ways in which pharmacists can support these activities. For example, ensuring full directions and explanations for the use of all products are easy to read and understand. Medication reviews should take into account the role of family carers, e.g. considering the feasibility of dosing schedules that require frequent attendance, attention to the number of formulations, simplification of dosing regimens to enable easy integration into daily routines. Pharmacists making themselves available to family carers as a source of advice and support for the hidden "clinical" roles that are frequently undertaken by family carers in the home such as advising on the need for "when required" (and sometimes regular) medicines, and identifying and responding to side effects, has been identified as important to family carers.

Fundamental to successful pharmaceutical care will be effective communication between family carers, the person for whom they care and pharmacists. As highlighted earlier, the first barrier to this communication may be the lack of awareness among pharmacists, and indeed of family carers themselves, in terms of each others' potential roles and opportunities for working together to better address the pharmaceutical needs of the person being cared for at home. Pharmacists should ensure they are available and accessible to discuss and review the administration and effectiveness of medicines, and provide an opportunity for family carers to express their views, observations and concerns. Equally, the pharmacist must bear in mind potentially differing perspectives and agendas of family carers and the person for whom they care. Depending on the relationship, caution may be required regarding sharing confidential information. It may be necessary to involve the person being cared for in discussions or expressly obtain their consent. Pharmacists are more familiar than most health care professionals with the barriers that third party consultations pose for good pharmaceutical care. However, recognizing and addressing this as an important feature of pharmacy services may lead to ways to support and empower family carers, who after all provide more health care than any group of professional carers. To date, there is very limited guidance for pharmacists regarding ethical legal contexts and expectations of providing information and support for carers who assist others with their medicines.

One of the most difficult areas for the development of pharmacy services is the integration between non-specialist and specialist services, with the associated complex drug therapy and pharmaceutical equipment. Greater communication between hospital-based and community-based (specialist and non-specialist) pharmacists may be one strand of improving the network of support for these patient/family carer groups, once they have left the specialist care providers. In the hospital setting, in-patients will often be able to identify others who will be assisting them with their medicines when they return home. Many will be visiting the patient in hospital. In most cases family carers and the person for whom they are caring will be happy to jointly discuss their medicines.[18] The period following hospital discharge has been identified in a number of studies as being problematic as changes to medication regimens commonly occur. There is often a delay and confusion in transferring information to the community setting, e.g. uncertainty regarding which pre-admission medicines are to be continued alongside any new ones. At the time of discharge from hospital, pharmacists could arrange their consultation for a time when the family carer can be present. This will ensure the family carer has the opportunity to hear explanations about medicines and their use, and ask questions.

It is also essential to recognise that some family carers and the people for whom they care are "experts" in the management of particular conditions. They are well-informed and have high levels of knowledge regarding the use of their medicines. They will also know what works for them in the context of their lives. It is important that pharmacists and other health professionals are ready to provide the support for these patients to enable them to maintain high quality pharmaceutical care, and perhaps individualise this according to their specific requests and agendas.

As populations age, all over the world, there is a need to develop health care interventions to support carers in their activities, to reduce carer-burden and enable them to be effective in their roles. It has been acknowledged that the views of carers themselves should be sought in developing and designing these interventions. In a study of family carers who provide assistance with medicines for people with dementia, the carers provided a number of practical suggestions that could be the focus of such interventions. These included improved processes of communication with health professionals, systems to improve timing and transfer of medicinesrelated information between health care settings and health professionals, and enhanced roles of pharmacy services in assisting in timely refills and information. Carers also high-lighted the need for greater training for health professionals.[34]

Increasingly health professionals are recognising the importance of providing effective support for family carers, and a number of studies are on-going, including in the pharmacy sector.[37] But, presently, while there has been research highlighting the important medicines-related roles of carers and the associated carer-burden, there is very limited evidence regarding effective interventions. The evaluation of such interventions also requires appropriate methods and measures for the assessment of outcomes from the perspectives of carers and the people for whom they care.

SUMMARY

This chapter has demonstrated the importance of identifying the perspectives and needs of family carers in the provision of pharmaceutical care. The involvement of family carers in medicines-management can be extensive and complex. Family carers undertake a wide-range of different activities and responsibilities in the context of their own perspectives, circumstances, and lives. The impact of pharmaceutical care will be seriously compromised until the medicines-related needs and perspectives or family carers are recognised as fundamental to its processes and outcomes. Appropriate legal and ethical frameworks, from the point of view of pharmacists and other health care professionals, are needed to help clarify the roles and responsibilities of pharmacists and pharmacy services to service users and their carers. The development of interventions to reduce associated carer-burden and enable carers to be effective, needs to be a priority for health professionals, and in their evaluation, carer-burden associated with medicines-management activities is an important outcome measure.

REFERENCES

1. Office for National Statistics. (1998). *Informal unpaid carers: results of an independent study carried out on behalf of the Department of Health as part of the 1995 General Household Survey.* London: The Stationery Office.

2. United Nations. (2014). *Population Facts No. 2014/4*—Population ageing and sustainable development. Available from www.unpopulation.org.

3. ONS. (2012). Population ageing in the United Kingdom, its constituent countries and the European Union. London: Office for National Statistics.

4. Department of Health and Human Services. (1998). *Informal caregiving: Compassion in action.* Washington, DC: Department of Health and Human Services. Based on data from the National Survey of Families and Households (NSFH), 1998 and the National Family Caregivers Association. (2004). *Random sample survey of family 20 caregivers*, Summer 2000. Unpublished and National Alliance for Caregiving and AARP, Caregiving in the U.S.

5. Feinberg, L., Reinhard, S.C., Houser, A., & Choula, R. (2011). *Valuing the invaluable: 2011 update, the growing contributions and costs of family caregiving, insight on the issues #51.* Washington, DC: AARP Public Policy Institute.

6. Australian Bureau of Statistics. (2012). *Survey of disability, ageing and carers.*

7. Mental Health Council of Australia and Carers Australia. (2000). *Carers of people with mental illness.*

8. National Alliance for Caregiving and AARP. (2004). *Caregiving in the U.S.*

9. Access Economics. *The economic value of informal care in 2010.* (2010.) Report for Carers Australia.

10. Unpaid carers UK. (2002). *Without us...? Recalculating the value of unpaid carers support.* London: Unpaid carers UK.

11. Department of Health. (2014). *Carers Strategy: Second national action plan 2014–2016.* London: Department of Health.

12. Ranelli, P.L. (1991). Exploratory study of caregivers' need and perceptions of pharmaceutical care for elder care-recipients. *Journal of Geriatric Drug Therapy* 6:75–84.

13. Mallet, L. & King, T. (1993). Evaluating family caregivers' knowledge of medication. *Journal of Geriatric Drug Therapy* 7:47–58.

14. Ranelli, P.L. & Aversa, S. L. (1994). Medication-related stressors among family caregivers. *American Journal of Hospital Pharmacy* 51:75–79.

15. Ranelli, P.L. & Hansen, R.W. (1994). Medication-related stressors and the family caregiver: a qualitative analysis. *Research in the Sociology of Health Care* 14:233–248.

16. Goldstein, R. & Rivers, P. (1996). The medication role of informal unpaid carers. *Health & Social Care in the Community* 4:150–158.

17. Boyle, E. & Chambers, M. (2000). Medication compliance in older individuals with depression: gaining the views of family unpaid carers. *Journal of Psychiatric and Mental Health Nursing* 7:512–522.

18. Gupta, D., Smith, F.J. & Francis, S-A. (2002). Supporting informal unpaid carers in their medication management activities: opportunities in the hospital setting. *Hospital Pharmacist* 9:55–58.

19. Francis, S-A., Smith, F., Gray, N., & Graffy, J. (2002). The roles of informal unpaid carers in the management of medication for older care-recipients. *International Journal of Pharmacy Practice* 10:1–9.

20. Smith, F.J., Francis, S-A., Gray, N.J., Denham, M.J., & Graffy, J.P. (2003). A multi-centre survey among informal unpaid carers who manage medication for older care-recipients: problems experienced and the development of services. *Health and Social Care in the Community* 11:138–145.

21. Slatter, A.J., Francis, S-A., Smith, F.J., Bush, A. (2004). Medication use in children with cystic fibrosis: The unpaid carers' perspectives. *British Journal of Nursing* 13:1135–1139.

22. Francis, S.A., Smith, F.J., Gray, N.J., & Denham. M. (2006). Partnerships between older people and their unpaid carers in the management of medication. *International Journal for Older People Nursing* 1:210–7

23. Newbould, J., Smith, F.J., & Francis, S-A. (2008). "I'm fine doing it on my own": partnerships between parents and young people in the management of medication for asthma and diabetes. *Journal of Child Health Care* 12: 116–128.

24. Gillespie, R., Mullan, J. & Harrison, L. (2014). Managing medications: the role of informal caregivers of older adults and people living with dementia: a review of the literature. *Journal of Clinical Nursing* 23: 3296–3308.

25. Alhaddad, B., Smith, F.J., Robertson, T., et al. (2015). Patients' practices and experiences of using nebuliser therapy in the management of COPD at home. *BMJ Open Resp Res* 2:e000076. doi:10.1136/bmjresp-2014- 000076

26. Travis, S.S., Bethea, L.S., & Winn, P. (2000). Medication administration hassles reported by family caregivers of dependent elderly persons. *Journal of Gerontology* 55A:M412–M417.

27. Travis, S.S., McAuley, W.J., Dmochowski, .J, Bernard, M.A., Kao, H-F., & Greene, R. (2007). Factors associated with medication hassles experienced by family care-givers of older adults. *Patient Education and Counselling* 66: 51–57.

28. Orlu-Gul, M,. Raimi-Abraham, B,. Jamieson, E., Wei, L., Murray, M., Stawarz, K., Stegemann, S., Tuleu, C., & Smith, F.J. (2014). Public Engagement workshop: How to Improve medicines for older people. *International Journal of Pharmaceutics* 459(1–2):65–9.

29. Department of Health. National Service Framework for Older People. (2001). *Medicines and older people: Implementing the medicines-related aspects of the NSF for older people.* London: Department of Health.

30. Rosin, A.J. & van Dijk, Y. (2005). Subtle ethical dilemmas in geriatric management and clinical research. *Journal of Medical Ethics* 31:355–9.

31. Atkin, K., Ahmad, W.I.U. (2000). Pumping iron: compliance with chelation therapy among young people who have thalassaemia major. *Sociology of Health and Illness* 22:500–524.

32. Alsaleh, Fm., Smith, Fj., Thompson, R., Al-Saleh, M.A., Taylor, Kmg. (2014). Insulin pump therapy: Impact on the lives of children/young people with diabetes mellitus and their parents. *International Journal of Clinical Pharmacy* Vol. 36(5), pp.1023–1030.

33. While, C., Duane, F., Beanland, C., & Koch, S. (2013). Medication-management: the perspectives of people with dementia and family carers. *Dementia* 12: 734–750.

34. Smith, F.J., Grijseels, M.S., Ryan, P., & Tobiansky, R. (2014). Assisting people with dementia with their medicines: Experiences of family carers. *IJPP* 23: 44–51.

35. National Family Caregivers Association. (2001). *Survey of self-identified family caregivers.*

36. Poland, F., Mapes, S., Pinnock, H., Katona, C., Sorensen, S., Fox, C., & Maidment, I. (2024). Perspectives of carers on medication management in dementia: lessons from collaboratively developing a research proposal. *BMC Research Notes* 7: 463.

37. http://psnc.org.uk/wp-content/uploads/2014/10/Carer-Friendly-Pharmacy-Pilot-Summary.pdf (accessed 03 February 2015)

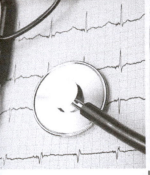
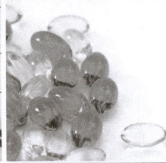
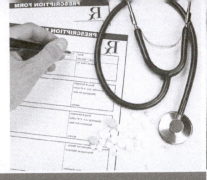
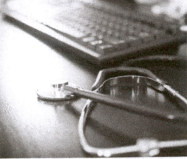
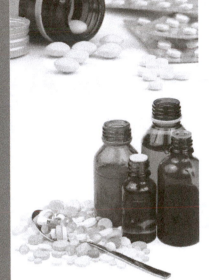
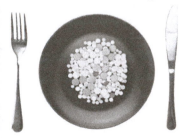
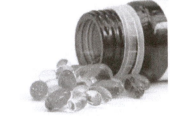
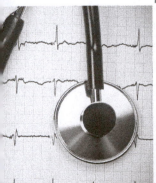
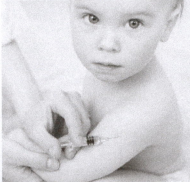
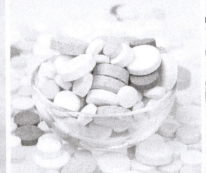
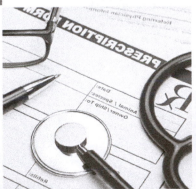

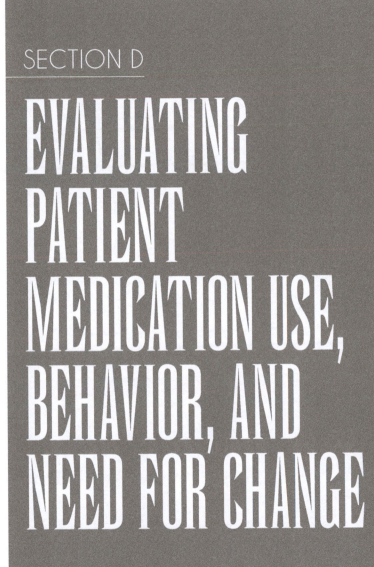

SECTION D

EVALUATING PATIENT MEDICATION USE, BEHAVIOR, AND NEED FOR CHANGE

CHAPTER 12

PSYCHOSOCIAL ASPECTS OF MEDICATION ADHERENCE

Nathaniel M. Rickles and Kevin C. Farmer

LEARNING OBJECTIVES:

1. Distinguish among different terms that describe various medication-taking behaviors.
2. Describe the consequences of medication non-adherence.
3. Compare and contrast among different methods to measure medication adherence and persistence.
4. Analyze the strengths and limitations of different types of interventions to improve medication adherence and persistence.
5. Summarize the different ways pharmacists can improve medication adherence and persistence.

KEY TERMS

Administrative support

Behavioral intervention

Direct methods

Educational intervention

Electronic monitoring device

Epidemiology of medication
non-adherence

Indirect methods

Medication adherence

Medication interest

Medication non-adherence

Medication persistence

Medication possession ratios (MPR)

Partial non-adherence

Pill counts

Primary non-adherence

Proportionate days covered ratios (PDC)

Refill record

Repeat non-adherence

Self-report

INTRODUCTION

Advancements in pharmaceutical research and development have created highly effective medications designed to improve and extend patients' lives. Patients can maximize the benefits and avoid some of the negative effects of these medications by taking the medications as prescribed according to clinical and research evidence. Medication adherence has been defined as the extent to which a patient acts in accordance with the prescribed interval and dose of a medication dosing regimen.[1] Therefore, medication non-adherence refers to a range of behaviors leading to non-prescribed use of a medication: failure to initially fill a prescription (primary medication non-adherence), failure to pick-up refills, taking an incorrect dose, forgetting to take doses, skipping doses, errors in dose timing, incorrect method of administration, and stopping the medication prematurely. Researchers have developed different terms to categorize such behaviors: primary medication non-adherence for not initiating medication use, partial non-adherence for behaviors related to missing 20% or less of prescribed doses, and repeat non-adherence for behaviors related to missing greater than 20% of prescribed doses.[2,3] While the same behaviors contributing to partial non-adherence can cause repeat non-adherence, it is not always the case. A patient may experience partial non-adherence due to forgetting but over months of taking a medication develop repeat non-adherence due to negative beliefs of taking the medication.

In general, many stakeholders in healthcare have moved away from the older term "compliance" since it tends to suggest patients are passive participants in the decision to take their medications. Terms such as "medication adherence" and "medication interest" suggest individuals are more proactive in their decisions to take medications.[4] The evolution of these terms illustrates the joint responsibility and relationship between the patient and healthcare provider in managing the patient's health, and recognizing that ultimately the patient actively manages and controls his or her health. For the purposes of simplicity and clarity, this chapter will use the term *medication adherence/non-adherence* as a general reference to the extent to which a patient adopts a prescribed medication regimen.

Medication non-adherence has been a long-standing public health problem. Poor adherence is associated with the unsafe use of medications and increased health costs. Specifically, the costs associated with patients not taking their medications as directed have been estimated to exceed $290 billion annually due to the additional healthcare services needed.[5] More than 25% of medication-related hospital admissions are reportedly due to poor adherence.[6] See Table 12-1 for additional examples of costs related to medication non-adherence. Further, over 100,000 patient deaths each year are linked to poor medication adherence.[7,8] The US. Surgeon General has stated that medication adherence is one of the country's most significant public health issues noting that medication non-adherence is a major contributor to the development of patient drug resistance and drug-resistant strains of infectious disease—a major public health crisis.[9] Medication adherence has been a topic discussed and investigated for more than 60 years and largely began from early research to understand the lack of patient engagement in tuberculosis screening in the 1950s. Much of this research has also yielded different theoretical models for explaining psychosocial factors associated with treatment adherence behavior. These models are reviewed in earlier chapters of this textbook. The Health Belief Model is one of the oldest and best researched models for understanding and predicting adherence behavior.[10] In this chapter, we will not focus on these theoretical explanations of medication adherence but rather examine the implications of medication adherence for clinical practice. Therefore, the chapter will explore the following topics: the epidemiology of non-adherence, causes/predictors of medication non-adherence, detection of medication nonadherence, measurement of medication adherence, and interventions to improve medication adherence.

TABLE 12-1: RISK OF HOSPITALIZATION AND TOTAL HEALTHCARE COSTS IN DIABETES AND HYPERLIPIDEMIA

		MEDICATION ADHERENCE LESS THAN 20%	MEDICATION ADHERENCE 80% OR GREATER
Diabetes	Total health costs	$8,867	$4,570
	Risk of hospitalization	30%	13%
Hyperlipidemia	Total health costs	$6,810	$3,124
	Risk of hospitalization	15%	12%

Adapted from: Sokol, MC, McGuigan KA, Verbrugge RR, Epstein, RS. Impact of medication adherence on hospitalization risk and healthcare cost. Med Care 2008;43(6):521–530.

EPIDEMIOLOGY OF MEDICATION NON-ADHERENCE

The degree to which an individual adheres with their medication differs by the person, the disease state, and the medication used. The rate of adherence with medications has been reported across a broad range of values from averages in the single digits to over 90%.[11,12] It is commonly reported that on average, across several disease states, that individuals adhere to their medication regimens about 50% of the time.[13] Recent reports of medication adherence indicate adherence rates in primary care populations of 46.2%, 60%, and 45.1% for depression, cardiovascular diseases, and diabetes respectively.[14-16] These adherence rates typically refer to partial or repeat non-adherence. Primary medication non-adherence rates are also relatively high with almost 30% of a newly prescribed medication never picked up at the pharmacy.[2] Even within disease states, there is much variability in reports of all adherence rates. This variability may be due to a number of factors including: various methods and time periods used to calculate adherence, the condition being treated, side-effects of the drug used, and other factors related to the patient which can significantly influence adherence. For example, adherence rates are often lower for chronic illnesses such as diabetes and higher for HIV. Adherence rates with acute conditions tend to be higher than chronic illnesses since acute conditions are associated with bothersome symptoms compared to ongoing and perhaps "silent" symptoms associated with chronic illnesses. Adherence rates also differed by the method of measurement used in adherence studies. The description and use of these methods can be found in the section on measurement of nonadherence in this chapter.

PREDICTORS OF MEDICATION NON-ADHERENCE

There are several patient, provider, and system-level factors and predictors that can help to identify those who may be at risk for medication non-adherence (see Table 12-2).[11,17-20] These indicators can then be used to target patients for further evaluation or need of interventions to improve adherence. Forgetfulness or the inability to remember the details of directions can be quite common. Memory issues are particularly a problem when the patient has a complex regimen involving receiving multiple medications, multiple doses/day, and/or requires devices for administration. Complicated regimens can be particular challenging for those with physical disabilities and/or requiring caregiver assistance and those with hectic lifestyles. In a similar fashion, a lack of understanding of specific instructions or details impedes the ability of the patient to execute directions. Patients may be bombarded with a large amount of verbal instructions and tend to forget a large amount of it unless written instructions are provided as reinforcements. These latter concerns about understanding of medication information are particularly notable with patients with low health literacy.

TABLE 12-2: MULTI-LEVEL FACTORS AFFECTING MEDICATION ADHERENCE

PATIENT LEVEL	PROVIDER LEVEL	SYSTEM LEVEL
• Memory/recall of regimen • Regimen comprehension • Medication Beliefs • Regimen complexity • Side effects • Caregiver support • Ability to pay/insurance coverage • Transportation • Type of illnesses • Cognitive limitations	• Quality of medication instruction and support • Relationship with patient • Knowledge about adherence • Communication skills • Quality of monitoring and problem-solving • Use of tools to improve consistency of care • Attitudes toward adherence management	• Access to insurance • Formulary coverage and complexity • Administrative barriers- Prior authorizations • Team integration and continuity • IT infrastructure and integration of multiple data systems • Use of guidelines/clinical pathways • Access to case management tools to optimize efficiency and effectiveness of care

Medication side effects can also lead to nonadherence, and can be particularly problematic when used for diseases in which side effects of the medication are more troublesome than the condition being treated. The asymptomatic nature of the disease also represents a significant factor contributing to medication nonadherence since patients can readily identify the benefits of therapy. The presence of depression or cognitive impairments has also been independently associated with nonadherence.[20] Race, gender, or socioeconomic status have not generally predicted adherence. However, the cost of the medication or the insurance copayment can be significant barriers in some individuals, depending on their current economic situation. One study showed that copayments above $50 were the strongest predictor of primary medication nonadherence; such high copayments made it 4.93% more likely prescriptions would not get filled.[21] Patient beliefs about medications such as addiction and the value of medications can affect their likelihood in starting and/or continuing medications. An often overlooked factor that contributes to medication nonadherence is patient satisfaction and relationship with the healthcare team.

DETECTION OF MEDICATION NON-ADHERENCE

Due to the many reasons noted in the previous section as to why individuals do not initiate and/or maintain prescribed medication use, healthcare professionals cannot simply assume the patient will use the medication as intended or directed by the prescriber. Healthcare providers often overestimate adherence and are not skilled in detecting poor adherence.[22] In addition, a recent study suggests community pharmacists are not consistently detecting and managing possible medication non-adherence.[23] There are many reasons why healthcare providers may have difficulty engaging consistently in non-adherence detection: (1) little time to explore non-adherence issues, (2) the lack of cues to remind to explore non-adherence, and (3) the lack of training on how to resolve non-adherence issues effectively and with sensitivity. For example, simple tools for pharmacists and healthcare providers include the use of a question "How do you take your medication?" and listening for red flags such as patients saying "I am supposed to take the medication once a day." This question is one of the three standard questions recommended by the Indian Health Service to detect non-adherence.[24] The other two questions are "What were you told the medication was for?" and "What were you told to expect from the medication?" Patient answers to these questions can give clinicians important insights on patient knowledge and concerns that might be causes for current or future medication non-adherence. Community pharmacists, unlike other healthcare professionals, have access to refill records, which can be helpful in detecting non-adherence by looking for gaps in medication use. The introduction of electronic prescribing has allowed pharmacists to identify individuals who are not picking up medications for the first time. There are several other screening tools available that have been shown to valid and useful in detecting non-adherence.[3,25-27] The differences between some of these tools are the extent of adherence concerns uncovered and for which can serve as the basis for interventions. Such tools are helpful, relatively quick guides to detecting non-adherence, but do not substitute for extended discussions exploring the roots of medication non-adherence. Regardless of tool used, how the information related to medication adherence is obtained and measured is critical to an accurate interpretation of adherence behavior and guiding interventions.

MEASUREMENT OF MEDICATION NON-ADHERENCE

Medication-taking behavior consists of two components: medication adherence and medication persistence.[1] Medication adherence can be measured as the extent to which a patient follows the prescribed interval and dose of a medication regimen. This could be specific to the frequency, dosage, or timing of a medication regimen. This represents dose taking in comparison to what was prescribed. In other words, how well did they take it compared to as recommended? This is commonly calculated by dividing the number of doses reportedly used by the number of doses prescribed and supplied during a specified time frame and expressed as a percentage. A patient taking 26 tablets of a once daily regimen in 30 days would have an adherence rate of 86.6% (26/30 X 100). Medication persistence refers to the length of time taking a medication. Persistence is defined as the duration of time from start of therapy until discontinuation. This measure may be expressed as the number of days or months of therapy. It can also be represented as a yes/no variable if one is interested in determining if a patient is still taking the medication at the end of a specified time.

Caution must be used when relating mean adherence values from studies to an individual patient. Mean values are calculated from groups or populations of individuals distributed around the mean. A specific individual's adherence value may not be close to the average. In a study evaluating adherence in diabetic patients using angiotensin-converting enzyme (ACE) inhibitors or angiotensin receptor blockers (ARBs), the mean adherence rate was 77%. However, upon closer examination of the data on an individual basis, only 60.4% of the patients had adherence rates considered "good" (> 80%), while 21.9% reported adherence categorized as "poor" (between 50% and 80%) and 17.7% had adherence categorized as "very poor" (< 50%).[28] In essence, 4 out of 10 patients in the study were classified as having poor or very poor adherence. As a result, one cannot rely on the mean adherence rates reported in clinical studies to give you information about an individual patient. An individual assessment of each patient is needed to ascertain their level of medication adherence.

Adherence rates also differ by the method of measurement used in adherence studies. In this section, we will explore the benefits or drawbacks of each method, and which would be the most appropriate for provider or researcher needs. Refer to Table 12-3 for a brief overview of the methods, how they are used, if they are used to determine adherence, persistence, or both, key strengths and limitations. Historically, methods have been categorized as either direct or indirect methods.

TABLE 12-3: METHODS FOR MEASURING MEDICATION ADHERENCE

MEASURE	USE IN CLINICAL PRACTICE OR RESEARCH STUDY	ADHERENCE (A) OR PERSISTENCE (P) ANALYSIS	STRENGTHS	LIMITATIONS
Direct Methods				
Blood/serum level	Research	P	Proof of use	Patient variability Invasive Expensive
Ingestible sensor	Practice Research	A P	Proof of use	Invasive Expensive Patient acceptability
Observation	Practice	A	Inexpensive Ease of use	Time intensive Patient may mimic use but not actually consume
Indirect Methods				
Patient interview	Practice Research	A	Inexpensive Ease of use May provide reasons for behavior	Social desirability Skill of interviewer Qualitative Patient recall Can overestimate
Patient diary	Practice Research	A	Inexpensive Can augment electronic monitoring	Patient must remember entries and return diary
Structured questionnaire(s)	Practice Research	A	Ease of use May provide reasons for behavior Many validated	Patient recall Can overestimate

Continued

TABLE 12-3: METHODS FOR MEASURING MEDICATION ADHERENCE

MEASURE	USE IN CLINICAL PRACTICE OR RESEARCH STUDY	ADHERENCE (A) OR PERSISTENCE (P) ANALYSIS	STRENGTHS	LIMITATIONS
Indirect Methods				
Pill count	Practice Research	A	Inexpensive Ease of use	Obtrusive Pill dumping Accuracy
Prescription refill records- (in same pharmacy or pharmacy system)	Practice	A P	Inexpensive Ease of use Accessible to pharmacists	All scripts must be filled in same pharmacy to see all records
Prescription insurance records-(large prescription databases)	Research	A P	Non-invasive Long term data Population data	Quality of data Captures refills regardless of which pharmacy patient goes to
Electronic monitoring devices	Research	A P	Data on dosing intervals Accuracy	Expensive Patient may use other bottles

DIRECT METHODS

BIOLOGICAL MEASURES

Direct methods are those which provide some type of "evidence" the medication was taken by the patient. These include detection of the drug in a biological fluid (usually blood or urine), a biological marker or "tag" attached to a medication, the use of an ingestible sensor, and directly observed administration. A positive biological assay does provide confirmation the patient received a dose of the medication within some limited time frame prior to analysis. Depending on the pharmacokinetic properties of the drug, it is possible for the patient to take just a few doses of the drug prior to the assay and achieve a detectable level of the drug, masking intentional nonadherence by the patient.[29,30] Many factors can also affect the therapeutic level of the drug including food and drug interactions which may make interpretation of the results very difficult. This type of adherence measure is generally impractical for several reasons since they are intrusive (i.e., requiring a blood draw), expensive, and basically provide a current "snapshot" with little information related to the individual's pattern of use.

Proteus Digital Health and the Otsuka Pharmaceutical Company have developed an ingestible sensor for which a patient swallows and sends a signal to a wearable sensor ("patch") that stores dates and times of when the ingestible sensor was swallowed, step counts, sleep duration, and patterns of rest and activity.[31] This data is then sent to a computerized device for display and transmission to a secure cloud-based server. Such technology may allow for greater estimation of medication adherence. While this could become a new gold standard of adherence estimation, it is likely to meet resistance with patient discomfort of "being watched" and ingesting a product with biosensor activity.

OBSERVATIONAL MEASURES

Another direct method of adherence measurement is the observation of patient medication use. This is an approach often used with specific medications for which require close adherence monitoring to ensure efficacy such as medications for substance abuse (methadone, disulfiram), HIV, and conditions for which patients are at high risk of non-adherence such as mental illness. The approach is considered impractical with large populations of individuals given it is time and resource intensive. Also, patients might act if they took the medication but didn't (i.e., hide tablets in the cheeks so it seems they took it).

INDIRECT METHODS

The majority of methods used to detect or analyze medication-taking behavior are indirect methods. The below section will present indirect methods in order from being most subjective to most objective self-reported medication use, pill counts, pharmacy and insurance claim refill records, and electronic monitoring. When indirect methods are used, the consumption or use of the medication by the patient is assumed.

SELF-REPORTED MEDICATION USE

Asking the patient to self-report their medication taking behavior is the simplest and most convenient method of evaluating medication adherence. This is frequently used in clinical practice for the healthcare provider to gauge the patient's medication-taking behavior. Patient self-reported adherence behavior may be conducted in several ways. The clinician interviews the patient with specific questions regarding how (and if) they are using their medication(s). The patient may also be asked to keep a diary of their medication use. The patient also can be given (in person, by mail, or other means) an adherence-specific questionnaire. Advantages to self-report instruments is simplicity and low cost. Limitations of self report methods has been unreliability in reporting accurate adherence and persistence since often subjective based on patient memory and other reporting biases.[32–35] Patients are generally reluctant to reveal they have not taken their medication as instructed and feel interrogated.[36,37] The lack of precision found with self-report methods is frequently due to the manner and language used in the interview, or poorly constructed questionnaires and surveys. The nature and orientation of the questions can influence the patient's response. Questions which make the patient appear responsible for nonadherence and blame the patient for not complying with instructions can bias the response.[38,39] In some cases, patients were asked if they had taken the prescribed number of doses, and if they did not, to estimate how many they had missed over a specific time period.[40]

The development and proliferation of validated structured adherence questionnaires has done much to address the unreliability issues noted with various patient self report methods. The tools previously referenced to be of value in the detection of non-adherence are also of value in the measurement of adherence.[3,25-27] In situations where it is desirable to use a self-report instrument, the use of a validated questionnaire provides a reliable, ready-to-use instrument that can be easily used in a practice or research setting. Several of these tools also explore reasons for patients' non-adherence and can assist with identifying patient-centered interventions.

PILL COUNTS

In addition to self-report, pill counts are another common, inexpensive, and easy method of assessing medication adherence. The patient brings their prescription bottle (or blister pack) with them during the next visit to the clinic or pharmacy. The number of pills returned is counted and compared with the date the prescription was filled and the number of pills which should have been taken during this period of time. Excess pills indicate the patient has taken less than the prescribed amount of medication. This method has a number of drawbacks that inhibit its reliability as an accurate measure of medication adherence. As the patient is aware that their medication is being counted, it is possible for the patient to "dump" unused pills prior to the visit to hide their non-adherence. Pill counts can also be perceived as obtrusive and perceived as a lack of trust, leading to an adversarial patient-provider relationship. The accuracy of pill counts can also be variable due to many other factors: accuracy of date and refill information. Studies have indicated pill counts tend to overestimate adherence behavior compared to prescription claims databases and electronic monitoring.[41,44,43] For non-oral dosage unit medications, clinicians can weigh devices such as metered-dose inhalers (MDIs) and estimate the number of inhalations used by the weight change of the canister.[45]

PHARMACY AND INSURANCE REFILL RECORDS

The use of pharmacy refill records has become a common tool to assess medication adherence and persistence. This can be used by a pharmacist to review an individual patient's medication record in the pharmacy (if all medications were obtained there) or more commonly by researchers using large administrative prescription claims databases. At the individual pharmacy level, it is critical to know that the patient obtained all medications through that pharmacy or associated pharmacies using the same computer system. Many pharmacies do not share common pharmacy records and therefore it is not possible to know if what appears to be nonadherence is really a situation of a patient refilling a medication at a different pharmacy. In a HMO pharmacy system, researchers studied patients on antihyperlipidemic medications and found a 32% probability that patients would discontinue their medication after one year.[46] Large administrative prescription claims databases have been used extensively to analyze medication adherence, and persistence.[47-48] As these databases are generated by pharmacy claims to health insurers, employers, Medicaid, Medicare, or the

Veterans Administration, all prescription activity by the patient is captured in that system regardless of the pharmacy used.

There are a number of different approaches for calculating medication adherence and persistence using pharmacy claims.[47-50] Many of the methods yield similar adherence rates. Some involve the examination of individual claims and the gaps between refills while other approaches focus on multiple refills of the medication creating a continuous measure of adherence. While there are several different ways to use claims data to define adherence rates, two major approaches to the calculations: medication possession ratios (MPR) and a proportionate days covered ratios (PDC). Both are ratios with numerators and denominators and often expressed as a number on a continuum of 0 to 1. A MPR or PDC of 0.8 is equivalent to 80% adherence.

MPR, in general, the numerator involves the summation of how many days of medication were supplied (amount of medication supplied through refills) over a particular time period. Some researchers will exclude the day's supply of the final fill while others will include the days for the final fill but cap the ratio at 1.0. Researchers often define the denominator in different ways. One example, the denominator is defined as the time interval as the time between the first and last fill of a medication. This approach focuses only on the time period that the patient remains on the medication, and does not account for a patient's discontinuation of the medication. A second approach defines the denominator as the time period from the first fill to the end of the measurement period (such as a calendar year). This latter approach does account for the discontinuation of the medication. The MPR can overestimate the true rate of medication adherence since it typically takes into account early refills during a defined measurement interval.

The PDC is calculated differently with the patient-level numerator defined as the number of days covered by the prescription refills during the denominator period. This approach considers early refills or days of overlap by adjusting the start dates of each fill of identical medication. The adjustment is made when the previous supply would have been used up and the start of the next available supply occurs the following day. This adjustment is based on the premise that when a patient refills a prescription before the preceding medication supply was exhausted (i.e., early refill), that the patient finishes the supply for the preceding fill before starting the new supply. Start dates of refills would not be adjusted given medications in the same therapeutic class since it is very likely the patient is expected to take multiple medication in a therapeutic class concurrently to control their illness. However, the PDC would reflect that the patient had received at least one of the therapeutic medications on a particular day. For example, if a patient is taking metformin and glipizide on the same day, then the day is only counted once as a covered medication day for diabetes.

Analyses of PDC data show that PDC provides a more conservative estimate of the adherence rate in situations when patients have switched medications within a class or concurrently uses more than one drug in a class.[51,52] Also, it was found that PDC and MPR provide nearly identical estimates when examining adherence to a single drug.

These researchers also found inpatient hospital stays (causing gaps in home medication use) did not significantly affect adherence estimates.

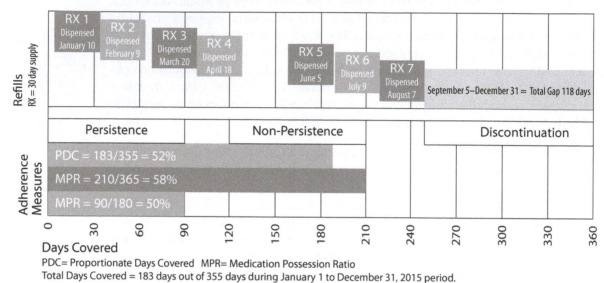

Observation Period—Jan 01, 2015 to December 31, 2015

PDC= Proportionate Days Covered, MPR= Medication Possession Ratio, RX = 30 day supply; RX1: Dispensed January 10th, RX2: Dispensed February 9th, RX3: Dispensed March 20th, RX4: Dispensed April 18th, RX5: Dispensed June 5th, RX6: Dispensed July 9th, RX7: Dispensed August 7th, September 5th–October 4th:30 day gap, October 5th–November 3rd: 30 day gap, November 4th–December 3rd: 30 day gap, December 4th–December 31st: 28 day gap, total gap 118 days; total days covered—183 days out of 355 days during January 1 to December 31, 2015 period.

FIGURE 12-1: SAMPLE MPR AND PDC CALCULATIONS

The use of pharmacy claims data has a number of advantages and limitations. The potential influence on patient behavior due to the feeling of being watched such as possibly felt by direct observation, pill counts, electronic monitoring, or patient report does not occur with prescription records data. Databases create the opportunity to study medication taking behavior at the population level, and generally do not have issues with small sample sizes which can influence statistical significance. The researcher should be familiar with the source of the claims data and how the data was compiled. The dataset should be complete and include patient eligibility information; otherwise the researcher may not know if the patient simply stops taking the medication, or may have been switched to another drug, changed insurance, or may have even died.

Electronic drug monitoring devices have gained wide acceptance among researchers evaluating medication-taking behavior and new devices are being developed to enhance adherence for patients. These devices are generally not used in clinical practice due to their costs. The device contains a microprocessor chip in the bottle cap that records the date and time the bottle is opened to obtain a dose. They can also be contained in pill boxes, blister packaging, inhalation devices, eye droppers, and topical formulations to record an administration of the medication.[53-55] This type of monitoring system has significant advantages over other adherence measures as it can provide continuous reliable data to capture not only medication adherence, but also can provide information on dosing schedule adherence for medications requiring precise dosing regimens. One of the most widely used electronic monitoring devices is the Medication Event Monitoring System (MEMS® unit APREX, a division of Aardex, LTD). A newer device using wireless technology is manufactured by AdhereTech (New York, NY). These bottle systems collect and send data on bottle openings in real time to a secure dashboard for subsequent analysis.

Electronic monitoring devices have several limitations. The recorded adherence activity (under or over adherence) may be influenced when the bottle is opened by mistake or used incorrectly by the patient. AdhereTech's bottles have multiple sensors, which measure both the open/close of the cap as well as the contents of the container, to avoid this pitfall. In any case, it's important for these technologies to not be overbearing for the patient. Thus, AdhereTech and others allow patients to remove more than one dose from the bottle at a time in situations where they plan to take the dose(s) later, or may transfer several doses to a smaller container. The use of a diary in conjunction with electronic monitoring allows the patient to document any opening of the device. There is also some evidence that similar to pill counts, the patient is acutely aware of the monitoring or surveillance. Electronic monitoring can cause an initial limited increase in adherence (patients wanting to initially please researcher) and/or feelings of anxiety or depression associated with being monitored.[56,57]

SELECTION OF A METHOD FOR MEASURING ADHERENCE

The choice of a measurement method to assess medication adherence or persistence should match the strengths of a method to the goals and needs of the clinician or researcher. No single method will be the best choice for all purposes. For the healthcare provider, the measures of choice would ideally be inexpensive, practical, easy to administer and interpret, and not interfere with the patient-provider relationship. What is important to the clinician is the ability to identify patients with nonadherence issues and then employ interventions to optimize the patient's medication-taking behavior. Physicians and other healthcare providers often believe they can identify and estimate medication adherence in their patients. However, research has found that clinicians tend to overestimate medication adherence and do not adequately detect poor adherence.[22] The clinician may then alter or change therapy on the basis that the drug was ineffective, when the patient was actually non-adherent with initial therapy. This can lead to the addition of unnecessary drugs, side-effects, and additional costs. In many cases, use of a structured questionnaire or patient interview (if the interviewer is skilled) is the most practical tool for the clinician. Prescription refill records can be very useful to identify potential adherence over the course of therapy, and can provide the pharmacist information before they see the patient again in a refill situation.

Measurement methods for adherence researchers and those conducting clinical trials require a reliable and accurate assessment of medication adherence or persistence. Electronic monitoring devices have become the standard measure of adherence in clinical trials. Detailed data of patient usage patterns can provide critical feedback to analyze the effectiveness and toxicities of medications and identify and correct misuse problems. One should not rely on a single method for adherence and persistence analysis, but use a combination of methods to augment potential weaknesses of the methods used.

INTERVENTIONS TO IMPROVE MEDICATION ADHERENCE

What could a health professional such as a pharmacist do after a patient has been identified with poor or inadequate medication adherence? The health professional is encouraged to work with the patient to help them understand the implications of their current medication use and explore for themselves ways to improve their medication adherence. A 2014 Cochrane analysis of 182 studies found vast differences in how studies design, measure and test the efficacy adherence interventions.[58] Such differences made it difficult for the authors to reach general conclusions based on inability to compare studies. In a small subset of high quality studies (n=17), adherence interventions were found to be complex involving multiple components. Only about a third of these high quality studies indicated the interventions improved medication adherence and other outcomes. The authors concluded that even the most effective interventions did not yield significant improvements. A older meta-analysis of adherence interventions also reported that comprehensive interventions involving multiple components were more successful than an intervention only using one approach.[59] Many of the interventions reviewed were aimed to overcome barriers through tailoring, provision of ongoing support by health professionals such as pharmacists and peers/families.[59-64] While interventions to improve medication use might be expensive initially, some research suggests that dollars spent on medications can reduce costs elsewhere. For example, Sokol and colleagues found that for every 1 dollar invested in diabetes medication approximately seven dollars could be saved in other services.[65] These strategies fall into three broad patient-centered categories; educational and behavioral interventions, and administrative supports.

EDUCATIONAL INTERVENTIONS

As the inability to learn and understand medication-related information may be a factor in the patient's nonadherence, provider education and the use of specific clear verbal and written information can be highly effective. This is of particular interest when the patient has complex regimens or requires strategies to deal with troublesome side effects. Information should be specific to the patient's condition and drug therapy. Information should be categorized and simplified to enhance patient understanding.

In addition, medication counseling should involve active assessment and tailoring based on what patients know, needs, and any barriers they may have to optimal medication use. Such patient-centered counseling will help foster a strong patient-provider relationship which is very likely critical to improve medication use. Providers might focus on empowering patients to engage in medication adherence as something they value and feel important.[64] Pharmacists should also encourage patient self-monitoring of their symptoms and how such changes in symptoms are related to the drug's effectiveness. The Health Collaboration Model (HCM) is one theoretical framework that supports the connection between pharmacist education and monitoring and improved adherence.[19] HCM states two main paths between pharmacist-guided patient education and medication adherence: (1) improved quality of pharmacist medication instruction and support can lead to improved patient comprehension, motivation, and initial medication adherence, and (2) improved pharmacist feedback on medication and medication problem-solving can lead to improved patient satisfaction, sustained medication adherence, and clinical outcomes. Chapters X and Y on communication and facilitating behavior change in this textbook will provide greater details on models and approaches to enhance patient-centered medication education.

BEHAVIORAL INTERVENTIONS

Numerous strategies and tools exist to provide behavioral support for the patient. This includes a variety of adherence aids including pill boxes, calendars, automated phone messages, text messages, various smart phone applications, or e-mail reminders.[61-63] Reminder cues can also be developed based on the patient's daily habits and activities to incorporate medication adherence into their daily lives. While these interventions show promise, there remains some concerns to the extent the smartphone applications are regulated, accurate, reliable, and accessible to different populations such as older and low income populations.[66-68]

It should be noted that there are several web-based and/or cloud-based platform solutions that are available to help pharmacists manage and monitor their educational and behavioral interventions to improve medications adherence.[69-71] Such interventions are typically a part of medication therapy management solutions to improve medication use. It is likely most cost effective for pharmacists to screen those at greatest risk for medication non-adherence at the population level and then target patient-centered interventions toward these specific individuals. These platforms allow for population-level initial screening and patient-level adherence management. Pharmacists can be reimbursed for many of these interventions, especially for specific patient populations at high risk, through federal, state, and private insurance initiatives.

Additionally, provider support must continue on a regular basis, otherwise adherence is likely to return to previous levels.[62] A number of resources are available to pharmacists and healthcare providers from health organizations, professional associations, and the pharmaceutical industry to assist with developing adherence intervention strategies. These include: The National Council on Patient Information and Education (NCPIE) http://www.talkaboutrx.org/, The American Pharmacist Association http://www.pharmacist.com, Adult Medication http://adultmeducation.com, a joint project of the American Society on Aging and the American Society of Consultant Pharmacists Foundation, and websites supported by pharmaceutical companies and chain pharmacies.

ADMINISTRATIVE SUPPORTS

The medication regimen should be tailored to the patient's lifestyle and needs whenever possible. Regimens that impinge on the patient's normal lifestyle will be difficult for the patient to adhere to. Dosing regimens should be simplified whenever possible, with once or twice daily regimens preferred or as the patient desires. Holdford and Inocencio recently showed the positive adherence effects associated with the process of enabling the pick-up of medications all at the same time (appointment-based medication synchronization, ABMS) vs. the pick-up of one medication on one date and the pick-up of other medications on different days.[72] Specifically, these researchers found that ABMS patients were 3.4 to 6.1 times more likely to be adherent than control patients not using ABMS. Another adherence promotion strategy involves the use of automated refill processes, which refill medication automatically without the patient's indication of need. A recent study showed that an automated refill program significantly improved medication adherence when compared to those not enrolled in the program.[73] This latter study also found the automated refill program significantly reduced the number of days of oversupply and possible amount of medication waste. There is also evidence that 90-day supplies of medication yield improved adherence compared to 30-day supplies.[74] A negative of 90-day supplies is that it has the potential to reduce the degree to which patients come to the pharmacy and have the opportunity to ask questions and receive more regular medication monitoring and follow-up.

Medication synchronization, automated refills programs, and 90-day supplies are all administrative supports that have been shown to reduce patient burden to pick up medications and, therefore, improve convenient access to prescribed medications. In addition to these administrative supports, researchers have also explored whether receiving medications through the mail order channel of distribution yields different outcomes than the community pharmacy distribution of medications.[75] More research is needed to confirm these findings and explore if findings remain consistent for different patient groups. In addition to these administrative strategies, pharmacists can also recommend to patients and prescribers alternate drugs if side effects are affecting optimal adherence.

SUMMARY

Medication nonadherence is a significant national and international public health concern since it contributes to poor health outcomes and greater utilization of healthcare resources. There have been several professional organizations and federal agencies expressing "a call to action" to reduce medication non-adherence.[9,60,76,77] For example, the *Script Your Future* was a public awareness campaign involving multiple stakeholders launched by the National Consumers League to increase discussions between practitioners and patients about medication adherence. The Centers for Medicare and Medicaid Services (CMS) uses three performance measures, adopted from measures developed by the Pharmacy Quality Alliance, to evaluate the efforts of Medicare Part D contractors to ensure high adherence to oral medications used for diabetes, high blood pressure, and high cholesterol.[78,79] These scores are on a scale of 1 to 5 stars with 5 stars being the highest rating. The star ratings are subsequently used to determine quality-related bonus payments for the Medicare Part D plans. Thus, there is considerable financial pressure for plans to improve medication adherence. We may see in the future that performance of community pharmacies to improve medication adherence may also be linked to financial incentives.

Our chapter describes the evolution of the term "adherence" and how medication-taking behavior is being viewed more as a joint cooperative effort between healthcare providers and patients, and not simply instructions the patient is expected to follow. The chapter also introduces the reader to common predictors of medication non-adherence predictors; these may be helpful in screening for those most vulnerable to non-adherence. There was an extensive discussion regarding the number of methods exist to identify or quantify medication nonadherence. Self-report instruments and pharmacy prescription records are used most commonly by pharmacists in their daily practice and often easy to use and interpret. More sophisticated methods are available to researchers who require quantitative information and greater precision for their needs.

Large meta-analyses and systematic reviews highlight that the most effective adherence interventions are those that are complex, using multiple approaches, and personalized to the patient's needs. Adherence interventions typically involve assessing patient barriers, targeting identified barriers using educational, behavioral, and administrative strategies, and providing ongoing follow-up and monitoring. We know the future will yield new adherence device or approaches that could initially improve adherence rates. However, the key to sustaining high adherence rates is the development of a positive and trusting provider-patient relationship involving several ongoing efforts to listen, engage, and remain connected. The short-term costs of building such relationships are significant but the long-term public health gain could be considerable with improved clinical, economic, and humanistic outcomes for patients and the entire healthcare system.

REFERENCES

1. Cramer, J. A., Roy, A., Burrell, A., Fairchild, J., Fuldeore, M. J., Ollendorf, D. A., & Wong, P. K. (2007). Medication compliance and persistence: Terminology and definitions. *Value in Health* 1–4.

2. Fischer, M.A,, Stedman, M.R., Li,l J., Vogeli, C., Shrank, W.H., Brookhart, M.A., et al. (2010). Primary medication non-adherence: Analysis of 195,930 electronic prescriptions. *J Gen Intern Med* 25(4):284–90.

3. Svarstad, B.L., Chewning, B.A., Sleath, B.L., & Claesson, C. (1999). The Brief Medication Questionnaire: A tool for screening patient adherence and barriers to adherence. *Patient Educ Coun* 37113–124.

4. Shea, S.C. (2006). *Improving medication adherence: How to talk with patients about their medications.* Philadelphia: Lippincott Williams and Wilkins.

5. New England Healthcare Institute. (2009). *Thinking outside of the pillbox: A system-wide approach to improve patient medication adherence for chronic disease.* Cambridge (MA): New England Healthcare Institute.

6. McDonell, P.J. & Jacobs, M.R. (2002). Hospital admissions resulting from preventable adverse drug reactions. *Ann Pharmacother* 36(9):1331–1336.

7. McCarthy, R. (1998). The price you pay for the drug not taken. *Bus Health* 16:27–33.

8. Simpson, S. H., Eurich, D. T., Majumdar, S. R., Padwal, R. S., Tsuyuki, R. T., & Varney, J. (2006). A meta-analysis of the association between adherence to drug therapy and mortality. *Br Med J* 1–6.

9. Benjamin, R.M. (2012). Medication adherence: helping patients take their medications as directed. *Public Health Rep* 127(1):2–3.

10. Janz, N.K. & Becker, M.H. (1984). The health belief model: A decade later. *Health Educ Q* 11(1):1–47.

11. Osterberg, L. & Blaschke, T. (2005). Adherence to medication. *N Engl J Med* 353:487–497.

12. DiMatteo, M.R. (2004). Variations in patients' adherence to medical recommendations. *Med Care* 42(3):200–209.

13. World Health Organization. (2003). *Adherence to long-term therapies. Evidence for action.* Geneva: World Health Organization.

14. Sansone, R.A., & Sansone, L.A. (2012). Antidepressant adherence: Are patients taking their medications? *Innov Clin Neurosci* 9(4-5):41–46.

15. Chowdhury, R., Khan, H., Heydon, E., Shroufi, A., Fahimi, S., Moore, C., et al. (2013). Adherence to cardiovascular therapy: a meta-analysis of prevalence and clinical consequences. *European Heart J* 34:2940–2948.

16. Curkendall, S.M., Thomas, N., Bell, K.F., Juneau, .PL., & Weiss, A.J. (2013). Predictors of medication adherence in patients with type 2 diabetes mellitus. *Curr Med Res Opin* 29(10):1275–86. Doi:10.1185/03007995.2013.821056. Epub 2013 Jul 23.

17. Burra, T.A., Chen, E., McIntyre, R.S., Grace, S.L., Robertson Blackmore, E., & Stewart, D.E. (2007). Predictors of self-reported antidepressant adherence. *Behavioral Medicine* 32(4):127–134.

18. Martin, L.R., Williams, S.R., Haskard, K.B., & DiMatteo, M.R. (2005). The challenge of patient adherence. *Therapeutics and Clinical Risk Management* 1(3):189–199.

19. Rickles, N.M. & Svarstad, B.L. (2012). The patient: behavioral determinants. In: Allen, L. (Ed.), *Remington: The science and practice of pharmacy*, 22nd ed. London: Pharmaceutical Press, 1893–1902.

20. DiMatteo, M.R., Lepper, H.S., & Croghan, T.W. (2000.) Depression is a risk factor for noncompliance with medical treatment. *Arch Intern Med* 160:2101–07.

21. Shrank, W.H., Choudhry, N.K., Fischer, M.A., Avorn, J., Powell, M., Schnee-weiss, S., et al. (2010). Epidemiology of prescriptions abandoned at the pharmacy. *Ann Intern Med* 153;633–40.

22. Miller, L.G., Liu, H., Hays, R.D., Golin, C..E, Beck, C.K., Asch, S.M., et al. (2002). How well do clinicians estimate patients' adherence to combination antiretroviral therapy? *J Gen Intern Med* 17(1):1–11.

23. Rickles, N.M., Young, G.A., Hall, J.A., Noland, C., Kim, A., Peterson, C., et al. Medication adherence communications in community pharmacies: a naturalistic investigation. *Pat Educ Counsel.* DOI: http://dx.doi.org/10.1016/j.pec.2015.10.003

24. Pfizer. (2003). *Pharmacist-patient consultation program: Promoting adherence.* New York: Pfizer.

25. Morisky, D.E., Green, L.W., & Levine, D.M. (1986). Concurrent and predictive validity of a self-reported measure of medication adherence. *Med Care* 24(1):67–74.

26. McHorney, C.A. (2009). The Adherence Estimator: A brief, proximal screener for patient propensity to adhere to prescription medications for chronic disease. *Curr Med Res Opin* 25(1):215–38.

27. Horne, R., Weinman, J., & Hankins, M. (1999.) The beliefs about medicines questionnaire: the development and evaluation of a new method for assessing the cognitive representation of a medication. *Psychol Health* 14(1):1–24.

28. Cooke, C.E. & Fatodu, H. (2006). Physician conformity and patient adherence to ACE inhibitors and ARBs in patients with diabetes, with and without renal disease and hypertension, in a Medicaid managed care organization. *JMCP* 12(8):649–655.

29. Feinstein, A.R. (1990). On white-coat effects and the electronic monitoring of compliance. *Arch Intern Med* 150(7)1377–1378.

30. Cramer, J.A., Scheyer, R.D., & Mattson, R.H. (1990). Compliance declines between clinic visits. *Arch Intern Med* 150(7)1509–1510.

31. Proteus Digital Health and Otsuka seek FDA approval for world's first digital pill. Accessed February 3, 2016. http://www.forbes.com/sites/robert-glatter/2015/09/14/ proteus-digital-health-and-otsuka-seek-fda-approval-for-worlds-first-digital-medicine/#7ceca3fc4b5c.

32. Straka, R.J., Fish, J.T., Benson, S.R., & Suh, J.T.(1997). Patient self-reporting of compliance does not correspond with electronic monitoring: An evaluation using isosorbide dinitrate as a model drug. *Pharmacotherapy* 17(1):126–132.

33. Park, L.C. & Lipman, R.S. (1964). A comparison of patient dosage deviation reports with pill counts. *Psychopharmacologia* 6209–302.

34. Inui, T.S., Carter, W.B., & Pecoraro, R.E. (1981). Screening for noncompliance among patients with hypertension: Is self-report the best available measure? *Med Care* 191061–1064.

35. Gordis, L., Markowitz, M., & Lilienfeld, A.M. (1969).The inaccuracy in using interviews to estimate patient reliability in taking medications at home. *Med Care* 749–54.

36. Cramer, J. A. & Mattson, R. H. (1991). Monitoring compliance with antiepileptic drug therapy. in: Cramer JA, Spilker B (Eds.) Patient Compliance in Medical Practice and Clinical Trials. Raven Press, New York;1991:123–137.

37. Myers, E.D. & Branthwaite, A. (1992). Out-patient Compliance with antidepressant medication. *British Journal of Psychiatry* 16083–86.

38. Ross, F.M. (1991). Patient compliance—whose responsibility? *Soc Sci Med* 2(1):89–94.

39. Sherbourne, C.D., Hays, R.D., Ordway, L., DiMatteo, M.R., & Kravitz, R.L. (1992). Antecedents of adherence to medical recommendations: Results from the medical outcomes study. *J Behav Med* 15(2):447–468.

40. Rickles, N.M., Svarstad, B.L. (2007). Relationships between multiple self-reported nonadherence measures and pharmacy records. *Res Soc Admin Pharm* 3/4:663–677.

41. Liu, H., Golin, C.E., Miller, L.G., Hays, R.D., Beck, C.K., Sanandaji, S., et al. (2001). A comparison study of multiple measures of adherence to HIV protease inhibitors. *Ann Intern Med* 134(10):968–977.

42. Grymonpre, R.E., Didur, C.D., Montgomery, P.R., & Sitar, D. S. (1998). Pill count, self-report, and pharmacy claims data to measure medication adherence in the elderly. *The Annals of Pharmacotherapy* 32(7-8):749–754.

43. Craig, H.M. (1985). Accuracy of indirect measure of medication compliance in hypertension. *Research in Nursing and Health* 861–66.

44. Matsui, D., Hermann, C., Klein, J.J., Berkovitch, M., Olivieri, N., & Koren, G. (1994). Critical comparison of novel and existing methods of compliance assessment during a clinical trial of an oral iron chelator. *J Clin Pharmacol* 34(9):944–949.

45. Rand, C.S., Wise, R.A., Nides, M.A., Simmons, M.S., Bleecker, E.R., Kusek, J.W. et al. (1992). Metered-dose inhaler adherence in a clinical trial. *Am Rev Respir Dis* 146(6):1559–1564.

46. Andrade, S.E., Walker, A.M., Gottlieb, L.K., Hollenberg, N.K., Testa, M.A., Saperia, G.M. et al. (1995). Discontinuation of antihyperlipidemic drugs - do rates reported in clinical trials reflect rates in primary care settings? *New Engl J Med* 332(17):1125–1131.

47. Steiner, J., Koepsell, T.D., Fihn, S.D., & Inui, T.S. (1988). A general method of compliance assessment using centralized pharmacy records. *Med Care* 26(8)814–823.

48. Hamilton, R.A. & Briceland, L.L. (1992). Use of prescription-refill records to assess patient compliance. *Am J Hosp Pharm* 49(7)1691–1696.

49. Peterson, A.M., Nau, D.P., Cramer, J.A., Benner, J., Gwadry-Sridhar, F., & Nichol, M.B. (2007). A checklist for medication compliance and persistence studies using retrospective databases. *Value in Health* 10(1):3–12.

50. Hess, L.M., Raebel, M.A., Conner, D.A., & Malone, D.C. (2006). Measurement of adherence in pharmacy administrative databases: A proposal for standard definitions and preferred measures. *Annals of Pharmacotherapy* 40:1280–1288.

51. Martin, B.C., et al. (2009). Contrasting Measures of Adherence with Simple Drug Use, Medication Switching, and Therapeutic Duplication. *Ann Pharmacother.* 43:36–44.

52. Campbell, K., et al. (July 2011). *FMQAI Reports on medication measures, July 2011.* Reports available at: http://www.fmqai.com/MedFiles/NQF0542_MIF.pdf and http://www.fmqai.com/MedFiles/Measure-527PC-508.pdf.

53. Hermann, M.M. & Diestelhorst, M. (2006). Microprocessor controlled compliance monitor for eye drop medication. *Br J Ophthalmol* 90(7):830–832.

54. Balkrishnan, R., Carroll, C.L., Camacho, F.T., & Feldman, S.R. (2003). Electronic monitoring of medication adherence in skin disease: Results of a pilot study. *J Amer Acad Dermatol* 49(4):651–654.

55. Kruse, W., Nikolaus, T., Rampmaier, J., Weber, E., & Schlierf, G. (1993). Actual versus prescribed timing of lovastatin doses assessed by electronic compliance monitoring. *Eur J Clin Pharmacol* 45(3):211–215.

56. Berg, K.M. & Arnsten, J.H. (2006). Practical and conceptual challenges in measuring antiretroviral adherence. *Acquir Immune Defic Syndr 43* (Suppl 1):S79–S87.

57. Elixhauser, A., Eisen, S.A., Romeis, J.C., & Homan, S.M. (1990). The effects of monitoring and feedback on compliance. *Med Care* 28(10)882–893.

58. Nieuwlaat, R., Wilczynsk,i N., Navarro, T., Hobson, N., Jeffery, R., Keepanasseril, A., et al. (2014). Interventions for enhancing medication adherence. *Cochrane Database of Systematic Reviews* Issue 11. Art. No.: CD000011. DOI: 10.1002/14651858.CD000011.pub4

59. Roter, D.L., Hall, J.A., Merisca, R., Nordstrom, B., Cretin, D., & Svarstad, B. (1998). Effectiveness of interventions to improve patient compliance: a meta-analysis. *Med Care* 36:1138–61.

60. National Council on Patient Information and Education. (2007). *Enhancing prescription medicine adherence: A national action plan.*

61. Schneider, P.J., Murphy, J.E., Pedersen, C.A. (2008). Impact of medication packaging on adherence and treatment outcomes in older ambulatory patients. *J Am Pharm Assoc* 48(1):58–63.

62. Lee, J.K., Grace, K.A., & Taylor, A.J. (2006). Effect of a pharmacy care program on medication adherence and persistence, blood pressure, and low-density lipoprotein cholesterol. *JAMA* 296(21):2614–2616.

63. Dayer, L., Heldenbrand, S., Anderson, P., & Gubbins, P. (2013). Smartphone medication adherence apps: Potential benefits to patients and providers. *J Am Pharm Assoc* 53(4):172–181.

64. Berger, B.A. & Villaume, W.A.(2013). *Motivational interviewing for health professionals: A sensible approach.* Washington, D.C.: American Pharmacists Association.

65. Sokol, M.C., McGuigan, K.A., Verbrugge, R.R., & Epstein, R. S. (2005). Impact of medication adherence on hospitalization risk and healthcare cost. *Med Care* 43:521–530.

66. Davies, M., Collings, M., Fletcher, W., & Mujtaba, H. (2014). Pharmacy apps: A new frontier on the digital landscape? *Pharm Pract* 12(3):453–464.

67. Lee, J.A., Nguyen, A.L., Berg. J., Amin, A., Bachman, M., Guo, Y., et al. (2014). Attitudes and preferences on the use of mobile health technology and health games for self-management: interviews with older adults on anticoagulation therapy. *JMIR mHealth uHealth* 2(3): e32. doi: 10.2196/mhealth.3196

68. Parker, S.J. Older adults are mobile too! Identifying the barriers and facilitators to older adults' use of mHealth for pain management. *BMC Geriatrics* 13(1):43.

69. http://www.mirixa.com. Accessed February 14, 2016.

70. http://www.outcomesmtm.com. Accessed February 14, 2016.

71. http://www.anthuriumsi.com/about-us/. Accessed February 14, 2016.

72. Holdford, D.A., Inocencio, T.J. (2013). Adherence and persistence associated with an appointment-based medication synchronization program. *J Am Pharm Assoc* 53:576–583.

73. Martin, O.S., Krynes, S.M, Averbukh, A., Choudhry, N.K., Brennan, T.A., Bunton, A. et al. (2015). Community pharmacy automatic refill program improves adherence to maintenance therapy and reduces wasted medication. *Am J Manag Care* 21(11):785–791.

74. Hermes, M., Gleason, P.P., & Starner, C.I. (2010). Adherence to chronic medication therapy associated with 90-day supplies compared with 30-day supplies [abstract]. *J Manag Care Pharm*. 16:141–142.

75. Khandelwal, N., Duncan, I., Rubinstein, E., Ahmed, T., Pegus, C., & Kudrak, K.E. (2011). Medication adherence for 90-day quantities of medication dispensed through retail and mail order pharmacies. *Am J Manag Care* 17(11):e427–e434.

76. Bosworth, H.B., Granger, B.B., Mendys ,P., Brindis, R., Burkholder, R., Czajkowski, S.M., et al. (2011). Medication adherence: A call for action. *Am Heart J* 162(3):412–424.

77. Script Your Future. National Consumers League. http://www.nclnet.org/health/106-prescription-drugs/234-ncls-medicationadherence-campaign. Accessed November 25, 2011.

78. Centers for Medicare and Medicaid Services. Medicare health and drug plan quality and performance ratings: 2012 Part C and Part D technical notes. Baltimore (MD): CMS; updated 2012 Jan 18.

79. Pharmacy Quality Alliance. Measures. http://pqaalliance.org/measures/cms.asp. Accessed February 15, 2016.

CHAPTER 13

FACILITATING BEHAVIORAL CHANGE

Jan Kavookjian, MBA, PhD

LEARNING OBJECTIVES:

1. Recognize the various ways and media types that a pharmacist can use to deliver educational or informational interventions for medication taking.

2. Explain why a pharmacist should explore patient literacy-related and cultural factors that may influence or impede medication taking behaviors.

3. List and describe the types of and examples for behavior stimulus interventions that have been used to influence patient medication taking behaviors.

4. Describe organizational or health system approaches that have been implemented to influence patient medication taking behaviors.

5. Describe the patient-centered principles, skills and micro skills of motivational interviewing that a pharmacist can use in counseling a patient about medication taking behaviors.

KEY TERMS

Social support

Adherence-challenging therapies/
 conditions

Behavior stimulus interventions

Cultural barriers

Decisional balance and internal
 motivation

Financial barriers and prescription
 assistance programs

Informational interventions

Literacy and health literacy

Medication taking behaviors

Motivational interviewing

Organizational or system-level
 interventions

Patient-centered communication

Patient-level interventions

Transtheoretical model of change
 (TTM)

INTRODUCTION

The evaluation of interventions aimed at influencing medication taking behavior is not a new topic. In fact, researchers and providers across most of the health professions have had an interest in studying medication adherence and non-adherence for the past several decades.[1,2] Because the expensive problem of non-adherence has not resolved itself or even improved remarkably, this field of interest continues to grow, incorporating new developments in what we know about patient and system barriers, in what we know about medication taking behavior and motivation, and even in the incorporation of technological tools.

The focus of this chapter will be to explore and summarize interventions that have been used to influence medication taking behavior. These include the general categories of educational interventions, specific behavioral stimulus interventions, social or support network initiatives, organizational approaches, technology tools, and structured communication or counseling strategies. It is important to point out that most behavior change initiatives use a combination of strategy types.[3,4] For example, education alone is often not enough to maintain behavior change. In addition to knowledge barriers, patients often have motivational or practical barriers to adherence that must be addressed through counseling or initiatives at the patient's healthcare system level.

Many landmark interventions for medication adherence have been explored in health care settings outside pharmacy and will be presented in this chapter along with interventions applied in pharmacy practice settings. In addition, while pharmacists engaging in disease management initiatives might intervene to help patients change a multitude of health behaviors (e.g., physical activity, healthy eating, monitoring, etc.), this chapter will primarily focus on interventions to influence medication taking behavior.

EDUCATIONAL INTERVENTIONS FOR MEDICATION TAKING BEHAVIOR CHANGE

Sometimes referred to as *informational* interventions,[3] educational interventions include cognitive strategies delivered through one or more avenues. This might include didactic instruction to an individual or a group; in recent years, diabetes education classes delivered in groups are reimbursable by CMS so the class or group format for this type of education is becoming more of the norm than one-on-one approaches for general diabetes education. The emergence of CMS requiring Medicare Part D payers to reimburse for a Medication Therapy Management (MTM) encounter for Medicare patients, requires a face-to-face encounter to talk about medication taking and problem solving. In pharmacy practice settings, verbal delivery is often accompanied by the provision of written material for the patient to take home for future reference. This is also an important way to later reinforce the decisions a patient might make while receiving the education. It is a tangible piece of "evidence" from the interaction that can serve as a resource and as a reminder. Other media for education delivery might include audio tapes or downloads to portable digital listening devices, DVDs, take-home or on-site computer programs, books (and coloring books for children), and other technologically based information delivery tools,[3-5] including mobile health (mHealth) applications (apps) readily accessible on smartphones.[6]

In educating patients, whether verbally or by using other media, there are important considerations in the development and delivery of an educational intervention. Education is only a part of an effective intervention process, but it is an essential part. A patient must first understand the illness and the medication before he/she will decide to take a medication appropriately.[4] Since the patient's understanding is such a crucial part of medication taking behavior, it is important to think about the target audience and characteristics that might pose as barriers to understanding an educational intervention. Among many characteristics to take into account, two important considerations are literacy level and cultural differences. While these topics are covered elsewhere in this book, it is important to briefly discuss their implications for selecting or designing educational interventions to influence medication taking behavior.

LITERACY AND HEALTH LITERACY

Health care providers are trained and rewarded for communicating in a highly scientific manner throughout their studies and professional interactions. It can be challenging for providers delivering education to patients to switch gears and tone down the literacy level of their communication to meet the comprehension needs of all of their patients. The "functional" reading level in the United States was established as being at the 8th grade level.[7] About 42 million US adults are considered functionally illiterate, and it is estimated that over 20% of US adults cannot read or comprehend at greater than the 5th grade reading level.

The concern about general literacy also extends to the more specific concept of health literacy. Health literacy has been a topic of recent emphasis from United States' entities like the Institute of Medicine, Agency for Healthcare Research and Quality, and the American Medical Association health literacy project. Recent reports from studies by these groups suggest that up to half of all US adults may lack the skills needed to function optimally in a healthcare environment, including skills like making appropriate decisions about dosing cold medicine for a child and understanding informed consent documents.[8]

CULTURAL BARRIERS MAY HINDER EDUCATIONAL INTERVENTIONS

In addition to literacy concerns, pharmacists educating patients about medication taking should be vigilant for cultural issues that might contribute to misunderstandings or mistrust. There may be language or cultural barriers that will hinder patient adherence with medication because of a misunderstanding about what the provider meant when delivering the message. Some of these may be related to traditions within a specific racial, ethnic or religious group, or may be present among patients for whom English is not their primary language.

Regional customs may also pose barriers to understanding, even where language of origin is not a barrier. For example, fried foods, including vegetables, are a mainstay in the dietary customs of the Southeastern United States. Encouraging uneducated patients in this region to eat more vegetables to improve their health should be clarified to include a discussion about ideas for preparing them in a healthy way. In addition, other cultures may have medication taking beliefs or restrictions that should be explored, including folk beliefs which may have little to no rational basis. Respectful discussion should take place in the face of such barriers in order to avoid offending the patient or risk having him/her become mistrustful and resistant to receiving education about medication taking.

USING VISUAL AIDS TO OVERCOME BARRIERS

It is important for pharmacists to become aware of the potential for literacy or cultural barriers among the population of patients they serve, particularly in the context of an educational intervention.[9] Some have focused on overcoming barriers to the delivery of education about medications by using visual aids that include pictures or universally recognized symbols to convey medication taking instructions. For example, the warning labels that are placed on prescription vials often include symbols along with text in an attempt to address these very issues. The use of symbols, like an ace of hearts to represent ace-inhibitor medications, has resulted in improved adherence and patient outcomes for undereducated inner city heart failure patients for whom health literacy was a major concern.[9]

Recent reviews of the medication adherence intervention literature suggest that studies of informational interventions alone sometimes contributed to improvements in self-reported adherence, but most did not produce improved clinical outcomes.[3] Authors concluded that most educational interventions for medication taking are delivered in a single episode and that multiple or follow-up deliveries would be more effective.[4,9,10] In addition, educational interventions are more often effective when delivered in combination with some of the other intervention methods discussed in the next several sections.[3,4,10–13]

BEHAVIOR STIMULUS INTERVENTIONS FOR MEDICATION TAKING BEHAVIOR CHANGE

Behavior change interventions include strategies that can be generally organized into three stimulus categories: 1) reminders (cues), 2) tailoring of medication regimen, or 3) reinforcement to encourage a patient to initiate and maintain change towards a desired behavior.

REMINDER STRATEGIES

Reminder strategies for influencing medication taking behavior have received a lot of attention in recent years. With the rise in technological sophistication, many simple and complex devices and services have been developed to help patients remember to take their medications. More complex developments include electronic reminder devices like pill boxes or watches or phone alarms, automated medication dispensers, smart phone apps, and even adherence reminder services. These services send a phone call, electronic mail (e-mail), or phone text message reminder at time to take the dose, or will send a phone call, email, phone text, or postal mail card/letter reminder for refills. Some systems have had significant influence on medication taking behavior when applied in controlled studies.[4,14]

In the everyday reality of some patients, cost, access, and lack of familiarity with technology can make these options unavailable. Simple, less expensive tools have also been developed. These include simple pillboxes, reminder packaging (blister), calendars, stickers, pamphlets, and others. An extensive review of medication memory aids available at that time (2005) is included in the Krueger review of medication adherence interventions.[4]

The use of adherence aids alone has not been very effective, producing a median impact of about 3%;[4] however, reminder systems by mail or telephone demonstrated consistent and significant improvements in adherence rates. As with other intervention strategies presented in this chapter, adherence aids and reminder systems are more effective when used in combination with other strategies, particularly education.

In conditions like schizophrenia and bipolar disorder, where non-adherence is prevalent and is impacted by illness-producing lack of insight, reminder systems can be important. One such intervention has produced improvements in adherence and reduction in relapse and hospitalization by using a systematic approach with large calendars and attached pen to track appointments, signs, medication containers with alarms, bus passes to assist patients in getting to their appointments, and notebooks for recording side effects to assist in discussion with the provider at the next appointment.[15,16]

TAILORING THE MEDICATION REGIMEN

It is well known that the more complex the dosing schedule of a medication, the less adherent a patient is likely to be with the regimen. The review by Krueger and colleagues suggested that the characteristics of complexity of a regimen and the effects of the regimen itself negatively affect adherence, particularly when a patient is taking more than four medications, has more frequent daily doses, is confused about the regimen, believes he/she cannot follow the regimen, and/or has a fear of side effects.[4] In addition, a recent review examining the impact of complexity of the dosing regimen compared adherence rates between once-daily to four-times-daily regimens. The researchers concluded that among 29 reviewed studies of once-daily dosing, the mean adherence rate was approximately 79%. This compares with 32 studies of twice-daily dosing (69% adherence rate), 13 studies of three-times daily dosing (65% adherence rate), and 11 studies of four-time-daily dosing (51% adherence rate).[17]

Similar conclusions have been presented in other adherence intervention reviews,[3,4,11] and reducing the dosing regimen and complexity have been often recommended as first-line adherence gaining strategies. By tailoring the dosing regimen to the patient's daily routine, the negative impacts of the illness may be minimized and the patient's sense of control over the illness may be increased. This includes not only simplifying the regimen, but also tying the medication taking process to other daily activities or routines to help the patient remember to take his/her medication. For example, suggesting that a coffee-drinking patient place his/her morning medication by the coffee pot will assist that patient in remembering to take the medication by tying it to another habitual behavior.

REINFORCEMENT FOR MEDICATION TAKING BEHAVIOR

Interventions aimed at reinforcing or rewarding medication taking have taken many forms across research studies and in practice. Providers who have given their patients skills-building types of training, or self care training and planning/contracts, have demonstrated significant increases in medication adherence rates,[3,4,11] particularly when delivered over time and when combined with other intervention strategies.

According to Kripalani and colleagues (2007) in a recent review of the adherence intervention literature, the most effective strategy in the reinforcement category includes assessing/monitoring adherence and giving feedback to the patient.[3] Studies involving this process had patients monitor and report their medication use and/or blood pressure. They were then given tailored feedback by their providers, including reinforcing statements. Improvements in adherence and clinical outcomes were more significant than in a study which only provided blood pressure readings to the patient and his/her provider. Other reviews reported similar findings.[11,18]

In recent years, employers have used the monitoring and feedback method in the form of Health Risk Assessments (HRAs) as part of a wellness initiative. HRAs use biometric assessment data to provide a report and feedback to employees, informing them of progress (or not), comparing their numbers to national standards, and encouraging them to engage in healthy behaviors including medication adherence.[19]

Recent studies among pharmacist-delivered adherence interventions have included ongoing monitoring and feedback.[9,10,20,21] The positive influence on adherence supports the role of pharmacists as providers in a unique position to deliver a medication adherence intervention that includes ongoing monitoring and feedback, particularly given the ongoing interaction with patients on maintenance medications for chronic illnesses.

It is possible that this method, which includes ongoing interaction, not only reinforces adherence but also actively involves the patient in the decision-making process. When a patient is involved in decision-making about his/her care, more opportunity exists for the development of the internal motivation that is necessary to maintain change on a target behavior.[11,18] Studies using other external rewards for adherence behavior had limited long-term impact.[11,12] This is perhaps due to the notion that external rewards generate extrinsic motivation, which is generally not sustained over time.[22,23] Patients tend to initially adopt either an approach or avoid coping style when they find out they have a chronic illness, and will stick with the early coping style throughout treatment, even in the face of additional information or stressors.[24] Getting patients involved early in the decision-making process for their care can help foster an approach coping style that may contribute to internal motivation and sustain behavioral movement towards medication adherence.

SOCIAL OR SUPPORT NETWORKS AND MEDICATION TAKING BEHAVIOR CHANGE

For many patients, the support of family, friends, caregivers, or lay/peer helpers, provides the necessary coping mechanism to engage in health behaviors.[4] Whether structured (with facilitation or counseling and an agenda) or unstructured (informal support group), in person or via chat rooms on the Internet, support can provide a sense of connection for individuals suffering with an illness or health condition.

Just as with the monitoring and feedback intervention described in a previous section, ongoing support is important to sustaining a behavior change like medication adherence. This is where a patient's health care provider can also have an important influence on medication adherence, particularly pharmacists who have an opportunity to regularly see patients when it's time to refill maintenance medications. Interventions that occur more than once foster a caring, collaborative relationship between a pharmacist and a patient.[4,20] Support for a patient partners with the concept of reinforcement to not only help a patient feel understood and less alone in the face of his/her illness and its care, but also to enable a patient to continue engaging in target behaviors and avoid engaging in undesired behaviors.

It is often difficult for patients to make changes that are unsupported in their social networks. Smoking cessation, for example, is particularly difficult for a patient whose primary social networks involve going out to bars and other settings where smoking is a prevalent social activity. Patients on medications that have an interaction with alcohol or certain foods may face the same challenge and may opt for non-adherence with the medication in order to maintain the social network and its contraindicated activities. It is important to explore these barriers with patients and help them to generate their own possible alternatives to the stimuli which may tempt them to be nonadherent.

Reviews of the literature on medication adherence include the notion of support as being important to successful intervention,[4,11] and even to the extent that family therapy may be warranted in some difficult cases.[11] This is particularly true for patients with severe mental illnesses like schizophrenia and bipolar disorder, where effects of the illness itself hinder a patient's ability to cognitively process (poor insight) and where non-adherence is prevalent, has very expensive consequences, and is particularly problematic. In severe cases of non-adherence with multiple relapses, a patient support intervention may even include a team of providers. Home visits from community services[13] are sometimes the nature of outpatient commitment orders, even on a weekly basis, for patients newly discharged from inpatient psychiatric hospital stays.

The key to successful intervention for such patients is highly dependent on the level of support, including listening to the patient and customizing the regimen in accordance with the patient's needs and wishes regarding treatment effects and side effects[13,25,] focusing on the positive aspects of medication use, focusing on enhancing insight, and fostering a therapeutic relationship with patients and their caregivers.[26]

ORGANIZATIONAL OR HEALTH SYSTEM APPROACHES TO MEDICATION TAKING BEHAVIOR CHANGE

Patients often cite health care system-related barriers and/or facilitators which influence their decisions about taking their medication as prescribed. This section will explore interventions at the system or organization level that have been employed to address issues under the patient's control as well as interactions between the patient and his/her provider and/or the health care delivery system.

Several have agreed that a factor of significant influence on a patient's adherence with medication taking and other health behaviors is the relationship with his/her health care provider.[3,4,11,13] The development of a therapeutic alliance between patient and health care provider is essential to this process. This includes an active effort on the part of the provider to listen and empathize with the patient in a nonjudgmental way, while empowering the patient to take a participative or shared role in the decision-making about his/her care. Several models of care and /or intervention are emerging in pharmacy practice that will fully engage pharmacists in patient counseling, with adherence counseling as a core feature for the purpose of helping patients achieve optimal outcomes. Some emerging contexts include a concerted focus on prevention of hospital readmissions in the face of CMS non-reimbursement for hospital admissions occurring within 30 days of a related discharge. Pharmacists may be part of the case management team conducting telephonic intervention with patients to help problem-solve with medications to prevent readmission. In addition, the emerging patient-centered medical home concept will expect pharmacists to be the care team member providing counseling about medication therapy problem-solving, including adherence. Other opportunities that are establishing an adherence intervention role for pharmacists include medication synchronization, a novel collaboration between pharmacist and prescribing physician of a patient on multiple medications to time all refills to a single day, with the patient arriving for an appointment that includes an MTM session and adherence monitoring and counseling, thus providing support for the patient while also removing a known system-level barrier to adherence. A goal relevant to counseling in any of these endeavors is to gain the patient's trust while facilitating his/her autonomy, and then assessing and monitoring adherence with the medication regimen. These contexts and concepts are at the core of topics that will be discussed in detail in the next section on counseling and communication interventions.

In addition to the therapeutic alliance with the health care provider, access to care (e.g., transportation, convenience and efficiency of follow-up visits, and parking) is important for getting patients back to the practice site to have prescriptions refilled.[13,18] Pharmacists should employ interventions aimed at reinforcing refills; running out of medication is an unfortunate opportunity for a patient to start a phase of non-adherence.

Interventions at this level might include refill reminder flags in the computer system or chart, with subsequent direct contact to remind the patient that a refill is due. Contracting with the patient for adherence, engaging health educators or patient advocates, scheduling appointments at a time and manner convenient to patients, collaboration among the patient's providers, and organizing the care into a disease-based clinic are also strategies providers can use at the practice level to influence medication adherence.[4,11,13,18] Krueger and colleagues also review organization-level technological initiatives (2005), such as adherence drug utilization review flags in the point of care patient chart, information/education kiosks or workstations, adherence incentives to providers, and public awareness campaigns, among others.[4]

Patients also engage in a variety of non-adherent behaviors to reduce medication dosing because of the financial burden of medications. It is often noted that senior adults on a fixed income may be faced with the dilemma of spending money on food or on medications. Sometimes patients will take fewer pills than prescribed, will stretch out the interval between doses, will skip days, will use a pill splitter and take a portion of the dose, and many other activities that reduce the cost but also the therapeutic benefit.

Patients who are insured, may or may not have a co-insurance payment (co-payment) ranging from $0 to actual cost of the drug, depending on whether there is a formulary, whether the drug is a generic, a formulary preferred brand, or a non-formulary preferred brand. Pharmacists in particular can watch for patients with potential financial limitations and check to see that the prescribed drug is one that will require the lowest co-payment for the patient; if this is not the case, the pharmacist should consider calling the prescriber to ask for a low-cost, therapeutically-equivalent switch.

Patients who are not insured or who are on federal assistance can find it very challenging to afford prescription drugs. Usually the co-payment for patients on Medicaid is very low (a few dollars), but for those uninsured Americans who live just above the poverty line, the cost of prescription drugs can be prohibitive, even in the newly emerging Affordable Care Act initiatives. Subsidized prescription drug programs exist and can influence adherence in a positive way.[27] Providers can become aware of programs that are available and how patients can qualify to use them. Table 13-1 includes a list of web sites that provide information about helping patients overcome financial barriers to acquiring medications. In addition, most of the pharmaceutical manufacturers have drug assistance programs known as patient assistance programs

(PAP); information can be found by visiting the manufacturer's home web site, or the web site designated for a specific medication. The links listed in Table 13-1 are only a few links to national initiatives; often, local resources are also available to assist in overcoming the financial barrier to taking medications.

TABLE 13-1: WEB ADDRESSES FOR PRESCRIPTION DRUG ASSISTANCE PROGRAMS/RESOURCES

www.rxassist.org	www.needymeds.org
www.pparx.org	www.xubex.com
www.rxoutreach.com	

COMMUNICATION OR COUNSELING STRATEGIES FOR MEDICATION TAKING BEHAVIOR CHANGE

The process of patient counseling by pharmacists has been studied ever since it was noted that pharmacists communicating with patients impact medication taking behavior. With the previous emphasis on pharmaceutical care and the current emphasis on medication therapy management and advanced care services like comprehensive disease management, accessible pharmacists are increasingly recognized as being in a unique position to intervene with medication-related problems. Many aspects of the interaction between patient and provider have been studied.

Research has suggested that providers can contribute to nonadherence when they have a poor therapeutic relationship with the patient;[13] this is particularly true with the complex and expensive adherence challenge for patients with schizophrenia and bipolar disorder.[25,26,28] Patients need to discuss and learn about their illnesses and medications in a safe, nonjudgmental interaction, regardless of the illness. When a patient feels listened to and understood, he/she will be more likely to trust the provider and receive information.

Not all providers understand how to build a therapeutic alliance with a patient and often don't realize how important it is. The traditional model of health care delivery, the biomedical model, has been driven by a provider mentality known as the "righting reflex."[29-31] Many who enter the health professions are motivated, at least in part, by a desire to help people. This often generates an overriding desire to fix what's "wrong" with patients, and a subsequent tendency to label patients by their illness or condition (e.g., "she is a diabetic, or an asthmatic...") rather than recognizing patients for their individual barriers and motivators regarding the management of their illnesses (e.g., "Mrs. Jones is a patient with diabetes who takes her medication as prescribed most days but finds healthy eating challenging").

The Miller and Rollnick analogy for the biomedical model is wrestling.[29] The biomedical model assumes a provider-centered mode of advising, persuading, arguing, demanding respect, and assuming that resistance to change is bad, among other characteristics. The biomedical model assumes that patients should be and are interested in their health once they are informed of their illness and risk of complications and that they will want to change to manage it. However, knowing about an illness is only one aspect of patient motivation.

Most behavior change that occurs with an approach based on the biomedical model involves temporary extrinsic motivation, or the external push or pull of the provider while in his/her presence. As mentioned previously, external motivation is typically not sustained. And, in fact, resistant patients who encounter providers who push or pull by threatening and shaming or by using scare tactics, may dig their heels in further and completely avoid change, thereby rendering the intervention more harmful than helpful.

The patient-centered model, on the other hand, takes into account an individual's motivators and barriers to change. Being patient-centered involves listening to the patient and collaborating for change by facilitating the patient's own internal motivation, engaging the patient in a shared role for decisions about his/her care, earning respect, and recognizing that resistance to change is important information to be explored. The Miller and Rollnick analogy for the patient-centered model is dancing.[29,30]

Many theories and models of behavior change intervention have been used to explain and predict patient medication adherence. Some of these have been explored in earlier chapters of this book. One theory or model which ties many other theories into a practical, brief method of intervention is the Transtheoretical Model of Change (TTM). The TTM has been used to explain and predict behavior change across many health behaviors like smoking cessation, substance abuse, weight control, exercise, diabetes diet adherence, medication adherence or discontinuation, and others.[32-38] The TTM suggests that people naturally change by moving across five sequential stages of motivation or readiness for change (precontemplation, contemplation, preparation, action, and maintenance), and that the primary objective of intervention is to facilitate movement from the current stage the patient is ready for to the next, with a focus on incremental change and not direct push or pull to action.

Motivational Interviewing (MI) is a patient-centered communication skills set and way of being that incorporates aspects of the TTM readiness concepts into brief encounters with patients. Most of the MI strategies involve efforts to influence another TTM construct, the decisional balance (DB) while also supporting self-efficacy. The DB is the individual's internal motivation mechanism for driving movement along the stages. Decisional balance[39,40] represents the influence an individual's pros (motivators) and cons (barriers) have on the decision of whether or not to engage in a target behavior. An individual who is more influenced by the cons will nearly always be in the pre-action stages of readiness for change and will be either resistant or ambivalent about change. Those more influenced by the pros are typically in preparation, action, or maintenance.[40]

Change in influence or salience of the pros and cons creates movement along the stages of change. This is the process of development of internal motivation and is at the core of the MI strategies. Table 13-2 presents possible pros and cons a patient may state for the medication adherence behavior; he/she may be more influenced by one or the other side of the balance and this will predict whether the patient is adherent or nonadherent.[40]

TABLE 13-2: EXAMPLE: DECISIONAL BALANCE PROS AND CONS FOR MEDICATION ADHERENCE

PROS	CONS
Control my own health	Inconvenient regimen
Prevent complications	The expense of co-payments
Have more energy	Side effects are unpleasant
Avoid hospitalization	Food interaction with my favorites
Make my family happy	Embarrassing for people to know
Peace of mind	Don't want to be reminded I am ill

One MI strategy for helping patients resolve ambivalence or resistance to a target behavior is to help them start thinking about the differences in their own stated pros and cons. This MI strategy is labeled Developing Discrepancy.[29] It involves a nonjudgmental, assertive, non-shaming reflection to the patient about the contrast between his/her own stated pros and cons, and is intended to create dissonance in the mind of the patient. Dissonance is motivating; the goal is to facilitate the patient's thinking about the discrepancy. Using the example in Table 13-2, a pharmacist's statement that uses the Developing Discrepancy strategy might look like this:

> "So on the one hand you want to have more energy and avoid being hospitalized, but on the other hand it's inconvenient to fit this drug regimen into your schedule."

There are several MI strategies that use DB to facilitate patient motivation; at the core of an MI intervention it's important to remember to allow the patient to express what his or her own pros and cons are. If the pharmacist feels a need to add to the list of pros or cons, he/she should first ask permission ("Mrs. Jones, do you mind if I tell you some additional benefits that other patients have said are important for them?"). It is important in an MI strategy to stay focused on the patient's pros, rather than arguing against their cons. When a provider argues against the patient's cons, this puts the patient in a position of defending the cons which only serves to reinforce the negative aspects of the target behavior, and can erode the patient's trust for the provider.

Motivational Interviewing strategies should consistently incorporate reflective listening and expressing empathy, exploring a patient's goals and barriers to change, and providing support and reinforcement of self-efficacy for making the change or even talking about making the change. The process is a style of counseling that helps patients explore and resolve their ambivalence or resistance to making a change.

The "spirit" of MI incorporates all of these concepts in a nonjudgmental manner while helping patients increase their readiness for change by focusing on the perceived discrepancy between a patient's actual behavior and ideal behavior and also focusing on incremental change to support self-efficacy.[29-31] The "spirit" of MI is about empathy and respect. Rather than pushing an agenda on a patient, the provider asks the patient to set goals for the encounter (e.g., "Mrs. Jones, today we need to talk about taking medication, healthy eating, and blood glucose monitoring. Which of these would you like to talk about first?"). To support autonomy in a shared decision-making endeavor, the provider also asks for permission to give information or advice (e.g., "May I share with you some things other patients have told me about what they do to remember to take their medications?").

The MI process has been adopted or endorsed by entities like the American Diabetes Association (ADA), the American Association of Diabetes Educators (AADE), the National Cancer Institute (NCI), the Case Management Society of America (CMSA), and others. The value of MI in health professions education has also been recognized at the international level.[41]

Applications of MI intervention to the problem of medication adherence are fairly recent, but have produced positive results. An intervention based on MI was successfully used among psychiatric patients to improve outpatient treatment adherence.[42] Another study by Liang and colleagues used a MI-based decision support software to intervene over the telephone with multiple sclerosis patients who are at risk for discontinuation of drug therapy. The mean rate of discontinuation in the MI intervention group was reduced from 13% to 1.2%, a statistically significant reduction.[43] A systematic review of the literature for MI as a medication adherence intervention with HAART therapy in HIV patients suggests that across systematically included well-conducted studies, MI was more effective than usual care in helping patients achieve medication adherence.[44] Additional research is needed to explore the impact of MI interventions on medication adherence for some of the challenging adherence topics presented in the next section.

CONSIDERATIONS FOR PATIENT CHALLENGES ABOUT ADHERENCE WITH MEDICATION

Getting to know a patient's response to his/her illness is an important first step in building rapport and in identifying potential barriers to adherence. Complex chronic illnesses may require change on multiple behaviors and this can be overwhelming. Consider the patient newly diagnosed with diabetes who is now being told to take medication and/or use insulin, to monitor blood glucose, and to change lifestyle habits regarding healthy eating and physical activity. This may also be in the face of other co-morbid conditions, and/or the debilitating effects of depression, a condition which often accompanies chronic illnesses like diabetes and negatively impacts medication adherence.

Considering all of these factors, a strategy of facilitating the patient to make decisions about which behavior to address first contributes to building trust by offering the patient the autonomy of deciding, rather than forcing a different agenda on him/her. Often, if the patient has successes on a behavior he/she is interested in working on, he/she will be more willing to address other related behaviors later. With particularly resistant patients, when targeting a multi-dimensional behavior like medication taking (e.g., right number of pills, right times/interval per day, right dose, etc.), if therapeutically possible, it may be helpful to choose one dimension to target at first, rather than the entire change all at once.

This is especially true of lifestyle change behaviors like healthy eating and physical activity where a provider should encourage small, incremental steps towards change (e.g., switching from whole milk to skim milk this week instead of addressing the entire diet, or parking farther out in the parking lot and taking the stairs instead of the elevator this week instead of taking on an extensive walking/running regimen). For an overwhelmed or resistant patient, having success on one aspect of a target behavior may reinforce the patient for taking on additional aspects of a target behavior. In light of this self-efficacy building incremental focus, it is also important to use incremental vocabulary like "healthy eating," "being active," or "cutting back," rather than words that imply big change like "diet," "exercise," or "quitting."

It is also important to emphasize again that all of the strategies described in this chapter are particularly challenging to use with patients experiencing psychosis, mental illness, impaired insight, and dementia.[25,26] Little is known about improving medication adherence in patients with these illnesses and conditions, partly because many studies specifically exclude patients with psychosis or dementia. It is also difficult to accurately assess adherence with medications for those conditions.

Another area of challenge for medication adherence intervention is among patients with HIV/AIDS. For patients with HIV/AIDS on highly active anti-retroviral therapy (HAART) the target level of medication adherence is greater than 95% in order to suppress replication of the virus and to prevent resistance.[45] This may require multiple, expensive medications in a complex dosing regimen with the potential for significant side effects and food interactions, although combined dosing options are increasingly available for the purpose of simplifying and supporting adherence. Unlike other more forgiving medication regimens, missing even one dose can be substantially detrimental and, with repeats over time, eventually can be fatal.

Little focus has been drawn in this chapter to the problem of nonadherence among pediatric patients with chronic illnesses (e.g., diabetes, asthma, rheumatoid arthritis, others). The challenge lies not only in understanding the patient's decision-making, but also that of the parent or caregiver. Many of the psychosocial issues discussed in previous chapters become more complex in the face of developmental and lifestyle changes that are a natural part of adolescence.

Most successful interventions in pediatric patients have involved a combination of interventions, including a behavioral intervention. The most common intervention used among pediatric patients is a token reinforcement process.[13] This reinforcement method gives pediatric patients the opportunity to earn tokens to be used to "purchase" items of interest, privileges/activities, or other rewards. The involvement of family, school personnel and other support networks have also been successful in reinforcing medication adherence behavior in pediatric patients.[13] Transition to adult medical care and self-management of a disease can be challenging for an emerging adult and is an area warranting further study.

AREAS FOR FUTURE EXPLORATION

It is difficult to fully know effectiveness of adherence interventions because of the challenges to study design and methods inherent in this type of research in human patients. Many of the adherence interventions tested have been complex and labor-intensive. It was suggested that more impact has been seen with interventions for adherence with acute medications, like antibiotics, than for maintenance medications for chronic illnesses.

Much of the adherence data is collected using self-report and it is known that patients overestimate (social desirability) self-report of health behaviors[36,46] and particularly medication taking.[47] In addition, the measures used and the ways they are implemented and interpreted varies considerably from study to study, making comparisons of results difficult.[3,4] In fact, recent literature[3,47,48,49] suggests that the studies on medication adherence exhibit substantial variability in design, measures and methods, making it difficult to compare findings, particularly in studies which also have varied duration of follow-up. The findings of several studies also suggest that once the intervention ends, the effect on adherence diminishes;[9] it is important to consider the implications of this in research and practice.

To thoroughly examine the impact of interventions for medication adherence in chronic illnesses, more research is needed and a more standardized methodology should be considered among researchers in this field.[49]

SUMMARY: MEDICATION TAKING BEHAVIOR CHANGE INTERVENTION IN PHARMACY PRACTICE

Development of a therapeutic alliance between pharmacist and patient has been shown to most significantly influence medication taking behavior and should be established as the initial part of any intervention. As trust is established, this is the gateway to other behavior change strategies. Within the context of the therapeutic alliance relationship, pharmacists should carefully listen, express empathy and engage in non-judgmental eliciting of patient knowledge deficits, health goals, and motivators/barriers to adherence.

First line strategies should attempt to facilitate shared patient decision-making about how to 1) simplify the regimen, and 2) tailor the regimen to other habitual activities in the patient's routine. This may include collaborating with the patient's other health care provider(s) and/or caregiver(s), while also helping the patient identify a support person or network to reinforce the commitment to medication adherence and other healthy behaviors. This may also include developing a therapeutic plan, which could include a contract between patient and provider, and should include application of adherence aids where needed.

Follow-up interactions with the patient are important to the reinforcement process and have clearly shown sustained impact on medication adherence. A follow-up telephone call in the early stages of intervention is optimal to reinforce behavior change while also providing support; direct contact at refill visits should include assessment and feedback about medication taking behaviors.

SUGGESTED ADDITIONAL READINGS

Kripalani, S., Yao, X., & Haynes, B. (2007). Interventions to enhance medication adherence in chronic medical conditions. *Arch Intern Med.* 167(6):540–549.

McDonald, H., Garg, A., & Haynes, R. (2002). Interventions to enhance patient adherence to medication prescriptions: scientific review. *JAMA* 288:2868–2879.

Rickles, N.M., Brown, T.A., McGivney, M.S., Snyder, M.E., & White, K.A. (2010). Adherence: A review of education, research, practice, and policy in the United States. *Pharmacy Practice* 2010; Jan–Mar;8(1):1–17.

Rollnick, S., Miller, W.R., & Butler, C.C. (2008). *Motivational Interviewing in Health Care.* New York, NY: The Guilford Press.

Miller, W.R. & Rollnick, S. (2013). *Motivational Interviewing, 3rd Edition: Preparing People for Change.* New York, NY: The Guilford Press.

REFERENCES

1. Marston, M. (1970). Compliance with medical regimens: a review of the literature. *Nursing Research* 19:312–323.

2. Sackett, D. & Snow, J. (1979). *Compliance in health care.* Baltimore, MD: Johns Hopkins University Press.

3. Kripalani, S., Xiaomei, Y., & Haynes, R. (2007). Interventions to enhance medication adherence in chronic medical conditions: a systematic review. *Arch Intern Med* 167:540–549.

4. Krueger, K., Berger, B., & Felkey, M. (2005). Medication adherence and persistence: a comprehensive review. *Advances in Therapy* 22(4):319–362.

5. Smith, S., Brock, T., & Howarth, S. (2005). Use of personal digital assistants to deliver education about adherence to antiretroviral medications. *J Am Pharm Assoc* 45(5):625–628.

6. Dayer, L,. Heldenbrand, S., Anderson, P., Gubbins, P.O., & Martin, B.C. (2013). Smartphone medication adherence apps: Potential benefits to patients and providers. *J Am Pharm Assoc* 53:172–181.

7. National Institute for Literacy: Fact Sheet: Adult and Family Literacy. Available at: http://lincs.ed.gov/facts/facts.html. Accessed November 30, 2014.

8. Weiss, B., Mays, M., Martz, W., et al. (2005). Quick assessment of literacy in primary care: The newest vital sign. *Ann Fam Med* 3:514–522.

9. Murray, M., Young, J., Hoke, S., et al. (2007). Pharmacist intervention to improve medication adherence in heart failure: a randomized trial. *Ann Intern Med* 146(10):714–725.

10. Lee, J., Grace, K., & Taylor, A. (2006). Effect of a pharmacy care program on medication adherence and persistence, blood pressure, and low-density lipoprotein cholesterol: A randomized controlled trial. *JAMA* 296(21):2563–2571.

11. Haynes, R., Yao, X., & Degani, A., et al. (2007). Interventions for enhancing medication adherence. *Cochrane Database Syst Rev* (2):CD000011.

12. McDonald, H., Garg, A., & Haynes, R. (2002). Interventions to enhance patient adherence to medication prescriptions: scientific review. *JAMA* 288(22);2868–2879.

13. Osterberg, L. & Blaschke, T. (2005). Adherence to medication. *NEJM* 353(5):487–497.

14. Sather, B., Forbes, J., Starck, D., & Rovers, J. (2007). Effect of a personal automated dose-dispensing system on adherence: a case series. *J Am Pharm Assoc* 47(1):82–85.

15. Maples, N., Velligan, D.I., Wang, M., et al. (2005). Cognitive adaptation training and adherence to medication. *Schizophr Bull* 31:528.

16. Bendle, S., Velligan, D.I., Mueller, J.L., et al. (2005). The MedeMonitor for improving adherence to oral medication in schizophrenia. *Schizophr Bull* 31:519.

17. Claxton, A., Cramer, J., & Pierce, C. (2001). A systematic review of the associations between dose regimens and medication compliance. *Clin Ther* 23:1296–1310.

18. Jacobson, T. (2004). The forgotten cardiac risk factor: noncompliance with lipid-lowering therapy. *Medscape Cardiology* 8(2). Available at www.medscape.com/viewarticle/496144. Accessed November 30, 2014.

19. Gurley, V. (2006). Leveraging health risk assessments for maximum effect. *J Managed Care Medicine* 10(1):12–17.)

20. Rickles, N., Svarstad, B., Statz-Paynter, J., et al. (2005). Pharmacist telemonitoring of antidepressant use: effects on pharmacist-patient collaboration. *J Am Pharm Assoc* 45(3):344–353.

21. Krass, I., Taylor, S., Smith, C., & Armour, C. (2005). Impact on medication use and adherence of Australian pharmacists' diabetes care services. *J Am Pharm Assoc* 45(1):33–40.

22. Murray, E. (1964). *Motivation and emotion.* Englewood Cliffs, NJ: Prentice-Hall, Inc.

23. Deci, E. (1985). *Intrinsic motivation and self-determination in human behavior.* New York: Plenum Press.

24. Lewis, F. & Daltroy, L. (2002). How causal explanations influence health behavior: Attribution theory. In K. Glanz, F.M. Lewis, & B.K. Rimer (Eds.), *Health behavior and health education: theory research, and practice*, third ed. San Francisco: Jossey-Bass.

25. Lacro. J., Dunn. L., Dolder, C., et al. (2002). Prevalence of and risk factors for medication nonadherence in patients with schizophrenia: A comprehensive review of recent literature. *J Clin Psychiatry* 63:892–909.

26. Kikkert, M., Schene, A., Koeter, M., et al. (2006). Medication adherence in schizophrenia: exploring patients', carers', and professionals' views. *Schizophr Bull* 32(4):786–794.

27. Spiker, E., Giannamore, M., & Nahata, M. (2005). Medication use patterns and health outcomes among patients using a subsidized prescription drug program. *J Am Pharm Assoc* 45(6):714–719.

28. Misdrahi, D., Llorca, P., Lancon, C., & Bayle, F. (2002). Compliance in schizophrenia: predictive factors, therapeutic considerations, and research implications. *Encephale* 28:266–272.

29. Miller, W. & Rollnick, S. (2013). Motivational interviewing: *Preparing people for change*, third ed. New York, NY: The Guilford Press.

30. Rollnick, S., Mason, P., & Butler, C. (2000). *Health behavior change: A guide for practitioners.* New York, NY: Churchill Livingstone.

31. Kavookjian, J. Motivational interviewing. (2011). In Richardson, M., Chant, C., Chessman, K.H., Finks, S.W., Hemstreet, B.A., Hume, A.L., et al (Eds.). *Parmacotherapy self-assessment program, 7th ed. Book 8: Science and practice of pharmacotherapy.* Lenexa, KS: American College of Clinical Pharmacy, 1–18.

32. DiClemente, C. & Prochaska, J. (1982). Self-change and therapy change of smoking behavior: a comparison of processes of change in cessation and maintenance. *Addict Behav* 7:133–142.

33. Prochaska, J. & DiClemente C. (1986). Common processes of self-change in smoking, weight control and psychological distress. In: Shiffman, S. & Wills, T. (Eds), *Coping and substance abuse.* New York, NY: Academic Press.

34. Moyers, T., Miller, W., & Hendrickson, M. (2005). How does motivational interviewing work? Therapist interpersonal skill predicts client involvement with motivational interviewing sessions. *J Consult Clin Psych* 73(4):590–598.

35. Resnicow, K., Davis, R., & Rollnick, S. (2006). Motivational interviewing for pediatric obesity: conceptual issues and evidence review. *J Am Diet Assoc* 106:2024–2033.

36. Kavookjian, J., Berger, B., Grimley, D., et al. (2005). Patient decision-making: strategies for diabetes diet adherence intervention. *Res Soc Admin Pharm* 1:389–407.

37. Willey, C., Redding, C., Stafford, J., et al. (2000). Stages of change for adherence with medication regimens for chronic disease: development and validation of a measure. *Clin Ther* 22:858–871.

38. Berger, B,. Hudmon, K., & Liang, H. (2004). Predicting treatment discontinuation among patients with multiple sclerosis: Application of the transtheoretical model of change. *J Am Pharm Assoc* 44:445–454.

39. Janis, I. & Mann, L. (1977). *Decision making: a psychological analysis of conflict, choice and commitment.* New York, NY: Free Press.

40. Prochaska, J., Velicer, W., Rossi, J., et al. (1994). Stages of change and decisional balance for 12 problem behaviors. *Health Psych* 13(1):39–46.

41. Martin, B., Plake, K., & Kavookjian, J. (2014, August). *Teaching and assessing motivational interviewing in US Schools of Pharmacy.* Workshop for the International Social Pharmacy Workshop, Boston, MA.

42. Swanson, A., Pantalon, M., Cohen K. (1997). Motivational interviewing and treatment adherence among psychiatric and dually diagnosed patients. *J Nerv Ment Dis* 187:630–635.

43. Liang, H. (2003). (2003). *Decreasing medication dropout: A study to develop and evaluate intervention software using the transtheoretical model of change and motivational interviewing* [dissertation]. Auburn, AL: Auburn University.

44. Hill, S. & Kavookjian, J. (2012). Motivational interviewing as a behavioral intervention to increase HAART adherence in patients who are HIV+: A systematic review of the literature. *Aids Care* 24(5): 583–592.

45. Ickovics, J., Cameron, A., Zackin, R., et al. (2002). Consequences and determinants of adherence to antiretroviral medication: results from Adult AIDS Clinical Trials Group protocol 370. *Antivir Ther* 7:185–193.

46. Clark, M., Abrams, D., Niaura, R., et al. (1991). Self-efficacy in weight management. *J Consult Clin Psych* 59:739–744.

47. Smith, S., Wahed, A., Kelley, S., et al. (2007). Assessing the validity of self-reported medication adherence in hepatitis C treatment. *Ann Pharmacother* 41.

48. Nichol, M., Venturini, F., & Sung, J. (1999). A critical evaluation of the methodology of the literature on medication compliance. *Ann Pharmacother* 33:531–540.

49. Rickles, N.M., Brown, T.A., McGivney, M.S., Snyder, M.E., & White, K.A. (2010.) Adherence: A review of education, research, practice, and policy in the United States. *Pharmacy Practice* Jan-Mar;8(1):1–17.

CHAPTER 14

PATIENT-CENTERED OUTCOMES ASSESSMENT IN HEALTH CARE

By Judith Barr, ScD, MEd

LEARNING OBJECTIVES:

1. Justify the economic and humanistic need for patient-centered outcomes in healthcare.

2. Identify at least five questions that should considered in the selection of an outcomes measure. Which do you think is the most important of the ones you selected? Justify why.

3. Describe the stages within the Wilson-Cleary model linking clinical variables to health-related quality of life outcomes. Given a clinical condition, develop a patient-centered, patient-reported outcomes assessment system that incorporates measures for each step in the model.

4. Describe the 2009 Food and Drug Administration's "Guidance for Industry on Patient-reported outcomes Measures" and potential impact on the development of any future patient-centered outcome measures. Identify characteristics of an outcome measure submitted for FDA Authorization that would likely i) be approved and ii) not be approved.

5. Contrast and compare the advantages and disadvantages of generic versus disease-specific health-related quality of life measures.

KEY TERMS

Donabedian Structure-Process-Outcome Model

Efficacy and clinical effectiveness

End result project

FDA Guidance for Industry. Patient-Reported Outcome Measures: Use in Medical Product Development to Support Labeling Claims and FDA qualified measure

FDA Patient Representatives

General versus disease-specific measures

Generic and disease-specific health status measures

Health

Health-related quality of life

Outcomes assessment

Patient-centered outcomes

Patient-Centered Outcomes Assessment Institute (PCORI)

Patient-focused drug development

Patient-reported outcomes

Reliability: intra-rater reliability, internal reliability, and inter-rater reliability

Systematic and random errors of measurement

Validity: content, construct, discriminate, convergent

Wilson-Cleary model

THE CASE:

Mrs. Wheeler is a 58-year-old former elementary school teacher with moderate chronic obstructive pulmonary disease (COPD). Ten years ago she first noticed some breathlessness after moderate exercise. These episodes then began to occur while in the classroom. Five years ago she was diagnosed with COPD. Her % of predicted forced expiratory volume (% pred FEV_1) was 75% and she was placed on albuterol 1–2 puffs every 4–6 hours as needed for shortness of breath. She quit her 35-year cigarette smoking habit and was stable with only rare exertion-related dyspnea attacks. Two years later however, her symptoms began to also include occasional coughing episodes and sputum production. After 30 years of teaching, Mrs. Wheeler retired because her symptoms although infrequent, were unpredictable and made managing a classroom of 20 nine-year-olds too challenging. Her % pred FEV_1 was now 62% and tiotropium 18 mcg inhaled daily was added to her therapy.

She lives at home with her husband, also retired. Their two adult children and four grandchildren live in nearby towns. Since retirement, her COPD has been stable with rare exacerbations. Mrs. Wheeler remained active—volunteering in several community organizations, participating in book and bridge clubs, knitting socks for the homeless with her church group, and helping her children with the needs of the grandchildren.

Nine months ago, Mrs. Wheeler developed the flu which led to an exacerbation of her COPD symptoms—increased breathlessness, coughing and production of sputum, and other chest symptoms. Oral prednisone 40 mg daily was added for five days. Although her acute flu symptoms resolved, she became progressively weaker, more physically limited, and moderately breathless in normal household activities. She was increasingly confined to home and unable to continue her volunteer activities or help with the care of her grandchildren. She was embarrassed by her chronic coughing and sputum production and no longer went to her book or bridge clubs. Her % pred FEV_1 dropped to 55% and indacterol 75mcg once daily was added to her previous tiotropium therapy.

Earlier this week, Mrs. Wheeler developed pneumonia and was admitted to your hospital. Although the infection has improved and she received a second course of corticosteroid therapy, this episode has further reduced Mrs. Wheeler's physical, social, and psychological status. Her % pred FEV_1 is now 42% and she is further weakened. Her family physician is aware of the hospital's interprofessional pulmonary rehabilitation (PR) program of which you are a member and recommends that she transition into this program. The patient-centered team, consisting of a pharmacist, physical therapist, occupational therapist, dietitian, nurse, psychologist, and pulmonologist, meets with Mrs. Wheeler who expresses exasperation with her condition, "There is nothing left that I enjoy doing."

What would be the measures included in an outcomes assessment system to measure her baseline condition, monitor her progress over time, and evaluate the effective of the PR program?

Outcomes assessment in general, and patient-centered outcomes in particular, are two of the most timely issues in American health care today. These two topics are interconnected, one a subset of the other. Broadly stated, outcomes assessment is a comprehensive and integrated system of assessments to measure the efficiency and effectiveness of health care services and interventions. Patient-centered outcomes is a more focused concept, included in an outcomes assessment system, that measures the impact of health care interventions on aspects of health that patients indicate are of importance to them.

Outcomes assessment asks the question: Are the services and therapies we provide patients improving their health status or at least preventing or slowing deterioration of their condition? In other words, are our medications, treatments, and other interventions effective (do they work?) and efficient (are they produced using only the necessary resources?)? Are patients better because they receive these services? Have we made a difference in patients' end results or "outcomes"? And, have we included during this assessment process, outcome measures that are valued by patients…have we included patient-centered outcomes? The answers to these questions will be used to shape broad health policies, reimbursement decisions, and patient treatment plans; therefore, outcomes assessment studies must be generalizable to the population to which the results will be applied. Unlike clinical trials or efficacy research that is conducted in ideal and controlled conditions, outcomes assessment or effectiveness research must be conducted in the "real world" by average practitioners under ordinary circumstance with typical patients.

Notice that the word "outcomes" in outcomes assessment is plural. This indicates that the outcomes assessment process generally uses more than one measure to determine the effectiveness of an intervention such as a specific pharmaceutical product or a complex PR program; it is an outcomes assessment system. A comprehensive battery of outcome measures, appropriate for the clinical condition and intervention being assessed, is included in the assessment. Outcomes assessment requires that more than a biologic or pathologic variable (biomarker) be measured to judge the effectiveness of treatments or interventions; it means more than lung function, blood pressure, or lipid profiles. It examines more than quantity of life; it also examines aspects of health that contribute to quality of life as perceived by patients.

In 1990 Epstein described outcomes assessment, effectiveness research, and the outcomes movement in the following way. Since that time the need for outcomes assessment, and now patient-centered and patient-reported outcomes, has only grown stronger:

> *Perhaps the most important effect of the outcomes movement has been a broadening of our focus to include a range of outcomes…We have seen a dramatic expansion in the range of outcomes that physicians and policy makers are willing to consider valid indicators of health. These go beyond traditional clinical indexes and include a series of variables assessed through [patient] interviews: functional status, emotional health, social interaction, cognitive function, degree of disability, and so forth. There is a growing appreciation in the medical community that instruments based on subjective data from patients can provide important information that may not be evident from physiologic measurements and may be as reliable as—or more reliable than—many of the clinical, biochemical, or physiologic indexes…[1]*

This chapter will examine why, 25 years later, the "outcomes movement" and now "patient-centered outcomes" and "patient-reported outcomes" are central topics in health care. We will review some early strategies to include measures of outcome in quality of care assessments. Then we will define the concept of "health" which serves as the foundation for the development of a comprehensive, and patient-centered, outcomes assessment strategy. We will describe the construct of health status measures, summarize the content of several of these measures, and review some operational characteristics which should be considered when selecting measures to assess Mrs. Wheeler's case as the interprofessional, patient-centered PR program team designs and later evaluates the effectiveness of the program. Recommendations from the 2012 and 2015 International Society for Quality of Life (ISQOL)[2,3] and the 2015 International Society for Pharmacoeconomics and Outcomes Research (ISPOR)[4] reports, and the 2009 U.S. Food and Drug Administration (FDA) *Guidance for Industry, Patient-Reported Outcomes Measures: Use in Medical Product Development to Support Labeling Claims[5]* will be incorporated into the description of outcome measures. The 2009 FDA Guidance will be explicitly examined in the selection of measures to evaluate symptoms in Mrs. Wheeler's case. Finally we will examine recent policies that codify the importance of patient-centered outcomes such as the establishment of the Patient-Centered Outcomes Assessment Institute (PCORI) and the Food and Drug Administration's Patient-Focused Drug Development (PFDD) program.

WHY IS THERE AN OUTCOMES ASSESSMENT MOVEMENT?

The outcomes assessment movement is a powerful force in health care today. It is fueled by two objectives—one economic and one humanistic. While these two objectives originate from different constituencies, they converge in a demand to evaluate our health care practices so that they provide cost-efficient and effective, patient-centered health care.

THE ECONOMIC OBJECTIVE

High American health care costs and the need to reduce these costs is the economic objective behind the outcomes assessment movement. In 2014, the United States spent more than $3.0 trillion on health care services, an increase of 4.5 % from 2014.[6] That averages to $9,523 for every man, woman, and child in this country[6] and more per person than any other country on earth.[7] The percentage of the US gross domestic product going to health care services is 17.5%.[6]

Perhaps if we as a country had the best health in the world, the expenditure could be justified. But, we don't. Compared to 34 other industrialized countries that are members of the member nations of Organization of Economic Co-operation and Development (OECD), in 2013 (nearest comparable data), the United States ranked 28 of 34 in "life expectancy at birth" of the OECD member nations at 78.8 years compared to the OECD average of 80.5 years. Japan led the countries with its citizens' life span averaging 83.4 years.[7] In another comparative health indicator, "infant mortality" (deaths per 1,000 live births), the United States was fifth from the top among the OECD member nations. The rate in the United States is 5.0 per 1000 live births, nearly four times higher than Iceland which has the lowest infant mortality (1.3 deaths per 1,000 live births). Unfortunately since 2004, infant mortality in the United States has gotten worse relative to the other OECD member countries; the United States moved from a lower than the OECD average to now being above the OECD average.[7]

These numbers document that the United States is investing more per capita in health care than any other country, but we may not be getting the most value in health outcome for our money. More than 40 years ago, Wennberg and colleagues suggested one possible reason for this problem—the United States was wasting money when unneeded health care services, or services of little value, were being performed. This conclusion was based on the discovery of huge variations in the rates of elective surgeries in different counties in New England without an associated variation in the morbidity and mortality of the population, even after adjusting for differences in population density, income and age.[8] Overall the quantity of health care inputs (and their associated costs) was not connected to the quality of patient outcomes. More surgeries (inputs) did not lead to decreased morbidity and mortality (outcomes). These findings implied that the same level of health could be achieved for the population with fewer surgeries, and therefore, lower cost. Every surgery that did not contribute to improved health resulted in wasted health care dollars.

Those early findings and subsequent studies from the Dartmouth Medical Atlas Group and its Institute for Health Policy and Clinical Practice have suggested that Medicare spending can be reduced by as much as 30% without patient harm if redundant health care practices or those of little or no value were eliminated.[9,10] Berwick and the RAND Corporation estimated 18–37% of the annual US health care expenses in 2012 were associated with wastes due to such factors as overtreatment, and failures of care delivery or care coordination.11 Third party payers argue that they should only pay for clinically indicated services of demonstrated effectiveness. Since many medical services have not been rigorously evaluated nor proven to be of clinical benefit, clinical effectiveness studies are needed. If a therapeutic intervention is found to be ineffective or a diagnostic procedure does not provide useful information, payments for those services should be discontinued. The lack of payment should lead to the discontinuation of ineffective health care services. Therefore, clinical effectiveness and outcomes assessment programs are a central tactic to reduce waste and associated health care costs. These topics will be covered in the next section.

A complementary strategy to reduce waste and associated costs in American health care services has been championed by the American Board of Internal Medicine (ABIM) Foundation. Launched in 2012, ABIM Foundation initiated the Choosing Wisely campaign and invited medical specialty groups to each develop its "Top 5" lists consisting of "five achievable practice changes to improve patient health through better treatment choices, reduced risks, and where possible, reduced costs."[12,13] Its purpose is to support initiatives focused on reducing utilization of inappropriate tests or treatments. Collectively the Choosing Wisely campaign now includes nearly 60 general and specialty medical, nursing, and other health professional organizations. The 2015 compilation of each organization's "Top Five Things Physicians and Patients Should Question," developed and supported by evidence-based recommendations, can be found on the Choosing Wisely web site.[14] Ninety-one of the recommendations relate to questionable medication use.

An important aspect of this effort is a patient-centered, patient education component supported by 34 consumers partner organizations led by *Consumer Reports*.[15] A series of videos have been developed to assist providers and patients make wise decisions about the most appropriate care based on their individual situation. Both American Academy of Family Physicians[16] and American Academy of Allergy, Asthma & Immunology[17] have produced videos illustrating how clinician-patient communications can be improved to prevent antibiotics use when they are not indicated for symptoms of viral rhinosinusitis.

Now you can see that cost reduction is the economic objective behind outcomes assessment—to follow the most efficient and effective, evidence-based health care practices that can be used to create a more cost-efficient, and clinically effective, national health care delivery system. Our nation is spending more on health care services than any other country, but it appears that we are not getting our money's worth. Variation analysis tells us there is waste in the system. Outcomes-based clinical effectiveness research and initiatives such as *Choosing Wisely* will tell us what health care services are of little or no value. Influenced by this information, third party payers such as insurance groups, self-insured businesses and federal and state governments will demand that clinically ineffective services and areas of waste be identified and eliminated. Outcomes assessment programs are essential for these decision. Then, health care expenses can be reduced by not paying for those services.

As present and future pharmacists, you are reading this chapter and asking: Why are economic issues of concern to me as I prepare to enter clinical practice? Because, either directly or indirectly, outcomes-based economic evaluation of health care practices will affect what services you provide, the frequency with which you provide those services, and the payment you will receive for them. As more health care is delivered through managed care and accountable care organizations and as more health clinicians are paid by capitation or other forms of prospective payment systems, there will be even further scrutiny of the value received for the health care dollar. Health care providers, including pharmacists and rehabilitation therapists, will have to demonstrate that the services they provide are clinically effective and that the recommended duration of therapy is necessary. If the effectiveness of a treatment is not established through well-designed outcomes assessment programs, clinicians will no longer refer patients for that service because third party payers will not pay for it. Over time, the economic pressure to reduce costs and the outcomes assessment pressure to demonstrate clinical effectiveness will modify health care practices.

THE PATIENT-CENTERED (HUMANISTIC) OBJECTIVE

The patient-centered or humanistic objective behind the outcomes movement is to include the patient's perspective when evaluating the clinical effectiveness of medications, procedures, or other interventions. Patients have their own opinions as to what are important outcomes to them as they agree to an intervention to improve their perception of their health. However, providers traditionally have selected their own outcome measures to judge the effectiveness of those services. They have relied heavily upon objective measures of physiologic biomarkers and physical functioning and have not incorporate subjective patient assessments of their health status. Rarely have patients been asked about the values they place on different aspects of their health state and about what changes in their clinical conditions would be of most importance to them. When patients are consulted, patient-reported and provider-reported priorities are frequently in conflict.

Further problems arise when effective communication within the health care team is inhibited by each health profession using its own discipline-specific assessment measures to evaluate the progress of the patient. This prevents providers from speaking a common assessment language and inhibits patient engagement in decision making and self-monitoring of clinical progress. Therefore, patient-centered outcome measures would serve three purposes: 1) introduce a patient perspective into patient management and clinical effectiveness studies, 2) provide a common assessment vocabulary for interprofessional discussion of patient needs, planning of treatment strategies, and assessment of clinical effectiveness, and 3) provide a mechanism by which patients can report standardized measures of symptoms and health status and be engaged in their clinical decision and management processes.

Patient-centered outcomes assessment builds upon the World Health Organization's (WHO) definition of health as "a complete physical, mental, and social well-being and nor merely the absence of disease."[18] From this perspective, health is a multidimensional concept consisting of at least three dimensions, also called domains. Therefore, to capture the impact of interventions on the full concept of "health," patient-centered outcomes assessment requires that clinical effectiveness studies evaluate these domains of health. This requires more than biologic biomarkers or physical function indicators be measured before, during, and after clinical interventions. In COPD, objective pulmonary function tests or exercise endurance tests no longer are sufficient outcomes measures, by themselves, to assess the impact of PR treatment on the multidimensional outcome of health, especially since neither are patient-reported nor from a patient-centered perspective.

Traditionally, as shown in Figure 14-1, three major considerations shape the decisions as to what pharmaceutical products are approved by the FDA, reach the market, and are then included on an institution's drug formulary. First, as judged through rigorous randomized and blinded clinical trials, the drug must prove to be efficacious; i.e., to produce the desired effect, usually on a physiologic biomarker. Second, it must prove to be safe in Phase I and II clinical drug trials, and that in Phase III and IV (post-marketing), the frequency and severity of adverse drug events does not outweigh the drug's benefit. Third, for formulary selection, the cost of the drug and associated expenses must be judged to be of sufficient clinical value to be included by each third party. To date, these criteria have been based primarily on objective biomarker outcomes not reported by the patient, have failed to include patient priorities, and have lacked patient-centered subjective measures.

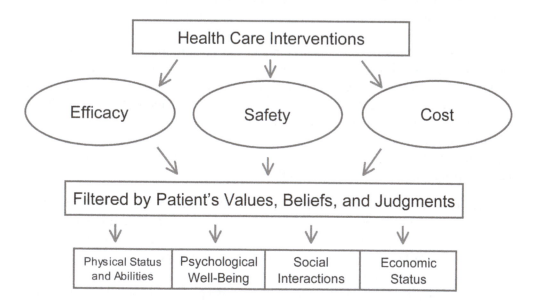

FIGURE 14-1: IMPACT OF HEALTH INTERVENTION AS TYPICALLY JUDGED BY THE HEALTH CARE SYSTEM, THEN FILTERED BY PATIENT'S VALUES, BELIEFS, AND JUDGEMENT

However, a patient-centered outcomes assessment system recognizes that patients have their own values, beliefs, and judgments which can filter the impact of an intervention in different ways. To patients, the effectiveness of an intervention, such as a new drug, is judged by its effect on their physical status, mental status, psychological well-being, social interactions, and economic stability. A clinician-selected, bio-marker-based outcome measure is unlikely to capture the outcomes of importance to patients. Therefore, conclusions about the effectiveness of a new drug may differ between clinicians and patients if only biomarkers, rather than a more patient-centered outcomes assessment system, are used in the evaluation.

For example, in Mrs. Wheeler's case, while medication adjustment and pulmonary rehabilitation may improve her % pred FEV_1 and some aspects of her physical function, the interprofessional PR team will also need to target her psychological and social functioning problems. To assess the effectiveness of these targeted efforts, patient-centered/patient-reported outcome measures assessing psychological and social functioning need to be added. Early in the current outcomes assessment movement, Ellwood described these broader measures as a "technology of patient experience designed to help patients, payers, and providers make rational medical care-related choices based on better insight into the effect of these choices on the patient's life. It would routinely and systematically measure the functioning and well-being of patients, along with disease-specific clinical outcomes."[20] Ellwood proposes that these types of measurements be central to the development of a longitudinal type of outcomes assessment based on patient-centered assessment. "The centerpiece and unifying ingredient of outcomes management is the tracking and measurement of function and well-being or quality of life across healthcare locations."[20]

In summary, there has been a convergence of two communities of interest: the economists' interest to reduce health care costs and the humanists' interest to incorporate patients' values and beliefs in the evaluation of health care services. The result is the patient-centered, outcomes assessment movement. When the two interests work in harmony, they produce a more cost-efficient and effective delivery system that directs attention specifically to individual patients and their well-being.

EARLIER APPROACHES TO MEASURING OUTCOMES

The measurement of patient outcomes was an important element in the evaluation strategies of two early pioneers of quality of care assessment. Neither was motivated by cost-reduction concerns: rather, they both were interested in measurement strategies to improve the quality, and standardize the delivery, of care. And both have important messages that we should consider as we develop cost-efficient, patient-centered, outcomes assessment programs.

THE "END RESULT" PROPOSAL: THE CODMAN APPROACH

In 1914 Dr. E. A. Codman proposed the "End Result" approach.[21] Codman, an early pioneer in quality of care measurement, was concerned with the lack of information about the effectiveness of medical practices, skill of practitioners, and the quality of American hospitals. He proposed that a hospital's annual report include data to document if procedures were effective and to measure if patients improved, that being the ultimate "end results."

Codman's "End Result" proposal was based on patient outcomes. If the mission of medical care was to cure patients, Codman reasoned that the evaluation of the care should not be based on outcome measures of the time; e.g., how many patients were admitted, whether surgery was performed, or what procedures the patient received. To Codman, the ultimate evaluation of the medical care provided was whether the "end result" included a "satisfied and relieved" patient, one who could resume function in the community after receiving medical treatment.

To operationalize the "end result" proposal, Codman trained a group of social workers who followed patients into the community after hospital discharge to measure the "end result" of care. If "satisfied and relieved" patients returned to their former function, then the treatment they received could be considered to be effective and the practitioners who provided that care were judged to be skillful. However, at the time, his proposal was judged by the medical community to be too radical and was never adopted by his hospital nor the broader medical community. Nearly 20 years later, he wrote "Although the End Result Idea may not achieve its entire fulfillment for several generations...I am able to enjoy the hypothesis that I may receive some honors from a more receptive generation."[22]

There are important lessons from the "End Result" proposal for our present outcomes assessment priorities. First is the need to evaluate the effectiveness of our practices by measuring the therapeutic impact on patients in their everyday functioning. That involves a broad assessment of functioning—not only physical functioning, but also psychological and social functioning. Now that valid and reliable, patient-centered and patient-reported outcome measures are available, we can perform this type of assessment; we just have to use them. However, if and when we do use them, the assessment frequently is performed within the health care setting immediately after the health intervention has been completed. Codman's End Result idea tells us that the timing is too soon and the assessment is in the wrong location. In addition to the discharge evaluations, ideally assessments also should be conducted in the home and work environments, in the "community" three to six months after the end of the treatment. That would provide enough time to determine the true effectiveness of the intervention. This measurement strategy is more challenging and more costly, but it would yield a more accurate reflection of the value of health care services to patients. Self-administered, multidimensional assessments may be an economical method to accomplish this goal.

OUTCOMES AS A COMPONENT OF QUALITY OF CARE: THE DONABEDIAN APPROACH

Avedis Donabedian is the father of the traditional quality of care measurement model, a model based on the evaluation of three components of care: structure, process, and outcome.[23] A solid *structure* must be present to provide care, the proper *processes* must be followed to deliver that care, and then appropriate *outcomes* must be measured to evaluate the effectiveness of the care.

In this model, the quality of the structural component includes factors related to the *structure* of a health care delivery system including its buildings, equipment, and staff. This can consist of an assessment of physical features such as the adequacy and quality of facilities and equipment and conformance to building codes and other standards, as well as the qualifications and experience of staff, personnel staffing patterns, organizational reporting, financing arrangements, other administrative elements. In pharmacy practices, examples of structural components could include equipment in and adequacy of pharmacy compounding areas, qualifications and organization of the pharmacy dispensing and clinical staff, and a pharmacy computer system integrated into the medical record and billing systems.

The *process* component consists of activities involved in the process of delivering health care services. These include the technical and interpersonal actions of health providers and patients, as well as operational/organizational processes within the health care system. If validated clinical pathways have been developed, the quality of the process of care can be assessed by determining how closely the health providers and patients have followed the designated course of care. Pharmacy-related process examples could include the provision of discharge counseling, processes for screening of drug interactions and adverse drug events, and processes for performing and assessing dispensing and quality checks.

The *outcome* component of the Donabedian model examines the effect of a health care intervention on patient and populations outcomes. If good structures are in place and good processes followed, then good outcomes should be produced. What outcomes are included in quality assurance or outcomes assessment programs are relative and are based on the goal of each system. Generally broad-based outcomes such as health status or patient satisfaction are considered "end" results. However, if, for example, the goal of a pharmacy program is to implement a focused effort to improve patients' diabetes control by increasing their medication adherence, then instead of a health status "end result," it would be appropriate to evaluate the effectiveness of this program by using an "intermediate" outcome of health such as "percent of patients with diabetes who are in glucose control." It is a relevant outcome for this pharmacy program, but it is not a broader measure of health such as "disease sequelae prevented." In Mrs. Wheeler's case, a goal of improving her %pred FEV_1 would be considered an "intermediate" outcome, but it is important to also consider broader end results such as improved functional status and quality of life outcomes.

Donabedian's structure-process-outcome model of quality of care assessment is useful in charting and measuring the impact of various components of health care delivery; however, emphasis has generally been placed on measuring structure and processes of care variables. Even when outcomes are measured, they tend to be easily collected intermediate outcomes such as objective physiologic or biologic markers, e.g. blood pressure or hemoglobin level. In pharmacy practice, outcomes have focused on improvements in the patient's physiologic biomarkers or improvement of symptoms. In the structure-process-outcome model, individual health professions tend to independently measure narrow profession-related elements rather than recognizing and assessing the interplay among the three components or across professions. A major advantage of an interprofessional PR program is its coordinated and holistic approach designed to impact the global outcome of "health" and its physical, social, and psychological elements. Its outcome assessment system need to be as comprehensive in its evaluation as in its design.

WHAT COULD BE THE COMPONENTS OF A COMPREHENSIVE, PATIENT-CENTERED OUTCOMES ASSESSMENT SYSTEM? THE WILSON-CLEARY MODEL[24]

How can we build a comprehensive, patient-centered outcomes assessment system to measure the effectiveness of drug therapy and other interventions? What type of model could capture the effect of such an intervention and create a reasonable progressive chain linking objective physiologic biomarkers with the objective multidimensional concept of health (physical, social, and psychological) and broader issues of health-related quality of life.

Wilson and Cleary[24] described the connection between biomarkers and health-related quality of life (HRQL) measures as composed of a chain of categories of outcomes, each more holistic and each more representative of overall health and well-being. By incorporating elements of the WHO's conceptualization of health, their five-part causal pathway can be used to explain both the relationships between biomarkers and HRQL measures as well as the effect of intervening variables that mediate these effects. The Wilson-Cleary (W-C) model (Figure 14-2) presents an integrated and comprehensive, patient-centered outcomes measurement system that can be used in three main stages of effectiveness research:

- to *measure initial* patient status at both the individual and group patient level
- to *monitor patient* progress during a treatment regimen to determine the effectiveness of care
- to *aggregate results* across patient populations to be used to *manage future* patients based on the comparative effectiveness of various structures and processes of care and patient characteristics

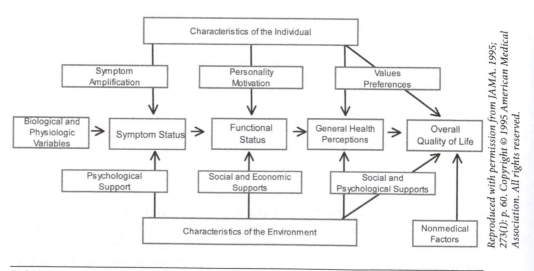

FIGURE 14-2: THE WILSON-CLEARY MODEL[24] OF PATIENT OUTCOMES LINKING CLINICAL VARIABLES TO HEALTH-RELATED QUALITY OF LIFE

The W-C model provides a taxonomy of outcome measures that links the biomedical world of disease causation to the social science world of complex behavior, feelings, and quality of life. As they state:

> *"We present a taxonomy of patient outcomes that categorizes measures of patient outcome according to the underlying health concepts they represent and proposes specific causal relationships between different health concepts, thereby integrating the two models of health described (biomedical and social science). Because our model focuses on relationships among aspects of health, the taxonomy we develop is not necessarily related to other classifications of health status measures. There is a conceptual difference between identifying the dimensions of health that are necessary to comprehensively and validly describe health and specifying a series of critical concepts on a causal pathway...The latter is our goal...It is not possible to create a one-to-one relationship between our levels and existing health-related quality of life measures because our causal model and the numerous existing measures have fundamentally different, though complementary goals."[24]*

In the causal model (Figure 14-2), measures of health are presented as existing on a continuum of increasing biological, social, and psychological complexity. Starting on the left, biomarkers can be measured by such traditional methods as laboratory tests that can be used to assess the functioning of cells, organs, and organ systems. Although there is not a direct relationship between the presence of abnormal biologic change and the presence and intensity of symptoms, some of these biological changes may progress to produce symptoms at the organism level.

Symptoms, the second level, are the patient's perceptions of an abnormal physical, emotional, or cognitive state and often bring the patient to the practitioner. The intensity of the subjective symptoms can be measured by pain scales, dyspnea indexes, and other measures that are specific for the disease symptom. In patient-centered outcomes assessment systems, these symptoms are reported by the patient (patient-reported outcomes or PROs) since it is the patient who experiences the symptoms. Other methods involve the clinician assessing and interpreting the patient's symptoms. These are clinician-reported outcomes and are only proxy measures of direct patient experiences.

The third level of the model is functional status measured by the ability of individuals to perform defined physical, social, psychological, and role tasks. The presence and intensity of symptoms can affect functional ability. For example, severe shortness of breath in individuals with COPD such as Mrs. Wheeler may reduce their ability to walk up stairs, play with their grandchildren, enjoy a good laugh, or continue in their job. The degree of functional decline can be shaped by "influencers" such a person's personality, tolerance for the symptoms, and motivation to perform the task. Also family and social support as well as economic and environmental factors can affect the individual's ability to perform selected functions. In COPD, the impact of shortness of breath on a person's functional status can be lessened if the individual is motivated to maintain function, if economic resources are available to modify the living and working space to prevent overexertion, and if family and coworkers are supportive in maintaining the individual's functional ability and sense of self-worth. Physical function is assessed by such objective measures as activities of daily living (assessing low levels of functioning; e.g., bathing, eating, toileting, continence), instrumental activities of daily living (assessing functioning within the community; e.g., mobility, shopping, cooking), and exercise tolerance tests such as the six-minute walking. Additional objective measures are available to determine social, psychological, and role functioning.

The fourth component assesses the impact of the disease on patients' perceptions of their health. General health perceptions are patient-reported, subjective ratings and are influenced by the cumulative effect and integration of the severity of the condition (as captured by the biomarkers), the intensity of the symptoms, the degree of functional limitation as well as other factors such as mental health. However, all of these factors can be moderated by the values and preferences of the patient as well as the amount of social and psychological support. For example, given two individuals with the same clinical symptoms and functional status, the person who also is a hypochondriac will have a lower subjective health perception than an individual who has a positive outlook on life in general, and health in particular.

The fifth and final component is overall quality of life. This encompasses not only health issues but life as a whole including economic viability, family matters, and spirituality. Following the causal model chain, patients' assessments of their overall quality of life depend on the severity of the physiologic problem, the amount of symptoms, whether the symptoms affect functional status, and patients' perception of their health. However, the overall quality of life also is influenced by three other groups of factors: the patients' values and beliefs, the social and psychological supports needed to help them to continue to function in all aspects of their lives, and nonmedical factors such as economic stability, family relationships, and spirituality. While instruments are available to assess overall quality of life, when evaluating the effectiveness of health care interventions, investigators generally do not assess these non-medical influences but rather use more focused, patient-reported, health-related quality of life (HRQL) measures to evaluate what physical, psychological, and social impact the disease has on patients as well to assess the effectiveness of health care services.

How can we use the W-C model to guide our selection of outcome measures to evaluate the effectiveness of Mrs. Wheeler's PR program? As one moves from left to right in this model, from objective physiological biomarkers to more subjective measures of symptoms, general health perception and quality of life, one moves outward from the cellular level to the individual, and then to the global interaction of the individual in society. A complete evaluation of a clinical intervention should include measures from each link of the causal model. Many measures could be used in each of the five stages. For example, a selection of measures for a comprehensive patient-centered COPD outcomes assessment package could include: % predicted FEV_1 and other pulmonary function tests for physiological biomarkers variables; a dyspnea scale as a symptom measure; six-minute walk as a functional measure; a health perception scale for the fourth phase; and general and disease-specific health status or HRQL measures for the final stage. For a comprehensive treatment of methods to measure Health, consult Ian McDowell's excellent text, *Measuring Health: A Guide to Rating Scales and Questionnaires, 3rd Edition.*[25]

Building on the W-C model, the considerations for selecting individual measures and for designing a comprehensive, patient-centered outcomes assessment program are described in the next section.

BUILDING A PATIENT-CENTERED OUTCOMES ASSESSMENT PROGRAM

What needs to be considered as you develop a patient-centered outcomes assessment program? First, what is the type of information that you need to know when considering the selection of an outcomes measure; i.e., what are the measurement, or psychometric, properties of each instrument? Is it reliable? Valid? Sensitive to change? These types of questions, and others reviewed below, have guided professional organizations,[2-4] governmental agencies,[5] and international consensus panels[26-27] in the development of guidelines for creating and assessing the quality of health-related outcome measures and for selecting measures to include in patient-reported outcomes assessment programs. In the second portion, the W-C model will provide the structure for, and guide the selection of, patient-centered outcome measures to evaluate the effectiveness of Mrs. Wheeler's PR program.

MEASUREMENT PROPERTIES TO CONSIDER IN THE SELECTION OF PATIENT-CENTERED OUTCOME MEASURES

As multidimensional, patient-centered outcomes assessment becomes recognized as an important component of quality of care evaluation, clinicians are beginning to include instruments to measure individual or composite multidimensional health-related factors in patient assessment batteries. However, the quality and administrative feasibility of the measures are quite variable; care must be taken when selecting outcome measures. While excellent measures are available, instruments may appear in the literature or be developed by local institutions that are conceptually incomplete or inadequately evaluated. Consider the following questions as you evaluate any instrument, but particularly multidimensional HRQL measures, for incorporation into a patient-centered, outcomes assessment program. Remember that while you are selecting measures to evaluate the effectiveness of a clinical program (its outcomes), as was mentioned earlier, patients must be evaluated with the selected measures at the beginning to establish a baseline, and at times during, the program. The pre-intervention measurement will capture the patient's baseline status which then serves as the value against which progress and outcome can be compared. A more complete taxonomy of applications of patient-reported outcome measures is summarized in Table 14-1.[28]

TABLE 14-1: A TAXONOMY OF APPLICATION OF PATIENT REPORTED OUTCOMES (PRO) IN PRACTICE[28]

INDIVIDUAL PRO DATA USED AT THE CLINICAL-PATIENT INTERFACE
Screening tools
Measuring tools
Patient-centered care

GROUP PRO DATA USED AT THE CLINICIAN-PATIENT INTERFACE
Decision aids
Facilitating communication among multidisciplinary teams

GROUP PRO DATA AWAY FROM THE CLINICAL-PATIENT INTERFACE
Evaluating the effectiveness of routine care and assessing the quality of care

1. *What is the goal of the assessment?* Before you begin searching for outcome measures, determine what is the goal of the assessment and what concepts or domains you want to assess in your patient population. Do you want a comprehensive assessment of all important elements associated with general health or only aspects of health adversely affected by a specific disease? Do you want to evaluate only physical functioning or do you want a more general and/or disease-specific HRQL measure? Besides the three health domains of physical, social, and psychological functioning, do you want the collection of assessment measures to include an evaluation of pain, wellbeing, or other concepts?

   For Mrs. Wheeler and PR program, you are interested in evaluating the impact the program has on the five components of health as captured in the W-C model. Therefore, a comprehensive assessment strategy should include one or more measures in each category including measures of physical, social, and psychological well-being. Additionally, since some general health status measures may not be sensitive enough to differentiate among levels of disease severity nor detect changes within an individual, disease-specific measures may need to be included.

2. *What is the population for which the instrument was developed?* Some measures have been developed for a general population, while others have been targeted for subpopulations or disease-specific populations. For example, a general population HRQL instrument could be used with geriatric patients, but a HRQL measure developed for a geriatric population should not be used in a general population study. The geriatric measure, while adequate for its intended population, may be limited in the extent of activities assessed by the instrument. You need to match your population to the population for which the instrument was developed.

   In Mrs. Wheeler's case, there are many patient-reported outcome measures developed to assess aspects of HRQL in individuals with pulmonary disease, but some of them have been developed only for use in asthma. Therefore, be sure the instruments you are considering have been validated in a COPD population.

3. *Is it a patient-reported measure?* Outcomes can be reported by clinicians, caregivers, or patients, but studies indicate differences may occur in subjective, and at times objective, valuations when assessed by different sources.[29] A *patient-centered* approach to assessment of health care interventions focuses on aspects of health that patients have identified to be of importance to them. Therefore, when assessing the effectiveness of programs, it is important to incorporate *patient-reported* outcome measures that capture the voice of the patient rather than clinicians or caregivers.

   For example, in Mrs. Wheeler's case, some dyspnea distress measures have been designed to be reported by clinicians. However, from a patient-centered approach, you would prefer to include patient-reported measures of the degree of dyspnea and the impact of that symptom on physical, social, and psychological function.

4. *Is the instrument reliable?* Three types of reliability should be considered: intra-rater reliability, internal reliability, and inter-rater reliability. First, in patient-reported, health-related surveys, this question asks "Would the survey capture the same patient responses if given to the same patient (rater) under the same conditions when the clinical status has not changed?" This measures test-retest or intra-rater reliability and is a measure of consistency of response. Second, in a multi-item, patient-reported survey measuring a specific factor such as "frequency of coughing," do correlations between different items indicate that the factor is measuring the same construct and producing the same scores across patients and across time. Are responses internally consistent —do they have high internal reliability? Third, if an instrument in a comprehensive, patient-centered, outcome assessment program requires a health professional for administration, then inter-rater reliability should be evaluated. For example, health professionals encourage patients to extend maximal excursion in pulmonary function tests and six-minute walks. Are different health professionals better at motivating patients to maximal exertion and does that make a difference in measured outcome? Inter-rater reliability asks the question: "Is the score of the measure reproducible when the test is administered by different staff members to the same patient, under the same conditions and without change in patient status (inter-rater reliability)?

5. *Is the instrument valid? Does the measure accurately assess what it is intended to measure?* For example, if it is a general HRQL measure, does it sample elements from the physical, psychological, and social dimensions that patients have indicated are important for their clinical state (content validity)? If it is a disease-specific health status instrument, have patient-reported health concerns associated with that specific disease been incorporated into the items in the survey (content validity)? Does the instrument discriminate among various levels of health or severity of illness (discriminate validity)? Does the instrument behave in a manner consistent with its theoretical properties (construct validity)? For example, do the patient scores or classification levels on the instrument agree with scores or classification levels of other validated measures covering the same concept (convergent validity, subset of construct validity)? The developer of the instrument you are considering should report this information in journal article and/or a User's Guide.

6. ***Do each of the sections within a multi-dimensional HRQL survey measure a unique concept or domain?*** If a HRQL outcomes measure is assessing multiple domains, such as both physical and psychological functioning, the developer of the survey should provide evidence that each section of the instrument measures a unique concept or domain and that items in one section do not overlap with concepts measured in other domains. Also the questions within a domain should have a higher correlation with that domain's score than those questions have with the scores of other domains. Factor analysis and Eigen values are part of a psychometric battery that generally are published by the developers of the survey. Again, the developer of the instrument you are considering should report this information in journal article and/or a User's Guide.

7. ***What is the expected distribution of scores of your target population with the measurement tool you are considering?*** This question is related to Question #2 above, but it is important enough to have you think about it separately. Will the instrument place your best patient near the top of the scale, but still allow room for improvement? Will the instrument place your worst patient near the bottom of the scale, but still allow detection of further deterioration if that occurs? You want the instrument's score to separate your patients based upon their health status. If you have a relatively healthy group, select a measurement tool that does not group them all near the top of the scale so you can not differentiate among them, nor detect further improvement (ceiling effect). Conversely, if you have a severely ill group, select an instrument does not group them all near the bottom of the scale so you can not differentiate among them, nor detect further deterioration (floor effect).

8. ***Is the scaling system sensitive enough to detect change within your population?*** Is the instrument sensitive enough to detect clinically significant changes across the range of illness severity? Instruments can have fine gradations, course gradations, and everything in between. If you expect large changes within your population, a fast and simple coarse scaled instrument may be adequate. However, if you expect small changes, you need a more sensitive, fine scaled instrument or you will not detect improvement.

9. ***Is the scoring system appropriate for your assessment goal?*** In an assessment of HRQL, do you want to detect change in each of the domains or are you more interested in improvement in an overall HRQL measure? Some instruments such as the SF-36[30-31] identify unique domain scores, and in aggregate, are called profile scores. This allows you to assess burden and track change in each of the eight SF-36 domains. Other instruments, such as the COPD Assessment Tool (CAT,[32-33] an eight-item summary measure of health status in COPD, but not endorsed for use in the United States[34]) yields a single, disease-specific impact summary score. If found to be valid and reliable, the CAT will be useful since it is easier than a longer profile tool for patients to complete and clinicians to score and follow. However, the SF-36 profile provides more information by tracking changes in each of the eight domains, while the CAT summary score only measures overall change. The SF-36 and CAT will be discussed in the Selection of Outcome Measures for Pulmonary Rehabilitation section.

10. ***Is the instrument acceptable to the patient population?*** Will the instrument be easy to understand by the intended patient population? Is it written for an

appropriate reading level? Will patients be comfortable answering the questions contained in the instrument? If it takes too long or is too complicated, this may create too much of a respondent burden for the patient who may refuse to complete it, skip questions within it, or answer indiscriminately. All these issues may create problems in scoring the measure that may invalidate the instrument.

11. ***Is it administratively and economically feasible to use the selected instrument?*** Different assessment measures require different administrative protocols. Some instruments are quite lengthy and require patient interviews administered by trained staff. At the other extreme, some measures can be completed independently by the patient in a short period of time. Also staff must determine the complexity and time required to process and scores the instrument. Therefore, the team must examine all aspects of the administrative burden posed by the instrument and determine if there is an adequate budget and properly trained staff to administer the selected measure.

12. ***Do you want to use an alternative administrative format?*** Most patient surveys were originally developed as self-administered paper-and-pencil questionnaires or as face-to-face interviews. Both methods carry administrative burdens. The paper and pencil method require scoring and the face-to-face method requires staff time. Alternative formats such as computer or smartphone platforms have great potential. They could be programmed to automatically score patient responses, enter results in patient e-records, and trigger clinician notification if results indicate action is needed. But before they are used in patient assessment programs, the equivalency of results from both methods of administration must be established.[35,36] Are the scores generated by a patient using a paper-and-pencil survey the same scores as those from an e-tablet format? Can the original survey format norms be used or are new format-specific norms needed?

Regardless of the administrative method, the developers of the original measure should provide directions for administration, usually in a User's Guide or in a journal publication. These have been developed to standardize the instrument so that results will have a consistent meaning. Staff must follow the instrument-specific directions and not modify in any way the administrative format without equivalency testing. Re-writing or re-phrasing any of the questions for your institutional setting or patient population. May compromise the measure's reliability and validity.

Particularly for an older population such as those with COPD, would the technology associated with an e-format be too intimidating? Or would a patient report symptoms more honestly on an anonymous e-tablet than to a clinician in a face-to-face interview? Does the formatting of the questionnaire on an e-device lead patient to respond differently than if a paper-and-pencil format was used? A review of published studies examining the equivalency between electronic and paper-based patient-reported outcomes indicate that 78% of studies indicate equivalency.[35] However, it is important to check the literature to determine if such a study has been published for your instrument before changing reporting format. Recommendations to establish the equivalency of different administrative methods have been developed by ISPOR's ePRO Good Research Practices Task Force.[36]

MRS. WHEELER, THE WILSON-CLEARY MODEL, AND PATIENT-CENTERED ASSESSMENT OF PULMONARY REHABILITATION

Since for this chapter, you are a member of an interprofessional PR team that will be selecting the outcome assessment measures for Mrs. Wheeler's PR program, a brief introduction to pulmonary rehabilitation is needed. As defined by the 2013 American Thoracic Society/European Respiratory Society Statement on Pulmonary Rehabilitation: Key Concepts and Advances in Pulmonary Rehabilitation, PR is "a comprehensive intervention based on a thorough patient assessment followed by patient tailored therapies that include, but are not limited to, exercise training, education, and behavior change, designed to improve the physical and psychological condition of people with chronic respiratory disease and to promote the long-term adherence to health-enhancing behaviors."[37] Comprehensive PR has been shown to improve physical strength and function and minimize dyspnea symptoms,[38] as well as reduce the burden of anxiety and depression and associated behaviors.[39,40] An interprofessional PR team, built upon and integrating the practice strengths of the professions included in the team, provides coordinated patient-centered care based on the expressed needs of patients such as reduction of physical and psychological symptoms and improvement in exercise tolerance and health-related quality of life.

COPD patients can benefit from PR at any stage in their illness, including during or directly after an exacerbation.[37] While in the hospital, Mrs. Wheeler meets with the PR team and indicates that she is eager to begin an eight-week PR program which will start two weeks after discharge when she is more stable. She expresses her frustration to the team about her shortness of breath which is limiting her physical activities. She says that even if she was strong enough, she won't go to her book or knitting club because she is embarrassed by her coughing and sputum production. But she also says that she misses her friends and would like to do more things with them and her family. To design patient-tailored therapies, the team asks what would be three goals for her PR program, and she replies: 1) to have less attacks of breathlessness (dyspnea) so she wouldn't be afraid to go out of the house, 2) to resume some of functions around the house, and 3) to resume activities with family and friends.

A day before Mrs. Wheeler is scheduled to start her PR program, she returns to the hospital for a battery of patient-centered assessments that will provide baseline data to determine the impact of her illness on each of the stages in the W-C model. Based on this information and her expressed goals, the team designs a patient-centered PR program tailored to Mrs. Wheeler's needs and selects outcomes measures following the Wilson-Cleary stages of physiologic to HRQ progressive impact.

ELEMENTS OF A PATIENT-CENTERED OUTCOMES ASSESSMENT SYSTEM (PRE/POST) FOR MRS. WHEELER

Physiologic Biomarkers: Pulmonary function tests evaluated by spirometry are physiologic biomarkers that indicate the degree of functional lung capacity or the volume of air that the patient can expel from the lungs after maximal inspiration and expiration. The American Thoracic Society (ATS) currently uses % pred FEV_1 as its primary staging metric for the severity of COPD.[41] During her acute episode, her %pred FEV_1 was 42% placing her in Stage 3 or "Severe" (30-50%). With her pneumonia resolved and other medication adjustments made, her %pred FEV_1 is 55%, placing her in Stage 2 or the low end of "Moderate" COPD (50-80%).

However, pulmonary function tests are only weakly correlated with a patient's physical function, mood states, and HRQL—patients with the same % pred FEV_1 can have varying limitations. The ATS acknowledges that using a single test, % pred FEV_1, for COPD staging is a limitation; "A composite picture of disease severity is highly desirable although it is currently unavailable."[42] The Global Initiative for Chronic Obstructive Lung Disease (GOLD) has proposed a multivariable, 4-quadrant COPD staging classification based on a combination of % pred FEV_1, exacerbation history, hospitalization history, and a choice among four different symptom measures.[43] However, the same patient may be placed in different severity categories depending on which of the four symptom measure is chosen.[44,45] The W-C model suggests that this problem (the inter-measure reliability of the GOLD classification strategy) could be associated with the effects of individual differences in personality and motivation that could be captured by different symptom measures. By basing your patient-centered outcomes assessment on the multiple stages of the Wilson-Cleary model, rather than on only a pulmonary function severity staging criteria, you will capture more of how the individual patient is affected by the condition.

THE LEARNING TIP

More than a biomarker is needed for patient-centered care.

Symptoms: Pathologic shortness of breath termed dyspnea is the most characteristic symptom of COPD, and one of the most troubling. As in Mrs. Wheeler's case, it is often the major factor forcing people to withdraw from the workplace and then further limiting their ability to function on a day-to-day basis. The fear of dyspnea leads individuals to avoid activities that could evoke breathlessness and contributes to their deepening physical limitations. It has long been known that the presence and magnitude of dyspnea is a subjective perception of each patient, affected by many physiologic and psychological factors such as degree of respiratory impairment, use of accessory muscles of respiration, and anxiety.[46,47] By quantifying the degree of dyspnea, the PR team can assess its baseline severity, develop treatment plans, and then evaluate the effectiveness of the program at discharge.

However, the severity of the symptom of functional dyspnea is influenced by many factors: What is the level of baseline functional impairment? What is the magnitude of the task that creates the dyspnea? What is the magnitude of the effort that the individual exerts to achieve the task? For example, if an individual with mild functional impairment slowly climbs stairs, dyspnea may not develop, but if the person has to rush and exert more effort for the same number of stairs, breathlessness occurs. While methods to standardize the assessment of dyspnea need further development,[48] the ATS statement on advances in pulmonary rehabilitation[37] lists eight dyspnea measures that are valid, reliable, and responsive to change that have been used in PR programs. One of the oldest and most widely used is the Medical Research Council (MRC) dyspnea scale,[49-51] a short patient-reported measure of perceived breathlessness given five levels of situational exertion. At her pre-PR testing session, Mrs. Wheeler's reports the highest level of dyspnea on this scale: "I am too breathless to leave the house or I am breathless when dressing."

Mrs. Wheeler has indicated that her bothersome symptoms include more than dyspnea. Heavy coughing and sputum production have made her too embarrassed to go to her book and bridge clubs, limiting her social functioning. Is there an outcome measure that can capture the intensity of all three of these symptoms, so common in many COPD patients, at baseline and then assess the improvement as a result of a pharmaceutical product or other therapeutic agent?

For pharmacists, this is a particularly interesting question. Many pulmonary medications for COPD are designed to reduce one or more of these three symptoms. But what patient-reported measure is valid and reliable, simple to administer and interpret, and sensitive to change? Not only are these questions of concern to the pharmacist and other members of the PR team, but they have occurred earlier to individuals involved in the drug development and FDA approval process for COPD medications. How can a pharmaceutical company justify to the FDA that a new pulmonary drug can reduce one or more of the three symptoms? What are the FDA's expectations for the characteristics of nonbiomarkers used to evaluate the efficacy of a new drug product? While clinical drug trials include biomarkers as efficacy measures, what measures can be used to evaluate improvements in patient-reported COPD symptoms?

Now begins an illustrative story of how the science of patient-reported/patient-centered outcomes measurement recently has been improved by the intersection of related interests among pharmaceutical companies, the drug regulators at FDA's Center for Drug Evaluation and Research (CDER), developers of patient-centered/patient-reported outcomes assessment measures, clinicians, and patients, in general but also specifically in COPD. In 2009, partially in response to growing concern about over-reaching quality of life claims and other poorly substantiated claims that were appearing in drug product advertisements, the FDA issued *Guidance for Industry. Patient-Reported Outcome Measures: Use in Medical Product Development to Support Labeling Claims*,[5] a document detailing standards that the FDA would apply to approval of drug product claims.[5] The Guidance stated "quality of life…is too general and undefined to be considered appropriate for a medical product claim,"[5] e.g., drug claim. It provided guidelines for PRO measure development; many of these quality concepts for outcomes measures were summarized in the 12 questions posed earlier in the chapter. In addition, the Guidance emphasized that the patient voice be included in measurement development so that the impact of the disease as *perceived by the patient* is included in the outcomes measure. For a product claim to state that a drug produced more than a biomarker treatment benefit, the FDA Guidance detailed that the effect must be documented by outcome measures that are reliable, valid and that especially include patient involvement during measurement development process.

However previous measures that have been used to evaluate COPD respiratory symptoms have not involved patients either to identify what they think should be measured about their symptoms nor to generate items that could be used to measure that concept. Up to this time, the collective impact of severe COPD symptoms has been estimated from financial charges associated with exacerbation care (e.g., hospitalization, ER visits, unscheduled clinic visits, additional medication) over a specified period. When patients were interviewed, their direct report of frequency of exacerbations had little correlation with the charge-based estimate with as many as 50–70% of the direct reported exacerbations being undetected by indirect means.[51]

Seeing a need for improvement, a consortium of experts in pulmonary medicine, clinical research, drug development regulatory issues, and instrument development was formed to develop a single, standardized instrument for evaluating the effects of treatment on acute exacerbations of COPD. The "concept"[1] to be measured was "acute exacerbation." This broad-based international effort, funded by unrestricted grants from four pharmaceutical companies, was called the EXAcerbations of Chronic pulmonary disease tool (EXACT)—Patient-Reported Outcome Initiative and the measurement tool it was developing was EXACT-PRO. It was the first consortium convened to develop a PRO instrument for use in medical product development trials and is the first such instrument, along with its later derivative measure, the EXACT-Respiratory Symptoms (E-RS:COPD), to undergo qualification review by the FDA."[52]

The coalition built its measurement tool around the concept of "exacerbations" and followed the principles of the FDA PRO guidance:[5] i) involved COPD patients with a history of exacerbations in focus groups to describe exacerbation attributes, care-seeking cues, and indication of progression and recovery,[53] ii) identified symptom items,[53] iii) conducted robust psychometric testing on a 23 symptom item prototype, yielding a 14 item instrument with three domains (breathlessness, cough and sputum, and chest symptoms),[54] iv) established validity, reliability, and sensitivity to change,[55] and v) prospectively evaluated its psychometric properties in three drug trials.[56] Based on conceptualization of "exacerbations," quality of evaluation design, and resultant characteristics of the EXACT-PRO measure, in 2014 the FDA gave its first qualification[2] to the EXACT-PRO.[58]

But more than accurate measurement of exacerbations are important to COPD management; the frequency and intensity of respiratory symptoms are also important to patients and clinicians. The consortium continued its work "to advance the science of chronic obstructive pulmonary disease through improved measurement methods."[52] Recognizing the need for a standardized instrument to assess the concept of "respiratory symptom" in stable COPD patients, the consortium created the EXACT-Respiratory Symptom (E-RS) from utilizing the 11 symptom questions, derived during

---

[1] Concept is defined by the FDA as "the specific measurement goal (i.e. the thing that is being measured by a PRO instrument). In clinical trials, a PRO instrument can be used to measure the effect of a medical intervention on one or more concepts. PRO concepts represent aspects of how patients function or feel related to a health condition or its treatment)[5]

[2] Qualification is a conclusion that within the stated context of use, the drug development tool can be relied on to have a specific interpretation and application in drug development and regulatory review[57]

development of the full 14-item EXACT-PRO.[52] Since "respiratory symptoms" was a different concept being measured, the development and documentation process was repeated. Qualitative input was derived from focus groups, this time with stable COPD patients who had no history of exacerbations over the previous 12 months.[59] Quantitative psychometric analyses were again conducted[60] incorporating principles of the FDA 2009 guidance document.[5] Data analysis supported the validity of the E-RS total score, evaluating respiratory symptoms overall, as well as scores for 3 domains: breathlessness (5 items), cough and sputum (3 items), and chest symptoms (3 items). In three prospective clinical trials, the total E-RS and domain scores correlated well with appropriate comparative measures.[60] In 2016 the FDA recognized the E-RS[61] as the second PRO instrument to receive its qualification under the PRO guidance. During the instrument FDA approval process, at the request of the FDA, the tool was retitled to Evaluating Respiratory Symptoms in COPD or E-RS:COPD to indicate that the measure was designed to assess respiratory symptoms specifically in COPD.

For both EXACT-PRO and E-RS:COPD, the patient answers the 14 or 11 items respectively each night using an e-dairy. The process takes an average of three minutes. While originally designed for use in drug trials, the E-RS:COPD would be an ideal PRO tool to use to follow COPD patients in PR programs as well as natural history studies.[60]

There is a reason the EXACT-PRO and E-RS:COPD development processes have been described in such detail—this process is likely to be the developmental path for future valid, reliable, and increasingly e-technology-based PRO measures, especially if the intent is to document the effect of new drugs on patient-reported symptom improvement. New, shorter, more precise and efficient measures that can utilize e-technology data collection and analysis may soon be the norm.

Let's step back from Mrs. Wheeler's COPD case and consider the broader implications of the 2009 FDA Guidance for the drug development process and also the practice of pharmacy. First, while the 2009 FDA Guidance targeted the need to improve PRO measures to support labeling claims, the document also discussed considerations about the selection of PROs to be included in the design of clinical drug trials. The implication was clear and signaled a paradigm shift. Broad statements about quality of life would no longer be acceptable. If more than biomarker claims were to be made, they now needed to be based on better PRO measures—measures developed with patient input, measures based on clearer conceptualization of the measurement goal, and measures that were psychometrically sound. If a PRO claim is desired at product launch, a pharmaceutical company needs to anticipate the drug's potential treatment benefit and associated product claims and incorporate FDA qualified outcomes measures throughout the drug development process.

But in prior drug submissions, individual pharmaceutical companies had approached the FDA with data from its own outcome measure (drug development tool-DDT) developed for its own product. In the 2014 *FDA Guidance for Industry and FDA Staff: Qualification Process for Drug Development Tools (DDT)*,[57] the FDA commented on this practice:

> *In the past, DDT acceptance in the drug development and regulation process was initiated on a sponsor- and drug-specific basis. Sponsors seeking to use a specific DDT typically developed only enough data to support its use in a specific case. Use in a different clinical setting or with other drugs would generally be left undetermined. Other drug sponsors or other parties would have little ability to build on that knowledge to expand the tool's use to additional settings.[57]*

What is ground-breaking about the EXACT-PRO Initiative is that four pharmaceutical companies agreed to collectively supported the effort. Pulmonary medicine clinicians, instrument development experts, and the pharmaceutical industry recognized that they all would benefit from their collaborative approach. The execution of the consortium's PRO measure design protocol has resulted in the success of EXACT-PRO[58] and E-RS:COPD[61] as the first two FDA approved qualified PRO measures to be used in drug development and, if appropriate, drug product claims. The consortium's goal was "to advance the science of chronic obstructive pulmonary disease through improved measurement methods."[52] The award of FDA qualification for their two PRO measures has met that goal assuring that they produce analytically valid measurements that can be relied on to have a specific use and interpretable meaning. Having a qualified PRO measure available to pharmaceutical companies "will help advance therapy development and evaluation in multiple cases and can more widely benefit patients."[57]

For pharmacists, there are two important implications of FDA PRO qualifications for clinical practice. First, a FDA qualified PRO provides a standardized measure that can be used as a common measure across clinical drug trials to evaluate the same concept/symptom. This means that a pharmacist or even a formulary committee can conduct a direct comparative effectiveness of different drugs using a common PRO. This makes it less likely that a pharmacist will have to interpolate the equivalency of different results based on different outcome measures. Second, a qualified PRO measure will be useful in the management and monitoring of individual response to medication regimens and other intervention programs. In Mrs. Wheeler's case, the pharmacist and PR team can feel confident that using the E-RS:COPD e-diary during the PR process will provide an accurate and reliable patient-centered and patient-reported measure to assess the impact of the respiratory symptoms that are a concern to her—breathlessness and coughing/sputum production as well as chest symptoms and combined (total) respiratory symptoms. She completes the 11-item e-tablet E-RS:COPD survey at baseline and then nightly during the PR program.

Functional status: Functional status refers to the ability to perform basic physical, social, and psychological activities needed for daily life. As pharmacists maximize the therapeutic benefit of medications, physical and occupational therapists concentrate on improving an individual's abilities to perform activities of daily living. While functional status is multidimensional, the most common outcome measure for this stage is generally a *physical* function measure—the six-minute walk or the distance an individual can walk in six minutes—is the tool used to assess this step. It is a simple, inexpensive, and safe "low-tech" method to measure one aspect of function and has three major advantages: 1) it does not require equipment, 2) it is a normal functional activity that corresponds more directly to the demands of everyday living, and 3) the patient can control the pace of the exercise.

With any type of measure, there are possibilities of errors that can occur in the measurement process.[62] The six-minute walk is a good example to illustrate this problem. Both systematic and random errors can reduce the accuracy and reliability of the walking test. Systematic errors occur consistently each time the test is performed and affect the accuracy of the test. Examples of this type of error are an incorrectly measured walking corridor distance creating inaccurately calculated distances or an incorrectly calibrated timing device resulting in a longer or shorter walk time than the desired period. The six-minute walking test also has sources of random error and variation that must be controlled to improve the reliability of patient results. For example, the use of encouragement during the walking test influences the distance covered by the subject. After an initial six-minute walk, patients were randomized to receive or not receive standardized encouragement during five additional walking tests. While the baseline walking distances were similar in both groups in the initial test, the group that received encouragement averaged 31.5 meters or nearly 8% further.[63] This example illustrates the need for standardized procedures used in a consistent manner during pre-and post-intervention assessment.

At baseline, Mrs. Wheeler's was able to walk 700 feet in an accurately measured corridor without encouragement during her six-minute walk. By comparison, a longitudinal sample of COPD patients averaged 1140 feet with a range of 480-1800 feet.[63] To accurately assess the impact of the PR program on her six-minute distance, at the completion of the program, the test should be conducted on the same corridor, again without encouragement.

But there are more than problems with walking that are affecting Mrs. Wheeler's ability to function in her daily life. She is not alone; up to one-third of COPD patients do not describe walking as an important goal in PR.[64] Individuals vary in their desired personal achievement goals, and while improvement in walking is desirable, Mrs. Wheeler is anxious that increased physical activity will trigger a dyspnea attack that will only make her more depressed. The team is concerned that her anxiety and depression will adversely affect her motivation to succeed and that may affect the outcome of the PR effort37. The team realizes that it will need to tailor specific psychological support to her unique needs and help her develop self-efficacy strategies.[65] It selects the Hospital Anxiety and Depression,[66,67] a 14-item self-completed scale, to assess her baseline psychological function.

THE LEARNING TIP

Assessment of function involves more than physical function. All forms of measurement must be standardized to achieve reproducible results.

General Health Perceptions: In the W-C model, the stage of general health perceptions represents a transitional state between functional status and health-related quality of life. Surveys measuring this stage capture patient-reported subjective assessments of a person's feeling and beliefs about their overall health, and thus, are not related to any one specific component of health. The concept of health perceptions fits well with the Health Belief Model of health behavior described in Chapter XX of this book. General health perceptions assessments have been known to be good predictors of future use of health care services[68] and even morbidity and mortality.[69] Many surveys have been designed to measure this subjective concept;[25] however, recent patient-reported outcome studies are more likely to evaluate it using the multi-dimensional SF-36v2™ Health Survey[70] which includes a five items of the General Health Perception scale within its 36-item, 8-scale instrument. The SF-36v2® will be described in the Overall Quality of Life: General (Generic) Health-Related Quality of Life section below.

THE LEARNING TIP

This is a transition stage in the W-C model and is more likely to be assessed in the HRQL stage.

Overall Quality of Life: The last stage of the W-C model is meant to summarize the progressive linkage across the previous stages by an overall, patient-reported, subjective assessment of health and well-being. However, there is concern that the use of the phrase "quality of life" is too broad a term; even the original 1990 Wilson-Cleary article stated that a review of this phrase was "beyond the scope of this article."[24] As you learned earlier in this chapter, the FDA directed attention to this controversy with its 2009 FDA Guidance[5] and its attempt to limit overreaching and unsubstantiated quality of life claims appearing in drug product labeling. In the 2009 FDA Guidance's "Index of Terms," *quality of life* is defined as:

> *Quality of life*—A general concept that implies an evaluation of the effect of all aspects of life on general well-being. Because this term implies the evaluation of nonhealth-related aspects of life, and because the term generally is accepted to mean *what the patient thinks it is*, it is too general and undefined to be considered appropriate for a medical product claim.[5]

The FDA also views a more limited *health-related quality of life* concept, limited to the three domains of the WHO's definition of health[18] (i.e., physical, social, and psychological), to be problematic and implies a restriction in its use in drug product claims. The FDA 2009 Guidance definition for this concept is:

> *Health-related quality of life (HRQL)*—HRQL is a multidomain concept that represents the patient's general perception of the effect of illness and treatment on physical, psychological, and social aspects of life. Claiming a statistical and meaningful improvement in HRQL implies: (1) that all HRQL domains that are important to interpreting change in how the clinical trial's population feels or functions as a result of the targeted disease and its treatment were measured; (2) that a general improvement was demonstrated; and (3) that no decrement was demonstrated in any domain.[5]

As a result of these FDA definitions and their direct impact on drug claims and indirect effects on types of measures used in drug development and clinical trials, it is unlikely that you will find pharmaceutical literature describing the effect of a new drug on the quality of life or HRQL of COPD patients. However, you as a pharmacist and a member of a PR team will find these terms used in the pulmonary rehabilitation literature to evaluate the effectiveness of PR programs. Both the 2013 ATS/ERS *Statement on Key Concepts and Advances in Pulmonary Rehabilitation*[37] and the 2015 Cochrane Collaborative meta-analysis of 65 randomized control trials of pulmonary rehabilitation[71] conclude that PR is beneficial in improving the **quality of life**[37] and **health-related quality of life**[71] of COPD patients. The Cochrane meta-analysis even concluded that "we believe that health-related quality of life should be considered the primary outcome in pulmonary rehabilitation."[71] Additionally, a 2015 systematic review of 70 Canadian studies[72] concluded that treating COPD improved **quality of life**. As an interprofessional team member, in order that the collective team can interpret the measures and evaluate the effectiveness of Mrs. Wheeler's PR program, it is important for you as the pharmacist to know about major PRO such as HRQL measures that are used by other health professions.

Although the FDA drug approval policies focus primarily on objective biomarkers and PRO symptom indicators, studies indicate that these measures may not be sensitive enough to detect changes in important functional, psychological, and social aspects of COPD that can occur as a result of an intervention.[37,72] Also, as was mentioned earlier in this chapter, within the same level of pulmonary function, patients may show considerable variation in impact of COPD on their daily functional activities, psychological status, and social interactions. That's why COPD was selected as the example to illustrate the need for a comprehensive, integrated outcomes assessment system. COPD is more than poor pulmonary function—it affects all aspects of health, but to different degrees for different people. Therefore, to differentiate among the varying impacts of COPD on different patients and to assess changes in the various W-C stages associated with a PR program, the team should incorporate patient-reported multidimensional health-quality of life measures to establish baseline status at the beginning of the PR program and at the end to assess the program's impact.

Health-Related Quality of Life Measures: Health-related quality of life (HRQL), also called more conservatively called health status, measures that capture disease impact over multiple domains will be used to illustrate the health-related quality of life stage in the W-C model. Again, they frequently contain subjective patient-reported items related to physical, social, and psychological health that are the target of health care interventions. Health status measures typically exclude economic, religious, work, and/or family factors.

Valid, reliable, and responsive HRQL measures include three important characteristics. The measures i) assess multiple dimensions of health; e.g., physical, mental/psychological, and social; ii) are a patient-centered form of assessment and are intended to measure the effect of the clinical condition on the patient as perceived and reported by the patient, not a health care provider or a relative of the patient, and iii) provide a standardized method of patient assessment that can be used by different health professionals in different patient populations at different times. These multidimensional, patient-centered, standardized HRQL measures offer new opportunities for more comprehensive patient assessments. For pharmacists, they provide a means to move beyond the traditional professionally grounded assessments of biomarkers and now incorporate the patient's individual perception (as influenced by the patient's values, beliefs, and expectations) of the impact of the disease on the physical, social, and psychological aspects of health, design an intervention, and then measure the effect of an intervention on HRQL.

These multidimensional HRQL measures can be designed to assess health *in general* or focus on the *disease-specific* consequences of a specific condition; e.g., how the clinical aspects of COPD have affected the HRQL of an individual. Because *general* (also called generic) HRQL measures can be used across all clinical conditions, they enable clinicians and policy makers to determine the relative impact of different disease states and treatment options on patient populations and resource allocation. On the other hand, *disease-specific* HRQL measures focus on those aspects of health that are most affected by characteristics of a specific clinical condition such as COPD, arthritis, cancer, or diabetes. Generally, *disease-specific* HRQL measures are more sensitive in detecting small changes in the disease's manifestations and the resultant impact on HRQL. However, by focusing only on the disease's features, the disease-specific HRQL may not detect other aspects of the patient's health that are undergoing change. Therefore, both types are frequently useful in a comprehensive outcomes assessment system to evaluate patient status and to measure the effectiveness of clinical interventions.

As examples of HRQL surveys that are patient-centered as well as patient-reported, one general HRQL (SF-36v2® Health Survey) and two disease-specific (Chronic Respiratory Questionnaire and the St. George's Respiratory Questionnaire) will be described. While clearly labeled domains of "physical," "social," and "psychological" are not present in these three, the comprehensive concept of "health" was included in the development of each.

GENERAL (GENERIC) HEALTH-RELATED QUALITY OF LIFE

The SF-36v2® Health Survey is the current version of the most widely used patient-centered, patient-reported, multidimensional assessment of health. Originally constructed in 1990 to survey health status, it was "designed for use in clinical practice and research, health policy evaluations, and general population surveys."[73] Its use has grown rapidly. It is brief (36 items), easy to take (5-10 minutes), patient-reported, and covers major domains of health making it ideal for use in general population as well as disease-specific assessments. As of March 2016, the SF-36 has been included in over 15,000 articles indexed in PubMed including 275 COPD publications. Optum®, a health technology/infrastructure company, presently holds the license for use of SF-36v2® Health Survey as well as two shorter versions—the 12-item SF-12v2® and the 8-item SF-8™. Optum® reports that thru early 2016 over 32,000 licenses have been issued for SF Health Surveys resulting in more than 14,000,000 surveys taken.[74] It is currently available in more than 170 translations.

Given its wide use, some background on the evolution of the SF-36v2® would be beneficial. In the 1980s, a comprehensive outcomes assessment was needed for the Medical Outcome Study (MOS), a multi-city research project to determine how different health systems and medical specialties (structure of care) and technical style and expenditures (processes of care) affected the health outcomes of patients with four chronic conditions (hypertension, diabetes, congestive heart failure, and recent myocardial infarction).[75,77] To monitor patient status over the 4-year MOS study, initially a comprehensive, but bulky, multidimensional, patient-reported MOS assessment package was created consisting of 40 physical and mental health concepts totaling 245 questions.[76] Not only did the MOS study provide valuable information about associations between structure and process characteristics and patient outcomes, but it also demonstrated that a self-reported patients' perspective concerning their health and satisfaction with care could be validly and reliably measured.

To enable health status measures to be used more widely, the length of the original MOS battery had to be shortened to reduce patient response burden and administrative complexity. Investigators created a conceptual framework to reduce the number of MOS health concepts and items by retaining the health concepts most frequently included in widely-used health surveys (physical, social and role functioning, mental health, general health perceptions), while modifying two concepts (splitting role function from both physical and mental concepts), and adding two concepts suggested by MOS data (pain and vitality).[73] Collectively the eight domains contain 35 items summarized in Table 14-2, plus an additional item asking patients to compare their present health to that of one year earlier.

TABLE 14-2: THE SF-36: PHYSICAL AND MENTAL COMPONENT SUMMARIES, 8 SCALES AND 35 ITEMS

PHYSICAL COMPONENT SUMMARY ITEMS
Limitations in physical functioning due to health (10 items)
Limitations in usual role activities due to physical health problems (4 items)
Bodily pain (2 items)
General health perceptions (5 items)

MENTAL COMPONENT SUMMARY ITEMS
Vitality (energy/fatigue) (4 items)
Limitations in usual social activities due to physical health (2 items)
Limitations in usual role activities due to personal or emotional problems (3 items)
General mental health (psychological distress and psychological well-being) (5 Items)

This design produced a shorter instrument that can discriminate among various levels of health and detect changes in health status over time. The result was a 36-item comprehensive, multidimensional representation of a full range of health states[77] with established validity,[78] internal consistency,[79] reliability,[79] and internal consistency checks.[78] Patients are asked to reflect on their health over the past four weeks when responding to the items. For scoring, the eight scales can be scored individually or aggregated into two summary measures: the physical component summary (PCS) and mental component summary (MCS).[80] Scoring for this first version of the SF-36® produces a profile of eight scale scores, reported as 0–100% for each with a higher score indicating a better health state. The two summary components, the primary placement of the eight scales between the summary components, and the number of question items in each scale, are listed in Table 14-2.

After 10 years of use, the SF-36 team made improvements to the SF-36® with revisions providing simpler layout for items and responses, changes in item wording to reduce colloquialisms and facilitate more straightforward translations, and expansion of levels of item responses. In the new SF-36v2®, the number of items, number and types of health domain scales, number and types of health component summaries remained the same.[81] The SF-36v2® represents an improved measurement tool that maintains comparability with the original version in terms of purpose and the psychometric rigor with which it was developed.[82] The revision also increased reliability and validity of scores and made the survey easier to read and understand.[82]

However, a major change occurred between how scales between the SF-36® and the new SF-36v2® are scored. Rather than the 0–100% scoring system used in the SF-36®, the new SF-36v2® uses a norm-based scoring algorithms for all of the 8 scales, transforming each patient's scale score to compare it to the population norm defined as a mean of 50 with a standard deviation of 10. A large sample of the US population was used to establish the population norm. Now using the SF-36v2® scoring algorithm, a patient's scores can be directly compared to a population mean. For example, using the SF-36v2® scoring system, a "social functioning" scale score of 40 means that this patient's is one standard deviation below the overall population mean of 50 for that scale. This survey provides a common metric that enables clinicians to compare the impact of disease for patients within a disease such as COPD, across other disease states, as well as the general population. When reading literature studies using a SF-36 measure, it is critical that you determine which version—the SF-36® or the SF-36v2®—was used in order to correctly interpret the results.

The SF-36 has become a family of surveys. In addition to the SF-36® Health Survey and SF-36v2® Health Survey, items from the SF-36v2® have been extracted to create a version with 12 items, the SF-12v2® Health Survey, and eight items, the SF-8™ Health Survey. Since the same scoring algorithm may be used for all SF-36 surveys, results from the physical and mental components can be roughly compared across all SF-36 surveys. The tradeoff in using the three versions of the Sf-36 surveys is a balance of respondent burden (36 items take more time than 12 or 8 items) and the precision of the scores (36 items creates more precision than 12 or 8 items).

The SF-36 is widely used in various settings including clinical trials, managed care organizations to monitor quality of care, and interventions and monitoring of chronic disease progression. Three recent studies illustrate the varied use of the SF-36 in COPD: :i) a comparison of functional capacity, biomarkers, and health status using the SF-36 in COPD[82] ; ii) comparative effectiveness of PR in pulmonary fibrosis and emphysema compared to COPD using the MRC dyspnea tool, six-minute walk, and SF-36;[83] and iii) evaluation of effectiveness of a home-based PR program as measured by walking test, hospital anxiety and depression scale, SF-36, and the chronic respiratory disease questionnaire (CRQ), a disease-specific health status survey described in the next section.[84]

Contact www.optum.com/optum-outcomes/what-we-do/health-surveys.html for information on the use of any of the surveys in the SF-36™ family and for the SF-36™ User's Manual.

DISEASE-SPECIFIC HEALTH-RELATED QUALITY OF LIFE (HRQL) MEASURES

Disease-specific HRQL measures are by definition measures that focus on the impact of the symptoms and limitations of a *specific disease* such as COPD, arthritis, cancer, or diabetes on the patient's perception of HRQL. The same general health concepts of physical, social, and psychological health underline the structure of both types of measures; however, within each health concept, the disease-specific survey items collect finer details related to the specific disease. Because of that focus, they are likely to be more sensitive to changes that are disease-specific than more general HRQL measures; they are not intended for comparisons across clinical conditions. As with the SF-36v2™, disease-specific HRQL survey results are generally reported as profile scores so that changes within each domain can be followed separately. When disease-specific surveys are given before and after an intervention, because of their disease-specific items, they are more likely to detect changes associated with the clinical trial. This was confirmed in an analysis of 43 randomized clinical trials in which disease-specific surveys were better able to detected HRQL changes associated with interventions than broader generic health measures.[85]

Three respiratory disease-specific health status instruments are described below. The first two are structured to generate domain and total scores profiles, while the third provides a summary score.

Chronic Respiratory Disease Questionnaire (CRQ)[86–91] Originally developed in 1987 as an interviewer-led (IL) questionnaire,[86] the 20-item CRQ-IL conceptualizes HRQL in respiratory disease as consisting of four domains of disease impact: dyspnea (5 items), fatigue (4 items), mastery of how well a patient feels control over the condition (4 items), and emotional functioning (7 items). These are reported as five separate scores—four domains and summary scores. In the original CRQ-IL methodology, a *patient-specific* dyspnea score is created when the interviewer asks each patient to self-identify five activities, important to each, that create shortness of breath and to quantify the degree of dyspnea associated with each activity. On average, this process requires 20–30 minutes of staff time for each administration. The patient-centered CRQ-IL approach enables a rehabilitation program to customize interventions that can be designed to improve the patient's ability to perform, and reduce the associated frequency and intensity of dyspnea with, each activity that was identified by the patient to be of importance. For the other three CRQ-IL domains, the interviewer asks patients standardized questions. While the CRQ-IL directly captures the patient's goal for PR interventions, this individualization of the dyspnea domain creates two problems: i) it is labor intensive by involving an interviewer to obtain responses from patients and ii) the individualized activities identified by patients are not the same for each patient; therefore, the same dyspnea domain score may not represent that same level of dyspnea impact across patients. While the pre-post PR dyspnea domain score may convey meaningful information to evaluate individual improvement, when conducting overall PR program effectiveness studies, aggregating patients' dyspnea scores across the program will result in imprecise and unstable measurement because the dyspnea items were not standardized. Now evaluation of overall PR treatment effectiveness is compromised due to poor properties, limiting comparisons across settings.

Revisions ensued. It is important to realize that multiple versions of the same parent survey may exist in the literature. One needs to be knowledgeable about what version of an outcome measurement you are considering and whether there is a more accurate, precise, and reproducible revision available. To illustrate: Initially, the CRQ survey was changed to a patient self-report, rather than the original interviewer-led format. For the first section, patients made a list of all activities that caused them breathless, selected the top five that were most important to them, and then indicated the relative intensity and importance of those five.[87] This created a reliable and stable self-reported survey (CRQ-SR)[88] that was sensitive to change,[89] but like the original CRQ-IL, it was not standardized since it was likely that every patient had a unique set of activities within the dyspnea scale. Next a second revision created a standardized, pre-determined set of items for the dyspnea domain. These developers reviewed activities that previous patients indicated had most frequently caused shortness of breath.[90] The top five activities from the broader population sample were converted into five standardized dyspnea items, while retaining the format of the other 15 CRQ items from the remaining three domains. Since patient-specific dyspnea issues were no longer identified, this version of the CRQ, entitled the CRQ-SA (CRQ self-administrated, with the standardized dyspnea items produces a narrower distribution of score compared to the individualized one.[90] Psychometric evaluation indicates that the CRQ-SA standardized 20-item survey is valid,[90] reliable,[90] stable,[90] and sensitive to change.[91] The patient-centeredness of self-identification of dyspnea concerns in the CRQ-IA and CRQ-SR has been traded for direct patient-reported information collected with a standardized CRQ-SA survey instrument. (Note: Unfortunately in the psychometric evolution of the CRQ, the two versions have different names/abbreviations. Self-reporting with individualized dyspnea items is the CRQ-SR[75-77] while the self-administered version with standardized dyspnea items is the CRQ-SA.[90-91])

Either CRQ can be used to structure the initial assessment of a COPD patient, to elicit patient-identified (individualized by the CRQ-IA/SR, group identified by CRQ-SA) degree of impact and rehabilitation goals, and then to measure the patient's progress and outcomes of the rehabilitation process over time. Now there is a choice —will you select the individualized method or the standardized method? A pharmacist will encounter such choices throughout practice. For example, will your hospital pharmacy department offer a support group for patients with diabetes or will individualized counseling be available for all? In the PR program, will the team provide individualized interventions that meet the specific functional needs of each patient or will a standardized PR program be followed. It's the same trade-off. Can a program be standardized and more time efficient while still meeting individualized patient needs? The answer lies within the themes of this chapter – conduct comparative effectiveness assessments of both approaches based on objective biomarkers and patient-centered outcomes measures that are valid, reliable, and perceived to be meaningful by the patient.

St. George's Respiratory Questionnaire for COPD Patients (SGRQ-C)[92-95] The other popular disease-specific HRQL instruments for COPD is the St. George's Respiratory Questionnaire (SGRQ), a self-administered survey taking approximately 8–10 minutes to complete. Developed in 1992 by the respiratory medicine department at St. George's Hospital in London, the SGRQ is a standardized, self-administered, health status instrument that was originally designed to measure the impact of both COPD and asthma on health impairment.[92] A 2007 re-analysis of the structure of the original SGRQ resulted in a COPD-specific instrument, the SGRQ-C,[93] consisting of 40 items in three components and organized into two parts: Part 1—Symptoms (patient perceptions of their recent COPD respiratory problems) and Part 2—Activity (disturbance of daily physical activity associated with shortness of breath) and Impact (disturbances of social and emotional functions). The items are weighted and require a manual or electronic method to convert individual items to component scores; an Excel-based scoring system is available.

Scores are available for each of the three components as well as a total score. As a result, the SGRQ-C can measure the impact of COPD on overall health, daily life, and perceived well-being. The instrument has good reliability and validity;[92] a minimally important difference of 4 units is associated with clinical improvement.[94] It has been used in over 200 published pulmonary rehabilitation studies as of March 2016 and has been translated into 77 languages, including an American English translation[95] of the original British version. The SGRQ-C Manual[96] contains additional information, including SGRQ scores in healthy subjects for comparative purposes.

COPD Assessment Test (CAT): As you can see, earlier health status measures have evolved to include patient-reported formats with fewer and more precise items. However the three health profiles discussed above maintained their original domain structure and still include 20–40 items resulting in a profile of scores for each of the domains/components.

But if one wanted to standardize the diagnosis and management of COPD, won't a shorter patient-reported, overall unified-score survey be helpful? That is the driving force behind the development of the short, 8-item COPD Assessment Test or CAT,[32] an effort affiliated with the Global Initiative for Chronic Obstructive Lung Disease (GOLD)[43] collaboration. Published in 2009, the CAT was developed with patient and clinician input to provide "a simple and reliable measure of health status in COPD and assist patients and the physicians in quantifying the impact of COPD on the patient's health."[33] Unlike earlier health profiles when each domain contains multiple items and generates its own score, the CAT consists of eight items, each intended to capture the characteristic or impact on a single feature of COPD (e.g., cough, sleep, limitations in activities at home, breathless in walking up a flight of stairs). Each of the eight questions has five levels, with the summary CAT score ranging from "8," no impact, to "40," most impact. The CAT has been reported to have good reproducibility,[32] to correlate well with the SGRQ,[32,97] to distinguish among patients with different degree of COPD severity,[97] and to be responsive,[98,99] and as responsive as more complex COPD health status measures,[99] when used as an outcome measure to evaluate group PR programs.

However a concern exists when an assessment measure includes questions covering multiple domains (multidimensional), but then collapses that information into a single summary score (unidimensional). If the purpose of CAT is to discriminate among COPD patients and to classify the degree of overall COPD impact on that patient relative to other patients, then the CAT may be a good tool. However, if the purpose is to identify and follow each patient's concerns about the individual eight COPD impacts, the summary CAT score is unlikely to be adequate. To design a patient-centered approach, the PR team needs more than a summary score; it needs to know how each patient rates each item. A mutual patient-clinician examination of a patient's response to each of the eight items will provide more information, and assist in a better design of a patient-centered PR program, than the summary CAT score. While CAT is easy to use and to score, it is unlikely the CAT score provides sufficient patient-specific information for the design and evaluation of a patient-centered PR program.

The American Thoracic Society 2013 pulmonary rehabilitation statement cites the summary score as a limitation of the CAT.[37] While the CAT is widely used in Europe,[97] in early 2016, the CAT web site (http://www.catestonline.org/) greets American COPD patients and clinicians with this message: "This website is not currently available to US residents." If you are interested in the CAT, consult the parent website for updates.

Generally generic HRQL measures provide a more comprehensive assessment of the patient's overall health status. While they may not be as sensitive to disease-specific changes, they can detect consequences of treatment that may be missed by more focused measures. What if physiologic and/or disease-specific quality of life measures show improvement as a result of treatment, but the general HRQL instrument indicates decline? This alerts the health professional to the possibility of side effects or other consequences of treatment that are adversely affecting the patient. In COPD, the CRQ or SGRQ could improve but the patient's SF-36v2™ could decrease as a result of drug-induced osteoporosis related to steroid use.

The learning tip: Revisions are being made to original HRQL instruments to make them shorter and to have better psychometric properties. However, this results in multiple versions in the literature which may lead to confusion when interpreting journal results. Also new shorter, more efficient HRQL-lite instruments may be developed, but may have limitations in effectiveness studies.

MRS. WHEELER'S OUTCOMES ASSESSMENT PACKAGE AND PR PROGRAM

With the results of the baseline assessment, the team then meets and develops a 8-week progressive PR program for Mrs. Wheeler. The pharmacist had maximized the pharmacologic effect of the medications prior to hospital discharge and also had ensured that she was using her inhaler correctly. Now the pharmacist will reassess the drug regimen based on the PR baseline values and monitor; the physical therapist will guide her in exercises to improve her breathing mechanics with inspiratory muscle training and pursed lip breathing techniques; the occupational therapist will help her perform her activities of daily living with less expenditure of energy; and the psychologist will provide behavioral counseling to help her reduce her anxiety about her dypsnea. All will provide education about COPD and ways to reduce stressors. Her case will be reviewed at weekly team meetings. It is anticipated that as Mrs. Wheeler feels more comfortable with her breathing; the physical therapist will work with her to improve her walking endurance; the occupational therapist will share strategies for functioning outside the home; the dietitian will provide dietary advice to help her to gain muscle mass; the pharmacist will continue to monitor and adjust her medication as she becomes more active; and the psychologist will monitor and provide support for her anxious and depressive states. Throughout this process, the team will assess Mrs. Wheeler's progress has on the outcome measures selected as well as the individualized goals she has selected.

CURRENT HEALTH POLICIES ILLUSTRATING THE IMPORTANCE OF PATIENT-CENTERED APPROACHES

Patient-centeredness and outcomes assessment have been the unifying themes of this chapter. At the individual practice level, it is vital that health professional, attend to patient-reported needs—not just their physiologic needs, but also their physical, social, and psychological needs—and that they be integrated into the design of an intervention plan; that valid and reliable patient-centered and patient-reported outcomes are used to monitor process; and that at the end of the intervention, they are used to assess the effectiveness of the program.

The reality of patient-centered involvement is not just occurring at the individual patient-clinician level, it is happening throughout the American health care system. Two recent national programs illustrate this: the Patient-Centered Outcomes Assessment Institute (PCORI) and the Food and Drug Administration's Patient Representative and Patient-Focused Drug Development programs.

PATIENT-CENTERED OUTCOMES RESEARCH INSTITUTE (PCORI)[100]

While patient-centeredness is not a new principle, its current importance has been catalyzed at the national level by the establishment of the Patient-Centered Outcomes Research Institute or PCORI. Authorized as part of the Patient Protection and Affordability Act of 2010, PCORI was established to fund patient-centered comparative clinical effectiveness research (CER)—research that can answer questions meaningful to patients and caregivers by comparing the effectiveness (outcomes) of different methods (including their structure and processes) to prevent, diagnose, and treat diseases and disorders. As stated in PCORI's Mission, by supporting comparative effectiveness research, answers can "help people make informed healthcare decisions and improve healthcare delivery and outcomes by producing and promoting high-integrity, evidence-based information that comes from research guided by patients, caregivers, and healthcare community."[101] These CER studies are intended to produce answers that can be used to help close the gaps in evidence needed to improve health care delivery and key health outcomes.

An underlying component of patient-centered comparative clinical effectiveness research is patient-centered outcomes research (PCOR)—"a relatively new research field that considers patient's need and preferences and focuses on outcomes most important to them. PCOR findings can help patients and other healthcare stakeholders, such as caregivers, clinicians, insurers, policymakers and others, make better-informed decisions about their health and health options."[102]

Patient centeredness is included in the processes of PCORI's internal functioning as well as in criteria and expectations for grant applications.[102] In its internal operations, patient-centeredness is a central PCORI tenet—patients are included on the PCORI Board of Directors, its decision-making bodies to identify funding priorities and to grant awards, and its efforts to disseminate and implement patient-centered outcomes and comparative effectiveness research. PCORI's strong emphasis on engaging patients is also incorporated into its grant criteria. For grant applications, meaningful patient involvement must be identified in a patient/stakeholder engagement plan detailing meaningful patient and stakeholder engagement strategies; e.g., patients are expected to be engaged in the framing of the research design and grant proposal, in the selection of patient-centered outcomes measures, in membership on steering committees and advisory boards to provide oversight for implementing and monitoring of the research process, in interpreting of results, and in disseminating findings. From December 2012 through early 2016, PCORI has awarded over $1 billion to fund nearly 700 CER/PCOR proposals.[100]

Two of many sources to provide examples of PCOR/CER research are: i) an April 2016 special issue of the journal *Health Affairs*, "Patients' and Consumers' Use of Evidence,"[103] includes several articles authored by PCORI awardees and ii) an article relevant for the COPD case: "Patient involvement in the design of a patient-centered clinical trial to promote adherence to supplemental oxygen therapy in COPD."[104]

PATIENT ENGAGEMENT AT THE FOOD AND DRUG ADMINISTRATION

While the FDA has previously sought patient input for some of its work, the 2012 Food and Drug Administration Safety and Innovation Act (FDASIA) created two mechanisms to ensure a more systematic process to provide an active patient voice throughout the drug development process and in the development of FDA policies: i) patient participation in medical product discussions under Section 1137—Patient Representatives and ii) patient-focused drug development under the reauthorization of Prescription Drug User Fee Amendments (PDUFA) Title I of FDASIA.

Patient participation in medical product discussions—FDA Patient Representatives: Section 1137 of FDASIA directs FDA "to solicit the views of patients during the medical product development process and consider the perspective of patients during regulatory discussions including: fostering participation of a patient representative who may serve as a special government employee in appropriate Agency meetings with medical product sponsors and investigators."[105] In response to this directive, the FDA's Office of Health and Constituent Affairs has developed the Patient Representative Program to prepare patients as special government employees to provide a knowledgeable patient voice in appropriate meetings during the medical product development process including the early stages of its regulatory processes. By 2015, the FDA had recruited and trained over 200 patient representatives who were able to provide first hand, disease-specific patient experiences to FDA advisory committees, divisional reviews, and meetings with drug developers.

Patient-focused drug development: As part of the 2012 PDUFA reauthorization, the FDA will be able to create a more systematic process to involving a broader voice for patients to shape its considerations. The FDA decision to approve a drug is primarily based on its assessment as to whether the benefits of the drug outweigh its risk. But do those decision makers understand the perspective of patients as to the impact of the disease on their lives and the risks patients are willing to accept to achieve some benefit? While the Patient Representative Program can provide a single patient voice at various FDA advisory committee meetings, a more comprehensive understanding of the impact of and treatment for specific diseases is needed. FDA is now systematically collecting patient input through a series of 20 disease-focused public meetings to obtain patient perspective on disease severity, unmet medical needs, impact of the disease on patients' activities and how has it changed over time, what are their greatest worries, and other impact questions. These will provide important well-grounded patient input into how the disease is affecting their lives and what would be most beneficial for therapeutic interventions; this in turn will shape drug development process and risk-benefit considerations. Also, systematically collected patient reports of important areas of desired disease relief may identify a need to develop new FDA qualified, patient-centered outcome measures that can be included in early drug trials. A series of reports, "The Voice of the Patient," summarizes the findings from each of the disease-specific, FDA Patient-focused Drug Development Initiative hearings.[107]

SUMMARY

While outcomes assessment is not new to health care, but it is now an important component of the nation's effort to reduce health care costs. At the same time, the voice of the patient has never been more important. The voice of the patient is being systematically integrated into individual patient treatment plans as well as clinical trial and comparative effectiveness research. Patient-centered drug outcomes measures evaluate aspects of health and health care that are important to the patient. Patient-reported outcomes directly capture patient perceptions of their health and function, but to be effective, they—as all outcome measures—must be valid, reliable, and responsive. When designing a comprehensive patient-centered and patient-reported outcomes assessment system, the causal link between physiologic biomarkers; through symptoms, function, and health perceptions; to multidimensional health-related quality of life including the World Health Organization components of health—physical, social, and psychological dimensions—must be measured.

AMPLIFYING THE PATIENT VOICE

Enhancing the patient's voice in the medical product approval and evaluation process is an important emerging area of product development, which we have embraced in a number of ways.

Those living with a disease are in a unique position to provide essential insights about life with their condition, its severity, and the adequacy of treatment options. We also recognize patients and caregivers have their own perspectives on benefits and risks of medical products, and we believe this input should be considered during regulatory decision-making.

In September 2015, FDA announced our first-ever <u>Patient Engagement Advisory Committee</u>, which will provide advice on complex issues related to the regulation of medical devices and their use by patients. This Advisory Committee will help ensure the needs, experiences, and perspectives of patients are considered in our work and incorporated in our decision-making. http://blogs.fda.gov/fdavoice/index.php/tag/patient-engagement-advisory-committee/

Acknowledgements: Many thanks to Danielle M. Miller, PharmD, RPh and Alexa Carlson, PharmD, RPh for their assistance with the patient case and to Gerald Schumacher, PhD, PharmD for comments on an earlier draft of this chapter.

Excerpts of this chapter appeared earlier in the monograph *Outcomes Assessment and Health-Related Quality of Life Measurement, 2ⁿᵈ Edition*. Barr J, Schumacher G, Ohman S. 2003, NERCOA Educational Series, National Education and Research Center for Outcomes Assessment in Healthcare (NERCOA), Northeastern University, Boston MA. Included with permission.

REFERENCES

1. Epstein, A.M. (1990). The outcomes movement: Will it get us where we want to go? *N Engl J Med* 323:266–270.

2. Snyder, C.F., Aaronson, N.K., Choucair, et al. (2012). Implementing patient-reported outcomes in clinical practice: a review of the options and consideration. *Qual Life Res* 21:1305–1314.

3. Aaronson, N., Elliott, T., Greenhalgh, J. et al. (2015). On behalf of the International Society for Quality of Life Research. *User's guide to implementing patient-reported outcomes assessment in clinical practice: version2: January 2015.* Accessed http://www.isoqol.org/UserFiles/2015UsersGuide-Version2.pdf

4. Walton, M.K., Powers, J.H., Hobart, J. et al. (2015). Clinical outcomes assessment: conceptual foundation—Report of the ISPOR clinical outcomes assessment emerging good practice for outcomes research task force. *Value in Health* 18:741–752.

5. U.S. Department of Health and Human Services, Food and Drug Administration. (2009). *Guidance for industry on patient-reported outcomes measures: Use in medical product development to support labeling claims.* Accessed at http://www.fda.gov/downloads/Drugs/Guidances/UCM193282.pdf

6. Martin, A.B., Hartman, M., Benson, J. et al. (2016). National health spending in 2014: Faster growth driven by coverage expansion and prescription drug spending. *Health Affairs* 35: 150–160

7. OECD. (2015). *Health at a glance 2015: oecd indicators.* OECD Publishing, Paris. http://dx.doi.org/10.1787/health_glance-2015-en

8. Wennberg, J. & Gittelsohn, A. (1973). Small area variations in health care delivery. *Science* 182:1102–1108.

9. Laillemand, N.C. (December 13, 2012). Health policy brief: Reducing waste in health care. *Health Affairs.*

10. The Dartmouth Atlas of Health Care. (2016). *Reflections on variation.* http://www.dartmouthatlas.org/keyissues/issue.aspx?con=1338

11. Berwick, D.M., & Hackbarth, A.D. (2012). Eliminating waste in US health care. JAMA 307:1513-1516.

12. Morden, N.E., Colla, C.H., Sequist, T.D., & Rosenthal, M.B. (2014). Choosing wisely—the politics and economics of labeling low-value services. *New Engl J Med* 370:589—592.

13. *Choosing Wisely: An initiative of the American Board of Internal Medicine Foundation.* (2016). http://www.choosingwisely.org/about-us/ Accessed March 15, 2016

14. *Choosing Wisely. Clinician lists: Complete lists of recommendations by society.* http://www.choosingwisely.org/clinician-lists Accessed March 15, 2016

15. *Choosing wisely: Consumer partners.* http://www.choosingwisely.org/about-us/partners/choosing-wisely-consumer-partners/ Accessed March 15, 2016

16. Schoof, B.K., Campos-Outcalt, D., & Duke, P.M. (2013). American Academy of Family Physicians' *Choosing Wisely*® Communication Module: Discussion with a patient with sinusitis who requests antibiotic. 2013. http://modules.choosingwisely.org/modules/m_02/videos/m02_1_sinusitis.html

17. Ledford, D. K. (2013). American Academy of Allergy, Asthma & Immunology's *Choosing Wisely*® Communication Module: Patient seeking antibiotics to treat viral sinusitis. http://modules.choosingwisely.org/modules/m_06/videos/m06_1_sinusitis.htm

18. World Health Organization. (1948). *Constitution of the World Health Organization.* Geneva: World Health Organization.

19. Spilker, B. (Ed.). (1996). *Quality of life and pharmacoeconomics in Clinical Trials,* 2nd edition. Philadelphia: Lippincott Raven.

20. Ellwood, P.M. (1988). Outcomes management: A technology of patient experiences. *N Engl J Med* 318:1549–1556.

21. Codman, E.A. (1914). The product of a hospital. *Surg Gynec Obst* 18:491–496.

22. Codman, E.A. (1934). *The shoulder: Rupture of the supraspinatus tendon and other lesions in or about the subacromial bursa.* Boston: Thomas Todd.

23. Donabedian, A. (1966). Evaluating the quality of medical care. *Milbank Q* 44:166–203

24. Wilson, I., & Cleary, P. (1995). Linking clinical variables with health-related quality of life: a conceptual model of patient outcomes. *JAMA* 273: 59–65.

25. McDowell, I. (2006). *Measuring health: A Guide to rating scales and questionnaires, 3rd edition*. Oxford: Oxford University Press.

26. Mokkink, L.B., Terwee, C.B., Patrick, D.L. et al. (2010.) The COSMIN checklist for assessing the methodological quality of studies on measurement properties of health status measurement instruments: an international Delphi Study. *Qual Life Res* 19; 539–549.

27. COSMIN. *Consensus-based Standards for the Selection of Health Measurement Instruments*. (at http://www.cosmin.nl/)

28. Greenhalgh, J. (2009). The application of PROs in clinical practice: What are they, do they work, and why? *Qual Life Res* 18: 115–123.

29. Barr, J.T., Schumacher, G.E., & Ohman, S. (2004). Client-reported outcomes: do they agree with objective staff-reported outcomes of individuals with schizophrenia residing in the community? *Value in Health 7*.

30. Ware, J.E. & Sherbourne, C.D. (1992). The MOS 36-item short-form health status survey. *Med Care* 30: 473–483.

31. Davies, A.R., Sherbourne, C.D., Peterson, J.R., & Ware, J.E. (1998). *Scoring manual: Adult health status and patient satisfaction measures used in the Rand's Insurance Experiment*. Santa Monica, CA: Rand Corporation.

32. Jones, P.W., Harding,G,. Berry, P., et al. (2009). Development and first valuation of the COPD Assessment Test. *Eur Respir J* 34:648–654.

33. Jones, P., Jenkins, C., & Bauerle, O. (February 2012). CAT COPD Assessment TestHealth. *Health Professional User Guide*. Accessed at http://www.catestonline.org/images/UserGuides/CATHCPUser%20guideEn.pdf

34. CAT: COPD Assessment Test http://www.catestonline.org/ and for U.S. residents. http://www.catestonline.org/US_residents.html

35. Campbell, N., Ali, F., Finlay, et al. (2015). Equivalence of electronic and paper-based patient-reported outcome measures. *Qual Life Res* 24:1949–61.

36. Coons, S.J., Gwaltney, C.J., Hays, R.D., et al. (2009). Recommendations on evidence needed to support measurement equivalence between electronic and paper-based patient-reported outcome (PRO) measures. ISPOR ePRO Good Practices Task Force report. *Value in Health* 12:419–429.

37. American Thoracic Society/European Respiratory Society Statement: Key concepts and advances in Pulmonary Rehabilitation. (2013). *Am J Respir Crit Care Med* 188:1011–1027 accessed at http://www.atsjournals.org/doi/pdf/10.1164/rccm.201309-1634ST

38. Ries, A.L., Kaplan, R.M., Limberg, et al. (1999). Effects of pulmonary rehabilitation on physiologic and psychosocial outcomes in patients with chronic obstructive pulmonary disease. *Ann Intern Med* 122:823–832.

39. Paz-Diaz, H., Montes de, O.M., Lopez, J.M., & Celli, B.R. (2007). Pulmonary rehabilitation improves depression, anxiety, dyspnea and health status in patients with COPD. *Am J Phys Med Rehabil* 86; 30–36.

40. Garuti, G., Cilione, C., & Dell'Orse, D., et al. (2003). Impact of comprehensive pulmonary rehabilitation on anxiety and depression in hospitalized COPD patients. *Monaldi Arch Chest Dis* 59:56–61.

41. American Thoracic Society. *Standards for the diagnosis and management of patients with COPD: Spirometric classification.* Accessed at http://www.thoracic.org/copd-guidelines/for-health-professionals/definition-diagnosis-and-staging/spirometric-classification.php

42. American Thoracic Society. (2015). *Standards for the diagnosis and management of patients with COPD: Assessment of severity.* Accessed at http://www.thoracic.org/copd-guidelines/for-health-professionals/definition-diagnosis-and-staging/assessment-of-severity-staging.php

43. *Global Strategy for the Diagnosis, Management and Prevention of COPD,* Global Initiative for Chronic Obstructive Lung Disease (GOLD). (2016). Available from: http://www.goldcopd.org/

44. Wilke, S., Smid, D.E., Spruit, M.A., et al. (2014). *The 2014 updated GOLD strategy: A comparison of the various scenarios.* J COPD F 212–220.doi: http://dx.doi.org/10.15326/jcopdf.1.2.2014.0135

45. Demeyer, H., Gimeno-Santos, E., & Rabinovich, R.A.(2016). Physical activity characteristics across GOLD quadrants depend on the questionnaire used. *PLoS ONE* 11(3):e0151255.doi.1371/journal.pone.0151255.

46. Gift, A.G., Plaut, S.M., & Jacox, A. (1986). Psychologic and physiologic factors related to dyspnea in subjects with chronic obstructive pulmonary disease. *Heart Lung* 15:595–601.

47. Gift, A.G. & Cahill, C.A.(1990). Psychophysiologic aspects of dyspnea in chronic obstructive pulmonary disease: a pilot study. *Heart Lung* 19:252–257.

48. American Thoracic Society. (2012). An official American Thoracic Society Statement: Update on the mechanisms, assessment, and management of dyspnea. *Am J Respir Crit Care Med* 185:435–452.

49. Fletcher, C.M. (1960). Standardized questionnaire on respiratory symptoms: A statement prepared and approved by the MRC Committee on the aetiology of chronic bronchitis (MRC breathlessness score). *BMJ* 2:1665.

50. Bestall, J.C., Paul, E.A., Garrod, R., et al. (1999.) Usefulness of the Medical Research Council (MRC) dyspnoea scale as a measure of disability in patients with chronic obstructive pulmonary disease. *Thorax* 54:581–586.

51. Langsetmo, L., Platt, R.W., Ernst, P. et al. (2008). Underreporting exacerbation of chronic obstructive pulmonary disease in a longitudinal cohort. *Am J Respir Crit Care Med* 177:396–401.

52. Leidy, N.K. & Murray, L.T. (2013). Patient-reported outcome (PRO) measures for clinical trials of COPD: The EXACT and E-RS. *COPD* 10:393–398.

53. Leidy, N.K., Wilcox, T.K., Jones, P.W. et al. (2010). Development of the EXAcerbations of Chronic obstructive pulmonary disease Tool (EXACT): a patient-reported outcome (PRO) measure. *Value Health* 13:965–975.

54. Jones, P.W., Chen, W.H., Wilcox, T.K. et al. (2011). Characterizing and quantifying the symptomatic features of COPD exacerbations. *Chest* 139:1388–94.

55. Leidy, N.K., Wilcox, T.K., Jones, P.W. et al. (2011). Standardizing measurement of chronic obstructive pulmonary disease exacerbations. Reliability and validity of a patient-reported diary. *Am J Respir Crit Care Med* 183:323–9.

56. Leidy, N.K., Murray, L.T., & Jones, P.W. (2014). Performance of the EXAcerbations of chronic pulmonary disease tool patient-reported outcome measure in three clinical trials of chronic obstructive pulmonary disease. *AnnalsATS* 11:316–325.

57. Food and Drug Administration. (January 2014). *Guidance for industry and FDA Staff: Qualification process for drug development tools.* Accessed at http://www.fda.gov/downloads/drugs/guidancecomplianceregulatoryinformation/guidances/ucm230597.pdf

58. Food and Drug Administration. (January 2014.) *Attachment to guidance for industry and FDA staff: Qualification process for drug development tools: Qualifications of exacerbations of chronic pulmonary disease tool for measurement of symptoms of acute bacterial exacerbations of chronic bronchitis in patient with chronic obstructive pulmonary disease.* Draft qualification guidance document. Accessed at http://www.fda.gov/downloads/Drugs/GuidanceComplianceRegulatoryInformation/Guidances/UCM380961.pdf

59. Leidy, N.K., Sexton, C.C., Jones, P.W. et al. (2014). Measuring respiratory symptoms in clinical trials of COPD: reliability and validity of a daily diary. *Thorax* 69:443–9.

60. Leidy, N.K., Murray, L.T., Monz, B. et al. (2014). Measuring respiratory symptoms of COPD: performance of the EXACT-Respiratory Symptoms Tool (E-RS) in three clinical trials. *Respiratory Research* 15:124–133.

61. Food and Drug Administration. (March 2016). *Attachment to guidance for industry and FDA Staff: qualification process for drug development tools:* evaluating respiratory symptoms in chronic obstructive pulmonary disease, a patient-reported outcome, for the measurement of severity of respiratory symptoms in stable chronic obstructive pulmonary disease: qualification for exploratory use. draft qualification guidance document for a patient-reported outcome (PRO) measure. March 2016. Accessed at http://www.fda.gov/ucm/groups/fdagov-public/@fdagov-drugs-gen/documents/document/ucm489526.pdf.

62. Guyatt, G.H., Pugsley, S.O., Sullivan, M.J., et al. (1984). Effect of encouragement on walking test performance. *Thorax* 39:818–822.

63. Casanova, C., Cote, C.G., Marin, J.M. et al. (2007). The 6-min walking distance: Long-term follow up in patients with COPD. *Eur Respir J* 29: 535–540.

64. Annegarn, J., Meijer, K., Passos, V.L., et al. (2012). CIRO1 Rehabilitation Network. Problematic activities of daily life are weakly associated with clinical characteristics in COPD. *J AmMed Dir Assoc* 13:284–290.

65. Coventry, P.A. (2009). Does pulmonary rehabilitation reduce anxiety and depression in chronic obstructive pulmonary disease? *Curr Opin Pulm Rehab* 15: 143–149.

66. Zigmond, A,S. & Snaith, R. P. (1983). The Hospital Anxiety and Depression Scale. *Acta Psychiatr Scand* 67:361–370.

67. Bjelland, I., Dahl, A.A., Haug, T.T., & Neckelmann, D. (2002). The validity of the Hospital Anxiety and Depressions Scale. An updated literature review. *J Psychosom Res* 52:69–77.

68. Connelly, J.E., Philbrick, J.T., Smith, G.R., et al. (1989). Health perceptions of primary care patients and the influence on health care utilization. *Med Care* 27:S99–S109.

69. Franks, P., Gold, M.R., & Fiscella, K. (2003). Sociodemographics, self-rated health, and mortality in the US. *Soc Sci Med* 56:2505–2014.

70. Maruish, M.E. (2011). *User's manual for the SF-36v2 health survey*. 3rd ed. Lincoln, RI: QualityMetric, Inc. https://www.optum.com/optum-outcomes.html

71. McCarthy, B., Casey, D., Devane, D. et al. (2015). Pulmonary rehabilitation for chronic obstructive pulmonary disease. *Cochrane Database of Systematic Reviews*. D0I:10.1002/14651858.Cd003793.pub3 as accessed at http://www.cochrane.org/CD003793/AIRWAYS_pulmonary-rehabilitation-for-chronic-obstructive-pulmonary-disease.

72. Dang-Tan, Ismaila, A., Zhang, S., et al. (2015). Clinical, humanistic, and economic burden of chronic obstructive pulmonary disease (COPD) in Canada: A systematic review. *BMC Res Notes* 8:464- DOI 10.1186/s13104-015-1424-y Accessed at http://www.ncbi.nlm.nih.gov/pmc/articles/PMC4578756/

73. Ware, J.E. & Sherbourne, C.D. (1992). A 36-item short-form health survey (SF-36): I. Conceptual framework and item selection. *Med Care* 30:473–83.

74. SF Health Surveys. https://www.optum.com/optum-outcomes/what-we-do/health-surveys.html

75. Tarlov, A.R., Ware, J.E., Greenfield, S., et al. (1989). The Medical Outcome Study: an application of methods for monitoring the results of medical care. *JAMA* 262:925–930.

76. Davies, A.R. & Ware, J.E. (1981). *Measuring health perceptions in the health insurance experiment.* Santa Monica, CA: The RAND Corporation, (publication no. R-2711-HHS).

77. Stewart, A.L. & Ware, J.E. (Eds.). (1992). *Measuring functioning and well-being: The medical outcomes study approach.* Durham, NC: Duke University Press.

78. McHorney, C.A., Ware, J.E., & Raczek, A.E. (1993). The MOS 36-item short-form health survey (SF-36): II. Psychometric and clinical tests of validity in measuring physical and mental health constructs. *Med Care* 31:247–263.

79. McHorney, C.A., Ware, J.E., Lu, J.F.R., et al. (1993). The MOS 36-item Short-Form Health Survey (SF-36): III. Tests of data quality, scaling assumptions, and reliability across diverse patient groups. *Med Care* 32:40–66.

80. Ware, J.E., Kosinski, M., & Keller, S.K. (1994). SF-36 *Physical and mental health summary scales: A user's manual.* Boston MA: The Health Institute.

81. Ware, J.E., Kosinski, Gandek, B. (2002). *The SF-36 Health Survey: Manual and interpretation guide.* Lincoln, Rhode Island: Quality Metrics Inc.

82. Kohli, P., Pinto-Plata, V., Divo, M., et al. (2015). Functional capacity, health status, and inflammatory biomarker profile in a cohort of patients with chronic obstructive pulmonary disease. *J Cardiopulm Rehabil Prev* 35:348–55.

83. Tomioka, H., Mamesaya, N., Yamashita, S., et al. (2016). Combined pulmonary fibrosis and emphysema: Effect of pulmonary rehabilitation in comparison with chronic obstructive pulmonary disease. *BMJ Open Respir Res* 22:3(1): e000099 doi:10.1136/bmjresp-2015-000099

84. Nikoletou, D., Man, W.D., Mustfa, N., et al. (2016). Evaluation of the effectiveness of a home-based inspiratory muscle training programme in patients with chronic obstructive pulmonary disease using multiple inspiratory muscle tests. *Disabil Rehabil* 38:250–9.

85. Wiebe, S., Guyatt, G., Weaver, B. et al. (2003). Comparative responsiveness of generic and specific quality-of-life instruments. *J Clin Epidem* 56:52–60.

86. Guyatt, G.H., Berman, L.B., Townsend, M., et al. (1987). A measure of quality of life for clinical trials in chronic lung disease. *Thorax* 42;773–8.

87. Williams, J.E., Singh, S.J., Sewell, L., Guyatt, G.H., & Morgan, M.D. (2001). Development of a self-reported Chronic Respiratory Questionnaire (CRQ-SR). *Thorax* 56:954–9.

88. Williams, J.E., Singh, S.J., Sewell, L., & Morgan, M.D. (2003). Health status measurement: sensitivity of the self-reported Chronic Respiratory Questionnaire (CRQ-SR) in pulmonary rehabilitation. *Thorax* 58:515–8.

89. Williams, J.E.A., Singh, S.J., Sewell, L., et al. (2003). Health status measurement: sensitivity of the self-reported Chronic Respiratory Questionnaire (CRQ-SR) in pulmonary rehabilitation. *Thorax* 58:515–518.

90. Schunemann, H.J., Griffith, L., Jaeschke, R., et al. (2003). A comparison of the original chronic respiratory questionnaire with a standardized one. *Chest* 124:1421–9.

91. Schunemann, H.J., Goldstein, R., Mador, M.J., et al. (2005). A randomized trial to evaluate the self-administered chronic respiratory questionnaire (CRQ-SA). *Eur Respir J* 25:31–40.

92. Jones, P.W., Quirk, F.H., Baveystock, C.M., et al. (1992). A self-complete measure of health status for chronic airflow limitation. The St. George's Respiratory Questionnaire. *Am Rev Respir Dis* 145:1321–27.

93. Meguro, M., Barley, E.A., Spencer, et al. (2007). Development and validation of an improved, COPD-specific version of the St. George's Respiratory Questionnaire. *Chest* 132:456–463.

94. Jones, P.W. (2002). Interpreting thresholds for a clinically significant change in health status in asthma and COPD. *Eur Respir J* 19:398–404.

95. Barr, J.T., Schumacherm G.E., Freeman, S., et al. (2000). American translation, modification, and validation of the St. George's Respiratory Questionnaire. *Clin Therap* 9:1121–41.

96. Jones, P.W. (2012). *St. George respiratory questionnaire for COPD Patients: Manual.* Accessed at http://www.healthstatus.sgul.ac.uk/SGRQ_download/sgrq-c-manual-april-2012.pdf

97. Jones, P.W., Brusselle, G., Dal Negro, R.W., et al. (2011). Properties of the COPD assessment test in a cross-sectional European study. *Eur Respir J* 38:29–35.

98. Dodd, J.W., Hogg, L., Nolan, J., et al. (2011). The COPD assessment test (CAT): response to pulmonary rehabilitation. A muticentre, prospective study. *Thorax* 66:425–429.

99. Jones, P.W., Harding, G., Wiklund, I., et al. (2012). Tests of the responsiveness of the Chronic Obstructive Pulmonary Disease (COPD) assessment Test™ (CAT) following acute exacerbations and pulmonary rehabilitation. *Chest* 142:134–140.

100. http://www.pcori.org

101. Patient-Centered Outcomes Research Institute. Mission Statement in PCORI Strategic Plan, November 2013. Accessed at http://www.pcori.org/sites/default/files/PCORI-Board-Meeting-Strategic-Plan-111813.pdf

102. Frank, L., Basch, E., & Selby, J.V. (2014). The PCORI perspective on patient-centered outcomes research. *JAMA* 312:1513–14.

103. Health Affairs. (2016). *Special issue patients' and consumers' use of evidence*, 35.

104. Holm, K.E., Casaburi, R., Cerreta, S., et al. (2015). Patient involvement in the design of a patient-centered clinical trial to promote adherence to supplemental oxygen therapy in COPD [published on October 31, 2015]. Patient doi: 10.1007/s40271-015-0150-z

105. Food and Drug Administration. (January 2016). Food and Drug Administration Safety and innovation Act (FDASIA) Section 1137: *Patient participation in medical product discussion report on stakeholder views*. Accessed at http://www.fda.gov/downloads/ForPatients/About/UCM486859.pdf

106. Mullins, T.M. *FDA invites patient organizations to take a place at the podium*. Accessed at http://blogs.fda.gov/fdavoice/index.php/tag/patient-focused-drug-development-pfdd-program/

107. Food and Drug Administration. *The Voice of the Patient: A series of reports from FDA's patient-focused drug development initiative*. Accessed at http://www.fda.gov/ForIndustry/UserFees/PrescriptionDrugUserFee/ucm368342.htm

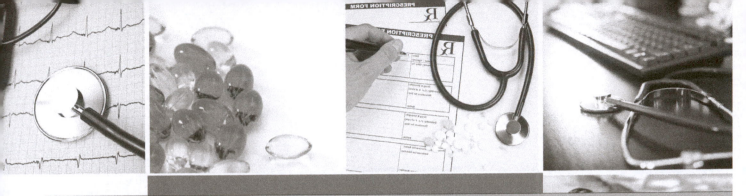

PART III TARGETING CARE OF SPECIFIC PATIENTS

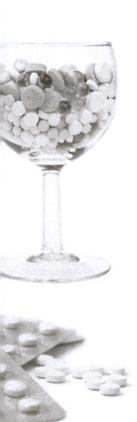

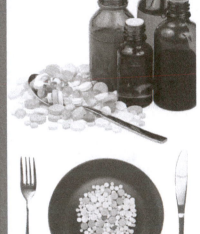

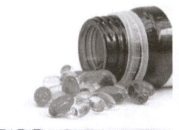

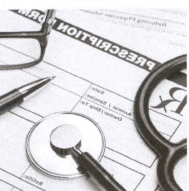

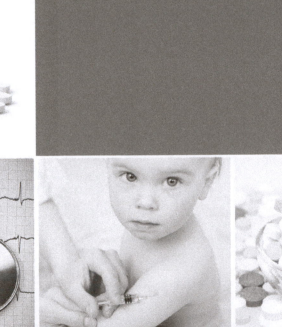

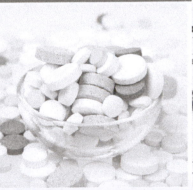

CHAPTER 15

CHILDREN AND ADOLESCENTS

Katri Hämeen-Anttila, PhD, Piia Siitonen, MSc, PhD (Cand), and Patricia J. Bush, MSc, PhD

LEARNING OBJECTIVES:

1. Identify the importance of empowering children as medicine users.
2. Explain how to provide information on medicines to children at different stages of cognitive development.
3. Describe the *Ten Guiding Principles for Teaching Children and Adolescents About Medicines*, A Position Statement of the United States Pharmacopeia, and determine to act accordingly.
4. Summarize the sources and variety of influences on children's and adolescents' medicine beliefs and behaviors.
5. Recognize that children and adolescents use medicines widely and that many factors determine their use autonomously.

KEY TERMS

Adolescents

Children

Cognitive development

Environmental influences

Medicine attitudes

Medicine autonomy

Medicine beliefs

Medicine education

Medicine knowledge

Medicine use

INTRODUCTION

Traditionally, relative to health and illness behavior, children have been viewed as passive, with adults making decisions for them and providing information about them to health professionals. However, children take medicines themselves, they are aware that medicines are stored at home, they observe medicine use by family members, and they view medicine promotion by the media on a regular basis. In addition, every trip to the drugstore and grocery store exposes children to the sight of medicines and sometimes to the sight of a pharmacist. In view of this exposure, it would be extremely unlikely that children would not be forming beliefs and attitudes about medicines. Moreover, these beliefs and attitudes should change as children gain more experience and develop more skills at interpreting what they observe.

During the past few decades there has been a gradual shift from viewing children as passive recipients of health information and health care to viewing them as active partners whose competence and information needs should be considered by health care professionals.[1,2,3] Some pharmacy organizations—United States Pharmacopeia (USP) and The International Pharmaceutical Federation (FIP)—have adopted statements emphasizing that children should be educated about their own medicines and also about medicine use in general during school health education.[2,4] (Table 15-1). Such education is crucial if we want to have a new generation of active and empowered medicine users who are competent in discussions with health care professionals. This is also the aim of the change in the health care approach from compliance to concordance.[5,6]

Studies from the United States and Australia show that parents of young children believe that 12 years is the age that a child should be able to start to take a medicine for common health problems, such as a headache or sore throat, without asking an adult.[7,8] This raises several questions. What should that average child know about medicines before assuming this responsibility? Do children know enough to take medicines on their own? How do children learn about medicines? Who should teach them?

No consensus exists among health professionals or health educators about the need for children to be educated about medicines, who should assume the responsibility for education, or what forms such education should take. Certainly no one profession is solely responsible. It is a matter of co-operation, where the role of the parents and the active involvement of the child should not be undermined.[9]

The fact that children are not simply little adults is important. It is not just that children have less experience than adults, it is that children's thinking progresses through stages and is *qualitatively* different from that of adults. For reasons of differences relating to knowledge, experience, autonomy, and developmental levels, children may view and understand health, illness, and treatment differently than adults. Thus, children should be treated differently with regard to pharmaceutical care and programs intended for teaching children about medicines should take into account what children already know, do, and want to know.

The goal of this chapter is to review what is known about children and medicines and to produce some pragmatic suggestions for health professionals and health educators. The remainder of this chapter presents information on how children learn, children's autonomy, knowledge, and attitudes relative to medicine use, and factors associated with children's medicine-related beliefs and behaviors. Next, a section deals with how health professionals and health educators can help children learn to use medicines wisely before the children bear some responsibility for doing so. A separate section deals with the special situation of adolescents and medicines.

HOW CHILDREN LEARN

COGNITIVE DEVELOPMENT STAGES

Adults not only know more than children, they are capable of processing what they know in a more complex way. Children progress through four stages as they develop more complex cognitive skills. The theory of cognitive development stages is credited to Jean Piaget.[10] Although the sequence of progression through the stages is the same, there is individual variation in the rate of progression, and the progression has been shown to vary with the specific topic area. For health in particular, even some adults do not operate at the highest stage. Thus, the age groups presented are rough estimations rather than specific indicators of different stages.

A value in being aware of the cognitive development stages of children is in appreciating that adults cannot provide children under cognitive stage four with information about health and illness and expect them to infer appropriate behavior. Moreover, in any given situation of health education addressed at a particular behavior, an adult may not be able to predict what a child will perceive.[11] Knowledge of Cognitive Development Theory may not help you to predict what a child thinks, but at least you should not be surprised to hear a 7-year-old child who, when asked to name some "bad" drugs, correctly did so, but then said that you get them at the "drug" store. That is perfectly logical. Another lovely example occurred when a 6-year-old was asked how likely she would be to take something special if she had trouble falling asleep. Her response, indicated by pointing to the largest bar on a graph: "Very likely." She was then asked, "What would you take?" Her response: "A teddy bear."

Stage 1: Sensory Motor

The first stage, lasting from birth to about two years, is known as the sensory motor stage. In this stage, the child learns through interacting with the environment, and cannot recall or imagine an object or person that is not present. Thus, learning about medicines does not (cannot) occur during this stage.

Stage 2: Preoperational

The second stage, roughly from 2–7 seven years, is known as the preoperational stage. During this stage, children begin to be able to recall past events, to understand symbols, and to use mental imaging. However, links from cause to effect are not understood, and magical thinking is often used to explain events. For example, an asthmatic child at this stage may not understand the connection between exercise and difficulties in breathing, i.e., link from cause to effect. Children in this stage are often "yea sayers." Here is an example from an interview with a 4-year-old child, illustrating both "yea saying" and magical thinking. "Did you ride an elephant to school today?" "Yes." "Do you have wings?" "Yes." "How do you know you have wings?" "The elephant told me."

Clearly, it is wise to avoid questions that call for a yes/no response when trying to get information from children in the preoperational stage. In addition, children at this stage are sensitive to what they perceive the interviewer—or a pharmacist in a pharmacy—wants to hear and will respond to please the interviewer. Thus, the interviewer must take great care not to provide either verbal or physical indicators of approval or disapproval of a young child's answers.

Stage 3: Concrete Operational

From roughly age 7–12 years, children's thinking becomes more logical and systematic. Children become problem solvers and are able to focus on several aspects of the same situation. They understand the difference between change and permanency. Compared to the previous stage, an asthmatic child at this stage will understand the connection between exercise and difficulties in breathing. Furthermore, if told, a child at a concrete operational stage is able to understand why two asthma medicines may need to be used.

Children use whatever is at hand within their sphere of knowledge and experience to explain an event, however illogical it may seem to an adult. For example, a 7-year-old urban boy, when asked, "Is that good, being on drugs?" responded, "No, you can mess up your mind and then you die." But, when next asked, "So what happens…?" the boy said, "…and then the police catch you and then they take you to the hospital and they gonna have to break your head open to get all the drugs out."[7] This 7-year-old represents a child entering the concrete operational stage and just beginning to apply logic and reasoning to events in his life. A sensitive adult, understanding this developmental process, can understand the child's logic. In this case, if drugs "mess up the mind," the child reasons that the mind is in the head and hospitals fix people. Thus, it follows, with compelling logic that the head must be broken open and the drugs removed to unburden the mind from its "messed up" state.

Stage 4: Formal Operational

This stage is considered to be from 12 years on. Children become more capable of hypothetical and abstract thought as they enter adolescence, but for formal operational thinking to occur in a particular area, attention and motivation are required. Thus, although individuals develop the capacity for this type of thinking—a capacity fully developed by late adolescence—the associated skills are not always applied. Understanding causal processes in health and illness is one of those content areas that seems to lag in some individuals through lack of interest or motivation, but certainly a better understanding of related processes and the relationships between internal and external factors is acquired. Someone trying to get information about health and illness from an adolescent (or an adult, for that matter) or to educate the adolescent cannot simply assume that the adolescent (or adult) is operating at this most advanced stage. In fact, the health literacy levels have been shown to be low also among adults worldwide indicating the need for concrete patient counseling also to adults.[12,13,14]

THEORIES AND MODELS

Four conceptual systems predominate in explaining how children learn and behave. One of these, Cognitive Development Theory (CDT) emphasizes the role of developmental processes that influence children's understanding. CDT has influenced studies of children's health beliefs and understanding of illness-related processes.[15,16,17] Behavioral Intention Theory (BIT)[18] is more often used for adults but is attractive for children because it emphasizes the influence of reference group norms and focusing on specific behaviors rather than inferences and abstractions for which children are often not cognitively prepared. Moreover, BIT posits that a behavior intention is the best predictor of an actual behavior. Social Cognitive Theory (SCT), a revision of Social Learning Theory (SLT), predominates.[19] According to SCT, behaviors are acquired and shaped through attention, retention, production, and motivation operating in three domains: personal, behavioral, and environmental. Personal factors include the child's own value system, and expectations derived from observation and experience; behavioral factors include performance skills; environmental factors include modeling and expressed opinions of peers, family, and media. Self-Determination Theory (SDT), often applied to education and health, is similar to

SCT as it also addresses the environment or social conditions that affect behavior motivation.[20,21] SDT puts greater emphasis on the type of motivation, whether autonomous or controlled, and what influences the type. SDT also recognizes amotivation, which means a lack of intention and motivation.

The Children's Health Belief Model (CHBM) was adapted from the classic Health Belief Model (HBM) to explain children's expectations of taking medicines.[22] (Figure 15-1) The CHBM is consistent with Gochman's[23] recommendation to place children's health behavior within their personal and social context, recognizing that their personal attributes are influenced by peers, families, and other social groups. This view of children's health behaviors supported the inclusion of the influence of the child's primary caregiver in the CHBM and also cognitive and psychological attributes that change with age and experience, such as knowledge, risk taking, and perception of control over health status (health locus of control).

In path analysis, the CHBM was very successful in predicting urban elementary schoolchildren's expectation to take medicines for five common health problems: cold, fever, upset stomach, trouble sleeping, and nervousness.[24] The child's perception of illness severity and benefit of taking medicines were the two strongest predictors, with Illness Concern and Perceived Vulnerability having weaker relationships.

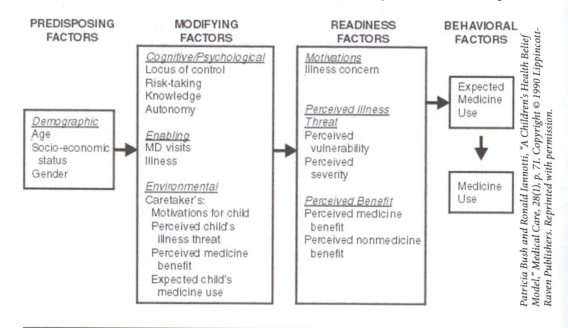

FIGURE 15-1: CHILDREN'S HEALTH BELIEF MODEL

Source: Adapted from Bush PJ, Iannotti RJ. A children's health belief model. Med Care 1990;28:69–86

From a developmental perspective, two findings were particularly noteworthy. Older children's variables were not more highly correlated with those of their mothers' than younger children's. Also, the children's own cognitions and attitudes appeared to develop independently of their mothers. The primary message was that mothers' health beliefs are correlated with those of their children but this effect was relatively small when compared with other developmental influences associated with the child. In fact, expected medicine use was not correlated between mothers and their children. Children's own motivational variables, influenced by their cognitive and affective processes, were more important in determining their expectations to take medicines than their mother's values, beliefs, and expectations. For example, Perceived Vulnerability, a strong predictor in adult models, was a weak predictor in the CHBM. The explanation is likely to be that children are not as cognitively prepared to predict events as are adults, due to lack of experience.

The variables in the CHBM were surprisingly stable.[24] Not only were most of the variables correlated over three years, but also expected medicine use among children about 8–12 years was predicted from variables measured three years earlier. These findings support educating children about medicines from an early age.

MEDICINE-RELATED BELIEFS AND BEHAVIORS

Factors likely to influence children's behaviors, beliefs, attitudes, and expectations regarding medicines, include the child's frequency of medicine use and environmental exposure. Some or all of these may interact.

MEDICINE USE FREQUENCY

Medicine use is common among children. In the United States, one survey found that half of the children under three years had been given an OTC (over-the-counter) medicine in the previous 30 days.[25] Similar and higher rates have been found in other countries for older children.[26,27,28,29,30,31,32,33,34,35] However, comparison of these studies is difficult since medicine use may be reported by parents[25,32,34,36,37] or by children themselves,[27,28,29,30,31,35] or by both the children and the parents.[22,33] Furthermore, the time during which medicines were used may differ considerably from two days,[22,34,37] one or two weeks,[28,30,32,33,35,36] to one month,[27,29] or even three months.[38] Although rates of medicine use, both OTC and prescription, tend to decrease after infancy and to begin to rise for females as they reach reproductive age, all surveys lead to the conclusion that medicine use is a common activity for children and adolescents.[25,26,27,28,29,30,31,32,33,34,35,36,37,38,39]

Girls use more medicines than boys and this trend increases with age.[27,28,30,33] Also socioeconomic class and ethnicity have been shown to have some influence on children's medicine use. Children in lower social classes and ethnic minorities reported using medicines more often than other children in some studies.[39,40] However, the association with ethnic background is not consistent between studies and some studies have shown that children with no immigration background use more self-medication.[33] Higher income and education level of the mother seems to be associated with the use of OTC drugs.[25,33,36] Furthermore, parents' perception of their children's state of health as poor[32,37] as well as parents' own medicine use[37] have been shown to be associated with higher medicines consumption.

Medicines are present in children's immediate and wider environment. Past research[41] found that the number of medicines in the household influences children's medicine-related expectations and behaviors and there is no reason to believe that has changed.

The number of medicines and ratio of OTC to prescription medicines has been found to vary widely among countries and subpopulations. In addition to the health status of family members, differences are most likely accounted for by culture, economic status, medicine advertising, and the places where medicines may be acquired which varies widely among countries.

Despite the admonition to parents to keep medicines locked up out of the reach of children, if the children are of school age, this admonition is rarely observed. In addition to medicine cabinets, medicines are all over the house, in drawers, purses, and cars. Most or all of the household medicines are accessible to most children of school age, a situation found in several European countries and the United States.[7,42,43,44] In fact, in many countries children report to knowing where the household medicines are kept and having physical access to them.[26,29,43,44] For example, in United States, 88% of 5–12-year-old[26] and 10–14-year old children[43] reported having access to household medicines. In Greece, 50% of the children 6–11 stated that they could easily find the household medicines and take them if they wanted to.[44] Also, 68% of Danish children (11–13 years) reported the availability of medicines for headaches at home, and 22% said they are allowed to take this medicine without asking permission.[29] In general, the accessibility to home medicines has shown to increase with age.[26,29,44] Asked of 8-year old Billy. "Billy, where are medicines in your house?" Billy: "Some are locked up in the medicine cabinet, but I stand on the side of the tub, I hold onto the shower curtain, and I swing across to get the key cause it's on the top of the medicine cabinet."[7]

Many children are afraid they will be given a grownup's medicine by mistake. USP has recommended that pharmacists or parents put a special sticker on children's medicines so that children will know they are not getting a grownup's medicine. Parents are also urged to keep their children's medicines in a separate place from those of adults to reduce the chance of a child being given an adult's medicine.

The medicine cabinet has also become a target of the message to students "Don't Do Drugs." Among 12–13 year olds in 2005 in the United States, prescribed medicines became the most commonly abused drugs. They were pain killers, depressants, and stimulants acquired from home medicine cabinets.[45] Motives vary from self-treatment for perceived problems, e.g., can't sleep, to recreation, e.g., getting high.[46] Concerns about prescription and over-the-counter drug use by students motivated D.A.R.E. (Drug Abuse Resistance Education) in the United States to develop and implement a school-based curriculum focused on these kinds of drugs in 2007–08. The curriculum has versions for 5th, 7th, and 9th grade students and includes a video for parents and community leaders.[47] D.A.R.E. is the largest school-based substance abuse curriculum in the U.S. and it is implemented by trained local police officers.

Increasingly, the wider community, including pharmacists, physicians, parent groups, and legal personnel, are being asked to cooperate with schools to educate children about medicines.[45,46,47]

CHILDREN'S MEDICINE KNOWLEDGE

Questionnaires using varying knowledge scales have been used to study children's medicine knowledge. In the United States, a medicine knowledge index containing items believed to include those fundamental to appropriate use of medicines was administered to urban schoolchildren in age 8–12,[7,26] and 7- and 10-years.[48] In general, children were found to have a poor[7,26] or only a medium level of knowledge.[48] The children scored best on questions relating to prescriptions and poorest on questions relating to the relationship between efficacy (i.e., how well a medicine works) and medicine characteristics such as size, color, taste, and place acquired.[7,26]

In Asia[49] and in Middle East,[50] schoolchildren aged 11–12 and 7–9 years, respectively, were found to have a medium but a limited level of medicine knowledge. The children knew best the storage of medicines[49] and poorest the adverse reactions and the usefulness of taking medicines when ill.[49,50]

Among adolescents in Europe, contradictory levels of medicine knowledge have been found. In Germany, adolescents age 15–17 years were found to have unsatisfactory level of knowledge,[28] while, in Malta and in Greece, children age 14–16 and 6–11 years, respectively, were found to have relatively good levels.[44,51] However, the Maltese had severe misconceptions in questions related to the relationship between the action and appearance of medicines, such as shape and color.

Young children often talk about medicines by referring to their appearance, e.g., color, form or taste, name, or therapeutic purpose.[26,42,52,53,54] Older children are more likely to refer to medicines by their brand names.[52,53,54] However, even 5–6-year-old children are aware of brand names.[26,55] However, the possibility that a particular medicine could have more than one name or more than one form is somewhat confusing to children.[51]

In general, children have limited ideas of how medicines work.[28,52,53,56,57] For example, no Finnish child aged 13–14 years[53] and only a third of German adolescents (15–17 years) were able to explain how antibiotics work.[28] In addition, the role of vaccines in the prevention of diseases was rarely known among children.[44,57] In general, children acknowledge that there are differences between medicines and the dose of medicines for children and adults.[49,51,52] However, in Finnish study, children 10–11 years disagreed on whether they could use the same medicines as adults or not.[57]

Children in various countries recognize the possibility that medicines may have harmful effects.[28,49,51,52,53,57,58,59] For example, children in Germany (15–17 years)[28] and in Finland (10–11[53,57] and 13–14 years[53]) were aware that medicines can cause adverse reactions. Older children are more likely to know that medicines may have harmful effects compared with younger children.[53,58] Furthermore, in the study of Almarsdottir et al.,[54] American children did not freely mention adverse reactions as possibly harmful.

On average, children view medicines cautiously. In several studies children have said that medicines should be taken only for sickness and when really needed.[53,59,60] Some studies have reported that some children have fears about getting the wrong medicine, especially an adult's medicine.[52] In other studies children have viewed medicines quite positively and have attributed recovery to them.[54]

Children's medicine knowledge has found to have interrelationships with different variables. Studies in the United States have found that the more internal a child's health locus of control, the more knowledgeable the child about medicines.[26,48] Also, children who knew the most about medicines and who had the most internal health locus were less likely than other children to perceive that medicines would help them for five common health problems and were less likely to expect to take medicines for them.[22] These relationships were also found in children in Spain.[48,61]

Furthermore, in many studies, child's knowledge of medicines has been found to be positively correlated with age,[26,44,49,50,62] socioeconomic status,[26,44,49] parent's educational level[48,49] and the presence of a first-degree relative working in a medical field.[49,50] For example, in Greece, older children and children with higher SES answered more frequently that when you are ill, you should not always take medicines than younger and those with lower SES.[44] Those children were also more knowledgeable about vaccines. However, in German study, the parents' educational level and parental employment in a medical field had no influence on their child's knowledge about medicines.[28] In addition, in some studies, female children had more knowledge about medicines than male children.[28,51,62]

CHILDREN'S MEDICINE AUTONOMY

Self-administration of medicines is quite common among children. In two American studies, 36% of 5–12-year-old children[26] and 36% of 10–14-year-old children[43] indicated they had taken medicine independently the last time they had taken one. Rudolf et al.[63] discovered that 44% of 9–16: year-old campers at a residential summer camp brought medicines with them. During the camp session, 25% of the younger (9–12 years) and 58% of the older (13–16 years) children self-medicated without consulting or informing an adult. Also, 58%–76% of Canadian children (12–15 years) reported having taken OTC pain medication over the previous three months without first checking with an adult.[38]

Furthermore, children may be more autonomous in medicine use than their caregivers indicate. On average, American mothers said that 12 years was the age when the average child could take a medicine for a headache independently; however, about one fifth of 3rd and 5th graders indicated they would do so, although most of them were younger than 12 years.[26] When Finnish children (10–11 years) were asked to evaluate the age suitable for a child or adolescent to independently take medicines, most children thought that children few years older than themselves could safely do so.[57]

Children are also quite independent in purchasing of medicines. In grades 3, 5, and 7, 14%–29% of American children indicated they had purchased a medicine independently, and 38%–44% of the children said they had picked up a prescription.[7,26] Furthermore, sharing and borrowing is quite a common among school-aged children. For example, in the United States, 20% of the girls (9–18 years) had borrowed or shared prescription medicines as did 13% of the boys.[64] In an American summer camp, 28% of the older children (13–16 years) shared medicines with others.[63] Also, 29%–48% of the Canadian children (12–15 years) reported that they had shared or borrowed medicines for different types of pain.[38] In addition, 33% of Danish 13 year-old girls reported that they have received medicine from friends or others.[65] In general, pain medicine is shared most often, and furthermore, used independently more often than other medicines.

HELPING CHILDREN LEARN ABOUT MEDICINES

Children rarely are learning about medicines in school and they are rarely learning about them from their health care providers. This leaves families and the media as the current main medicine "educators" of children.

Pediatricians, and likely other health care professionals as well, usually seek some information from children about their illness and symptoms. However, when giving information about diagnosis and treatment, physicians tend to address the parent.[66,67] The age of the child influences the situation with older children given more information than younger children. However, even young children are interested in and often anxious about their medical condition, and they retain some information better than adults. It is important to talk to the children, if for no other reason than that the quality of communications to children affects adherence and treatment outcomes, probably through reducing anxiety.[68,69]

It is not enough simply to have good intentions and to decide to educate children about medicines. Most health care professionals are poor judges of what children at various levels can comprehend.[70] However, most can be taught how to recognize the child's developmental level and to communicate at that level effectively.[71] Moreover, if a health professional communicates with children at an appropriate level, a bonus is that their parents are more likely to understand.

For communicating with children, the first step is to make a commitment to do it. The second step is to learn how to communicate with children at their cognitive development levels,[71] to do it consistently, and to not give up if not every child responds. The third step is to decide where. The fourth step is to prepare developmentally appropriate materials to augment communications.

ONE-ON-ONE COMMUNICATION

1. Immediately focus on the child.

Engaging the child immediately will reduce the probability that a parent will respond for the child and will help the child recognize that you are interested in her or him. Bring yourself to the child's eye level and make eye contact. A good way to start communicating is to ask what kind of experiences the child has had with medicines. If you get a positive response and the child starts a discussion, first address the topics that the child raises. For example, for a preschool child, the taste and the way the medicine is taken, e.g., swallowing difficulties may be the most important things. You should respect that and address the child's concerns even if at the end of the meeting that has been the only thing that you discussed.

Remember that the child can also be asked to find solutions. For example, in a Finnish study one child said that she learned to swallow tablets by swallowing blueberries.[53] If you get any response from the child it is a MUST to react to it, to answer the child's questions, and to encourage the child to be active in future communications with health care professionals.

2. Attempt to communicate at the child's developmental level.

Here are developmentally different responses to the same question, "What makes a cold go away?" from three children, ages 6, 8, and 10 years.[71] The 6-year-old and 8-year-old both replied, "A medicine." The 10-year-old said, "By taking the right medication from your doctor." When asked, "What kind of medicine?" the 6-year-old replied, "Medicine that helps you." The 8-year-old replied, "Tylenol, Dimetapp." The next question was, "How does that help?" The 6-year-old responded, "It takes the coughing away so you won't have a cold anymore." The 8-year-old said, "It helps fight the germs away." The 10-year-old replied, "If you take it and it goes in your system and it clears away the fluids and stuff that is in your body, like the mucus in your nose or something when it is stuffed up."

Although there is a general correlation with age, children develop at different rates that vary with the subject. The skills may be present but not applied within a content area, or a child may appear more advanced during a transitional phase. For example, another 8-year-old exhibited formal operational thinking when asked how a medicine would help cancer: "Well, the medicine kind of helps your immune system and white blood cells and from what I've heard kind of sterilizes the germs."

For a child in the preoperational stage with otitis media, you might say, "This medicine will go into your body to make your ear feel better. It will only work if you take it three times every day. Your mom will help you to know when to take the medicine. Be sure to use up all the medicine, even if your ear feels better." For a child in the concrete operational stage, you might say, "This medicine will go into your body to help fight off the germs that are causing the infection in your ear. The medicine will only work if you take it three times a day until (date). If you don't take it that way, your ear infection is likely to come back. So keep taking it even if you feel better. Work with your mom so you both know you have taken the medicine at the right time." For a child in the formal operational stage, you might say, "This medicine goes into your system to help your immune system fight off the bacteria that are causing your ear infection. The medical name for your ear infection is otitis media. The medicine used to fight the bacteria is an antibiotic. Its name is (name). What time do you usually get up? You must take this antibiotic every eight hours, that is, three times a day at (times) for the next ten days. If you don't, the bacteria may not all be killed and your ear infection can return. Keep taking it until it is all gone, even if you think your ear infection is cured. Let's look at the label together. What does it say? What time will you be taking it? What would you do if you miss a dose?"

3. Ask open-ended questions rather than those requiring only a "yes" or "no" response.

Ask follow-up questions to make sure the child understands and have the child repeat what you said. A child may parrot back a correct response or read the label correctly without real understanding.

4. Use simple declarative sentences for all children.

This is good advice when talking to adults as well. The goal is not to empower the child with total responsibility but to build a partnership between parent and child, to work with the parent to begin to grant autonomy coupled with proper patient education and information. Modeling an appropriate communication style will help the parent continue communicating with the child about medicines and other health issues and to grant appropriate autonomy.

5. Ask children to ask you questions.

Be a medicines educator. Try to empower the child to feel comfortable asking you questions about his or her health problem, the particular medicine, or medicines in general. Tell what kind of questions are important to ask, such as what is this medicine for, how much do I take it, for how long do I take it, how do I know it works and what should I do if I have side-effects or other problems.

6. Augment oral communications with written material.

Average adults only recall about 30% of what they are told by a doctor. You should not expect more from children. Written materials can be reviewed at home after the hospital, clinic, or pharmacy visit. Written materials should be tailored to the child's stage of cognitive development, focus on action-oriented tasks, and be clinically sound[72] (Table 15-2). Well-designed medicine leaflets can be a useful tool for pharmacists when communicating with children about their treatment.[73] An experimental pilot study assessing children's understanding of how to take an antiepileptic medicine revealed that children presented with an age-appropriate medication leaflet had a better understanding of the indication and frequency of administration of the medicine compared to children presented with a standard leaflet.[74] They also were more likely to find the leaflet easy to read and understand.

TABLE 15-1: RECOMMENDATIONS FOR DEVELOPING MEDICATION LEAFLETS FOR CHILDREN[72,73]

INFORMATION

Contains accurate, valid and up to date information on the topic of the leaflet

Information is at an appropriate depth and breadth to address the issue. It contains information on:

- what the medication is for
- how to administer
- common side effects
- what to do if dose is missed
- what to have the child tell the caregiver and /or
- when the parent should call the physician

Can also recommend additional reputable resources for patients to acquire more information

MESSAGES

Contains messages that are action-oriented, addressing what to do not just what to know

Medical jargon is avoided and replaced with lay-terms

MATERIALS

Contains materials that are not too busy (does not affect readability)

An appropriate font size is used to enhance readability for intended population

The mix of written text and graphics is appropriate for the child's age

The graphics reinforce the corresponding text

The reading level is appropriate for the intended audience

ORGANIZATION

Leaflet is organized in such a manner as to promote understanding of the topic

7. Give the children tasks.

Have the child put a colored sticker on the medicine so the child will know it's hers or his at home. For antibiotics, a calendar can be given to the child with times and dates to be taken noted. The child can be asked to cross off each dose and to bring the calendar to the next visit. The date for a follow-up visit can also be on the calendar. The child could be given the task of reminding mother in the morning and in the evening to give the child the medicine. The child might be told to eat something, e.g., some bread, before taking the tablet. By committing children to such tasks and giving them a feeling of ownership, potential problems, e.g., a bad taste, may not be important.

In addition to parents and health professionals, an innovative school-based program has shown that fellow students can be medicine educators of their peers and parents. In 2003–04, a student peer-taught program, whose goal was to decrease antibiotic use for colds and flu, but also included information on basic medicine use, was implemented in one school district (21 schools) in the capital of Moldova, with a second school district (20 schools) serving as the control. Students (12–13 years old) and adults most responsible for the family's health care completed surveys pre-post intervention asking about the incidence of colds and flu during the past winter, treatment, beliefs about cause, and usefulness of antibiotics. In addition to peer-taught sessions in school, the program included parents' meetings, a booklet, a vignette video, newsletters, a poster, and a poster contest. The intervention was successful. The relative reported use of antibiotics for colds and flu dropped from 50.5% to 37.6% for intervention students and from 72.5% to 38.3% for intervention adults. All relative responses related to beliefs about the cause of colds and flu and the usefulness of antibiotics to treat them changed in a positive direction.[75]

The success of this student-taught program supported the World Health Organizations' (WHO) efforts to decrease inappropriate antibiotic use. WHO supported the 2004 Second International Conference on Improving Use of Medicines' (ICIUM) recommendation "...children can be effective change agents in improving community medicine use. Countries should consider school-based educational programs that involve children as a way for key messages to reach parents."

But how old do the children have to be to be medicine use educators? It appears that school children as young as seven years can do it. In 2006–07, 21 kindergartens in Tiraspol and Briceni in Moldova presented educational interactive performances to educate their audiences about unnecessary antibiotic use for colds and flu.[76,77] A questionnaire given to the children's parents had indicated that 72% of the children had had a cold or flu the previous winter, and 76% of them had been given an antibiotic, with 69% obtained via a doctor's prescription.

After holding focus groups with ministers of health, educators, and parents of kindergartners, the schools independently prepared their presentations. Involved were 85 teachers, 54 health care workers, 1200 family members and community leaders, and 548 children.

The kindergarten children presented the primary message in various entertaining ways with some adult participation. Follow-up workshops concluded that the "edutainment" was successful, that learning can be fun, and that children can serve as conduits to carry important health messages. Attendees will never forget the message, "Don't take antibiotics for colds and flu."

CHILDREN WITH SPECIAL NEEDS

Chronically ill children need special attention. Many, e.g., children with asthma, are responsible for taking their own medicines.[7,78] Older children in large families and urban children also may have more autonomy at an earlier age than other children.

Illustrated materials are particularly important for those chronically-ill children who use devices such as inhalers, patches, or syringes to take their medicines. The children can demonstrate their proper use.

MEDICINE EDUCATION IN SCHOOLS

Considering the pervasiveness of medicines in society, it is surprising that school health education relative to medicines, has been almost completely restricted to prevention of poisoning among young children and prevention of abusable substance use among older children. It is most certainly possible to begin to educate children about medicines as early as preschool as recommended by the United States Pharmacopeia and American School Health Association.[72]

The USP assembled an international panel of health professionals and educators. This panel developed a USP Position Paper which became known as "the golden rule" as it was distributed on a yellow plastic ruler imprinted with "Ten Guiding Principles for Teaching Children and Adolescents about Medicine."[2] (See Table 15-1.) In addition to the American School Health Association, these Principles were adopted by the American Academy of Pediatrics and distributed in other countries such as Moldova, Sweden, and Ireland.[77,79,80]

To become active participants in their own medication, children need to learn knowledge and skills about rational medicine use. The underlying ideology of empowerment is thus present. In the context of medicine education, the empowerment approach would mean first, giving sufficient information about medicines, e.g., what should be known before taking medicines; second, teaching the skills needed to use medicines, e.g., the steps needed for taking medicines rationally, or what to do to avoid possible adverse reactions; and third, facilitating active involvement in discussions concerning the child's own medicines with health care professionals, e.g., by teaching the right questions to be asked. This kind of approach would build up the skills and competencies needed for children to gradually take more responsibility over their own medicines.

In practice, after selecting a target grade, your first task is to learn what these children already know, do, and want to know about medicines. The second task is to set out learning objectives, a task that involves clarifying what you think these children should know. Children's interest in medicines at different ages has been studied. It was found that children are quite similar in various countries in their desires for information about medicines, and that children are eager to learn about medicines.[52,81]

As for what to teach children of different ages, the USP *Guide to Developing and Evaluating Medicine Education Programs for Children and Adolescents*[72] is helpful. It presents 10 Key Behaviors for taking medicines and links them to specific behaviors for children by their ages from 3–12 years. It also includes lists of what children said they want to know about medicines at different ages.

After deciding what to teach, the third task is to prepare a teaching plan. For example, for 3rd grade children (about 8-years-old), you might decide that you want to address attributes of medicines that are unrelated to medicine efficacy such as color, taste, size, dose form, cost, and name. Examples can be brought to the class. To illustrate that the same medicine can be different colors, two tablets of different colors that are bioequivalent can be shown along with two M&Ms that are different colors. The children understand that the M&Ms have the same "active" ingredient inside, and the analogy can be made with the tablets. Labels can be read to teach that the same medicine can have different names and may also vary in cost.

For older children, you may want to develop a lesson about antibiotics and the importance of completing the course, with the lesson including the differences between viruses and bacteria. Or read patient information leaflets with the children and try to find ways to avoid side effects that children could try at home. This could be as easy as taking an antibiotic with food; however, the main point is that the children themselves find such ideas and have an opportunity to try them in practice. Children from the early grades can role-play going to a pharmacy where they first decide on some important questions that can be asked from a pharmacist, and then act as pharmacist and customer.

Some particular points that you may want to make include how to understand and counteract media promotion of medicines and understand that legal drugs may be as dangerous as illegal drugs and should not be taken without restraint. Also counterfeit medicines may be discussed and stressed that medicines should always be bought from a legal pharmacy and how legal medicines can be recognized. However, it is important that the children understand that even though every medicine has its side-effects, everyone must sometimes use medicines and that they are almost always safe to use when used as instructed. Studies have found that most school age children have a healthy respect for (and sometimes fear of) medicines. To induce fear of using them is definitely not a goal of medicine education.

In practice, the empowerment approach is reflected in the way the educator addresses children. If you genuinely want to involve children, you should appreciate their competence and give them power even during classes. You will find that the children have more autonomy and competence than adults usually expect! Find out what the children know, do, and want to know regarding medicines before you start telling them what you think they should know.

ADOLESCENTS

Some recommendations regarding communicating with adolescents can be made. Adolescents need privacy, and they need to know that their communications are confidential. Adolescents need to talk with adults who are absolutely comfortable talking with them about any subject, including abortion, acne, birth control, sexuality, steroids, and STDs (including HIV+ and AIDS). This must be done in a completely non-judgmental way and without letting the adolescent perceive that you find his or her beliefs foolish, irrational, or amusing. Adolescents have a great deal of misinformation about how their bodies work and how they should be maintained. Many adolescents are distrustful of information provided by older persons. If you cannot be completely comfortable when talking with adolescents, you can at least provide appropriate written materials and referrals.

When communicating with adolescents, you should remember that they may be embarrassed very easily—even when discussing very common medicines, like painkillers. This is why you should explain carefully that the questions you ask are necessary to help you choose the correct medicine. Furthermore, remember that the adolescent might be alone in the pharmacy for the first time and might not know how to behave.

There are some typical features of cognitive development that may affect the counseling situation: the invincibility fable, the personal fable, and the imaginary audience.[82] The invincibility fable means that an adolescent may feel that she or he never will be harmed, and consequently may take all kinds of risks, falsely secure in the belief in his or her own immunity. This explains a lot of teen risk taking. Such risk taking may be, e.g., taking medicines with alcohol. The personal fable means that an adolescent may imagine his or her own life and feelings as unique. For example, a teen may complain to his or her mother, "Mom, you don't know what it is like to be in love!" The imaginary audience means that adolescent typically fantasizes about how others react to his or her appearance and behavior. Adolescents may feel that everyone around them is just as concerned with, and as critical of their actions and appearance, as the adolescents themselves. This explains why a small pimple may seem catastrophic to a teenager.

Another concern is medicine sharing and taking medicines belonging to a parent or other relative without their permission. If adolescents have had a grounded medicines education, they will understand when sharing is dangerous, e.g., sharing a tranquilizer, and when it is probably not, e.g., sharing an acetaminophen tablet. As for taking someone's medicine without permission, i.e., stealing, such behavior should also be addressed in medicines education long before the child reaches adolescence.

SUMMARY

This chapter has sought to provide health professionals and health educators with the tools necessary to both plan medicine education programs for children and to communicate with children when counseling them about their own medicines. For those who are further interested in multicultural perspectives on children and medicines, a book *Children, Medicines, and Culture* is recommended.[83]

REFERENCES

1. Kalnins, I., McQueen, D., Backett, K., Curtice, L., & Currie, C. (1992). Children, empowerment and health promotion: some new directions in research and practice. *Health Promot Int* 7:53–9.

2. Bush, P.J., Ozias, J.M., Walson, P.D., & Ward, R.M. (1999). Ten guiding principles for teaching children and adolescents about medicines. US Pharmacopeia. *Clin Ther* 21:1280–4.

3. Croom, A., Wiebe, D.J., Berg, C.A., Lindsay, R., Donaldson, D., Foster, C., Murray, M., & Swinyard, M.T. (2011). Adolescent and parent perceptions of patient-centered communication while managing type 1 diabetes. *J Pediatr Psychol* 36:206–15.

4. International Pharmaceutical Federation. (2001). *FIP Statement of Principle. The pharmacist's responsibility and role in teaching children and adolescents about medicines.* http://www.fip.org/www2/uploads/database_file.php?id=180&table_id=

5. Britten, N. & Weiss M. (2004). What is concordance? In Bond, C. (Ed.). *Concordance*. London: Pharmaceutical Press, 9–28.

6. McKinnon, J. (2014). Pursuing concordance: Moving away from paternalism. *Br J Nurs.* 23:677–84

7. Iannotti, R.J. & Bush, P.J. (1992). The development of autonomy in children's health behaviors. In Susman, E.J., Feagans, L.V., & Ray, W. (Eds.). *Emotion, cognition, health, and development in children and adolescents: A two-way street.* Hillsdale, NJ: Lawrence Erlbaum, 53–74.

8. Halim, M., Vincent, H., Saini, Hämeen-Anttila, K., Vainio, K., & Moles, R. (2010). Validating the Children's Medicine Use Questionnaire (CMUQ) in Australia. *Pharm World Sci* 32:81–9.

9. Hämeen-Anttila, K. (2006). *Education before medication. Empowering children as medicine users.* Kuopio University Publications A. Pharmaceutical Sciences 89. University of Kuopio, Kuopio. (Academic dissertation).

10. Piaget, J. (1932). *The moral judgement of the child.* Gabain, M., trans. New York: Harcourt, Brace, World.

11. Bush, P.J. & Davidson, F.R. (1982). Medicines and "drugs": what do children think? *Health Educ Q* 9:113–28.

12. HLS-EU consortium. *Comparative report of health literacy in eight EU member states.* The European health literacy survey HLS-EU 2012 (www.health-literacy.eu)

13. United Nations Economic and Social Council (ECOSOC). (2010). Health literacy and the Millennium Development Goals: United Nations Economic and Social Council (ECOSOC) regional meeting background paper (abstracted). *J Health Commun* 15 Suppl 2:211–23.

14. White, F. (2013). The imperative of public health education: A global perspective. *Med Princ Pract* 22:515–529.

15. Bibace, R., & Walsh, M.E. (1980). Development of children's concepts of illness. *Pediatrics* 66:913–7.

16. Burbach, D.J., & Peterson, L. (1986). Children's concepts of physical illness: a review and critique of the cognitive developmental literature. *Health Psychol* 5:307–25.

17. Perrin, E. & Gerrity, S. (1981). There's a demon in your belly. *Pediatrics* 57:841–9.

18. Fishbein, M. & Ajzen, I. (1975). *Belief, attitude, intention, and behavior: An introduction to theory and research.* Reading, MA: Addison-Wesley.

19. Bandura, A. (1986). *Social foundations of thought and action: A social cognitive theory.* Englewood Cliffs, NJ: Prentice-Hall.

20. Vallerand, R.J. (1999). A hierarchical model of intrinsic and extrinsic motivation. In: Zanna, A. Advances in experimental social psychology. New York: Academic Press, 271–360.

21. Deci, E.L. & Ryan, R.M. (2008). Self-determination theory: A macrotheory of human motivation, development, and health. *Can Psychol* 49:182–85.

22. Bush, P.J. & Iannotti, R.J. (1990). A children's health belief model. *Med Care* 28:69–86.

23. Gochman, D.S. (1982). Labels, systems and motives: some perspectives for future research and programs. *Health Educ Q* 9:167–74.

24. Bush, P.J. & Iannotti, R.J. (1988). The origins and stability of children's health beliefs relative to medicine use. *Soc Sci Med* 27:345–55.

25. Kogan, M.D., Pappas, G., Yu, S.M., & Kotelchuk, M. (1994). Over-the-counter medication use among U.S. preschooll-age children. *JAMA* 272:1025–30.

26. Bush, P.J., Iannotti, R.J., & Davidson, F.R. (1985). A longitudinal study of children and medicines. In Breimer, D.D., & Speiser, P. (Eds.). *Topics in pharmaceutical sciences*. Amsterdam, NY: Elsevier Science Publishers, 391–403.

27. Hansen, E.H., Holstein, B.E., Due, P., & Currie, C.E. (2003). International survey of self-reported medicine use among adolescents. *The Ann Pharmacother* 37:361–6.

28. Stoelben, S., Krappweis, J., Rossler, G., & Kirch, W. (2000). Adolescents' drug use and drug knowledge. *Eur J Pediatr* 159:608–14.

29. Holstein, B.E., Hansen, E.H., Due, P., & Almarsdottir, A.B. (2003). Self-reported medicine use among 11- to 15-year-old girls and boys in Denmark 1988–1998. *Scand J Public Health* 31:334–41.

30. Dengler, R. & Roberts, H. (1996). Adolescents' use of prescribed and over-the-counter preparations. *J Pub Health Med* 18:437–42.

31. Westerlund, M., Brånstad, J.O., & Westerlund, T. (2008). Medicine-taking behavior and drug-related problems in adolescents of a Swedish high school. *Pharm World Sci* 30:243–250.

32. Carrasco-Garrido, P., Jimenez-Garcia, R., Barrera, V.H., de Andres, A.L., & de Miguel, A.G. (2009). Medication consumption in the Spanish paediatric population: related factors and time trend, 1993–2003. *Br J Clin Pharmacol* 68:455–461.

33. Du, Y. & Knopf, H. (2009). Self-medication among children and adolescents in Germany: results of the National Health Survey for Children and Adolescents (KiGGS). *Br J Clin Pharmacol* 68:599–608.

34. Ylinen, S., Hämeen-Anttila, K., Sepponen, K., Kettis Lindblad, Å., & Ahonen, R. (2010). The use of prescription medicines and self medication among Finnish children under 12 years. *Pharmacoepidemiol Drug Saf* 19:1000–1008.

35. Moraes, A.C., Delaporte, T.R., Molena-Fernandes, C.A., & Falcao, M.C. (2011). Factors associated with medicine use and self medication are different in adolescents. *Clinics (Sao Paulo)* 66:1149–1155.

36. Oliveira, E.A., Bertoldi, A.D., Domingues, M.R., Santos, I.S., & Barros, A.J. (2012). Factors associated to medicine use among children from the 2004 Pelotas Birth Cohort (Brazil). *Rev Saude Publica* 46:487–96.

37. Hämeen-Anttila, K., Lindell-Osuagwu, L., Sepponen, K., Vainio, K., Halonen, P., & Ahonen, R. (2010). Factors associated with medicine use among Finnish children under 12 years. *Pharmacoepidemiol Drug Saf* 19: 400–407.

38. Chambers, C.T., Reid, G.J., McGrath, P.J., & Finley, A. (1997). Self-administration of over-the-counter medication for pain among adolescents. *Arch Pediatr Adolesc Med* 151:449–55.

39. Holstein, B.E. & Hansen, E.H. (2005). Self-reported medicine use among adolescents from ethnic minority groups. *Eur J Clin Pharmacol* 61:69–70.

40. Holstein, B,E., Hansen, E.H., & Due, P. (2004). Social class variation in medicine use among adolescents. *Eur J Public Health* 14:49–52.

41. Sanz, E.J., Bush, P.J., & Garcia, M. Medicines at home: The contents of medicine cabinets in eight countries. In Bush, P.J., Trakas, O.J., Sanz, E.J., Wirsing, R., Vaskilampi, T., & Prout, A. (Eds.), *Children, medicines, and culture.* Binghamton, NY: Pharmaceutical Products Press, 77–104.

42. Trakas, D.J. & Sanz, E. (Eds.). (1996). *Childhood and medicine use in a cross-cultural perspective: A European concerted action.* Brussels: European Commission Report EUR 16646 EN.

43. Sloand, E,D. & Vessey, J.A. (2001). Self-medication with common household medicines by young adolescents. *Issues Compr Pediatr Nurs* 24:57–67.

44. Bozoni, K., Kalmanti, M., & Koukouli, S. (2006). Perception and knowledge of medicines of primary schoolchildren: the influence of age and socioeconomic status. *Eur J Pediatr* 165:42–9.

45. Jones, B.A., Fullwood, H., & Hawthorn, M. (2012). Preventing prescription drug abuse in adolescence. *Prev Res* 19:13–16.

46. McCabe, S.E. & Boyd, C.J. (2012). Do motives matter? Nonmedical use of prescription medications among adolescents. *Prev Res* 10–12.

47. Darnell, A.J. & Emshoff, J.G. (2008). *Findings from the evaluation of the D.A.R.E. prescription and over-the-counter drug curriculum.* Emstar Research, Inc. Atlanta, Georgia, USA.

48. Almarsdottir, A.B. & Zimmer, C. (1998). Children's knowledge about medicines. *Child: Glob J Child Res* 5:265–81.

49. Dawood, O.T., Ibrahim, M.I.M., & Abdullah, A.C. (2011). Factors influencing children's knowledge and attitudes toward medicines in Malaysia. *J Mens Health* 8:288–29.

50. Sharaideh, R., Wazaify, M., Albsoul-Younes, A.M. (2013). Knowledge and attitude of school children in Amman/Jordan toward the appropriate use of medicines: A cross-sectional study. *Saudi Pharm J* 21: 25–33.

51. Darmanin Ellul, R., Cordina, M., Buhagiar, A., Fenech, A., & Mifsud, J. (2008). Knowledge and sources of information about medicines among adolescents in Malta. *Pharm Pract* 6:178–186.

52. Menacker, F., Aramburuzabala, P., Minian, N., Bush, P.J., & Bibace, R. (1999). Children and medicines: what they want to know and how they want to learn. *J Soc Adm Pharm* 16:38–52.

53. Hämeen-Anttila, K., Juvonen, M., Ahonen, R., Bush, P.J., & Airaksinen, M. (2006). How well can children understand medicine related topics? *Patient Educ Couns* 60:171–8.

54. Almarsdottir, A.B., Hartzema, A.G., Bush, P.J., Simpson, K.N., & Zimmer, C. (1997). Children's attitudes and beliefs about illness and medicines: triangulation of open-ended and semi-structured interviews. *J Soc Adm Pharm* 14:26–41.

55. Pradel, F.G., Hartzema, A.G., & Bush, P.J. (2001). Asthma self-management: The perspective of children. *Patient Educ Couns* 45:199–209.

56. Aramburuzabala, P., Garcia, M., Polaino, A., & Sanz, E. (1996). Medicine use, behaviour and children's perceptions of medicines and health care in Madrid and Tenerife (Spain). In Trakas, D. & Sanz E. (Eds.), *Childhood and medicine use in a cross-cultural perspective: A European concerted action.* Brussels: European Commission Report EUR 16646 EN, 245–68.

57. Kärkkäinen, S., Hämeen-Anttila, K., Vainio, K., Kontturi, S., Patrikainen, R., & Keinonen, T. (2014). Fourth graders' perceptions about medicines and medicine use. *Health Educ* 114: 43–57.

58. Whatley, B., Williams, S.E., Gard, P.R., & MacAdam, A.B. (2012). Healthy children's identification and risk perception of medicines in England. *Res Social Adm Pharm* 8: 478–483.

59. Garcia, M., Sanz, E., Aramburuzabala, P., Almarsdottir, A.B. (1996). Concepts of adverse drug reactions among children in eight countries. In Bush, P.J., Trakas, D.J., Sanz, E., Wirsing, R.L., Vaskilampi, T., & Prout, A. (Eds.), *Children, medicines, and culture.* New York: Pharmaceutical Products Press, 193–208.

60. Vaskilampi, T., Kalpio, O., Ahonen, R., & Hallia, O. (1996). Finnish study on medicine use, health behaviour and perceptions of medicines and health care. In Trakas, D. & Sanz, E. (Eds.), *Childhood and medicine use in a cross-cultural perspective: A European concerted action*. Brussels: European Commission Report EUR 16646 EN, 191–219.

61. Almarsdottir, A.B., Aramburuzabala, P., Garcia, M., & Sanz, E.J. (1996). Children's perceived benefit of medicines in Chapel Hill, Madrid, and Tenerife. In Bush, P.J., Trakas, D.J., Sanz, E.J., Wirsing, R., Vaskilampi, T., & Prout, A. (Eds.), *Children, medicines, and culture*. Binghamton, NY: Pharmaceutical Products Press, 127-153.

62. Ramzan, S., Hansen, E.H., Nørgaard, L.S., Arevalo, L.C., & Jacobsen, R. (2014). Validation of the Danish translation of the   Medicine Knowledge Questionnaire among elementary school children. *Res Social Adm Pharm* (article in press).

63. Rudolf, M.C., Alario, A.J., Youth, B., & Riggs, S. (1993). Self-medication in childhood: observations at a residential summer camp. *Pediatrics* 91:1182–4.

64. Daniel, K.L., Honein, M.A., & Moore, C.A. (2003). Sharing prescription medication among teenage girls: Potential danger to unplanned/undiagnosed pregnancies. *Pediatrics* 111:1167–70.

65. Holstein, B.E., Andersen, A., Krolner, R., Due,P., & Hansen, E.H. (2008). Young adolescents' use of medicine for headache: Sources of supply, availability and accessibility at home. *Pharmacoepidemiol Drug Saf* 17:406–410.

66. Pantell, R.H. & Lewis, C.C. (1986). Physician communication with pediatric patients: a theoretical and empirical analysis. *Adv Develop Behav Pediatrics* 7:65–119.

67. Tates, K., Meeuwesen, L., Bensing, J., & Elbers, E. (2002). Joking or decision-making? Affective and instrumental behaviour in doctor-parent-child communication. *Psychol Health* 17:281–95.

68. Iannotti, R.J. & Bush, P.J. (1992). Toward a developmental theory of compliance. In Krasnegor, N., Epstein, S., Johnson, S., & Yaffe S. (Eds.), *Developmental aspects of health compliance behavior*. Hillsdale, NJ: Lawrence Erlbaum, 59–76.

69. Sanz, E. (2003). Concordance and children's use of medicines. *BMJ* 327:858–60.

70. Perrin, E.C. & Perrin, J.M. (1983). Clinicians' assessments of children's understanding of illness. *Am J Dis Child* 137:874–8.

71. O'Brien, R.W. & Bush, P.J. (1993). Helping children learn how to use medicines. *Office Nurse* 6(3):14–9.

72. United States Pharmacopeia and American School Health Association. (1999). *Guide to developing and evaluating medicine education programs and materials for children and adolescents.* United States Pharmacopeial Convention. Rockville, MD, USA. http://www.usp.org/pdf/EN/consumers/guide.pdf

73. Morgan, J.A., Huynh, D., & Pradel, F.G. (2011). *Developing medicine information leaflets for children.* 20th Pediatric Pharmacy Conference and Annual meeting (PPAG), Memphis, TN, March 16, 2011. Poster.

74. Tromm, N.E., Biggs, J.M., Dario, A., Heavner, K., Pradel, F.G., & Morgan, J.A. (2014). *Assessment of the understanding of pediatric oriented medication education materials versus standard available education materials.* 23rd Annual PPAG Meeting, Nashville, TN, May 2, 2014. Poster

75. Cebotarenco, N. & Bush, P.J. (2007). Reducing antibiotics for colds and flu: A student taught program. *Health Educ Res* 23:137–145.

76. Bush, P.J. (2007). Can kindergartners help decrease inappropriate antibiotic use? *J Sch Health* 77:650–650.

77. Bush, P.J. & Cebotarenco, N. (2010). It's time children learned about medicines. *J Pharm Health Serv* Res 1:1–6.

78. Ayala, G.X., Yeatts, K., & Carpenter, D.M. (2009). Factors associated with asthma management self-efficacy among 7th and 8th grade students. *J Pediatr Psychol* 34:862–8.

79. Bush, P.J. (2005). *Children, youth & medicines.* KILEN. Stockholm, Sweden. 31 May–3 June.

80. Bush, P.J. (2005). *Let's teach children about medicines.* Irish Centre for Continuing Education, Dublin, Ireland, 15 Oct, 2005.

81. Hämeen-Anttila, K., Juvonen, M., Ahonen, R., Bush, P.J., & Airaksinen, M. (2005). What schoolchildren should be taught about medicines: combined opinions of children and teachers. *Health Educ* 105:424–436.

82. Stassen, B.K. (1998). *The developing person through the life span.* New York: Worth.

83. Bush, P.J., Trakas, D.J., Sanz, E.J., Wirsing, R.L., Vaskilampi, T., & Prout, A. (Eds.). (1996). *Children, Medicines, and Culture.* Binghamton, NY, Pharmaceutical Products Press.

CHAPTER 16

MEDICATION USE AMONG OLDER ADULTS

Denise L. Orwig, PhD, Rasheeda Johnson, Emma Sheldon Gentry, Linda Gore Martin, PharmD, MBA, BCPS, Nicole J. Brandt, PharmD, MBA, CGP, BCPP

LEARNING OBJECTIVES:

1. Identify current population trends and needs of older adults in the United States.
2. Describe the nature and extent of prescription and non-prescription medication use among older adults.
3. Summarize the different physical, cognitive, economic, and social factors associated with aging.
4. Compare and contrast the different types of living environments for older adults.
5. Evaluate the psychosocial considerations associated with providing optimal medication management to older adults.

KEY TERMS

Adverse Drug Events (ADEs)

Assisted Living

Board and Care Homes

Communication

Complementary and alternative medicine (CAM)

Concordance

Continuing Care Retirement Communities (CCRCs)

Health literacy

Independent Housing Arrangements

Long-term care

Medicaid

Medicare

Medication counseling

Medication nonadherence

Medication Therapy Management (MTM)

Nursing Homes

Pharmacodynamics

Pharmacokinetics

INTRODUCTION

The topic of aging in humans has become increasingly important, especially as the number of older adults continues to increase. By 2050, the number of Americans aged 65 and older will more than double to 88 million, comprising roughly 20% of the United States population.[1,2] In addition to the increase in both number and proportion of people over age 65, people over age 85 (and especially those over age 100) will comprise the fastest growing group. In 1900, the average life expectancy was 47 years and it had increased to a little more than 68 in 1950. By 2010, humans could expect to live 78 years. Extraordinary breakthroughs in healthcare were largely responsible for the increase in average life expectancy, which included decreased death rates of infants and children and eradicated infectious diseases through better sanitation, vaccinations, and antibiotics. Although the changes in prevention of death from chronic diseases have not had such a large numerical impact, it is anticipated that the average life expectancy will reach 80 years by 2050.

With a larger proportion of the population living longer, the issue of health in older adults becomes more relevant. The last years of life are often accompanied by illness. At least 85–90% of persons aged 65 and over have at least one chronic illness, 60% have two or more, a third have three or more, and 25% have four or more.[3] The cost of providing healthcare for an older American is three to five times greater than the cost for someone younger than 65.[1,4] By 2030, the projected US healthcare spending will increase by 25% due to the aging of the population unless improving and preserving the health of older adults is more actively addressed.[5]

There is great variability among people as they age (individually, and by gender and ethnicity), both with respect to the age at which age-related changes are noticed and also the rate at which these changes occur. Each individual is subjected to a unique combination of factors that affect aging. It is subsequently difficult to define an age at which a person becomes "elderly." There are different types of aging including chronological age, functional age, cosmetic age, and economic age. Many of the biological age changes that occur do not become significant until after age 50, although age 65 is commonly used to define older adults since the Social Security Administration began using it in 1935 to denote retirement age.[6] There have been further classifications of older adults referring to 65–74 as "young old," 75–84 as "middle old" or "old old," and 85 plus as the "oldest old."[7]

The shift in demographics, namely a maturing society living longer with more heterogeneity, is creating an undeniable imperative regarding the healthcare practitioner's knowledge of medication therapy in the older patient. This knowledge is especially important since older adults have a higher rate of medication use compared to the general population. The healthcare delivery system will be challenged to meet the needs of the growing aging population that will incur problems of comorbid diseases, dependency, and functional loss. The healthcare delivery system needs to focus on preventing hospitalizations and premature mortality, reducing disease morbidity, minimizing institutionalization and inappropriate utilization of services, and maximizing the appropriate use of medications. Since medications are a significant part of the healthcare for older adults, the unique aspects of medication use among older adults will be the topic of the remainder of this chapter. Pharmacists need to be more proactive in improving the use of medications through reducing adverse drug events, identifying adherence issues, and ensuring appropriate therapeutic use and effect. In order to be successful in these endeavors, pharmacists and other healthcare providers should be aware of the biological, social, economic, and behavioral factors that can impact medication use.

MEDICATION USE

PRESCRIPTION AND OVER-THE-COUNTER MEDICATIONS

The most common health problems affecting older adults are often treated with medications, which provide valuable, if not lifesaving, therapy but also a risk of an adverse response. Persons 65 and older are the leading consumers of drugs, accounting for 34% of prescription medications and 50% of over-the-counter medications.[8–11] This is most likely due to increasing level of chronic disease conditions with age such that 85% of persons in this age group have at least one chronic illness and a third have three or more.[10] Roughly 28% of adults 65 and older take more than five medications per week,[12] and approximately 12% take 10 or more different medications, making polypharmacy a common problem among older adults.[13] The average older community dweller takes four medications concurrently.[14,15] Medication use is even more pronounced in the nursing home setting where on average residents are taking approximately nine medications on a daily basis.[16,17] As the average life expectancy increases so does the incidence of chronic diseases and the number of persons receiving long-term drug therapy. The continued growth of the older adult population means the burden on the healthcare system and society will also increase. There will be a greater number of people with multiple chronic conditions and with a diminished physiological reserve who are likely to be treated with medications.

The medications that are used most commonly by older adults are not surprising. The top three categories represent cardiovascular medicines (e.g., antihypertensives), central nervous system (CNS) agents (e.g., antidepressants), and treatments for musculoskeletal and joint diseases (e.g., non steroidal anti-inflammatory agents). Overall, there is no real difference in the number of prescription medicines taken by elderly men and women; however, they do differ in the therapeutic categories of medicines they take. In addition to using more diuretics and CNS medicines (hypnotics, anxiolytics, and antidepressants), women take more thyroid medication, drugs for immunosupression, and treatments for nutrition and blood disorders.[18]

The pharmacist needs to obtain a medication history and make sure that the older adult is asked about all medications including over-the-counter (OTC) products as well as herbal remedies. In addition to tobacco use, an index of suspicion needs to be maintained both for alcohol abuse and illicit drug use, which can confound diagnoses as well as the risks and benefits of medications. Targeted questions concerning medication use and "brown bag" assessments, where the patient brings in all medications, may help to identify potential problems.

ALCOHOL

Alcohol use, misuse and abuse among older individuals is a growing healthcare concern. Although less common when compared to younger adult populations, rates of alcohol use and abuse in the aging baby boomer population is a problem that is projected to increase likely due to a history of heavier drinking habits in this older cohort.[19] In the 2010 National Survey on Drug Use and Health (NSDUH), 38.2% of individuals over the age of 65 in the community consume alcohol daily, 7.6% of this population were "binge drinkers," and 1.6% were heavy drinkers.[20] Alcohol use in older adults has a more pronounced effect due to physiologic changes. This predisposes an older adult to greater adversities such as confusion or falls. Chronic abuse of alcohol can lead to numerous effects on the body such as liver damage, gastrointestinal bleeds, anemia, and dementia.

Alcohol has the potential to adversely interact with numerous prescribed medications, OTC medications and herbal remedies. Moreover, age-related pharmacodynamics and pharmacokinetic changes may increase the risk of such adverse alcohol-to-medication interactions.[21,22] Although some of the interactions occur mostly among people who drink heavily, many of the interactions can occur with smaller amounts of alcohol (e.g., light to moderate drinkers) due to decreases in cellular, organ, and body system reserves as a person ages.[22] The prevalence of alcohol and medication interactions among older adults who consume alcohol ranges from 19%–38%.[23-25] A recent survey noted that there are numerous medications that interact with alcohol and patients indicated that 48% of them did not receive any advice regarding an interaction of their medication with alcohol.[26] All of these reasons stress the importance of pharmacists educating the patient not only to the deleterious effects of alcohol but to the potential interactions. This is why it is vital for pharmacists to educate, screen and empower all patients but especially older adults who are at greater risk for adverse events.

OTHER DRUGS OF ABUSE

Illicit drug use describes the use and misuse of marijuana, cocaine, inhalants, hallucinogens, heroin, or any prescription-type psychotherapeutic drug use that is not clinically warranted.[27] Although drug misuse and abuse is less common in older adults, the fact that many older adults see more than one prescriber and often have family members who have prescriptions for or use abusable drugs, obtaining these medications can be relatively easy.

The combined 2002 and 2003 NSDUH data estimated that 1.8% of older adults used an illicit drug in the previous month prior to the survey, notably, marijuana (1.1%), prescription drug misuse (0.7%) and cocaine (0.2%).[28] Data from the 2103 NSDUH indicates that among adults aged 50 to 64, the rate of current illicit drug use increased from 2.7 % in 2002 to 6.0 % in 2013, with the highest increase among those who were 50–54.[29] Furthermore, use of any illicit drug is estimated to increase from 2.2% (1.6 million) to 3.1% (3.5 million) by 2020 and nonmedical use of prescription drugs (opioids, sedatives, tranquilizers, and stimulants) is projected to increase from 1.2% (911,000) to 2.4% (2.7 million).[30]

The implications of this drug abuse, increased health-related problems as the body ages, and drug interactions with prescribed medications are enormous. Studies have found that older patients are more motivated and likely to continue in treatment for substance abuse than younger patients, but treatment is often complicated by multiple chronic illnesses. Pharmacists can be the central healthcare professional to help manage these patients and their medication use.[31]

COMPLEMENTARY AND ALTERNATIVE MEDICINE

There are recent statistics that indicate that Americans are increasingly replacing prescription medications with not only vitamin and mineral supplements, but also with herbal and other natural products referred to as complementary and alternative medicine (CAM); thus, the use of CAM is receiving increasing attention in the medical community. It is estimated that 38%–53% of older adults in the United States use a variety of CAM.[32] In 2010, the most common reasons for CAM use were illness prevention or overall wellness (77%) and/or pain reduction (73%).[32] An estimated $20.5 billion were spent on herbal products, botanicals, and dietary supplements in 2004.[33] The rising popularity of alternative therapies may reflect attempts to augment formal medical care as well as the belief that "natural" preparations are safe.[34,35] Quite the contrary, the number of adverse events, drug interactions, and deaths involving these products have been on the rise.[36–40] In a recent survey on the use of herbal products among older adults, 21% were currently taking at least one herbal product or dietary supplement while the potential for adverse drug reactions was apparent in 19% of the users. A supplemental questionnaire to the 2002 National Health Interview Survey showed that the most commonly used herbal products reported by older adults were Echinacea, garlic, ginkgo biloba, ginseng, and saw palmetto.[41] Most patients are reluctant to share their use of CAM with their healthcare providers, with only 40% indicating they told their physician.[42,43] It is imperative for physicians and pharmacists to create a supportive environment for open communication to learn about CAM use and advise on possible interactions.

BIOLOGICAL ISSUES

AGE-RELATED PHYSIOLOGIC CHANGES

An important aspect of medication use among older adults is an increased physiological vulnerability to medications and an impaired ability to recover from drug-induced side effects. Even though humans age at different rates, they all have decreasing physiologic reserves over time. The series of physiologic alterations in the aging body affects how drugs produce their effects on the body (pharmacodynamics) and how a drug is absorbed, distributed, metabolized, and excreted from the body (pharmacokinetics). These changes affect renal, hepatic, gastrointestinal, pulmonary, cardiovascular, and neurological function.[44] This loss of function and reserve leads to both an increase in drug utilization (to treat disease and dysfunction) as well as the potential for increased adverse effects and intolerance. The inadequacy of homeostatic control mechanisms in older adults greatly increases the likelihood that an exaggerated response or drug interaction will assume clinical importance or require lower doses. There are additional biological changes with age that can also impact the appropriate use of medications, including hearing and vision changes as well as cognitive decline.

HEARING AND VISION LOSS

In 1990, approximately four million people in the United States had severe vision impairment. Vision impairment is the most common sensory deficit in the older population. The prevalence of vision impairment increases significantly with age (rates are from 1990 and per 1000); persons age 0–54 have a rate of 6.1, 55 and over 104, and 85 and over 216. Watson states that vision loss is the third major reason older adults need assistance with activities of daily living (ADLs) (after arthritis and cardiac disease).[45] Most of these persons are not blind and, therefore, can use devices and techniques to help them with medication use. The normal aging of the eye becomes apparent about age 45 when near and far vision is affected by the decreased ability to focus (presbyopia). Most older adults have similar acuity to younger adults under high contrast conditions, but have major decreases when illumination or contrast is decreased; this is especially important in glare conditions. Color discrimination, adaptation to dark, and field of vision (which depends on higher-order processing) decline with age. The major diseases that increase the loss of vision include cataracts, glaucoma, macular degeneration, and diabetic retinopathy. Persons with low vision need spacing between words more than those with normal vision and this may have important implications for providing medication literature.[46] Vision loss may eliminate the use of written material altogether and make medication labels difficult to read, particularly on a glossy surface.

Helzner found an overall prevalence of hearing loss of 59.9% in their cohort aged 73–84. White men had the highest rate of 64.9% followed by white women, black men, and black women (59.3, 58.1, and 55.0% respectively). Men (white or black) had the highest rate of high-frequency loss, experiencing a loss of 91.8% and 76.1%, respectively. Also, for each five-year increase in age, the prevalence rate of hearing loss doubled. Hearing loss has been associated with several systemic diseases, including cardiovascular and diabetes mellitus, as well as ototoxic drugs used for other disorders.[47] Hearing impairment could greatly impact the medication counseling process.

Since both hearing and vision loss involve changes at both the organ system level and within the nervous system, the association between hearing and vision loss and cognition has been investigated. A study by Anstey et al., found that decrease in vision over two years was positively associated with memory decline (but not verbal ability or processing speed) while hearing decline was not associated with any cognitive domain.[48]

COGNITION AND MEMORY

Medication management skills decrease with advancing age regardless of whether measurable cognitive decline exists. However, the concurrent existence of cognitive decline exacerbates the problem.[49] Aging causes a decline in short-term memory, particularly for information that is presented quickly and verbally. On average, the decline is gradual and slow until approximately age 60–70. Information about completely unfamiliar things also becomes much harder to remember with age. Declines in working memory, especially when the tasks have high levels of executive control are also seen with aging. However, Kramer et al. found that older adults have a better memory for previously identified objects, indicating that some memory processes are preserved or improved with age.[50] Decreased cognitive levels have been associated with an increased risk of hearing loss (23% for each standard deviation decrease in the modified Mini-Mental State Examination). A decline in hearing may affect understanding or the two may have a common vascular cause.[47]

Dramatic increases in the number of people with cognitive impairment will have a tremendous impact on the healthcare system and the need for supportive services, particularly when it comes to medication management.[51] With an increase in age also comes an increase in incidence and prevalence of Alzheimer's Disease (AD) and other dementias so that by 2050, there will be more than 14 million patients with AD.[52] In addition, depending on the definition, the prevalence of mild cognitive impairment (MCI) is 3% to 53%, with a reasonable estimate of 19% in persons over 75 years.[53] In 2000, AD and other dementias (of which AD is the most frequent) constituted the third most expensive health condition in the US, after heart disease and cancer.[54,55] The Alzheimer's Association and the National Institute on Aging estimate that current direct and indirect costs of caring for AD patients are at least $100 billion annually. Medicare costs for beneficiaries with AD, at $91 billion in 2005, are expected to increase 75%, to $160 billion in 2010. Medicaid expenditures on residential dementia care will increase 14%, from $21 billion in 2005 to $24 billion in 2010.[16]

A study by Maioli et al. found that although MCI has been considered prodromal to dementias, in a mean follow-up of 1.2 years (range 0.23–3.1), only 28.6% of the 52 patients converted to dementia (and 17.3% reverted to normal). Of those who converted, AD was diagnosed in 53.3%, with the remaining percentage due to other causes.[56] The differentiation between MCI related to pseudodementia (or reversible forms) is critical since many of these patients are experiencing medication-related impairment or disorders that can be treated (such as depression).

CHRONIC AND COMORBID DISEASE

As mentioned earlier, as people age they are more likely to experience acute illnesses and suffer from chronic conditions. The existence of more than one condition or comorbidity is common. Joyce and colleagues[57] examined the Medicare Current Beneficiary Surveys (MCBS) from 1992–1999 and Medicare Claims for individuals 65 years old and found that only a small % had no comorbidities. Less than 20% of 65-year-olds with hypertension or cancer did not have another comorbidity. Ninety percent of older adults with COPD or diabetes had at least one additional comorbid condition. Patients with coronary heart disease or stroke have comorbidities over 95% of the time. Hypertension, osteoarthritis, and heart disease are the most common comorbid diseases among older adults and of those with hypertension, at least 20% also have diabetes.

Many older adults do not remember all of their disorders unless prompted with a checklist or other method.[58] Wetzels et al. found that underreporting of health problems is frequent particularly in people without pain.[59] This underreporting may increase the chance that medications are also underreported (especially OTC or herbal products) or that patients with treatable conditions are not receiving medications. Knowledge and understanding of diseases has been associated with increased adherence. Beliefs, especially about the severity of disease (or when symptoms exist), are also important. Number of comorbidities is highly correlated with number of medications and complexity of drug regimen.

SOCIAL ISSUES

CULTURAL

The United States has always been a melting pot of cultures. For centuries the population was primarily of European descent, but today's culture represents a diversity of people from around the world. Increasing diversity brings possible disparities in healthcare that include access to quality healthcare, inappropriate or suboptimal treatments, and underutilization of preventive and specialty services. The Institute of Medicine (IOM) in 2002 issued a nearly 800-page report on disparities in healthcare related to cultural characteristics, which can be accessed at http://www.nap.edu/catalog.php?record_id=10260#toc.[60] All aspects of cultural differences are covered in this report, showing that disparities can occur between age groups, racial or ethnic groups, gender, socioeconomic groups, geographical locations (north versus south), or between urban and rural groups.

Despite recent progress, disparities persist in access to healthcare in the United States.[61-63] In particular, blacks are less likely to have regular sources of healthcare. They receive less preventive care, see physicians less often, visit fewer specialists, and receive services later in the course of many diseases than whites.[62,64-66] Minority elderly may be more likely to consider health conditions to be part of the normal aging process, which may inhibit appropriate health service utilization.[67-69] Disparities in medication use have been reported for some conditions (e.g., depression, diabetes, hypertension, hypercholesterolemia), with whites being more likely to receive treatment.[70] Even when similarities exist in rates of medication use among racial groups, the issue of appropriateness or quality of treatment is still not clear.

Recent emphasis in older adult research has been on the differences between the rural and urban resident. Rural older adults, however, are not homogenous; local cultures are often based on ethnicity.[71] Gesler et al. stated, in summarizing three rural studies, that, regardless of what belief is prevalent, health professionals must be aware of it in order to be culturally sensitive. For example, in a cultural context, rural residents have been shown to allow their religious beliefs to play a greater role in their health behavior. Pharmacists who are aware of these differences may be better equipped to establish rapport with the patient and to determine whether they are telling the provider what they think that person wants to hear as opposed to expressing their true feelings, beliefs, and symptoms.[72]

HEALTH LITERACY

An estimated 90 million Americans have low health literacy, defined by the IOM as "the degree to which individuals can obtain, process, and understand the basic health information and services they need to make appropriate health decisions."[73]

A systematic review of health literacy in the United States found an overall low health literacy rate of 26% and a marginal literacy rate of an additional 20%. The lower health literacy levels are associated with increasing age, ethnicity, and lower levels of education. Studies that had an average age over 50 showed a low literacy prevalence of 37.9%.[74] Wolf et al. found that older adults with significant deficits in health literacy had higher rates of hypertension, diabetes mellitus, heart failure and arthritis. They also had significantly lower physical and mental health functioning with increased limitations on activities.[75]

Factors in low literacy levels and the resultant adherence to medications may involve changes in cognition and memory in the older adults. Older adults have reduced processing resources (attention and working memory).[76] This change means that extra time should be spent on counseling to allow the older adult to comprehend the messages being presented about their medications. In order to maximize working memory capacity in older adults, unique education efforts should be designed to provide repeated information.

Other factors that may be associated with reduced health literacy in the older adult may be changes in vision and hearing. Decreased visual acuity reduces the ability to read prescription labels and to tell colors apart (especially yellows and greens). The decreased ability to see, in association with decreased hearing, can lead to errors in interpreting printed instructions, even if verbal instructions are also given.

Medication counseling may be impacted by the "cultural" aspects of hearing loss. A small study that interviewed groups of hard of hearing (some elderly) and deaf patients, found that deaf patients believe that physicians do not appreciate their full lives and have misconceptions about how to communicate with them. Because of the grammatical differences between American Sign Language and spoken English, the patients feel like the healthcare providers think they are stupid. The providers often also fail to maintain eye contact. This is especially a problem if the patient is trying to lip read, but the patient also feels left out if the contact is with an interpreter. The deaf would like more time and accommodations other than writing notes; this may be significant in older adults who often have problems writing due to vision loss or arthritis.

The hard of hearing did not have as strong of feelings as the deaf; but are often ashamed, frustrated, and in denial. Older adults with impaired hearing felt that providers did not understand how hard it was to communicate and thought that speaking louder would be helpful. However, the providers usually do not slow down or take any more time to determine whether or not the patient understood. The hard of hearing frequently have problems with staff and with automated phone systems.[77] Jacobson gave some advice on how to counsel hearing impaired patients: (a) Respect their intelligence, sensitivity and confidentiality; (b) Rephrase and clarify if the patient does not appear to understand; (3) Ask the patient about preferences using any assistive devices or interpreters; and (4) Arrange for a quiet area to decrease competing sounds.[78]

COMMUNICATION

With the aging population in the United States becoming more ethnically diverse, communication is going to become even more of a concern. Not only are there physical limitations such as decreased hearing and impaired vision, which can impede effective communication, but now there is the potential for language and cultural barriers. Communication issues in addition to all of the other issues discussed can ultimately decrease adherence to interventions such as medications. More attention has been given to concordance, which is "an agreement reached after negotiation between a patient and a healthcare professional that respects the beliefs and wishes of the patient in determining whether, when and how medications are to be taken"; essentially, concordance hinges on the ability of a provider to effectively communicate with his or her patient.[79] Miscommunication and unresolved patient concerns result from information gaps in the patient education process and the inability of the patient to express and resolve personal concerns. Studies suggest that effective communication between patients and healthcare providers improves self-management of medications.[80]

Communication is not only critical between the patient and healthcare provider but also the caregiver. Often, the inability to manage medications is not identified until a crisis happens, such as a hospitalization. The principal of empowering and supporting the caregiver is evident from individuals caring for people with Alzheimer's Disease. Evidence has shown that providing support to the caregiver through education ultimately results in the patient remaining longer in the community.[81]

ECONOMIC ISSUES

HEALTHCARE SYSTEM

Ability to pay is a major factor in being able to obtain necessary treatment and services, including medications. In general, older adults pay for their medications either through insurance or self-pay; insurance usually has a patient contribution for services (e.g., co-payment, co-insurance or deductible) in addition to a premium. There are three major types of insurance coverage available to older adults: Medicare, Medicaid, and private insurance. The Medicare Program (Social Security Act Title XVIII, a Federal program) has several parts. The three parts that are relevant to nearly all US citizens age 65 and older are Part A (the hospital insurance coverage), Part B (the supplemental insurance coverage for items such as physician visits and other outpatient services), and Part D (the prescription drug program). The Medicaid program is health insurance coverage for the poor; Medicaid is a joint program which is managed by the individual state with additional funding from the federal government. Older adults who have Medicaid benefits to cover medical costs not covered by Medicare are called "dual eligibles."[82]

Medicare Part D was enacted with the implementation of the Medicare Prescription Drug, Improvement and Modernization Act of 2003 (MMA).[83] In addition to the prescription plan, there are regulations requiring pharmacists as well as other qualified healthcare providers to provide medication therapy management (MTM) to targeted beneficiaries. Targeted beneficiaries are defined as individuals with Medicare Part D who have multiple Part D medications or multiple chronic disease states and are likely to incur annual costs for Part D medications that exceed a level set by the Department of Health and Human Services. Although the spectrum of services is extremely broad, the aim of this program is to optimize therapeutic outcomes related to medications, improve medication use, reduce the risk of adverse events and drug interactions and increase patient compliance with prescribed regimens. This initiative has increased the role of the pharmacist as an active member of the interdisciplinary team. Furthermore, MTM services (i.e. Comprehensive medication reviews (CMRs) have consistently and substantially improved medication adherence as well as quality of prescribing of evidence-based medications for CHF, COPD and Diabetes.[84]

TYPES OF ENVIRONMENTS

The elderly in the United States may be living in one of a variety of arrangements (see Table 16-1 for summary). Most older adults continue to live in the community (either in their own home or with a caregiver; who may or may not be a relative) until they need significant supervision that warrants having a higher level of care such as a nursing home or assisted living facility. As older adults live longer they move out of their homes later in their life. With the growing availability of assisted living facilities and increased services for home care, the residents of nursing homes commonly have more progressed illness than residents of the 1970s and 80s. Much of this shift in living arrangements is due to the implementation of the Medicaid home and community-based waiver programs that provide funding for some types of care so that older adults can stay at home.[82]

TABLE 16-1: TYPES OF LONG-TERM CARE

TYPES OF LONG-TERM CARE	HELP WITH ACTIVITIES OF DAILY LIVING	HELP WITH ADDITIONAL SERVICES	HELP WITH CARE NEEDS	RANGE OF COSTS
Community-Based Services	Yes	Yes	No	Low to medium
Home Health Care	Yes	Yes	Yes	Low to high
In-Law Apartments	Yes	Yes	Yes	Low to high
Housing for Aging and Disabled Individuals	Yes	Yes	No	Low to high
Board and Care Homes	Yes	Yes	Yes	Low to high
Assisted Living	Yes	Yes	Yes	Medium to high
Continuing Care Retirement Communities	Yes	Yes	Yes	High
Nursing Homes	Yes	Yes	Yes	High

From the Centers for Medicare and Medicaid Services. Types of long-term care. April 10, 2007 (Accessed February 26, 2015, at http://www.medicare.gov/LongTermCare/Static/TypesOverview.asp.)

LONG-TERM CARE

Long-term care encompasses a variety of services that includes medical and non-medical care to people who have a chronic illness or disability. The services address the health, personal care and social needs of the older adult. Long-term care services can be provided in a variety of locations with the ultimate goal of restoring and/or maintaining the health and function of the individual. The level and type of services required depends on the extent of the person's disability and co-morbidity profile. A majority of long-term care services are provided in community settings and a smaller % is provided in nursing homes. Annually 8,357,100 people receive support from the five main long-term care service systems; home health agencies (4,742,500), nursing homes (1,383,700), hospices (1,244,500), residential care communities (713,300), and adult day service centers (273,200).[85] By 2050, the number of individuals using paid long-term care services in any setting (e.g., at home, residential care such as assisted living, or skilled nursing facilities) will likely double from the 13 million using services in 2000, to 27 million people.[86] Generally, Medicare does not pay for long-term care. Medicare pays only for medically-necessary skilled nursing facilities or home healthcare. Most long-term care assists people with support services such as activities of daily living and Medicare does not pay for this "custodial care" or non-skilled care including care that most people do for themselves; for example, diabetes monitoring. Medicaid may pay for certain health services and nursing home care for older people with low incomes and limited assets. In most states, Medicaid also pays for some long-term care services at home and in the community. Eligibility criteria and what services are covered vary from state to state.[82]

Approximately 14% of those over 65 need help with one or more activities of daily living or instrumental activities of daily living (ADL or IADL, long-term care needs) and 50% of those 85 and over.[87] However, at least 75% of these people live in the community (61% for those 85 and over).[87] Of these community-based older adults, as many as 28% receive no needed care, while 47% receive care only from non-paid caregivers.[87] Of the older adults living at home, about 10% in the 65- to 74-year-olds and about 35% over age 85 require help from a caregiver.[88] It is estimated that two out of three (66%) older people with disabilities who receive long term care services at home get all their care exclusively from their family caregiver, which is primarily wives and daughters. Another quarter (26%) receives some combination of family care and paid help while, only 9% receive paid help alone.[89]

Formal long-term care may be given through community or home care, adult day care, assisted living or nursing homes. Those with terminal illnesses may be under the care of hospice organizations; most hospice care (80%) for those 65 and over is paid for by Medicare.[82] Acute situations that require more medical services may involve hospitals, in-patient rehabilitation facilities, skilled nursing units, and long-term acute care hospitals; the latter three may involve months of care. The Research Triangle Institute has tried to define the long-term acute care facilities. The long-term care hospital is similar to the step-down unit of an intensive care unit in the hospital for medically complex patients. The in-patient rehabilitation facility cares for less medically complex, but acutely functionally-impaired patients. The skilled nursing facility is reserved for the least medically complex patients. These facilities are all covered under Medicare Part A.[90]

Many communities provide services and programs to help older adults and people with disabilities with a variety of personal activities. These services include Meals-on-Wheels, transportation services, personal care, chore or errand services, adult day care, and a variety of activities in senior centers (including case management). These services are usually free or at low cost to individuals who qualify. Local organizations, called Area Agencies on Aging, coordinate these services to promote the independence and dignity of older adults.[91]

Often, older adults get help with personal activities (for example, help with the laundry, bathing, dressing, cooking, and cleaning) at home from family members, friends, or volunteers. Some home care can only be given by licensed health workers, such as skilled nursing care and certain other healthcare services that you get in your home for the treatment of an illness or injury. Medicare only pays for home care if the individual meets certain conditions. The state Medicaid program may pay for home health services including skilled nursing care, home healthcare, personal care, chore and errand services, and medical equipment. Home care costs can vary depending on where the person lives, the type of care needed, and how often care is needed. Usually home care payment is based on charges by the hour.[91] In 2012, the total spending (i.e. public, out-of-pocket and other private spending) for long-term care was $219.9 billion, or 9.3% of all US personal health care spending. This is projected to increase to $346 billion in 2040, causing concern about how this will be sustained financially.[92]

The following information on types of Long-Term Care can be accessed at https://www.caregiver.org/print/45. The majority of long-term care service users were aged 65 and over: 94.5% of hospice patients, 93.3% of residential care residents, 85.1% of nursing home residents, 82.4% of home health patients, and 63.5% of participants in adult day services centers. Generally, when differentiating based on age by sector: residential care communities (50.5%), hospices (46.8%), and nursing homes (42.3%) serve more persons aged 85 and over, and adult day services centers (36.5%) serve more persons under age 65 than other sectors.[93]

INDEPENDENT HOUSING

Independent Housing Arrangements may include staying in the former home, moving into an in-law apartment or obtaining housing through "low-income housing for the elderly and disabled" programs. An in-law apartment is a separate housing arrangement within a single-family home or on the same lot; it may also be referred to as a second unit, accessory apartment, or accessory dwelling unit. An in-law apartment is a complete living space and includes a private kitchen and bath. The Federal Government and most states have programs that help pay for housing for older people with low or moderate incomes. Residents usually live in their own apartments in the complex; waiting lists for units are common. Some of these housing programs also offer help with meals and other activities like housekeeping, shopping, and doing the laundry.

BOARD AND CARE HOMES

Board and Care Homes are group living arrangements that provide help with activities of daily living for those who cannot live on their own, but do not need nursing home services. It is sometimes referred to as a "group home" with one to five residents. In some cases, private long-term care insurance and other types of assistance programs may help pay for this type of living arrangement. Many of these homes do not receive payment from Medicare or Medicaid, exist with regulations varying by state, and are often not strictly monitored.

ASSISTED LIVING

Assisted Living Facilities are state-regulated group living arrangements that provide help with activities of daily living, including taking medicine and getting to appointments. Residents often live in their own room or apartment within a building or group of buildings and have some or all of their meals together. Social and recreational activities are usually provided. Some assisted living facilities have health services on-site. Nearly a million individual assisted living units now exist in the United

States. Funding is nearly always private pay. Medicare does not pay for assisted living and Medicaid (in the 41 states where authorized) pays only for the services and not room and board.[94] Residents usually pay a monthly rent and then pay additional fees for the services that they get.

CONTINUING CARE RETIREMENT COMMUNITIES (CCRCs)

Continuing Care Retirement Communities are housing communities that have different levels of care based on the individual needs. In the same community, there may be individual homes or apartments for residents who still live on their own, an assisted living facility for people who need some help with daily care, and a nursing home for those who require higher levels of care. Residents move from one level of care to another based on their needs, but still stay in the CCRC. The contract usually requires the individual to use the community's assisted living facility or nursing home. CCRCs generally charge a large payment before you move in (called an entry fee) and then charge monthly fees.

NURSING HOMES

Nursing Homes are facilities that provide care to people who cannot be cared for at home or in the community. Due to the decrease in disabilities and the alternatives, the total numbers are decreased and the percentage of older adults age 85 and over in nursing homes is 11%. (2012, compared to 21.1% in 1985).[95] A study by the US Department of Health and Human Services reports that people who reach age 65 will likely have a 40 % chance of entering a nursing home. About 10% of the people who enter a nursing home will stay there five years or more. Payment is through private funds or Medicaid. Medicare will pay for skilled rehabilitative care for limited periods (100 days total, most of which have a co-pay).[94] Nursing homes provide a wide range of personal care and health services. For most people, this care generally is to assist people with custodial care services. Medicare does not pay for these types of services; approximately 48% of nursing home care is paid by Medicaid.[94] Some nursing homes may provide skilled care after an injury or hospital stay; Medicare pays for such skilled nursing facility care for a limited period of time and for those who meet certain conditions.

As noted in this chapter, older individuals may reside in various setting such as nursing home. When looking at the presence of pharmacy or pharmacist services, it is estimated that nearly all nursing homes (97.4%) and residential care communities (92.6%) offered pharmacy or pharmacist services, while fewer adult day services centers (34.9%) and home health agencies (5.5%) provided these services.[93] Medication Therapy Management services (MTMS) can potentially be available across the continuum of care for those that are eligible. However, it is imperative that this service is integrated into the existing care delivery and builds on existing clinical initiatives to improve medication safety and utilization. The American Society of Consultant Pharmacists has published guidelines on how to provide Medication Regimen Reviews (MRRs) as well as MTMS within long term care facilities legitimately.[96]

MEDICATION ADHERENCE

Nonadherence or errors in taking medications correctly are disturbingly common, with over half of the 1.6 billion prescriptions written annually in the United States taken incorrectly.[97,98] Studies have reported nonadherence rates in older adults that range from 26% to 59%[99] Larger nonadherence rates tend to occur when the patients do not have symptoms.[100] The medical and economic consequences of older patients' nonadherence to drug therapy may include lack of drug efficacy, treatment failure, disease progression, emergence of resistant bacteria, medication overdose, otherwise avoidable hospitalizations, and unnecessary medical expenses.[101,102] It is estimated that 30% to 50% of prescribed medications fail to produce their intended results.[97] Medication management is a complicated process, involving selecting the right drug, insuring that the patient can obtain it and take it correctly, and evaluating its action on the patient.[103] Older adults are often responsible for taking their own medications despite physical dependence and cognitive impairment.[14,104] Compounding this situation, up to half of persons in the community and up to 60% of hospitalized elders have trouble comprehending medication information.[102,105] For patients with chronic conditions, adherence with ongoing medications is often a problem.

Medication nonadherence can take many forms such as failure to fill the original prescription, failure to refill a prescription, failure to take the dose as prescribed, failure to take it at the appropriate time, failure to follow directions for taking the medication, and failure to follow warnings. The barriers causing medication nonadherence vary widely and are especially relevant for older adults. They fall in the realm of prescription issues, patient-provider communication issues, and disability issues. Some of the barriers to correct medication use reported in the literature for older adults are regimen complexity, miscommunication (gaps in patient education process), unresolved patient concerns[97] (inability of patient to express concerns), hearing impairments[106] (interferes with patient counseling process), vision impairments[107,108] (may make medication labels difficult to read and lack of color discrimination may lead to administration errors), functional impairments[109] (difficulty opening containers or administering the medication as prescribed, e.g., bronchodilators), and cognitive impairments[110] (memory problems). Table 16-2 summarizes the various factors contributing to nonadherence in the older patient as derived from Bero et al.[111]

There has been a recent focus on delineating medication nonadherence due to intentional versus non-intentional nonadherence. Older adults exhibit more problems with both intentional and non-intentional nonadherence than do younger cohorts due to higher frequency of cognitive problems, more erroneous beliefs about illness and treatment, worries about polypharmacy, and issues of cost.[112]

TABLE 16-2: FACTORS INFLUENCING THE ABILITY TO COMPLY WITH A MEDICATION REGIMEN*

> 3 chronic conditions
> 5 prescription medications
> 12 medication dosages per day
Medication regimen changed > 4 times during past 12 months
> 3 prescribers involved
Significant cognitive or physical impairments (e.g., memory, hearing, vision, child-resistant containers)
Living alone in the community
Recently discharged from the hospital
Low literacy
Medication Cost

*Adapted from Bero, L.A., Lipton, H.L., and Bird, J.A. Characterization of geriatric drug-related hospital readmissions. Medical Care 29 (1991):989–1003.

In general, drug-related admissions secondary to nonadherence have been reported to occur in 3% to 28% of elderly patients.[113-115] Nonadherence was the most common cause of avoidable hospitalizations (6%).[116] Col and colleagues[115] found that 11% of the admissions were related to nonadherence with the mean cost per admission associated with medication nonadherence being $2150. Up 10% of total US health care costs can be attributed to nonadherence in the United States every year.[117] Even preventing half of the avoidable serious adverse events related to medication noncompliance would result in significant savings.

ADVERSE DRUG EVENTS (ADEs)

When used appropriately, drugs may be the single most important intervention in the care of an older patient, but when used inappropriately they no longer provide therapeutic benefit, and may even endanger the health of the older patient by causing an adverse drug event. Since the use of medications increases with age, older patients are at greater risk for developing adverse events which are often incorrectly attributed to the aging process or to a progression of the disease.[116] It is estimated that between 5–35% of older community dwelling individuals experience an ADE.[118] Factors believed to be responsible for increased adverse events in elderly patients are polypharmacy (including prescription, over-the-counter, and herbal medications), increased drug-drug interaction, pharmacokinetic factors, pharmacodynamic factors, the pathology of aging and noncompliance.[119] ADEs can have serious consequences for the elderly. The mildest form of an ADE could be an unanticipated side effect of a medication, such as nausea. More ominous ADEs have been documented in many published reports.[111,120-124] Appropriate use of medications is such an important issue for older adults it was targeted in the Healthy People 2000 report.[125] The Joint Commission[126] specifically recommends that institutions establish programs to monitor, track, and prevent adverse drug events and medication errors.

COSTS OF ADEs

It has long been established that drugs may cause or contribute to negative adverse events such as significant morbidity and increased costs of care in this population by increasing healthcare utilization.[121,127-130] It is estimated that drug-related morbidity and mortality costs $76.6 billion annually (1994 dollars) in the ambulatory setting in the United States. The largest component of this total cost is associated with drug-related hospitalizations,[128] with 28% of these adverse drug events being preventable.[121] Preventable costs account for an estimated 47% of the total annual costs.[131] Classen et al.[132] found that patients with adverse drug events had a significantly prolonged length of stay, increased costs and a two-fold increased risk of death compared to matched controls. A GAO study indicated that hospitalizations due to ADEs in the elderly account for $20 billion dollars each year.[133]

PHARMACEUTICAL CARE

Pharmacists are in a pivotal role to help improve communication as well as medication adherence among older adults. Pharmacists interact with a variety of individuals including patients, family members, healthcare professionals and other pharmacists. Due to the presence of pharmacies in many community settings, pharmacists are viewed as the most accessible healthcare provider. That is why it is critical that pharmacists play an active role in providing pharmaceutical care to older adults.

It is well known that older adults see multiple providers and utilize multiple medications. Due to the fragmentation of healthcare leading to poorly coordinated care, there is an associated increase in rate of hospitalization as well as other healthcare costs.[134] This is one of the reasons why the American Geriatrics Society published a position statement on the role of interdisciplinary care for older adults with complex needs.[135] This position statement supports the interdisciplinary care model because it can meet the complex needs of older individuals with multiple medical comorbidities; improves healthcare processes and outcomes for geriatric syndromes (e.g. falls), benefits the healthcare system as well as caregivers of older adults and provides training and education of future healthcare providers to care for the needs of older adults.

SUMMARY

As healthcare professionals, there are obvious opportunities to improve healthcare of older adults through health promotion strategies and strategies that target primary, secondary, and tertiary prevention. There have been ongoing initiatives to increase public awareness and to set objective measurements through "Healthy People 2020," (www.healthypeople.gov/) a set of health objectives for the United States which builds on initiatives pursued over the past two decades. The initiatives include 1979 Surgeon General's Report, *Healthy People*, and *Healthy People 2000: National Health Promotion and Disease Prevention Objectives*. These national health objectives serve as the basis for the development of state and community plans and recently have been utilized to generate a report, *The State of Aging and Health in America 2013.* (www.cdc.gov/aging/saha.htm) This report has provided a report on the 15 key indicators of older adult health at the national and state levels related to health status, health behaviors, preventive care and screening and injuries in adults over the age of 65. These guidelines and tools can be accessed at www.cdc.gov/aging/help/dph-aging/state-aging-health.html.

Pharmaceutical care (or patient-directed pharmacist care) for the older adult requires the pharmacist to have an understanding of the differences in this current population with respect to diversity, education level, health status, and the variety of medications (prescription, OTC, herbal/supplements) available. The "Baby Boomer" generation will bring a new type of older patient who will be a more educated consumer of healthcare services, have different expectations of the healthcare system and its practitioners, and have access to an unprecedented number of treatment options. There will be ongoing drug development for conditions of "aging," providing new medications on the market along with prescription medications becoming increasingly available over-the-counter. In addition to billions of dollars spent annually on research and development of new medications, pharmaceutical companies spent $5 billion in 2008 on direct-to-consumer advertising. It is not only the medications themselves that are important, but where they are purchased. Virtual pharmacies are a growing market on the Internet with pharmaceuticals being the 4th largest product category advertised. Medications purchased through virtual pharmacies accounted for 45% of e-healthcare transactions in 2004 (producing $349 million). Online prescription drug sales increased from $4 billion in 2007 to $12 billion in 2008 and it is expected to continue to rise exponentially in the coming years. The prospect of cost savings and convenience with the internet is appealing to older adults, but they could also be putting themselves at risk.

It is anticipated that healthcare reform will likely result in an increase in managed care environments with an expected reduction in costly services like inpatient care. As the delivery of healthcare continues to evolve, more emphasis will be directed towards lower cost alternatives like home care and assisted living arrangements. In this ever-changing climate, the challenges and opportunities for experts in geriatric pharmacotherapy will increase dramatically and will be necessary in order to serve the needs of the growing older adult population.

REFERENCES

1. Trends in aging—United States and worldwide. (2003) *MMWR Morb Mortal Wkly Rep.* 52(6):101–104, 106.

2. Wan, H., Sengupta, M., Velkoff, V.A., DeBarrow, K.A., & Bureau, U.S.C. (2005) *65+ in the United States: 2005 [Current Population Reports].* Washington, D.C.: U.S. Government Printing Office.

3. Schraeder, C., Dworak, D., Stoll, J.F., Kucera, C., Waldschmidt, V., Dworak, M.P. (2005). Managing elders with comorbidities. *J Ambul Care Manage* 28(3):201–209.

4. Alemayehu, B. & Warner, K.E. (2004). The lifetime distribution of health care costs. *Health Serv Res.* 39(3):627–642.

5. Agency for Healthcare Research and Quality CfDCaP. (2002). Physical activity and older Americans: Benefits and strategies. http://www.ahrq.gov/ppip/activity.htm.

6. The origins of the retirement age in social security. http://www.ssa.gov/history/age65.html.

7. Susman, R. & Riley, M.W. (1985). Introducing the oldest old. *Millbank Memorial Fund Q* 63:177–186.

8. Avorn, J. (1990). The elderly and drug policy: Coming of age. *Health Aff (Millwood)* 9(3):6-19.

9. Salom, I.L. & Davis, K. (1995). Prescribing for older patients: How to avoid toxic drug reactions. *Geriatrics* 50(10):37–40, 43; discussion 44–35.

10. Mueller, C., Schur, C., & O'Connell, J. (1997). Prescription drug spending: The impact of age and chronic disease status. *Am J Public Health* 87(10):1626–1629.

11. Patterns of medication use in the United States. (2006). *Slone Survey* http://www.bu.edu/slone/files/2012/11/SloneSurveyReport2006.pdf

12. Patterson, S.M., Hughes, C., Kerse, N., Cardwell, C.R., & Bradley, M.C. (2012). Interventions to improve the appropriate use of polypharmacy for older people. *The Cochrane database of systematic reviews* 5:Cd008165.

13. Kaufman, D,W., Kelly, J.P., Rosenberg, L., Anderson, T.E., & Mitchell, A.A. (2002). Recent patterns of medication use in the ambulatory adult population of the United States: The Slone survey. *Jama* 287(3):337–344.

14. Ruscin, J.M. & Semla, T.P. (1996). Assessment of medication management skills in older outpatients. *The Annals of Pharmacotherapy* 30(10):1083–1088.

15. Nikolaus, T., Kruse, W., Bach, M., Specht-Leible, N., Oster, P., & Schlierf, G. (1996). Elderly patients' problems with medication. An in-hospital and follow-up study. *Eur J Clin Pharmacol* 49(4):255–259.

16. Lewin Group. (2004). CMS review of current standards of practice for long-term care pharmacy services: Long-term care pharmacy primer. http://www.cms.hhs.gov/Reports/downloads/LewinGroup.pdf. Accessed March 27, 2015.

17. Lau, D.T., Kasper, J.D., Potter, D.E., & Lyles, A. (2004). Potentially inappropriate medication prescriptions among elderly nursing home residents: their scope and associated resident and facility characteristics. *Health Serv Res* 39(5):1257–1276.

18. Roe, C.M., McNamara, A.M., & Motheral, B.R. (2002). Gender- and age-related prescription drug use patterns. *Ann Pharmacother* 36(1):30–39.

19. Aira, M., Hartikainen, S., & Sulkava, R. (2005). Community prevalence of alcohol use and concomitant use of medication--a source of possible risk in the elderly aged 75 and older? *Int J Geriatr Psychiatry* 20(7):680–685.

20. Results from the 2010 National Survey on Drug Use and Health: Summary of National Findings. (2010.)

21. Cusack, B.J. (2004). Pharmacokinetics in older persons. *Am J Geriatr Pharmacother* 2(4):274–302.

22. Mallet, L., Spinewine, A., & Huang, A. (2007). The challenge of managing drug interactions in elderly people. *Lancet* 370(9582):185–191.

23. Pringle, K.E., Ahern, F.M., Heller, D.A., Gold, C.H., & Brown, T.V. (2005). Potential for alcohol and prescription drug interactions in older people. *J Am Geriatr Soc* 53(11):1930–1936.

24. Forster, L.E., Pollow, R., & Stoller, E.P. (1993). Alcohol use and potential risk for alcohol-related adverse drug reactions among community-based elderly. *J Community Health* 18(4):225–239.

25. Adams, W.L. (1995). Potential for adverse drug-alcohol interactions among retirement community residents. *JAGS* 43(9):1021–1025.

26. Brown, R.L., Dimond, A.R., Hulisz, D., et al. (2007). Pharmacoepidemiology of potential alcohol-prescription drug interactions among primary care patients with alcohol-use disorders. *J Am Pharm Assoc* 47:135–139.

27. Farkas, K. & Drabble, L. Prevalence of alcohol, tobacco, and other drug use problems among older adults. In Council on Social Work Education G-EC, ed. *Advanced MSW curriculum in substance use and aging.* Vol 42008.

28. Substance use among older adults: 2002 and 2003 update. (2005). http://www.nevadaprc.org/docs/olderadults.updated.pdf.

29. Results from the 2013 National Survey on Drug Use and Health: Summary of National Findings. (2013). http://www.samhsa.gov/data/sites/default/files/NSDUHresultsPDFWHTML2013/Web/NSDUHresults2013.htm#2.1.

30. Wu, L.T. & Blazer, D.G. (2011). Illicit and nonmedical drug use among older adults: A review. *J Aging Health* 23(3):481–504.

31. Lantz, M. (2005). Prescription drug and alcohol abuse in an older woman. *Clin Geriatr* 13(1):39–43.

32. AARP, NCCAM. (2011). What PEOPLE AGED 50 AND OLDER DISCUSS WITH THEIR HEALTH CARE PROVIDERS. https://nccih.nih.gov/sites/nccam.nih.gov/files/news/camstats/2010/NCCAM_aarp_survey.pdf.

33. Bagchi, D. (2006). Nutraceuticals and functional foods regulations in the United States and around the world. *Toxicology* 221(1):1–3.

34. Bouchayer, F. (1990). Alternative medicines. *Compl Med Res* 4:4–8.

35. Astin, J.A. (1998). Why patients use alternative medicine: results of a national study. *Jama* 279(19):1548–1553.

36. Marinac, J.S., Buchinger, C.L., Godfrey, L.A., Wooten, J.M., Sun, C., & Willsie, S.K. (2007). Herbal products and dietary supplements: a survey of use, attitudes, and knowledge among older adults. *J Am Osteopath Assoc* 107(1):13–20; quiz 21-13.

37. Huxtable, R.J. (1992). The myth of beneficent nature: The risks of herbal preparations. *Ann Intern Med* 117(2):165–166.

38. Hasegawa, G.R. (2000). Uncertain quality of dietary supplements: history repeated. *Am J Health Syst Pharm* 57(10):951.

39. Miller, L.G. (1998). Herbal medicinals: Selected clinical considerations focusing on known or potential drug-herb interactions. *Arch Intern Med* 158(20):2200–2211.

40. Fugh-Berman, A. (2000). Herb-drug interactions. *Lancet* 355(9198):134–138.

41. Arcury, T.A., Grzywacz, J.G., Bell, R.A., Neiberg, R.H., Lang, W., & Quandt, S.A. (2007). Herbal remedy use as health self-management among older adults. *J Gerontol B Psychol Sci Soc Sci* 62(2):S142–149.

42. Kuo, G.M., Hawley, S.T., Weiss, L.T., Balkrishnan, R., & Volk, R.J. (2004). Factors associated with herbal use among urban multiethnic primary care patients: A cross-sectional survey. *BMC Complement Altern Med* 4:18.

43. Kennedy, J. (2005). Herb and supplement use in the US adult population. *Clinical therapeutics* 27(11):1847–1858.

44. Sawhney, R., Sehl, M., & Naeim, A. (2005). Physiologic aspects of aging: impact on cancer management and decision making, part I. *Cancer J.* 11(6):449–460.

45. Watson, G.R. (2001). Low vision in the geriatric population: Rehabilitation and management. *J Am Geriatr Soc* 49(3):317–330.

46. Sass, S.M., Legge, G.E.,& Lee H.W.(2006). Low-vision reading speed: Influences of linguistic inference and aging. *Optom Vis Sci* 83(3):166–177.

47. Helzner, E.P., Cauley, J.A., Pratt, S.R., et al. (2005). Race and sex differences in age-related hearing loss: The health, aging and body composition study. *J Am Geriatr Soc* 53(12):2119–2127.

48. Anstey, K.J., Luszcz, M.A., & Sanchez, L. (2001). Two-year decline in vision but not hearing is associated with memory decline in very old adults in a population-based sample. *Gerontology* 47(5):289–293.

49. Lieto, J.M. & Schmidt, K.S. (2005). Reduced ability to self-administer medication is associated with assisted living placement in a continuing care retirement community. *J Am Med Dir Assoc* 6(4):246–249.

50. Kramer, A.F., Boot, W.R., McCarley, J.S., Peterson, M.S., Colcombe, A., & Scialfa, C.T. (2006). Aging, memory and visual search. *Acta Psychol (Amst)* 122(3):288–304.

51. Cooper, C., Carpenter, I., Katona, C., et al. (2005). The AdHOC Study of older adults' adherence to medication in 11 countries. *Am J Geriatr Psychiatry* 13(12):1067–1076.

52. Hebert, L.E., Scherr, P.A., Bienias, J.L., Bennett, D.A., & Evans, D.A. (2003). Alzheimer disease in the US population: Prevalence estimates using the 2000 census. *Arch Neurol* 60(8):1119–1122.

53. Rosenberg, P.B., Johnston, D., & Lyketsos, C.G. (2006). A clinical approach to mild cognitive impairment. *Am J Psychiatry* 163(11):1884–1890.

54. Fillit, H. & Hill, J. (2005). Economics of dementia and pharmacoeconomics of dementia therapy. *Am J Geriatr Pharmacother* 3(1):39–49.

55. Kirchstein, R. *Disease specific estimates of direct and indirect costs of illness and NIH support. Fiscal year 2000 update.* [website]. http://ospp.od.nih.gov/ecostudies/COIreportweb.htm. Accessed March 27, 2015.

56. Maioli, F., Coveri, M., Pagni, P., et al. (2007). Conversion of mild cognitive impairment to dementia in elderly subjects: A preliminary study in a memory and cognitive disorder unit. *Arch Gerontol Geriatr* 44 Suppl 1:233–241.

57. Joyce, G.F., Keeler, E.B., Shang, B., & Goldman, D.P. (2005). The lifetime burden of chronic disease among the elderly. *Health Aff (Millwood)* 24 Suppl 2:W5R18–29.

58. MacLaughlin, E.J., Raehl, C.L., Treadway, A.K., Sterling, T.L., Zoller, D.P., & Bond, C.A. (2005). Assessing medication adherence in the elderly: which tools to use in clinical practice? *Drugs Aging* 22(3):231–255.

59. Wetzels, R., van Eijken, M., Grol, R., Wensing, M., & van Weel, C. (2005). Self-management is not related to lower demand for primary care in independent-living elderly. *J Am Geriatr Soc* 53(5):918–919.

60. *Unequal treatment: confronting racial and ethnic disparities in health care.* (2002). Washington, D.C.: The National Academic Press.

61. Dunlop, D,D., Manheim, L.M., Song, J., & Chang, R.W. (2002). Gender and ethnic/racial disparities in health care utilization among older adults. *J Gerontol B Psychol Sci Soc Sci* 57(4):S221–233.

62. Lavizzo-Mourey, R. & Knickman, J.R. (2003). Racial disparities—the need for research and action. *N Engl J Med* 349(14):1379–1380.

63. Shi, L., Green, L.H., & Kazakova, S. (2004). Primary care experience and racial disparities in self-reported health status. *J Am Board Fam Pract* 17(6):443–452.

64. Bach, P.B., Pham, H.H., Schrag, D., Tate, R.C., & Hargraves, J.L. (2004). Primary care physicians who treat blacks and whites. *N Engl J Med.* 351(6):575–584.

65. Blustein, J. & Weiss, L.J. (1998). Visits to specialists under Medicare: Socioeconomic advantage and access to care. *J Health Care Poor Underserved* 9(2):153–169.

66. Gornick, M.E., Eggers, P.W., Reilly, T.W., et al. (1996). Effects of race and income on mortality and use of services among Medicare beneficiaries. *N Engl J Med* 335(11):791–799.

67. Michielutte, R., Diseker, R.A., Stafford, C.L., & Carr, P. (1984). Knowledge of diabetes and glaucoma in a rural North Carolina community. *J Community Health* 9(4):269–284.

68. Ontiveros, J.A., Black, S.A., Jakobi, P.L., & Goodwin, J.S. (1999). Ethnic variation in attitudes toward hypertension in adults ages 75 and older. *Prev Med* 29(6 Pt 1):443–449.

69. Goodwin, J.S., Black, S.A., & Satish, S. (1999). Aging versus disease: The opinions of older black, Hispanic, and non-Hispanic white Americans about the causes and treatment of common medical conditions. *J Am Geriatr Soc* 47(8):973–979.

70. Crystal, S., Sambamoorthi, U., Walkup, J.T., & Akincigil, A. (2003). Diagnosis and treatment of depression in the elderly medicare population: Predictors, disparities, and trends. *J Am Geriatr Soc* 51(12):1718–1728.

71. Gesler, W., Arcury, T.A., & Koenig, H.G. (2000). An introduction to three studies of rural elderly people: Effects of religion and culture on health. *J Cross Cult Gerontol* 15:1–12.

72. Gallo, J.J., Bogner, H.R., Morales, K.H., & Ford, D.E. (2005). Patient ethnicity and the identification and active management of depression in late life. *Arch Intern Med* 165(17):1962–1968.

73. Committee on Health Literacy. (2004). *Health literacy: A prescription to end confusion.* Washington, D.C.: National Academic Press.

74. Paasche-Orlow, M.K., Parker, R.M., Gazmararian, J.A., Nielsen-Bohlman, L.T., & Rudd, R.R. (2005). The prevalence of limited health literacy. *J Gen Intern Med* 20(2):175–184.

75. Wolf, M.S., Gazmararian, J.A., & Baker, D.W. (2005). Health literacy and functional health status among older adults. *Arch Intern Med* 165(17):1946–1952.

76. Baudouin, A., Vanneste, S., Pouthas, V., & Isingrini, M. (2006). Age-related changes in duration reproduction: involvement of working memory processes. *Brain Cogn* 62(1):17–23.

77. Lezzoni, L.I., O'Day, B.L., Killeen, M., & Harker, H. (2004). Communicating about health care: observations from persons who are deaf or hard of hearing. *Ann Intern Med* 140(5):356–362.

78. Jacobson, J. (1999). Counseling the deaf and hearing-impaired. *Am J Health Syst Pharm* 56(7):610–611.

79. Chewning, B., Wiederholt, J.B. (2003). Concordance in cancer medication management. *Patient Educ Couns* 50(1):75–8.

80. Peterson, M.A. & Dragon, C.J. (1998). Improving medication adherence in patients receiving home health. *Home Healthcare Consultant* 5(9):25–27.

81. Mittelman, M.S., Ferris, S.H., Shulman, E., Steinberg, G., & Levin, B. (1996). A family intervention to delay nursing home placement of patients with Alzheimer disease. A randomized controlled trial. *Jama* 276(21):1725–1731.

82. Dual Eligibility. [website]. http://www.cms.hhs.gov/DualEligible/. Accessed March 27, 2015.

83. Summary of H.R.1: Medicare Prescription Drug, Improvement and Modernization Act of 2003; Public Law 108-173. *CMS Legislative Summary* 2004; http://www.cms.hhs.gov/MMAUpdate/downloads/PL108-173summary.pdf. Accessed March 27, 2015.

84. Perlroth, D., Marrufo, G., Montesinos, A., et al. (2013) Medication Therapy Management in Chronically Ill Populations: Final Report. Prepared for CMS by Acumen, LLC and Westat.

85. Center for Disease Control and Prevention. (2013). *Long-term care services.* http://www.cdc.gov/nchs/data/nsltcp/long_term_care_services_2013.pdf.

86. The future supply of long-term care workers in relation to the aging baby boom generation: Report to Congress Washington, DC: Office of the Assistant Secretary for Planning and Evaluation. (2003).

87. Schneider, E.L. & Guralnik, J.M. (1990). The aging of America. Impact on health care costs. *Jama* 263(17):2335–2340.

88. Lamy, P.P. (1993). Institutionalization and drug use in older adults in the U.S. *Drugs Aging* (3):232–237.

89. Doty, P. (2010). The evolving balance of formal and informal, institutional and non-institutional long-term care for older Americans: A thirty- year perspective. *Public Policy & Aging Report* 20(1):3–9.

90. Mihalich, L.K. (2007). The role of long-term care hospitals. *Dennis Barry's Reimbursement Advisor* 22(7):6–9.

91. Medicare. Long-Term Care. [website]. http://www.medicare.gov/LongTermCare/Static/Home.asp?dest=NAV%7CHome%7CWhatIsLTC#Tab Top. Accessed March 27, 2015.

92. Forum NHP. (2014). The Basics: National Spending for Long-Term Services and Supports. http://www.nhpf.org/library/the-basics/Basics_LTSS_03-27-14.pdf.

93. Harris-Kojetin, L. SM., Park-Lee, E., & Valverde, R. (2013). *Long-term care services in the United States: 2013 overview.* Hyattsville, MD: National Center for Health Statistics.

94. Tumlinson, A. & Woods, S. (2007). *Long-term care in America: An introduction.* Washington, D.C.: Avalere Health LLC.

95. 2012 Profile of Older Americans Administration on Aging Administration for Community Living U.S. Department of Health and Human Services. http://www.aoa.gov/Aging_Statistics/Profile/2012/docs/2012profile.pdf.

96. ASCP. *Guidelines for medication therapy management services in long-term care facilities.* Alexandria, VA: American Society of Consultant Pharmacists; 2007.

97. Berg, J.S., Dischler, J., Wagner, D.J., Raia, J.J., & Palmer-Shevlin, N.(1993). Medication compliance: a healthcare problem. *Ann Pharmacother* 27(9 Suppl):S1–24.

98. Whitney, H.A. (1993). Medication compliance: A healthcare problem. Ann *Pharmacother* 27 (Suppl).

99. van Eijken, M., Tsang, S., Wensing, M., de Smet, P.A., & Grol, R.P. (2003). Interventions to improve medication compliance in older patients living in the community: a systematic review of the literature. Drugs Aging 20(3):229–240.

100. Loghman-Adham, M. (2003). Medication noncompliance in patients with chronic disease: issues in dialysis and renal transplantation. *Am J Manag Care* 9(2):155–171.

101. Greenberg, R.N. (1984). Overview of patient compliance with medication dosing: a literature review. *Clinical therapeutics* 6(5):592–599.

102. Notenboom, K., Beers, E., van Riet-Nales, D.A., et al. (2014). Practical problems with medication use that older people experience: a qualitative study. *J Am Geriatr Soc* 62(12):2339–2344.

103. Garrard, J., Harms, S., & Hanlon J. (1998). *Medication management of community based elderly people in managed care organizations.* Paper presented at: How Managed Care Can Help Older Persons Live Well with Chronic Conditions; Oct. 27–28, 1998; Washington D.C.

104. Campbell, N.L., Boustani, M.A., Skopelja, E.N., Gao, S., Unverzagt, F.W.,& Murray, M.D. (2012). Medication adherence in older adults with cognitive impairment: A systematic evidence-based review. *Am J Geriatr Pharmacother* 10(3):165–177.

105. Royall, D.R., Cordes, J., & Polk, M. (1997). Executive control and the comprehension of medical information by elderly retirees. *Exp Aging Res* 23(4):301–313.

106. Uhlmann, R.F., Larson, E.B., Rees, T.S., Koepsell, T.D., & Duckert, L.G. (1989). Relationship of hearing impairment to dementia and cognitive dysfunction in older adults. *JAMA* 261(13):1916–1919.

107. Luscombe, D.K., Jinks, M.J., & Duncan, S. (1992). A survey of prescription label preferences among community pharmacy patrons. *J Clin Pharm Ther* 17(4):241–244.

108. Jinks, M.J., Evenson, L.M., Campbell, R.K., & Kreager, M.C. (1989). Prescription labels for aging eyes. *Am Pharm* NS29(5):31–33.

109. Meyer, M.E. & Schuna, A.A. (1989). Assessment of geriatric patients' functional ability to take medication. *DICP* 23(2):171–174.

110. Maddigan, S.L., Farris, K.B., Keating, N., Wiens, C.A., & Johnson, J.A. (2003). Predictors of older adults' capacity for medication management in a self-medication program: A retrospective chart review. *J Aging Health* 15(2):332–352.

111. Bero, L.A., Lipton, H.L., & Bird, J.A. (1991). Characterization of geriatric drug-related hospital readmissions. *Med Care* 29(10):989–1003.

112. Mukhtar, O., Weinman, J., & Jackson, S.H. (2014). Intentional non-adherence to medications by older adults. *Drugs Aging* 31(3):149–157.

113. Dartnell, J.G., Anderson, R.P., Chohan, V., et al. (1996). Hospitalisation for adverse events related to drug therapy: incidence, avoidability and costs. *Med J Aust* 164(11):659–662.

114. Tafreshi, M.J., Melby, M.J., Kaback, K.R., & Nord TC. (1999). Medication-related visits to the emergency department: a prospective study. *Ann Pharmacother* 33(12):1252–1257.

115. Col, N., Fanale, J.E., & Kronholm, P. (1990). The role of medication noncompliance and adverse drug reactions in hospitalizations of the elderly. *Arch Intern Med* 150(4):841–845.

116. Courtman, B.J. & Stallings, S.B. (1995). Characterization of drug-related problems in elderly patients on admission to a medical ward. *Can J Hosp Pharm* 48(3):161–166.

117. Iuga, A.O. & McGuire, M.J. (2014). Adherence and health care costs. *Risk management and healthcare policy* 7:35–44.

118. Hajjar, E.R., Hanlon, J.T., Artz, M.B., et al. (2003). Adverse drug reaction risk factors in older outpatients. *Am J Geriatr Pharmacother* 1:82–89.

119. Beyth, R.J. & Shorr, R.I. (1999). Epidemiology of adverse drug reactions in the elderly by drug class. *Drugs Aging* 14(3):231–239.

120. Lindley, C.M., Tully, M.P., Paramsothy, V., & Tallis, R.C. (1992). Inappropriate medication is a major cause of adverse drug reactions in elderly patients. *Age Ageing* 21(4):294–300.

121. Bates, D.W., Cullen, D.J., Laird, N., et al. (1995). Incidence of adverse drug events and potential adverse drug events. Implications for prevention. ADE Prevention Study Group. *JAMA* 274(1):29–34.

122. Lazarou, J., Pomeranz, B.H., & Corey, P.N. (1998). Incidence of adverse drug reactions in hospitalized patients: a meta- analysis of prospective studies. *JAMA* 279(15):1200–1205.

123. Lesar, T.S., Lomaestro, B.M., & Pohl, H. (1997). Medication-prescribing errors in a teaching hospital. A 9-year experience. *Arch Intern Med* 157(14):1569–1576.

124. Cullen, D.J., Sweitzer, B.J., Bates, D.W., Burdick, E., Edmondson. A., Leape, L.L. (1997). Preventable adverse drug events in hospitalized patients: A comparative study of intensive care and general care units. *Crit Care Med* 25(8):1289–1297.

125. U.S. Department of Health and Human Services. (1991). *Healthy People 2000: National health promotion and disease prevention objectives.* Washington D.C.: Government Printing Office.

126. Organizations JCoAoH. Section I: Treatment of patients. Medication use. *Accreditation manual for hospitals.* Oakbrook Terrace, IL:1–25.

127. Walker, J. & Wynne, H. (1994). Review: The frequency and severity of adverse drug reactions in elderly people. *Age Ageing* 23(3):255–259.

128. Johnson, J.G., Spitzer, R.L., Williams, J.B., et al. (1995). Psychiatric comorbidity, health status, and functional impairment associated with alcohol abuse and dependence in primary care patients: findings of the PRIME MD-1000 study. *J Consult Clin Psychol* 63(1):133–140.

129. Atkin, P.A. & Shenfield, G.M. (1995). Medication-related adverse reactions and the elderly: a literature review. *Adverse Drug React Toxicol Rev* 14(3):175–191.

130. Hanlon, J.T., Schmader, K.E., Koronkowski, M.J., et al. (1997). Adverse drug events in high risk older outpatients. *JAGS* 45(8):945–948.

131. Bootman, J.L., Harrison, D.L., & Cox, E. (1997). The health care cost of drug-related morbidity and mortality in nursing facilities. *Arch Intern Med* 157(18):2089–2096.

132. Classen, D.C., Pestotnik, S.L., Evans, R.S., Lloyd, J.F., & Burke, J.P. (1997). Adverse drug events in hospitalized patients. Excess length of stay, extra costs, and attributable mortality. *JAMA* 277(4):301–306.

133. GAO. (1995). *Prescription drugs and the elderly: Many still receive potentially harmful drugs despite recent improvements.* Washington D.C.: U.S. General Accounting Office.

134. Wolff, J.L., Starfield, B., & Anderson, G. (2002). Prevalence, expenditures, and complications of multiple chronic conditions in the elderly. *Arch Intern Med* 162(20):2269–2276.

135. Mion, L., Odegard, P.S., Resnick, B., & Segal-Galan, F. (2006). Interdisciplinary care for older adults with complex needs: American Geriatrics Society position statement. *J Am Geriatr Soc* 54(5):849–852.

CHAPTER 17

DEATH AND DYING

Albert I Wertheimer, PhD, MBA and Xiaohan Hu, MD, MPH

LEARNING OBJECTIVES:

1. Define death and describe the evolution of the understanding of death over time.
2. Identify different perspectives of death.
3. Describe the current views on death and life.
4. Apply examples of bioethics in clinical practice.
5. Integrate the role of the pharmacist in helping patients recognize the dying process sooner and be able to provide optimal end of life care.

KEY TERMS

Denial

Acceptance

Anger

Bargaining

Various cultural views of death

HISTORICAL DEVELOPMENT OF THE FIELD

In the 19th century it was quite common to learn that an individual had died from "natural causes." When there was a death of a person aged 50 years or more and there was no obvious violence or criminal activity or observable pathology, it was reported that the patient had died of natural causes. Today, of course, we would not be satisfied with this cause of death as we are able to learn a great deal more about the pathology involved. Similarly, death was handled as a family activity. The patient was displayed for a few days in the parlor of the house of a relative and a burial took place shortly afterwards. That quaint phenomenon no longer exists as there have been a number of developments in both the clinical medical practice as well as in the commercial world.

Today in the 21st century, no one would think of having a funeral and the visitation take place without the involvement of a funeral parlor or mortuary. The funeral director has taken over and arranges everything regarding the disposition of the newly departed. However, there are a number of matters that are not solved or provided by the funeral director. Since diagnosis has become more precise, it is often possible to learn well in advance of the actual time of the impending event. It can even be two or three years in advance. The signs of imminent death have also been discovered in a cancer study recently, for example, nonreactive pupils, bleeding complications after major surgeries, etc.[1] Although physical signs of death may differ in impending death with other causes, studying this information enables doctors, nurses, and pharmacists to recognize the dying process sooner, and thus adjust the treatment focus to hospice and end-of-life care. In addition, recognizing the signs gives the families more time to accept and cope with the grief and an opportunity to make a better use of the final days of life with their beloved one. Naturally, the patient has an opportunity to react to this news and that is exactly what happens. Thanks to the work of Dr. Elizabeth Kubler-Ross, we know a great deal more about the phases and activities involved in the dying process.[2]

Dr. Kubler-Ross began receiving widespread recognition for her work in 1969. Before that time, and even today, there is a great deal of fascination with the topic of death and dying in the lay press. We have all heard or read about the remembrances of persons with near death experiences. We still have no definitive evidence of whether there is an after-life, or whether one can communicate following death.

The practicing pharmacist is often able to determine that a patient is in a terminal situation when the prescriptions for narcotic analgesics call for ever-increasing dosages and when the patient appears to be in deteriorating health status. What does the pharmacist say to the patient or to family members picking up the medications? Fortunately, through the work of Kubler-Ross,[3] Moody,[4] Woodson[5] and other pioneers in this discipline, we have some information that enables us to assist the dying patient and his or her family.

Kalish[6] tells us that the dying process is like any other stage in human development; it is influenced by numerous decisions and other variables. Well, what do we know? Actually, there is quite a robust literature on this topic. We find that there are numerous articles prior to the work of Kubler-Ross that dealt with death and dying but this was considered to be a morbid topic or a taboo area. In fact, some studies indicated that the terminal patient was stigmatized[7] and that nurses and other healthcare workers attempted to avoid them. An early study (1963)[8] indicated that nurses took longer to respond to call lights or messages from terminal cases when compared to non-terminal cases, and Kastenbaum reported that the lives of younger people are considered to be worth more in time and expense than the lives of the elderly, since they have more social value. Glazer and Strauss reported the treatment of children and adolescents elicits more sympathy and attracts more workers than does treatment of the aged.[9]

Numerous reports in the literature indicate differential treatment of persons of different races and ethnic groups in all age groups. Even gender plays a role as society expects women will seek medical care when there is a need, while men are expected to be stoic. Some feel that men may die sooner, partially as a result of their adherence to the male role model "to tough it out" and not seek care from a physician promptly. One's financial situation can influence whether one will seek care immediately or postpone a decision and that case is replicated in situations where one may or may not have adequate health insurance.

Since the late 1980s, palliative care, which aims at alleviating pain, reducing symptoms, and lessening stress of patients with advanced or life-threatening illness or their caregivers, has emerged in some of the hospitals in the United States. This program should be distinguished from the traditional hospice services. Hospice services are usually provided to those who have decided not to pursue further treatment options and been certified by two physicians that they will have less than six months of life. In contrast, palliative care can be delivered to patients without restrictions of prognosis. Studies have shown that early palliative care, as a multidisciplinary approach delivered by a team of physicians, nurses, and pharmacists, is significantly superior than standard care in terms of improving quality of life in a group of lung cancer patients.[10] Palliative care is also associated with reduced health resource utilization and better outcomes of patients and their caregivers.[11] There are more than 1240 hospitals in the United States have a palliative care program in order to address the physical, emotional and social needs of patients with serious illness.[12]

WHAT IS DEATH

Death always has been and always will be with us. It is an integral part of human existence and has always been a subject of deep concern to all of us. Since the dawn of human kind, the human mind has pondered death, searching for the answer to its mysteries. For the key to the question of death unlocks the door of life. Now, when humankind is surrounded by death and destruction as never before, it becomes essential that we study the problems of death and try to understand its true meaning.

RELIGIOUS PERSPECTIVE

Long before we had information or inferences from scientists and clinicians about death, what we knew or thought about death and dying came from religious teachings and from the writings of ancient philosophers. The variations in the conception of death will have a particular influence on people's lifestyles, how much people fear death, and the expression of grief and mourning towards their beloved one's departure.

Full acceptance of the fact of death is seen as required in both Buddhism and Hinduism. It is felt that one robs oneself of a purposeful live if one attempts to ignore death or deludes oneself into believing that he or she will endure forever. Only he who accepts death as an integral part of life, calmly and courageously, gains a purposeful life.

Eastern philosophy relies on the concept of afterlife to cope with the agony of the death of beloved ones.[13] Buddhist teaching sees death as the cutting-off of the life force of a physical body, which is then transformed or displaced to continue functioning in another form. In this way, every birth is really a rebirth.[14] Some people would also think of the death of their beloved one as a blessed thing if he/she ended his/her journey peacefully and has lived a happy life.

With Hindus, the belief is that there are differences in the quality of deaths; depending on the degree of disciplined versus undisciplined living. There is praying for mercy at the hands of Yama, the God of Death, but universal recognition that after death, all persons are born again in the next world in a situation related to their deeds in this world. It is believed that one aspires toward the Supreme Person, when he finds the "self," understands the self and all worlds and desires. He gains immortality, which is understood to be freedom from the continuous chain of rebirth. For most Hindus, death is seen as a necessity and as a blessing. It is necessary because, otherwise, the world would run out of space and resources if no one died, and it is a blessing as it is an opportunity to move to a higher level of incarnation.[15]

Judaism teaches facing death in a straight-forward manner, and encourages the family to be present to support the dying person. Moreover, the deathbed confessional is considered most important in the transition to the world to come. The dying person is expected, if possible, to seek repentance, to go through confession, to put his/her material matters in order, and to provide ethical instruction and blessing of the family. This enables the patient to express fears, find comfort and inner strength, and communicate meaningfully with those close to him or her. The Orthodox discuss an afterlife, but this is not a central tenet of the religion.[16]

The Christian view of death is probably most well known to the readers of this book. In contrast to eastern philosophy, Christians believe that people will only live and die once. However, Christians do not believe that everything will come to a cessation at death. The spirit of the departed one will continue to influence the living ones. Also, the concept of leading a good life in order to be admitted to heaven and in seeking rewards for the good or pure life on earth is recognized widely. The Catholic "Last Rites" administed when death is imminent are meant to assist in a path to heaven. The concept of hell, where "bad" people end up, is the subject of numerous stories, jokes, and myths.

SCIENTIFIC PERSPECTIVE ON DEATH

In 1969 Kubler-Ross published her book, *Death and Dying*, which became a catalyst for an enormous body of subsequent work on this topic. She provided a grid or structure to the phases in the attitudes and behavior of the patient upon learning of the diagnosis of a terminal illness.

The five phases are:

- Denial
- Anger
- Bargaining
- Depression
- Acceptance

Denial is often accompanied by shock. Maybe the lab tests were wrong, perhaps the medical charts got mixed up. It can't be me—last week I was completely healthy. There is quite often a sensation of loneliness, recognizing that no one else can help and that one is in this dilemma alone. There is considerable internal conflict while the patient ponders their new reality and health status. Guilt enters the consciousness. Did I do something to deserve this? I should have treated my parents/neighbor/teachers better or with more respect. There may be some degree of meaninglessness, where one wonders if any efforts might postpone the inevitable and whether it would make any difference in the world, even if that were to be possible.

Eventually, these emotions turn into anger. I worked so hard and never had that dreamed of vacation. I won't be able to spend that money I've been saving for a comfortable retirement. I will not be able to meet my grandchildren, see graduations or weddings. It was a mistake to spend so much time on my career (or business) at the expense of family activities.

Some feel that it is not fair; and become angry because they are a "good" person, but that crook down the block is perfectly healthy at age 89. Anger can be directed at one's loved ones, caregivers, and business associates, or randomly at persons he or she encounters as he or she is reminded by the vitality and energy in them or when he or her hears others making plans for the future. Anger is a phase that eventually fades and dissipates when the dying person realizes that it is not productive in changing the inevitable future course or in enhancing relationships with those he or she deals with.

At some point, the anger recedes, while not totally disappearing, being taken over by the bargaining phase. The wise or sensitive person comes to realize that others will avoid him if he can talk only about his problems. This whining makes others uncomfortable and contributes nothing toward a solution to the basic problem. It is a natural human instinct to attempt to bargain in an effort toward self preservation.

The patient says to his God: If you spare me, I will go to church every Sunday for the rest of my life, or if you let me live, I will volunteer my skills to poor or homeless persons, or I will be better at doing this or that. Many of us have met people who no longer eat candy or who teach Sunday, religious school as a volunteer because "their prayer was answered or fulfilled."

It goes beyond the focus of this chapter to discuss the effectiveness of such offered bargains. The religiously devout will probably endorse them and suggest that a prayer might not have been fulfilled because the supplicant's life until that point in time was not sufficiently worthy. For those who tend to trust science and facts for the most-part, the bargaining may appear to be a waste of time, but an activity that causes no harm.

Assuming that the prognosis remains bleak, next comes a gradual but steady realization of the actual consequences ahead and one's powerlessness to modify that eventuality. This leads to a phase of depression. One's life is about to end shortly and the quality of life between now and then may be most undesirable and limited. Most terminal patients conquer this depression and move toward the final phase prior to death; that of acceptance. These persons redevelop an increased self-awareness and entry to this stage is observable as contact with others increases or as broken contacts are re-established.

During acceptance, there is increased self-reliance and pro-active efforts towards benefiting from the limited few days available ahead. Financial matters are put into final order; instructions to family and colleagues are given, and pending matters are closed. The patient may want to learn about his disease in greater detail; he may volunteer his time for worthy causes (not as in the earlier bargaining phase) so some more people will remember him as a kind and generous person. Patients often want to assist others with the same condition or to help prevent it. For example, it might mean speaking to young people's groups about the dangers of cigarette smoking.

During acceptance, it may include comforting those in one's immediate family, telling them to move on with their lives, and informing them that the patient is prepared for this finality.

But clearly, this model, as is the case with all models, is not accurate for all terminal persons or at all times. It is possible that someone might remain in the anger phase until the end, or until the final day. A lot of people will experience anxiety in the last days as well. The anxiety may come from the fear towards death and also is dependent on the cultural background of one person, i.e., how he or she conceptualizes death. Alvarado et al. studied the association between religious belief and anxiety to death, and the results showed that people with greater strength of conviction tend to have less anxiety towards death as they might have a belief in afterlife.[17] Therefore, those with ultra strong religious views may act and feel different from a non-religious individual or from a devout believer in science. Many other factors may modify the application of this five stage model.

The United States is comprised of a large number of diverse ethnic and racial groups with origins from all over the world. And, as one might expect most of these numerous ethnic and racial groups have culturally learned practices and beliefs about death and dying. There are too many of these to permit us to go into detail about any one of them, but the major differences lie in whether death is seen as a transition to another existence or as an end, and whether death is a type of punishment or whether it is a recognition that the individual might be ready for the next, possibly higher life. Between these extremes, many different practices and beliefs all co-exist. To us as objective scientists and practitioners employing evidence-based treatments, it is frustrating, because we will not be able to know what is best, if anything is best.

Those same attitudes and beliefs that shaped the practices of Americans who immigrated to the United States are still alive and well in the areas from where they emigrated.

Lynn Payer described a difference between British and American care for the terminally ill, which should have great significance for us. "The lesser belief in medicine's ability to prolong life and the greater belief in medicine's role in making life nicer are undoubtedly the reason that hospices for the dying grew up first in Britain, not America. To accept the idea of hospice, one must accept the fact that people die… American physicians seem to regard death as the ultimate failure of their skill. British doctors frequently regard death as physiological, sometimes even devoutly to be wished."[18]

Now in the 21st century, and with the benefit of religious scholars, scientists, philosophers, psychologists, clinicians and laypersons having near-death experiences, we still ask: What is death and how should we think about it? Do we fear it or welcome it? Is death the end or a transition? For all of these questions, there are no definitive answers. Toynbee[19] has described how humans have sought to reconcile themselves to the fact of death. One strategy is hedonism; to enjoy life as much as possible before death comes into the picture. Another mechanism is through the use of pessimism; to convince oneself that life is so distasteful that death is a relief from the unfortunate state of living. Suicide is an operationalization of such pessimism. Some may attempt to circumvent death through physical countermeasures such as serious exercise, proper nutrition, stress reduction, and healthy lifestyles. And there are several other avenues that have been mentioned or attempted in the past.

Sandra M. Gilbert explored the relationship between us and death in her book: *Death's Door: Modern Dying and the Ways We Grieve*. Infusing her own life stories into her research on academic literatures, Gilbert used a poetic, humanistic, and meticulous way to depict the inevitability of death. And from the psychology of our reactions to death (mourning, grief, etc.), to how this has changed over the last century, and finally how this change has influenced our recognition of death, Gilbert delivered a penetrating analysis of life and death in a both elegant and critical way.[20]

One area of special interest is in the death of children and young people. Death is seen as a natural consequence of aging. We're one to observe the obituary notices in any city newspaper, it is most likely the case that most of the deceased will have been in their late 60s, or in their 70s or 80s. However when we read about the death of a 12-year-old child, we have additional feelings of loss and remorse, that such a young and "unlived" life was lost so soon. It is said that the greatest source of pain and anguish to a parent is the death and burial of their child.

In all of the pages of this chapter to this point, death has been understood to mean the loss of life to some disease, or from the sequalae of an automobile accident or other unintentional event. Yet, we all know that not all deaths are passive events. There are numerous examples of suicide or euthanasia (assisted suicide) and, of course, there are vastly different cultural reactions to the taking of one's own life. That, as well as death from military hostile activities or capital punishment by the civil authorities are also specific cases that will not be directly addressed in this chapter.

Perhaps, one of the most difficult situations for a pharmacist to understand is the intentional lack of medication persistence or adherence when the proper use of the medication can keep a life-threatening disease or condition at bay indefinitely. When poor persistence or adherence will surely lead to early health status decline and death, we ask how someone might elect to destroy themselves in such a way. The most vivid example is the intentional lack of adherence with anti-retroviral drugs for patients with HIV/AIDS. With the proper use of the drugs, patients today can live fairly normal lives for an extended period of time; perhaps for 10 or more years. Yet, we ask, why would someone fail to take their medications knowing that such behavior is a certain death sentence? In some cases, multiple doses per day or frequently adjusting dosing frequency are required for treating serious illness, and such complexity may play a negative role in patient's persistence and adherence, which will further influence the therapy's effects. And some drug therapy may also cause a decline in the quality of life due to drug reactions, as a result the patient may decide that life with painful drug side effects is too uncomfortable and that there is little or no hope for the future.

Guilt may play a role, where one may have unknowingly infected other persons with this life-threatening condition, and rather than living with the guilt, the patient may elect to end their possibly pitiful existence. We have vastly different feelings about the imminent death of persons who have caused their own problems through risky behaviors; the motorcycle driver without a helmet in an accident, the injectable drugs abuser who contracts hepatitis or HIV, the liver cancer patient who contracted the disease from risky sexual activity, etc.

BIOETHICS AND NEW TECHNOLOGIES

It seems strange that there can be anything new about death. It has been present since the existence of the first living being. Yet, scientific developments have raised new issues that did not require attention in earlier days. First of all, there is debate about the definition of death. As is widely known, one may still have the heart functioning in a coma or be in a permanent vegetative state. Persons can be maintained nearly indefinitely by life-supporting technology. There have been cases where this has been done for nearly two decades. However, in recent time, this has raised increasing awareness among medical community that the concept of "brain death" should be strictly distinguished from a coma or vegetative state. As family members or friends, they may think if their beloved one is still breathing then there might be a miracle, so they hope to continue the life-supporting machines to keep the patient "alive." But the truth is that if a patient is properly diagnosed as "brain death," then he or she is dead. Also the respiratory function of the patient could be maintained by advanced ventilators, the loss of capacity and consciousness are irreversible.[21] There is no way to treat death, and to continue the life-supporting technology is not only useless, but also disrespectful to the patient. The question of the time or definition of death has particular meaning for the families of those who are or might be deceased, and to the medical community as well. This latter interest comes to importance when the patient at or near death is an organ donor.

The matter of new technologies to maintain life must be considered. Today, the medical armamentarium includes agents that are expected to extend the lives of terminal cancer patients by two months, at enormous expense and with a very limited quality of life. Should that therapy be undertaken and who should make that decision? In recent times, some of these decisions are made by the payers; the health insurance company or managed care organization that decides whether to pay for the therapy or not. Society will have to come to grips with these issues and questions.

The mirror image of that question is the matter of euthanasia. While it is garnering headlines these days, it has most likely been around, at least informally, for centuries, when the kind and empathetic physician decided to increase the morphine level on a terminal patient in excruciating pain. Most often the request came from the patient him or herself or from close family members.

The legalization of euthanasia (mercy killing) has been the source of passionate battles in the States where it has been considered. The law must provide a protection to the caregiver who follows such a request so that he is not prosecuted for murder under existing laws.

It appears that the Europeans have made more strides in the euthanasia debate than the Americans. In the Netherlands, for example, a patient, who is determined to be sane and aware of his decision, can try to persuade his physician and a panel of other physicians that the prognosis is totally hopeless and that he can no longer endure with the pain and suffering he must endure, the financial drain of his continued custodial, palliative care on him and his surviving family. The panel then reaches a decision to find a respectful response to his request so that he may die with dignity.[22] A recent nation-wide study in Netherlands has shown that an euthanasia request is associated with age, diagnosis, and involvement of palliative teams and psychiatrist in care.[23] Although only a small proportion of patients requested euthanasia, the researchers found that younger age, more advanced diagnosis (cancer, nervous system), and no or less involvement of palliative teams and psychiatrists in care might be linked with an euthanasia request from a patient. We as healthcare providers need to provide best quality end-of-life care and make careful decision regarding such requests.

SUMMARY

After thousands of years of recorded history, we still know very little of what happens during death and what follows it, if anything. The social sciences have given the pharmacist important facts, findings and techniques to assist the terminal patient and the family in dealing with the process of dying. Understanding the different cultural and religious perspectives on death, the psychological and physical phases of the death and dying continuum, and the philosophical challenges patients and families experience regarding during the dying process can assist pharmacists in optimizing their support and care to a dying patient and his/her caregivers at the end of life.

REFERENCES

1. Hui, D., Dos Santos, R., Chisholm, G., et al. (2015). Bedside clinical signs associated with impending death in patients with advanced cancer: preliminary findings of a prospective, longitudinal cohort study. *Cancer* 15;121(6):960–7.

2. Kubler-Ross, E. (1969). *On death and dying.* New York: Macmillan.

3. Mody, R.A. (1976). *Life after life.* New York: Bantam Books.

4. Woodson, R. (1976). Concept of hospice care in terminal disease. In J.M. Veath (Ed.), *Breast cancer.* Karger, Basle, 16–179.

5. Kalish, R.A. (1975). Death and dying in a social context. In R.H. Binstock & E. Shanas (Eds.), *Handbook of aging and the social sciences*, 2nd Edition. New York: VanNostrand, 149–170.

6. Feifel, H. (Ed.). (1959). *The meaning of death.* New York: McGraw-Hill.

7. Aldrich, C.K. (1963). The dying patient's grief. *JAMA* 184, 329.

8. Glaser, B. & Strauss, A. (1968). *Time for dying.* Chicago: Aldine.

9. Temel, J.S., Greer, J.A., Muzikansky, A. et al. (2010). Early palliative care for patients with metastatic non-small-cell lung cancer. *N Engl J Med.* 19;363(8):733–42.

10. Fawole, O.A.1., Dy, S.M., Wilson, R.F., et al. (2013). A systematic review of communication quality improvement interventions for patients with advanced and serious illness. *J Gen Intern Med.* 28(4):570–7.

11. National Consensus Project for Quality Palliative Care. (2009). *Clinical practice guidelines for quality palliative care*, Second Edition. Pittsburg: National Consensus Project.

12. Lee, S.K. (2009). East Asian attitudes toward death: A search for the ways to help east asian elderly dying in contemporary America. *Perm J.* Summer;13(3):55–60.

13. Kubler-Ross, E. (1975). Death: The final stage of growth. Englewood Cliffs: Prentice Hall, 66.

14. Ibid., 68.

15. Shneidman, E.S. (1980). *Death: Current perspectives.* Palo Alto: Mayfield, 36. on

16. Alvarado, K.A., Templer, D.I., Bresler, C., et al., (1995). The relationship of religious variables to death depression and death anxiety. *J Clin Psychol* 51(2):202–4.

17. Payer, L. (1989). *Medicine and culture.* New York: Penguin, 120.

18. Toynbee, A. (1968). The relation between life and death, living and dying. In Toynbee, A., Mant, A.K., Smart, N. et al., *Man's concern with death.* New York: McGraw-Hill.

19. Gilbert. S.M. (2007). *Death's door: Modern dying and the ways we grieve.* New York: W W Norton Publishers.

20. Wijdicks, E.F. (2001). The diagnosis of brain death. *N Engl J Med.* 19;344(16):1215–21

21. vd Heide, A., Onwuteaka-Philipsen, B., Rurup, M. et al. (May 10, 2007). *End of life practices in the Netherlands under the Euthanasia act.* NEJM, 356, 19, 1957.

22. Onwuteaka-Philipsen, B.D., Rurup, M.L., & Pasman, H.R. (2010). The last phase of life: Who requests and who receives euthanasia or physician-assisted suicide? *Med Care.* 48(7):596–603.

CHAPTER 18

PSYCHOSOCIAL ASPECTS OF CARING FOR INDIVIDUALS WITH MENTAL ILLNESS

Nathaniel M. Rickles, PharmD, PhD, BCPP

LEARNING OBJECTIVES:

1. Identify the key factors in the development of the US mental health service delivery system.
2. Describe the role of labeling and stigma in the treatment of individuals with mental illness.
3. Explain the recovery process of individuals with mental illness.
4. Analyze the factors that affect current prescribing and dispensing of psychotropic medications in the United States.
5. Differentiate between the various roles pharmacists can have in caring for individuals with mental illness.

KEY TERMS

Asylum

Chlorpromazine

Collective responsibility

Community mental health centers (CMHCs)

Deinstitutionalization

Deviant

Diagnostic and Statistical Manual of Mental Disorders (DSM)

Diathesis stress model

Empowerment

Etiology of mental illness

General adaptation syndrome (GAS)

Hill Burton Act of 1946

Institutionalization

Medicalization

Mental Health Systems Act of 1980

Mental illness

Moral treatment

National Alliance on Mental Illness (NAMI)

National Committee for Mental Hygiene (NCMH)

Program for Assertive Community Treatment (PACT)

Revolving door phenomenon

Social Security Act of 1965

Stigma

Stress

Internal conditions of recovery

External conditions of recovery

Human rights

Supportive culture

Recovery-oriented services

College of Psychiatric and Neurologic Pharmacists (CPNP)

INTRODUCTION

Every day, in practically every pharmacy setting, a pharmacist will interact with an individual who has a mental illness. We may not know with certainty whether the individual has a mental illness because physical and mental illnesses share the same properties of being associated with conditions that are both observable and not observable. Mental illness affects millions of Americans and has no demographic boundaries as it affects the young, the old, males, females, different ethnic groups, different educational levels, and different geographic areas. Certain mental illnesses may be more common in one group than another, such as depression is twice more prevalent in women than men.[1] The care of those with mental illness is the subject of a booming pharmaceutical industry and a wide range of psychological services aimed at controlling symptoms and reducing societal costs associated with uncontrolled symptoms. In a 2009 study, researchers reported that the percentage of antidepressant treatment nearly doubled during the 10-year period from 1996 to 2005.[2] At the onset, it is important to note that the reader be conscious of efforts being made throughout this chapter to avoid labeling individuals as "schizophrenic" or "mentally ill" and, rather to refer to this population as "individuals with mental illness." The identity of an individual is much more than their illness; the illness should not define them but rather be a part of them. Individuals with mental illness are mothers, fathers, sisters, brothers, friends, employees, etc. A discussion about labeling and its consequences and why this change in language is important will be discussed later in this chapter.

In order to fully appreciate the current mental health system and pharmacy's role in it, it is important to spend the first part of this chapter understanding the historical development of the United States' mental healthcare system. Such history will also bring forward the key psychosocial issues that affect all stakeholders in the mental health system including pharmacists. It is this historical context that will form the basis of the second part of the chapter focusing on current issues in mental healthcare and the third part on the roles of pharmacy in interprofessional mental healthcare.

COLONIAL AMERICA

Many of the attitudes and behaviors of the early Colonists toward individuals with mental illness stem from European attitudes that developed over centuries. European society identified individuals with mental illness as deviant, persecuted these individuals, and burned them at the stake for being "Satan's representatives."[3] Based on such origins, it is not surprising that the Colonists believed mental illnesses flowed from natural and supernatural sources such as the devil.[4] The Colonists would eventually come to believe individuals with mental illness were no longer seen as passive recipients of the spirits but that they had individual control over these impulses.

In general, individuals who were "distracted" and "lunatick" were perceived as an individual rather than a societal problem. There were no social policies to deal with the individuals with mental illness.[4] Subsequently, individuals with mental illness were viewed as the primary responsibility of the family. Based on British principles of collective responsibility, both the poor and individuals with mental illness who threatened public safety and were not cared for by their families were helped by local communities.[4] This latter civic philosophy of the Colonists led to the development of institutional care for individuals with mental illness. Institutional care for individuals with mental illness came largely in four forms during the mid and late 1700s: general hospitals, private institutions, public hospitals, (the first public hospital for individuals with mental illness was founded in Virginia in 1769), and prisons.[4] Due to a low population density in the Colonial and early American period, the number of individuals identified with mental illness was low.

19TH CENTURY AMERICA

As the population of the new America grew and the industrial revolution led to shifts from farms to factories, individuals became more geographically mobile and less likely to remain home. Such transformations led to the need for more institutions to care for relatives with mental illnesses. The 1800s brought about a surge in the number of public and private institutions (asylums) caring for individuals with mental illness. This increase in asylums was also supported by two other factors: (1) the thinking that therapeutic approaches for mental illnesses required a well-ordered institution and (2) beliefs from the religious arrival of the Second Great Awakening suggesting individuals are capable of overcoming their weaknesses and being cured.[4]

Since the government saw itself as having an obligation to care for all its citizens, more and more individuals were entered into the local asylums. City asylums became overcrowded and poorly staffed. These conditions and the efforts of advocate Dorothea Dix led to the development of more state-funded asylums in the geographic centers of different states to ensure "equal" access to all citizens.[4] These early asylums were focused on "moral treatment," which consisted of religious exercises, recreation, and mechanical restraint. The institutionalization of individuals with mental illness was largely made by family members with the small role of the legal system. The asylums were generally comprised of diverse patient populations with multiple diagnoses and cultures; some asylums were segregated along racial and ethnic lines. In particular, the number of older adults committed to asylums also grew since local authorities saw the benefit of redefining problems in the elderly as psychiatric in nature and having the state pay for such care. As the size and diversity of the asylums grew, the social organization and treatment philosophy of the asylums became more rigid and coercive. For example, overworked attendants would often respond to behavioral problems with force and heavily resort to straightjackets and seclusion rooms. In contrast, there were also some cases where close interpersonal relationships were formed between patients and staff.

THE RISE OF AMERICAN PSYCHIATRY

Many of the early physicians treating the mentally ill saw their role to largely cure mental illnesses through two main mechanisms: guiding patients regarding appropriate behaviors and correcting imbalances in the physical-mental system through the use of chemicals and/or biological procedures. The lack of consensus on how asylums should optimally provide care to those with mental illness, few curative treatments, and the growing numbers in the asylums all contributed to the characterization of asylums as depressing, hopeless "snake pits" where staff members were focused on maintaining the patient's daily routines.

The first approach to treating mental illnesses, and guiding patients toward appropriate behaviors, grew out of a growing scientific interest during the late 19th century in understanding psychological and social roots of human behavior. It is hard to identify precisely the birth of the psychotherapy. Such confusion about the origins of psychotherapy came largely by how the media and textbooks have popularized Sigmund Freud's early 20th century use of psychoanalysis and "lying on the couch" techniques to investigate the meanings of hidden or subconscious impulses and dreams. Today, there are over 400 known approaches to psychotherapy.[5] These psychotherapeutic approaches range in extent to which they apply behavioral, cognitive, and emotional modalities to helping improve patient functioning. Multi-modal approaches that use a combination of psychotherapeutic techniques are commonly used. For example, cognitive-behavioral therapies are one of the more widely used and effective psychotherapeutic modalities for the care of individuals with various mental health concerns (i.e., life adjustments, role conflicts, stress management) and psychiatric illnesses.

During the late 1800s, the second mechanism of treating mental illnesses, biological treatments, become more widely used as physicians began exploring the possibility that there are biological causes of mental illness. It is during this time that the field of neurology began to emerge and individuals such as Dr. Emil Kraepelin began to scientifically explore what later became known as schizophrenia.[3] This period was also marked by clinicians and researchers identifying areas and functions of the brain as reflected in the works of Drs. Alois Alzheimer, Carl Wernicke, and Alfred Meyer. Psychiatry was seen on a dynamic continuum between normal to abnormal and its scientific study took place more and more in research institutes and psychiatric hospitals.

Mental illnesses were beginning to be seen as hereditary and thus occurred from one generation to the next.[4] Thus, supporters of the eugenics movement called for laws regulating marriage and involuntary sterilization of the mentally ill. Another aspect of this movement was its focus on prevention of mental illnesses, which gradually developed greater predominance in mental health services. In 1909, a National Committee for Mental Hygiene (NCMH) was formed with the goals of protecting individuals with mental illness, improving hospitals for the mentally ill, promoting research on treatment and prevention, and establishing state societies of mental health.[4]

TRANSITION TOWARDS COMMUNITY-BASED MENTAL HEALTHCARE

The economic depression of the 1930s and World War II brought about reductions in hospital funding to carry out services, to provide staffing, and to add physical facilities. Such reductions and growing numbers of patients led to poor treatment conditions such as lack of cleanliness and abusive staff. These conditions contributed to growing tensions regarding the amount of professional autonomy and accountability between the state governments and asylum psychiatrists.

World War II also brought about changes in how psychiatrists viewed the treatment trajectory of many mental illnesses. Military psychiatrists came from the battlefields reporting brief treatment of such symptoms as irritability, anxiety, and nightmares and then sending soldiers back into the battlefields. Such reports helped the mental health treatment community begin to think that more treatment of individuals with mental illness could occur in the community and not necessarily require hospitalization. Psychiatrists were beginning to think that early treatment might even prevent hospitalization.

It is also during the 1930s and 40s that new biological treatments were being explored such as insulin shock treatments, electric shock therapy, fever therapy, and pre-frontal lobotomies. Although these approaches were found to have serious side effects and risks, they were important steps by psychiatry to explore how changes in body chemistry and structure lead to potential therapeutic changes in patient behavior. Psychiatrists were beginning to explore the use of existing medications to treat symptoms of mental illness. Chlorpromazine, an antihistamine, was used typically to relax surgical patients experiencing surgical trauma. Psychiatrists examined chlorpromazine's benefits in helping to sedate patients with schizophrenia. The success of chlorpromazine in schizophrenia made many physicians realize the potential for drugs that affect behavior to treat the symptoms of mental illnesses. As a result, many more drugs began to be developed to manage psychiatric symptoms such as the tranquilizer reserpine and antidepressants such as iproniazid and imipramine.

In conjunction with the increase in biological treatments of mental illnesses, there was also a shift towards greater diagnostic specificity classification of symptoms in mental disorders. The American Psychiatric Association's first edition of the Diagnostic and Statistical Manual of Mental Disorders (DSM) was developed in 1952 and identified 128 diagnostic categories. In 1994, the DSM-IV had 357 categories/diagnoses of mental illnesses and was organized according to five main axes: Axis 1: Clinical disorders, other conditions that may be a focus of clinical attention; Axis 2: Personality disorders, mental retardation; Axis 3: General medical conditions, Axis 4: Psychosocial and environmental problems, and Axis 5: Global assessment of functioning. Since the first DSM edition, there have been numerous changes in what and how illnesses are classified.[6] In 2013, DSM-V was published with such changes including how intellectual disabilities, communication disorders, autism spectrum disorders, schizophrenia, bipolar illness, and depressive disorders are defined and evaluated.[7] In some cases, new disorders were identified such as disruptive mood dysregulation disorder and premenstrual dysphoric disorder.

The increase in biological treatments and a diagnostic classification of mental illnesses were both part of a growing movement toward the "medicalization" of mental illness in which doctors targeted patients' symptoms with treatments and failed to view the psychosocial aspects of the patient's experience.[8] The promise of psychopharmacology in managing psychiatric symptoms and the poor conditions in state hospitals were contributors to the realization that the country needed greater federal resources to ensure greater scientific research and training involving these new treatments and improvements in hospital care. The National Institute of Mental Health was founded in 1949 and pledged to train more mental health professionals through fellowships and grants and support research relating to the cause, diagnosis, and treatment of mental illness.[4] In addition, President Kennedy's 1961 Joint Commission on Mental Illness and Health called for larger investments in basic research, more training programs and guidelines for treatments, and greater public education about mental illness.[3] Such federal initiatives led to rapid expansions in various mental health occupations such as clinical psychology, psychiatric social work, and psychiatric nursing.

There was also a growing focus towards community healthcare that was stimulated in part by the Hill Burton Act of 1946 that brought about a general increase in community hospitals and their development of psychiatric units.[4] These inpatient units admitted patients with severe and persistent mental illnesses. The 1960s brought greater development in community psychiatry through the construction of community mental health centers (CMHCs). These CMHCs largely provided care to those with substance abuse and life issues such as marital problems and other personal stressors. The increase in community-based sites for mental healthcare helped improve access to early intervention services and avoided long-term psychiatric hospitalizations. At the same time community-based psychiatry was taking shape, the Social Security Act of 1965 encouraged the states to reduce costs by shifting the care of older adults with mental illnesses from state-operated psychiatric hospitals to federally-funded nursing homes. This combination of changes led to four major points of access to mental health services and, thus, the types of patients served by the setting: CMHCs for individuals with less severe illnesses, inpatient community-based hospitals for individuals with more severe but requiring limited treatment, state-based psychiatric facilities for young and middle-age individuals with mental illness requiring more extensive treatment, and nursing homes for older adults with mental illnesses.

TRANSITION TOWARDS GREATER INDIVIDUALISM IN MENTAL HEALTHCARE

During the 1960s and 70s, there were significant challenges to the medicalization of mental illnesses. Erving Goffman's 1961 book *Asylums* highlighted how prolonged psychiatric hospitalizations led to individuals losing their self-identity and esteem and contributed to acts of deviance.[9] Goffman describes how individuals living for months and years in psychiatric hospitals became "institutionalized" and lost critical skills and abilities to function outside hospital life. Others during this time, psychiatrists such as R.D. Laing and Thomas Szasz, and philosopher Michel Focault, questioned the diagnosis and treatment of mental illnesses. They saw such medical diagnoses and treatments as a way for society to label and control people who may think and behave differently than those in the mainstream culture. One example of their argument is the American Psychiatric Association's decision to include homosexuality as a psychiatric illness in the DSM until 1980, when it was removed from the third edition of DSM.

Additional challenges to psychiatry were seen in the courts and on television. The court case of Rouse vs. Cameron (1966) supported the expectation that individuals with mental illness who were committed to psychiatric hospitals had a right to adequate treatments.[4] Ken Kesey's book *One Flew Over the Cuckoo's Nest* and subsequent 1975 movie powerfully presented the unjust and involuntary treatment of individuals with mental illness.

Due to these challenges to the mental healthcare system, the National Alliance on Mental Illness (NAMI) was formed in 1979 and became the largest national grassroots mental health organization dedicated to "building better lives for the millions of Americans affected by mental illness."[10] This organization publishes brochures, books and other materials to promote awareness about mental illnesses and their consequences. The Mental Health Systems Act of 1980 provided protection of patient rights and support services for vulnerable groups.[3] In particular, mental health advocates were concerned that commitment procedures were often vague and arbitrary, individuals have a right to refuse treatment, and care would be provided in a confidential manner.

MODERN PSYCHIATRIC CARE

In the late 1970s concerns mounted about the quality of institutional care and individual rights. Concurrently, several effective medications were being brought to market that targeted the symptoms of various mental illnesses. These factors led to the government perceiving the need and value of releasing long-term institutionalized persons from state facilities and having them enter the community. This "deinstitutionalization" process resulted in many state psychiatric hospitals closing and individuals with mental illness being released into the streets without follow-up care, shelter, and other resources to be successfully integrated into their communities. Many of these individuals would return to the hospital quickly due to poor follow-up and inadequate management of symptoms. These individuals would go in and out of the psychiatric hospitals multiple times (known as the "revolving door" phenomenon) and often leave clinicians and hospital staff frustrated.[11]

In response to these concerns, the National Institute of Mental Health initiated a federal/state partnership to develop programs for those with severe and persistent mental illnesses related to housing, financial assistance, treatment and support services. One program that served as a model for several outpatient mental health programs is the Program for Assertive Community Treatment (PACT) founded in Madison, Wisconsin in 1980.[12] PACT was designed to prevent hospitalizations by teaching individuals with mental illness skills and provide support services for these individuals to live in the community. Some of these services included on-going monitoring, crisis intervention, and family involvement in care. Results showed PACT enabled individuals with mental illness to have better personal relationships, have greater satisfaction with care, and lower rates of hospitalizations. Today, there are several community-based programs that attempt to better target exacerbation of symptoms and reduce hospitalizations.

The current mental health system involves a mix of state psychiatric facilities, private psychiatric facilities, inpatient psychiatric units in community hospitals, community mental health centers, and a variety of clinic and short-term stay facilities. Since the 1950s revolution in psychiatric medicines, hundreds of psychiatric medicines have come to the market to treat a variety of mental illnesses. Newer psychotropic medicines have fewer side effects, fewer drug interactions, and are useful in targeting specific symptoms of illnesses. Much of the literature recommends ideal treatments for a variety of psychiatric illnesses involves both cognitive and behavioral therapies along with medications. Also numerous public health efforts have improved the screening and detection of mental illnesses. The historical context of the first part of this chapter lays the foundation for appreciating the development of the modern mental healthcare system in the United States. Such context also shapes some of the key contemporary trends and issues in mental health such as the focus on labeling and reducing stigma, searching for etiologies of mental disorders, facilitating patient recovery, establishing parity in mental health insurance, and psychotropic prescribing practices.

CONTEMPORARY ISSUES
IN MENTAL HEALTHCARE

LABELING AND REDUCING STIGMA OF MENTAL ILLNESS

Labels identify or define who we are. How do we define mental illness? What does such a person with mental illness look like and how are they different from a physically ill person? People typically respond to such questions that individuals with mental illness look odd, unkempt, talk to themselves, and act strangely. They will also respond that physically ill individuals have a broken leg, look pale, and appear weak. While these generalizations of individuals (stereotypes) with mental and physical illness hold true in many cases, there are many situations when it becomes difficult to distinguish who has mental or physical illness. For example, in both cases of high blood pressure and depression and/or anxiety, the symptoms may not be present and thus difficult to identify that the individual has either or both illnesses. Individuals also confuse the distinctions between developmental disorders such as Down's Syndrome or autism and mental disorders. Definitions of mental illness also change depending on clinical or socio-cultural perspectives. For example, the American Psychiatric Association[6] defines mental illness in clinical terms as:

> A clinically significant behavioral or psychological syndrome or pattern that occurs in an individual and that is associated with present distress (e.g., a painful symptom) or disability (i.e., impairment in one or more important areas of functioning) or with a significantly increased risk of suffering death, pain, disability, or an important loss of freedom.

Conversely, Eaton[3] uses a socio-cultural perspective and defines mental illness as including two components: "(1) a collection of emotions or behaviors that meet all three conditions: rare, culturally deviant, inexplicable and (2) leads to one or more of following consequences: loss of control over environment, detachment from social networks, and interference with the individual's sense of biography/self."

Regardless of which definition and perspective we wish to accept and the extent to which we include various illnesses as a part of the spectrum of mental illness, we are faced with the question as to what it means to label someone as having mental illness. The signs and symptoms of most mental illnesses are often viewed as "deviant" since they fall outside the typical boundaries of expected human cognition and behavior. For example, most people would not report a symptom of schizophrenia that one's thoughts are being broadcasted on television and would consider this symptom as deviant thinking. Any form of deviance is dependent on culture as norms are defined by the culture. Some cultures may view individuals with mental illness as possessing special powers. In other words, an individual acting bizarre is only considered deviant if the culture that surrounds that individual believes the behavior is deviant. Why does society develop such labels for acts considered deviant? Society determines what is deviant in large part so it can ensure structure, order, and context to daily living and expectations.

Stigma is a negative consequence of labeling and associated with three components: (1) sets a person apart from others, (2) links the marked person to undesirable characteristics, and (3) rejects and avoids the labeled individual.[13] A person may have consciously or unconsciously expressed stigma towards a mentally ill person when he/she has seen a poorly dressed man talking angrily to himself and think he is acting strange, potentially dangerous, and avoid going near him. Stigma, however, is a matter of degree since it depends often on how much the individual being marked is linked with the undesirable characteristics. One may attribute less stigma towards a person who acts a little strange but quietly sits on a bench than toward a person who acts angrily to himself since they may be perceived less dangerous.

While scales measuring stigma have been developed and validated,[14] one hears and sees stigma with words such as "nut," "crazy," "cuckoo," "psycho," and "sicko" communicated on a daily basis throughout our culture. One key source of stigma is through the portrayals of individuals with mental illness in television, movies, and novels. Hollywood has often presented individuals with mental illness as deranged, dangerous, impulsive, and uncontrollable.[15] Examples of such movies are: *Friday the 13th—A New Beginning* (1985), *Psycho III* (1986), *Misery* (1990), and *Silence of the Lambs* (1991). There have been some more positive images of individuals with mental illness such as *Rain Man* (1988) and *A Beautiful Mind* (2001). Novels such as William Heffernan's *Ritual* (1988) and Jeff Raines' *Unbalanced Acts* (1990) both describe murderers with significant psychopathology. Although clinicians are thought to be unconditional and not affected by such negative attitudes, the literature provides evidence that clinicians also express similar discomfort with those with mental illness as the general public.[16]

In recent years, there have been numerous local, state, and national campaigns by advocacy organizations to increase the screening and reduce stigma of mental illnesses. There have been numerous direct-to-individual advertisements regarding mental illnesses and treatments for mental illnesses. Further, the National Institute of Mental Health has and continues to encourage research regarding the study and reduction of stigma of mental illnesses. These combined efforts may be associated with the significant increases in the number of individuals receiving various psychotropic medications such as antidepressants and anti-anxiety agents.[17] All these changes would presumably reduce stigma associated with mental illnesses. In particular, since most individuals know of one or more individuals taking antidepressants, it would be expected that depression is one of the mental illnesses where stigma would be much less prevalent than in previous years.

SEARCHING FOR ETIOLOGIES OF MENTAL ILLNESS

While there has been much progress in mental healthcare over the last century, we are still unclear on the role of many structures in the brain, and how various mental illnesses develop and respond to treatments. Mechanisms of action of most psychotropics also remain unknown. To answer these and other questions about the etiology and treatment of mental illnesses, neuroscientists have been actively engaged in considerable research exploring the use of brain imaging technologies and radioactive lab techniques to help link brain structures and functions with behavior and patient outcomes. Another important area of research in the etiology of mental illness has explored the concept of stress and how stress contributes to mental illness.

This latter research area has yielded both biological and social definitions of stress. In Hans Selye's *The Stress of Life*, he described stress biologically as a disruption in the normal homeostasis of organisms and described three phases of the stress response or also known as the general adaptation syndrome (GAS): a general and widespread alarm stage, a specific response stage involving defense of tissues, and exhaustion if the stressor has not been removed.[18] In related work, Seligman[19] reported that individuals who are ineffective in terminating a stressor will eventually give up and accept the stressor (he called this learned helplessness). Selye also found that many different stressors or mental representations of stressors led to the same GAS, that the entire organism was affected, and that GAS could lead to exhaustion in the absence of the stressor.[18] It is believed that these consequences of GAS explain in large part some of the symptoms of depression and anxiety.

In addition to these biological conceptualizations of stress, most social scientists have defined stress as it relates to feelings of being overwhelmed by circumstances. For example, Mechanic[20] defines stress as "a discrepancy between the demands imping- ing on an individual, and his/her potential responses to those demands." Wheaton[21] defines stress as "conditions of threat, demands, or structural constraints that, by the very fact of their occurrence or existence, call into question the operating integrity of the organism." Although there is general agreement on what defines stress socially or biologically, individuals vary considerably on how they interpret various stressors with some events being more or less stressful. There has been considerable research in mental healthcare on identifying how different life events in isolation and cumu- latively contribute to the risk for mental illnesses. The diathesis stress model is a well- known model that has added considerably to how researchers and clinicians think stressors result in mental illnesses.

In this context, diathesis refers to genetic or inherited vulnerability to respond to stress in maladaptive ways.[3] The model demonstrates that the manifestation of men- tal illness is a combined result of stress, a genetic risk for mental illnesses (such as schizophrenia, bipolar illness, depression, anxiety, etc.) and how severely those dis- orders get manifested based on stress, and the protectiveness of one's environment. At high levels of stress (such as prolonged combat or a new transition) or having a significant genetic predisposition to mental illness, many individuals may meet the criteria for having a mental disorder. Individuals exposed to a high level of stress and possess a strong genetic predisposition to mental illness may be more likely to experience the more severe forms of a mental illness. Only those individuals who have little genetic predisposition to an illness or exposed to low environmental stress may avoid symptoms of mental illness. It is possible that individuals who have high genetic predisposition to a mental illness may avoid meeting criteria for the disorder if they live in a protective environment providing adequate support. While the dia- thesis stress model is a useful way to conceptualize the interaction of genetics and stress in predicting the likelihood of mental illness, Kendler[22] notes the model is built on the questionable assumption that genes and the environment act additively and independently of each other. This assumption is problematic since individuals often select their own environments and such environments then act differently with their genetic predispositions and, therefore, it becomes unclear how much of the vulnerability to mental illness is associated with environmental stress and due to genetic predisposition.

FACILITATING PATIENT RECOVERY

The concept that individuals can recover from mental illnesses is not new as it has been around since the 1980s when studies and first-person accounts highlighted that individuals with mental illness can come out of the system relatively intact and return to one's sense of self and self-worth.[23,24] This concept of recovery is central to many of the current outreach and public education efforts of organizations advocating for individuals with mental illness and their families. Jacobson and Greenley's[25] model of recovery suggests recovery refers both to the internal and external conditions that enable a person to return to fuller functioning in society.

The internal conditions of recovery include hope, healing, empowerment, and connection. Hope refers to the individual's belief that recovery is possible. Having such a belief often means that the individual has accepted that there is a problem, committing to change, focusing on the positives, and avoiding the negative aspects of their past experiences. Jacobson and Greenley[25] indicate that healing means not necessarily a return to baseline functioning but rather overcoming internalized stigma towards oneself for having mental illness and regaining one's self-esteem, self-respect, control over symptoms, and/or managing the social and psychological effects of stress. These authors refer to empowerment as an internal capacity to take greater control and responsibility for themselves. Connection is that part of recovery in which the individual reconnects with the social world by filling various roles in society including employment, family, religion, and community participation.

External conditions of recovery refer to those conditions outside the individual that help the individual achieve recovery. These conditions include human rights, a supportive culture, and the availability of recovery-oriented services. Human rights include those efforts to: (1) reduce and eliminate stigma and discrimination against persons with psychiatric disabilities, (2) promote and protect the rights of those in the mental health system, (3) provide equal opportunities for individuals in education, employment, and housing, and (4) ensure access to needed resources such as food, shelter, and services that facilitate recovery (job training, subsidized housing, health services, etc.). A supportive culture highlights the need to incorporate individual rights into all decisions and informed consent as a part of daily practice. The need for informed consent has been especially important given past media reports that individuals with mental illness were not adequately informed of being put on placebos in clinical trials evaluating drug efficacy and toxicity. Another aspect of a supportive culture is the development of collaborative relationships regarding all aspects of care between individuals with mental illness, their families, and the healthcare team. This approach views the individual with mental illness as capable of active participation in decision-making.

The provision of recovery-oriented services is typically directed at symptom relief, crisis intervention, case management, rehabilitation, protection of rights, and support. Models of psychiatric rehabilitation integrate services provided by professionals, individuals with mental illness, and collaboratively between providers and individuals with mental illness.[25] Professionals often provide such services related to medication management, therapy, and case management. Individual-run services are developed and implemented by individuals with mental illnesses for individuals with mental illnesses and include peer support programs, hospitalization alternatives, hotlines, online support groups, and other programs involving role modeling and mentoring. Collaborative services are provided by and for individuals with mental illnesses, professionals, family members, friends, and other members of the community. These latter services include recovery education and training, crisis planning, development of recovery and treatment plans, individual rights, etc.

The internal and external conditions of recovery are interdependent on one another. A movement towards facilitating an external condition can help bring about positive change in an internal condition of recovery and likewise a change in internal conditions can lead to a change in the external conditions of recovery. Two examples illustrate this interdependence. First, a local community's effort to reduce stigma can help individuals with mental illness heal and gain a better sense of self. Second, as more individuals enter recovery, they will provide more models for policy-related efforts to facilitate recovery services and a larger supportive culture for healing.

ESTABLISHING PARITY IN MENTAL HEALTH INSURANCE

Since the birth of the managed healthcare movement in the 1970s and 80s, health insurance companies have explored multiple ways to increase their profit margins by controlling the rising costs of healthcare. Such cost-containment approaches include setting up restricted lists of medications that are less expensive (formularies), restricting the number of office visits and procedures, and sharing costs with individuals through co-payments and deductables. While these approaches have been applied to both physical and mental healthcare, there is evidence that the health insurance industry has not applied these and other approaches equally across physical and mental illnesses. Some of these inequities may be due in part to the fact that physical and mental healthcare have been handled separately by many health insurance plans. That is, many health insurance plans, including government-based plans, have outsourced ("carved out") the management of mental health services to behavioral healthcare organizations in an effort to identify more cost efficient systems to specifically manage growing mental health costs. These contracted service providers or managed behavioral healthcare organizations are under significant pressures to contain mental healthcare costs to maximize profits.

These pressures and the stigma around mental illnesses are thought to be some of the key reasons for the insurance industry's greater health coverage for physical illnesses than mental illnesses. Such actions have left individuals with mental illness with restricted access to mental healthcare, i.e., limited number of psychotherapy visits, medication management visits, and days of psychiatric hospitalization. Research has shown that limits in mental health insurance have caused individuals to limit their use of medications and other treatments, which put them and the health system at risk for negative outcomes including worsening symptoms and higher health costs.[26] Individuals with mental illnesses and their families have advanced numerous successful efforts to local, state, and federal policymakers to enact legislation requiring greater parity in health insurance between physical and mental illnesses. Until more national health reforms are made, this debate over parity of coverage will likely remain a significant concern for individuals and providers throughout the mental health system.

PSYCHOTROPIC PRESCRIBING PRACTICES

Psychiatrists, medical doctors specializing in mental health, have been traditionally the main prescribers of psychotropic medications. In the last two decades, there have been significant changes in psychotropic prescribing. First, psychiatrists are not the only medical doctors prescribing medications for individuals with mental illness. There have been significant increases in prescribing of antidepressants and anxiety medications by primary care physicians.[2,17] It is not entirely clear whether this increase is due to an increase in public recognition of depression and anxiety disorders (via direct-to-individual advertising), primary care physicians having a better understanding of depression and greater comfort with antidepressants and their relatively safer medication profiles than in years past, or the insurance industry's effort to limit patient access to specialists such as psychiatrists, and/or pharmaceutical industry sales efforts. In addition, physicians of all practice types are also using psychotropic medications for medical conditions such as pain management and sleep disorders. There is growing concern that psychotropic medications are being prescribed without clear and documented indication that the individual needs the medication.

Second, nurse practitioners and physician assistants are two professions within the allied health professions that have prescribing privileges throughout the United States and thus contribute to a significant amount of psychotropic prescribing. Third, pharmacists in several states have collaborative practice agreements with physicians that allow them to prescribe under limited situations. Pharmacists have prescribing privileges in Veteran Affairs Medical Centers and in specialized settings such as state facilities for individuals with developmental disabilities. Fourth, psychologists have lobbied in several states to have prescribing privileges for psychotropic medications. These individuals are typically required to take courses and pass certification requirements to be allowed to prescribe these medications.

The American Psychiatric Association and the American Medical Association have initiated successful lobbying efforts to thwart many of these legislative initiatives for other practitioners to have prescribing privileges. Physicians may feel threatened that other professionals are encroaching on their roles as prescribers and affecting their ability to generate income from prescribing. They also argue that these other health professionals lack the education and training to prescribe safely. Pharmacists interested in prescribing privileges have argued persuasively through a growing number of demonstration projects and published interventions showing that pharmacist management of medication therapy can have a significant impact on many patient outcomes including lower costs, improved clinical outcomes, adherence, etc.[27-29] The literature is filled with several studies demonstrating the value of pharmacists in both primary and specialty healthcare. The next section of the chapter focuses more specifically on how pharmacists engage the mental healthcare system.

PHARMACY ROLES
IN MENTAL HEALTHCARE

Pharmacists in mental healthcare have been involved in numerous collaborative services with physicians including (1) monitoring and reducing side effects, (2) assessing drug serum concentrations, (3) identifying drug interactions, (4) assisting in the development of treatment plans, and (5) identifying ways to improve medication adherence. Over the past three decades, clinical pharmacists performing these kinds of collaborative services to individuals with mental illness have shown to have a significant and positive impact on several patient and health system outcomes.[30-32] These studies have specifically demonstrated that psychotropic monitoring by clinical pharmacists was significantly associated with reductions in the number and doses of medications, hospitalizations, side effects, and improved medication adherence and clinical symptoms. Community pharmacists have also been shown to have a significant and positive impact on psychotropic education and monitoring.[27,31,32] These latter studies have shown that community pharmacists can significantly improve patient knowledge, beliefs, and sense of treatment progress. More multi-center, cost-effectiveness trials are needed to further demonstrate the role of pharmacists in mental healthcare.[30]

Since the late 1970s and early 1980s, there have been several postgraduate opportunities in pharmacy practice, psychiatric pharmacy residencies and fellowships, throughout the country to increase the number of trained pharmacists in mental healthcare. These psychiatric residencies and fellowships provide pharmacists an opportunity to train specifically in the area of mental healthcare. In the late 1990s, pharmacists who had extensive experiences in mental healthcare and/or had completed specialty residencies in psychiatric pharmacy became eligible to demonstrate their competencies in national certification exams on psychiatric pharmacy. A successful completion of these certification exams allows individuals to become board certified in psychiatric pharmacy (BCPP) for a seven-year period until they are required to meet requirements for recertification. The number of psychiatric pharmacists has grown considerably since the late 1990s and was the impetus for the development of an association in 1998, the College of Psychiatric and Neurologic Pharmacists (CPNP), dedicated to the "advancing the reach and practice of neuropsychiatric pharmacists" on the lives of individuals with mental illness.[33]

PHARMACY ATTITUDES TOWARD MENTAL ILLNESS

There has been some research exploring the attitudes of those in pharmacy toward individuals with mental illness. Several studies show pharmacists and pharmacy students have generally positive views towards those with mental illness.[34-38] Studies also show community pharmacists are uncomfortable with mental illness and such may affect the provision of services to those with mental illness.[36,39]

CPNP and NAMI collaborated on a 2012 national survey characterizing the relationship between individuals with mental health conditions and community pharmacists.[40] In this survey of 1,031 individuals with mental illness and caregivers, it was found that 91% felt very comfortable going to their community pharmacies, and 83%

felt respected by their pharmacist. A little more than half of the respondents reported a strong professional relationship with the pharmacist; over 40% indicated having no such relationship with the pharmacist. Survey results also revealed that 75% of respondents reported not receiving effectiveness and/or safety monitoring assistance from the pharmacist. Such results are congruent with findings the earlier studies showing the association between negative attitudes toward mental illnesses and provision of services to those with these mental illnesses.[36,39] This brief review suggests community pharmacists may not be consistently engaging individuals with mental illness and individuals with mental illness are reporting this lack of consistent pharmacist engagement. There have some pilot efforts involving individuals with lived experience of mental illness to reduce stigma among pharmacy students and pharmacists.[41-44] More research is needed to test educational and behavioral interventions to change pharmacist attitudes toward the caring for those with mental illnesses.

SUMMARY

This chapter has hopefully enlightened the reader to the rich and complex history of care provided to individuals with mental illness in the United States. Much of this history shows a field struggling with definitions of what it is to have mental illness and how we as a culture should respond to these definitions in terms of diagnosis, treatment and prevention. The mental health system is still considered by many to be quite fragmented, leaving individuals with mental illness with critical gaps in care. Current and future pharmacists should view themselves as a part of an interprofessional solution that resolves these gaps by helping to provide continuity in medication-related services and maximizing pharmacotherapy outcomes that facilitate the recovery of individuals with mental illness.

REFERENCES

1. Depression Guideline Panel. (April 1993). *Depression in primary care: volume 1. Detection and diagnosis.* Clinical practice guideline, number 5. Rockville, MD. U.S. Department of Health and Human Services, Public Health Services, Agency for Healthcare Policy and Research. AHCPR Publication No. 93–0551.

2. Olfson, M. & Marcus, S.C. (2009). National patterns in antidepressant medication treatment. *Arch Gen Psychiatry* 66(8):848–856.

3. Eaton, W.W. (2001). *The sociology of mental disorders,* Third Edition. Westport (CT): Praeger Publishers.

4. Grob, G.N. (1994). *The mad among us: A history of the care of America's mentally ill.* New York: The Free Press.

5. Corsini, R.J. (1995). Introduction. In Corsini, R.J. & Weddig, D. (Eds.). *Current psychotherapies,* fifth edition. Itasca (IL): F.E. Peacock Publishers, Inc.

6. American Psychiatric Association. (1994). *Diagnostic and statistical manual of mental disorders*, fourth edition, revised. Washington, DC, American Psychiatric Association.

7. American Psychiatric Association. (2013). *Diagnostic and statistical manual of mental disorders*, fifth edition, revised. Washington, DC, American Psychiatric Association.

8. Conrad, P. & Schneider, J.W. (1980). Looking at levels of medicalization: a comment on Strong's critique of the thesis of medical imperialism. *Soc Sci Med* 14A:75–79.

9. Goffman, E. (1961). *Asylums: Essays on the social situation of mental patients and other inmates.* New York: Random House.

10. National Alliance for the Mentally Ill, NAMI [homepage on the Internet]. Arlington, VA: National Alliance for the Mentally Ill; cited January 22, 2016]. About NAMI; [1 screen].Available from: http://www.nami.org/Content/NavigationMenu/Inform_Yourself/About_NAMI/About_NAMI.htm.

11. Glazer, W.M. & Ereshefsky, L. (1996). A pharmacoeconomic model of outpatient antipsychotic therapy in "revolving door" schizophrenic patients. *J Clin Psychiatry* 57:337–345.

12. Stein, L.I. & Test, M.A. (1980). Alternative to mental hospital treatment. I. Conceptual model, treatment program, and clinical evaluation. *Arch Gen Psych* 37:392–397.

13. Jones, E., Farina, A., Hastorf, A.H., Markus, H., Miller, D.T., & Scott RA.(1984). *Social stigma: The psychology of marked relationships.* New York: Freeman.

14. Link, B.G., Cullen, F.T., Struening, E., Shrout, P., & Dohrenwend, B.P. (1989). A modified labeling theory approach in the area of the mental disorders: an empirical assessment. *Am Soc Rev* 54;400–423.

15. Wahl, O.F. (1995). *Media madness: Public images of mental illness.* New Brunswick: Rutgers University Press.

16. Chin, S.H. & Balon, R. (2006). Attitudes and perceptions toward depression and schizophrenia among residents in different medical specialties. *Acad Psych* 30:262–263.

17. Pincus, H.A., Tanielian, T.L., Marcus, S.C., Olfson, M., Zarin, D.A., Thompson, J., et al. (1998). Prescribing trends in psychotropic medications: primary care, psychiatry, and other medical specialties. *JAMA* 279(7):526–531.

18. Selye, H. (1956). *The stress of life.* New York: McGraw-Hill.

19. Seligman, M.E.P. (1975). *Helplessness: On depression, development, and death.* San Francisco: W.H. Freeman.

20. Mechanic, D. (1978). *Medical sociology* second edition. New York: Free Press.

21. Wheaton, B. (1996). The domains and boundaries of stress concepts. In Kaplan, H.B. (Ed.), *Psychosocial stress: Perspectives on structure, theory, life course, and methods.* New: Academic Press.

22. Kendler, K.S.L.E. (1986). Models for the joint effect of genotype and environment on liability to psychiatric illness. *Am J of Psychiatry* 143(3):279-89.

23. Harding, C.M., Brooks, G.W., Ashikaga, T., Strauss, J.S., & Breier, A. (1987). The Vermont longitudinal study of persons with severe mental illness: II. long-term outcome of subjects who retrospectively met DSM-III criteria for schizophrenia. *Am J Psychiatry* 144:727–735.

24. Deegan, P.E. (1998). Recovery: The lived experience of rehabilitation. *Psychosocial Rehab J* 11(4):11–19.

25. Jacobson, N. & Greenley, D. (2001). What is recovery? A conceptual model and explication. *Psychiatr Serv* 52:482–485.

26. Soumerai, S.B., McLaughlin, T.J., Ross-Degnan, D., Casteris, C.S., & Bollini, P. (1994). Effects of limiting Medicaid drug-reimbursement benefits on the use of psychotropic agents and acute mental health services by patients with schizophrenia. *N Engl J Med* 331:650–5.

27. Rickles, N.M., Brown, T.A., McGivney, M.S., Snyder, M.E, & White, K.A. (2010). Adherence: a review of education, research, practice and policy in the United States. *Pharmacy Practice* (Internet) Jan-Mar;8(1):1–17.

28. Tan, E.C., Steward, K., Elliott, R.A., & George, J. (2014). Pharmacist services provided in general practice clinics: a systematic review and meta-analysis. *Res Soc Admin Pharm* 10: 608–622.

29. Chishom-Burns, M.A., Graff Zivin, J.S., Kim, J.K., Spivey, C.A., Slack, M., Herrier, R.N. et al. (2010). Economic effects of pharmacists on health outcomes in the United States: A systematic review. *Am J Health-Syst Pharm* 67:1624–34.

30. Finley, P.R., Crismon, M.L., Rush, A.J. (2003). Evaluating the impact of pharmacists in mental health: a systematic review. *Pharmacotherapy* 23(12): 1634–1644.

31. Rickles, N.M., Svarstad, B.L., Statz-Paynter, J., Taylor, L.V.,& Kobak, K. (2005). Pharmacists' telemonitoring of antidepressant use: Effects on patient feedback and other outcomes. *Journal of the American Pharmacists Association* 45(3): 344–353.

32. Rubio-Valera, M., Serrano-Blanco, A., Magdalena Belio, J., Fernandez, A., Garcia-Campayom, J., Pujo, M., et al. (2011). Effectiveness of pharmacist care in the improvement of adherence to antidepressants: a systematic review and meta-analysis. *Ann Pharmacother* 45:39–48.

33. College of Neurologic and Psychiatric Pharmacists (c. 2003-2016). [homepage on the Internet]. Lincoln, NE: College of Neurologic and Psychiatric Pharmacists; cited January 24, 2016]. About CPNP; [1 screen]. Available from: https://cpnp.org/about.

34. Bryant, S.G., Guernsey, B.G., Pearce, E.L., & Hokanson, J.A. (1985). Pharmacists' perceptions of mental healthcare, psychiatrists, and mentally ill patients. *Am J Hosp Pharm* 42;1366–9.

35. Crismon, M.L., Jermain, D.M., & Torian, S.J. (1990). Attitudes of pharmacy students toward mental illness. *Am J Hosp Pharm* 47:1369-73.

36. Phokeo, V., Sproule, B., & Raman-Wilms, L. (2004). Community pharmacists' attitudes toward and professional interactions with users of psychiatric medication. *Psychiatr Serv* 55:1434–1436.

37. Cates, M.E., Burton, A.R., & Woolley, T.W. (2005). Attitudes of pharmacists toward mental illness and providing pharmaceutical care to the mentally ill. *Ann Pharmacother* 39:1450–5.

38. Bell, J.S., Johns, R., Chen, T.F. (2006). Pharmacy students'; and graduates' attitudes toward people with schizophrenia and severe depression. *Am J Pharm Educ* 70(4):1–6.

39. Rickles, N.M., Dube, G.L., McCarter, A., & Olshan, J.S. (2010). Relationship between attitudes toward mental illness and provision of pharmacy services. *J Am Pharm Assoc* 50:704–713.

40. College of Psychiatric and Neurologic Pharmacists Foundation [Internet]. Omaha: The Foundation; [updated 2015]. Caley CF, Stimmel GL. Characterizing the relationship between individuals with mental health conditions and community pharmacists. Available at: https://cpnpf.org/_docs/foundation/2012/ nami-survey-report.pdf. Accessed January 24, 2016.

41. Buhler, A.V. & Karimi, R.M. (2008).Peer-level patient presenters decrease pharmacy students' social distance from patients with schizophrenia and clinical depression. *American Journal of Pharmaceutical Education* 72(5):article 106.

42. O'Reilly, C.L., Bell, J.S., & Chen, T.F. (2010). Consumer-led mental health education for pharmacy students. *American Journal of Pharmaceutical Education* 74(9):article 167.

43. O'Reilly, C.L., Bell, J.S., & Chen, T.F. (2012). Mental health consumers and caregivers as instructors for health professional students: a qualitative study. *Social Psychiatry & Psychiatric Epidemiology* 47:607–613.

44. Rickles, N.M & DaCosta, A. (n.d.). A consumer-led intervention to improve pharmacists' attitudes toward mental illness. *Mental Health Clinician*. In press.

CHAPTER 19

CULTURAL INFLUENCES ON MEDICATION USE

Jeri J. Sias, PharmD, MPH, Amanda M. Loya, PharmD, Abigail E. Strate, PharmD, Ilene Abramson, PhD

LEARNING OBJECTIVES:

1. Summarize how demographic shifts in the United States and social determinants of health shape disparities found in healthcare and the health workforce.
2. Explain how education, legal and accreditation expectations regarding culturally competent care influence pharmacy education and pharmacy practice.
3. Explore how attitudes and values shape patient care across cultures.
4. Apply patient explanatory, acculturation and cultural competency models to healthcare and medication use.
5. Describe the influences of cultural beliefs, behaviors, and culture-bound syndromes in patient care and medication use.

KEY TERMS

Cultural competency

Cultural influences

Culture

Health disparities

Medication Use

Social determinants of health

OVERVIEW OF CULTURAL INFLUENCES IN PHARMACY

CULTURE, CULTURAL COMPETENCY, COMMUNITY COMPETENCY

In recent years, pharmacists across healthcare settings have expanded their roles as providers to improve health outcomes and address public health disparities. For example, pharmacists have been advocating for and providing immunizations across cultures in inpatient and outpatient settings. To improve transitions of care for appropriate and safe medication use from the hospital to the home, pharmacists are increasingly and pro-actively collaborating across the healthcare team. Through Medication Therapy Management (MTM) and chronic Disease State Management (DSM), pharmacists are addressing more complex medication regimens, complementary alternative medicine (CAM) use, and access to medications—issues which cut across cultures.

The success of these services, however, depends heavily on practitioners' ability (attitudes, values, knowledge and skills) to interact with a variety of patient groups including the ever-increasing multi-national and diverse religious populations across North America. To explore cultural influences on medication use, this chapter provides an introduction to the terminology, disparities, education, legal, and accreditation matters and then transitions to models geared toward improving cultural competency in pharmacy practice with examples of diverse cultural beliefs and practices.

An abstract term, *culture* escapes a precise definition. Culture is dynamic and encompasses the ways that groups of people communicate, believe, relate, and pass on similar patterns of behavior. These social groups are often based on a common identity such as age, sex, religion, sexual orientation, race or ethnicity.[1] Pharmacists who strive for *cultural competency* recognize that "patients (and providers) have diverse values, beliefs, and behaviors. To address the health and medication issues facing diverse populations, pharmacist should be able to tailor their therapeutic choices and education to meet patients' social, cultural, and linguistic needs."[2]

A pharmacist with *community competency* understands that a patient's health may be influenced by constructs such as the history, context, culture, and geography of communities.[3] For example, the outbreak of the Ebola virus in 2014 with isolated cases in the United States shaped the process for screening certain populations for Ebola and for hospitals responding to potential virus outbreaks. On an individual, family, and community level, persons traveling to and from West Africa were concerned about discrimination and access to care.[4] There are community (e.g., history, context) as well as cultural influences that shape health care.

Certainly, a pharmacist's knowledge of specific cultural beliefs can be helpful. For example, if a pharmacist learns that the Cambodian healing practice of *coining*, which involves dipping coins in mentholated oil and vigorously rubbing them on the skin, can cause bruising and other mild skin abrasions, they are less likely to view a child with these markings as a victim of physical abuse.

Pharmacist providers however, must avoid the false sense of total competency inadvertently created by learning "a little" about a given population. In the following example, Melanie Tervalon and Jane Murray-Garcia illustrate the results of overestimating one's knowledge of patient characteristics:

> An African American nurse is caring for a middle-aged Latina woman several hours after the patient had undergone surgery. A Latino physician…commented to the nurse that the patient appeared to be in a great deal of postoperative pain. The nurse summarily dismissed his perception, informing him that she took a course in cross-cultural medicine and "knew" that Hispanic patients "over express the pain they are feeling." The physician had a difficult time influencing the perspective of this nurse, who focused on her self-proclaimed cultural expertise.[5]

The nurse provider was armed with some information about a culture that then could be potentially harmful to the patient. But, what other knowledge and skills about diverse cultures, communities, and disparities could help shape the attitudes and values that the nurse had?

CASE FOR UNDERSTANDING CULTURAL INFLUENCES

HEALTH AND HEALTHCARE DISPARITIES

While having the knowledge of cultures and the competency to work in diverse populations are important, there are compelling health disparities and pharmacy workforce issues that further highlight the importance of culture in health. A *health disparity* occurs when one segment of the population experiences a higher burden of illness, morbidity, and mortality in comparison to another group. A *healthcare disparity* is when there are differences between segments of the population in access to healthcare, health insurance, and quality of care.[6] Dr. Martin Luther King, Jr. once said, "Of all the forms of inequality, injustice [disparities] in health care is the most shocking and inhumane."[7]

The Institute of Medicine (IOM) released a report on the prevalence of healthcare disparities in 2003 which stated that racial and ethnic minority groups in the United States have decreased access to care and receive lower quality care compared to their white counterparts. Then, in 2012, the IOM took another look at healthcare disparities in the United States to determine progress since their initial report. Their first key finding was that healthcare disparities continue.[8] David Satcher, the former U.S. Surgeon General, reminds us that although "it is in our interests as a nation to make sure that all of our people are as healthy as they can be," many populations are far from this goal.[9]

Kathleen Sebelius, Secretary of the U.S. Department of Health and Human Services (DHHS) once remarked, "It is time to refocus, reinforce, and repeat the message that health disparities exist and that health equity benefits everyone."[10] And in 2010, the DHHS released a report with their action plan to reduce healthcare disparities.

The action plan was designed to complement other ongoing activities, including the Healthy People 2020 goals and objectives.[10] Healthy People 2020 serves as the most recent national health agenda for the United States.

The Healthy People 2020 goals related to health disparities have expanded over time. The 2000 Healthy People goal was to "reduce health disparities." Today, the 2020 goal is "to achieve health equity, eliminate disparities, and improve the health of all groups." The goals recognize that disparities occur across many varying groups related to race, gender, sexual orientation, disability, and location.[11]

EXAMPLES OF HEALTH DISPARITIES IN RACIAL AND ETHNIC GROUPS

There are substantial health disparities that exist between different cultural groups in the United States. The U.S. Department of Health and Human Services Office of Minority Health provides more details on health disparities faced by the following race and/or ethnic populations in the United States.

African-Americans (or Blacks per census reporting), are individuals originating in any of the black racial groups from Africa.[12] As of 2012, the US Census reports the number of persons identifying as African American to be 43.1 million, or second among racial and ethnic minority populations in the United States.[13] The overall prevalence and mortality rates for African Americans as compared to non-Hispanic whites is higher for several diseases including (but not limited to):

- Diabetes (80% more likely to have a diagnosis of diabetes)
- Heart Diseases (30% more likely to die from heart disease, 2010)
- HIV/AIDS (8.6 times more likely to be diagnosed with HIV, 2011)
- Infant Mortality (2.2 times infant mortality rate, 2009)

American Indian and Alaska Natives (AI/AN) are individuals with roots in one of the original populations of the Americas and who maintain tribal or community affiliation.[14] In 2012, 5.2 million persons (about 2% of population) reported their race as AI/AN (alone or combined with other races) to the US Census. There are 566 federally-recognized tribes whose members have access to health and education services provided through the U.S. Indian Health Service. Diseases that disproportionately affect AI/AN patients as compared to non-Hispanic Whites include:

- Asthma (children 80% more likely to have asthma)
- Chronic Liver Disease (2.4 times higher mortality rate)
- Infant Mortality Rate (1.6 times higher infant mortality rate)

Asian Americans are residents with origins ranging from the Far East to Southeast Asia and to India.[15] As of 2012, this group accounted for 15.5 million people in the United States (approximately 5% of US population). This group has historically often evaluated for health along with Native Hawaiian and Pacific Islanders, but has begun to be assessed separately as population groups. Although Asian American women have the highest life expectancy (85.5 years) as a group compared to all other racial and ethnic populations, health disparities still exist. Compared to non-Hispanic white Americans, Asian Americans are at higher risk for the following:

- Diabetes (20% more likely to have diagnosis of Diabetes)
- Hepatitis B (3 times more like to develop chronic Hepatitis B)
- Tuberculosis (24 times more likely to contract Tuberculosis)[15]

Hispanic or Latino are terms for individuals from Mexico, Central or South America, the islands of Cuba or Puerto Rico, or from other Spanish cultures or origin.[16] According to the 2012 Census, this population comprises 53 million in the United States, or nearly 17% of the total population, and is the highest among racial and ethnic minority populations in the United States. Hispanic/Latino populations have experienced lower mortality rates of heart disease than non-Hispanic Whites (30% less likely to die, 2008). However, health disparities faced by Hispanics vary within Hispanic subgroups, but in general, disease burden and mortality found in Hispanics when compared to non-Hispanic whites in the United States are:

- Cervical Cancer (women 1.4 times more likely to die from cervical cancer)[16]
- Diabetes (1.5 times as likely to die from diabetes, 2010)
- Pneumococcal Vaccination (65 years and older 40% less likely to have been vaccinated, 2010)

Native Hawaiian and Pacific Islanders (NH/PI), though a smaller portion of the population at 1.2 million as of 2012 (approximately 0.5% of the United States), face their own distinct health care challenges.[17] Because data for this population has not been studied as long, information is not as robust. This group is composed of the original populations from the Pacific Islands including, but not limited to, Hawaii, Guam, and Samoa. This group is more likely to contract tuberculosis and have higher infant death rates than other racial and ethnic groups. In comparison to non-Hispanic whites, NH/PI populations have experienced higher rates of:

- Asthma (two times as likely to have asthma)
- Heart Disease (three times more likely to be diagnosed with coronary heart disease, 2009)
- Obesity (30 % more likely to be obese, 2011)[17]

With these health disparities among racial and ethnic minority populations, there are compelling opportunities for pharmacists to expand access and care for the public. However, it is also important to recognize other social and environmental factors that influence health when approaching working across diverse cultures.

SOCIAL DETERMINANTS OF HEALTH

Since 1948, according to the World Health Organization (WHO), health has been defined as "a state of complete physical, mental and social well-being and not merely the absence of disease or infirmity."[18] And, within some cultures, health is also linked to spiritual well-being. However, in what manner does health connect with culture and what cultural influences exist related to medication use?

To explore the influence of culture in health care and causes for health disparities, pharmacists should understand the concept of *Social Determinants of Health*. Social Determinants of Health have been described as "the social and physical environments that promote good health" for individuals, families, and communities.[19] In Healthy People 2020, an approach (Figure 19-1) provides a five-part framework for Social Determinants of Health including "economic stability, education, social and community context, health/health care, and neighborhood/built environment."[19]

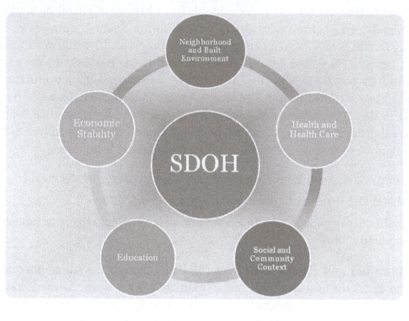

FIGURE 19-1: SOCIAL DETERMINANTS OF HEALTH[19]

1. Neighborhood and Built Environment

A population's neighborhood and environment have a significant impact on that population's health. Factors that can negatively affect a person's health include a lack of access to healthy foods, a lack of quality housing (or any housing), a high rate of crime and violence, and poor environmental conditions.[19]

2. Social and Community Context

Key underlying factors affecting a population's social and community context include the social cohesion of that population, their civic participation, their perceptions of discrimination, and rates of incarceration or institutionalization. Each of these factors plays a role in impacting a person's health.[19]

3. Education

Factors that affect a population's education, and, in turn their health, include high school graduation rates, enrollment in higher education, early childhood education, and language and literacy.[19]

Literacy: As pharmacists participate more in the overall health and wellness of individuals, they should understand the role that language and literacy play in the overall health of a person. There are 36 million people (more than 10% of the population) in the United States whose reading skills are estimated to be no higher than 3rd grade.[20]

In the United States, approximately 50% of adults experience challenges in the interpretation and use of health information.[20] Low literacy has far reaching consequences in a person's life including having a significant impact on the state of their health.

Perhaps a future pharmacist has difficulty understanding the emotional trauma of low literate or semi-literate individuals. As the Russian proverb goes, "the well-fed person can never comprehend how the hungry person feels." Imagine being forced to interpret medical handouts quickly in the presence of busy healthcare staff and a growing line of impatient strangers behind you at the pharmacy counter. A patient in this situation would understandably nod in understanding rather than clarify questions.

Also keep in mind:

- Key risk populations affected by limited literacy are the elderly, low income, unemployed, high school dropouts, minority groups.[21]
- Those with low general literacy often report lower self-reported health status.[22]
- Low health literacy alone costs the US healthcare system between $106 billion to $238 billion annually.[22]

Language Assistance: Across the United States, an estimated 20% of the population does not use the English language at home.[23] Further Limited English Proficiency (LEP), need for assistive hearing devices, or sight impairment can cause other challenges in healthcare. The lack of linguistically/culturally appropriate exchanges impairs interaction between limited English speakers and any clinician, including the pharmacist. Insufficient verbal and non-verbal interaction readily leads to misunderstanding of medication use and to potentially fatal outcomes.[24] Glen Flores, national expert on language barriers in healthcare, cited an example of misunderstandings in a medical setting:

"In a case that cost a Florida hospital a $71 million malpractice settlement, Flores said an 18 year-old who said he was "intoxicado," which can mean nauseated in Spanish, spent 36 hours in a hospital being treated for a drug overdose [due to similarity to the English word "intoxicated"] before doctors realized that he had a brain aneurysm."[24]

If this person had come to the pharmacy and spoken to someone unfamiliar with those Spanish words superficially resembling terms in English, staff members might have accidentally offered an inappropriate over-the-counter remedy for a hangover. In the end, the family of this young man could have sued the pharmacy as well.

4. Economic Stability

According to the Healthy People 2020 description of the Social Determinants of Health, the factors that influence the economic stability of a person include poverty, employment, food security, and housing stability. While each of these factors play a role in a person's health, another related factor, and one that a pharmacist should be particularly aware of, is the coverage of health insurance.[19] The Center for American Progress reports the absence of insurance covering clinical services and medications to be the primary access barrier to healthcare.[7]

The Agency for Healthcare Research and Quality (AHRQ) annually releases the Healthcare Quality and Disparities Report assessing the state of healthcare in the United States. Since 2000, the report has consistently shown increases in the percentage of people in the United States without health insurance. The 2014 report, however, was the first to show a significant drop in the number of uninsured. From 2010 to early 2014 the percentage of adults without insurance fell from 22.3% to 15.6%. The AHRQ attributes this decline to the opening of the Affordable Care Act marketplace exchanges in 2013.[25] The AHRQ report also notes that insurance coverage increased for Black and Hispanic Americans from 2010 to 2014. However, disparities still exist between these racial groups and White Americans with Hispanics having the worst coverage rates.[25]

5. Health and Healthcare

Factors that affect a population's health and healthcare include their access to health care (previously discussed), access to primary care (including culturally competent and diverse care), and their health literacy. As pharmacists, it is important to recognize the significant impact of health literacy and the cultural diversity of the healthcare workforce on patients' health.[19]

Health Literacy: While literacy is the ability to read and understand written material, health literacy is the ability to obtain, process, and understand health-related material in order to make correct healthcare choices. Health literacy is affected by the language of healthcare professionals, education levels, cultural barriers, and English literacy.[26] However, education levels do not necessarily correlate with health literacy levels for all patients. Contemporary medical and technological advances can baffle even the most educated patient and compromise their understanding of medications. Perhaps the most important fact to remember is that pharmacists, like all other clinicians, cannot know if their patients have high health literacy levels. Given this reality, the best response is to provide clear, understandable data to all patients.

DIVERSITY IN THE PHARMACY WORKFORCE

In 2003 the report from the American Society of Health-System Pharmacists (*ASHP*) recommended the need for more diversity in the pharmacy workforce: "Healthcare organizations should implement strategies to recruit, retain, and promote at all levels of the organization a diverse staff and leadership that are representative of the demographic characteristics of the service area."[27] However, according to pharmacy school enrollment data, the diversity of pharmacy students based on reported race or ethnicity since 2000 has shown some fluctuations through 2013 (Figure 29-2).28 While there have been increases in the percentage of students identifying as Asian (13.8% in 2000 to 19.2% in 2013) with doubling in the percentage of students identifying themselves as Black or African American (5.3% in 2000 to 10.5% in 2013), the percentage of students identifying themselves as Hispanic or Latino has remained relatively stable. Persons identifying as American Indian have not been reported. In general, the percentage enrollment does not represent the overall racial and ethnic diversity of the United States (highlighted in health disparities).

The IOM connects workforce diversity to "improved access to care for racial and ethnic minorities, greater patient choice and satisfaction, better patient-clinician communication, and improved educational experience for allied health students."[29] Unfortunately, healthcare settings lag behind the general national workforce already staffed (50%) by minorities.[27] But consumers often patronize an establishment whose culture and values resemble their own. In short, keeping a diverse pharmacy workforce is more than a response to the climate of the 21st century.

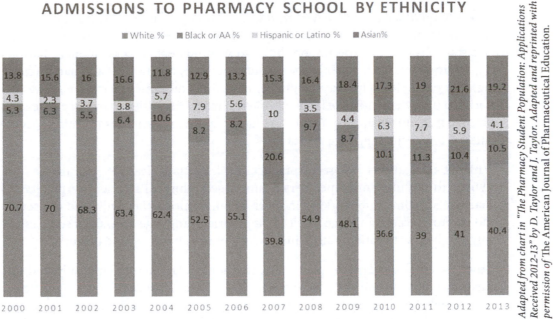

ADMISSIONS TO PHARMACY SCHOOL BY ETHNICITY

■ White % ■ Black or AA % ■ Hispanic or Latino % ■ Asian%

Adapted from chart in "The Pharmacy Student Population: Applications Received 2012-13" by D. Taylor and J. Taylor. Adapted and reprinted with permission of The American Journal of Pharmaceutical Education.

FIGURE 19-2: ADMISSIONS TO PHARMACY SCHOOL BY ETHNICITY[28]

EDUCATION, LEGAL AND ACCREDITATION EXPECTATIONS

CHANGING LANDSCAPE FOR PHARMACY EDUCATION

Accreditation standards and goals for pharmacy education have become more specific regarding the importance of training the next generation of pharmacy professionals who can address and problem solve care for patients from diverse communities. According to the 2016 Guidance for Standards of the Accreditation Council for Pharmacy Education (ACPE) and the CAPE Outcomes (Center for the Advancement of Pharmaceutical Education), pharmacy students should have opportunities for developing skills to communicate with, assess, educate, and care for patients from diverse socioeconomic and cultures across populations.[30,31] Further, pharmacy education standards highlight the importance of not only working with patients from different cultures, but also emphasize the necessity to have the inter-professional skills to communicate and collaborate with providers from diverse cultures and disciplines.

According to Title VI of the U.S. Civil Rights Act and Executive Order 13166 signed in 2000, persons with Limited English Proficiency (LEP) who receive federal support are eligible for language assistance.[32] The U.S. Department of Health and Human Services "requires all recipients of federal financial assistance from HHS to provide meaningful access to LEP persons."[33] These federal programs affect pharmacies with more cities and states mandating language access from the pharmacy to the patient.[34,35]

Access to qualified and trained interpreters and bilingual personnel is not uniformly available in pharmacies across the country. However, the bar is being raised for pharmacists to have increasing responsibility to serve patients across language barriers (e.g., trained interpreters, language assistance devices for the deaf and hard of hearing). For example, an increasing number of chain community pharmacies have networks to provide immediate language interpretation for patients. In some cities and states (e.g., California, New York), laws have required pharmacies (meeting specific criteria) to provide language assistance.[36,37]

While it may always not seem practical or financially feasible, pharmacists are advised to not use family members or untrained bilingual staff as interpreters. As pharmacists commit to working in diverse communities, they will need to provide and improve access language services. Appropriate language access and services not only can help with patient safety and understanding, but it is good business.

Other national standards support the provision of care across culturally and linguistically diverse populations. The National CLAS (Culturally and Linguistically Appropriate Services) Standards have been updated (2013) to include one overarching principle and an additional[14] action items (Table 20-1) to assist organizations and health care leaders to improve health equity across populations.[38] The principle standard is to "provide effective, equitable, understandable, and respectful quality care and services that are responsive to diverse cultural health beliefs and practices, preferred languages, health literacy, and other communication needs."[38] The 2013 CLAS standards provide a blueprint for how to provide leadership, communication assistance, community involvement, and continuous improvement when providing services for diverse cultures and languages.

TABLE 19-1: NATIONAL STANDARDS FOR CULTURALLY AND LINGUISTICALLY APPROPRIATE SERVICES (CLAS) IN HEALTH AND HEALTH CARE (2013)[38]

PRINCIPAL STANDARD:

1. Provide effective, equitable, understandable, and respectful quality care and services that are responsive to diverse cultural health beliefs and practices, preferred languages, health literacy, and other communication needs.

GOVERNANCE, LEADERSHIP, AND WORKFORCE:

2. Advance and sustain organizational governance and leadership that promotes CLAS and health equity through policy, practices, and allocated resources.

Continued

TABLE 19-1: NATIONAL STANDARDS FOR CULTURALLY AND LINGUISTICALLY APPROPRIATE SERVICES (CLAS) IN HEALTH AND HEALTH CARE (2013)[38]

GOVERNANCE, LEADERSHIP, AND WORKFORCE:

3. Recruit, promote, and support a culturally and linguistically diverse governance, leadership, and workforce that are responsive to the population in the service area.

4. Educate and train governance, leadership, and workforce in culturally and linguistically appropriate policies and practices on an ongoing basis.

COMMUNICATION AND LANGUAGE ASSISTANCE:

5. Offer language assistance to individuals who have limited English proficiency and/or other communication needs, at no cost to them, to facilitate timely access to all health care and services.

6. Inform all individuals of the availability of language assistance services clearly and in their preferred language, verbally and in writing.

7. Ensure the competence of individuals providing language assistance, recognizing that the use of untrained individuals and/or minors as interpreters should be avoided.

8. Provide easy-to-understand print and multimedia materials and signage in the languages commonly used by the populations in the service area.

ENGAGEMENT, CONTINUOUS IMPROVEMENT, AND ACCOUNTABILITY:

9. Establish culturally and linguistically appropriate goals, policies, and management accountability, and infuse them throughout the organization's planning and operations.

10. Conduct ongoing assessments of the organization's CLAS-related activities and integrate CLAS-related measures into measurement and continuous quality improvement activities.

11. Collect and maintain accurate and reliable demographic data to monitor and evaluate the impact of CLAS on health equity and outcomes and to inform service delivery.

12. Conduct regular assessments of community health assets and needs and use the results to plan and implement services that respond to the cultural and linguistic diversity of populations in the service area.

13. Partner with the community to design, implement, and evaluate policies, practices, and services to ensure cultural and linguistic appropriateness.

14. Create conflict and grievance resolution processes that are culturally and linguistically appropriate to identify, prevent, and resolve conflicts or complaints.

15. Communicate the organization's progress in implementing and sustaining CLAS to all stakeholders, constituents, and the general public.

As of 2015, five states require (California, Connecticut, New Jersey, New Mexico, and Washington) and one state strongly recommends (Maryland) cultural competency or multicultural training for health care professionals. Eight additional states (stretching from the Southwest to the Midwest and Southeast and up to the New England States) have had similar legislation under consideration.[38,39]

INCREASING EXPECTATIONS BY NATIONAL ACCREDITING BODIES

In 2010, the Joint Commission, the national accrediting body for many healthcare institutions, completed a report for area hospitals regarding culture and language services. The primary recommendations in the report highlight the importance of using trained interpreters, ensuring that staff understands the scope of available services for patients from diverse cultures, as well as pro-actively gathering information about the served community through recognizing the patient demographics served and recruiting community input and data.[40]

On a broader scale, the Joint Commission has provided a "roadmap" for hospitals to incorporate more culturally competent practices. These practices focus on improving effective communication from admission of the patient through assessment and treatment to discharge or transfer of the patients. Health care personnel and organizations have increasing responsibility to ensure that the appropriate barriers (e.g., culture, religion, language) are assessed and addressed through the continuum of care. Further, the Joint Commission recognizes that the environment of care is important to creating the physical space in the healthcare setting that is welcoming to persons of diverse backgrounds (e.g., signs in languages appropriate to demographic served).[41] Increasingly, national accreditation bodies recognize the value of culture and its influence on patient safety and overall care.

ROLE OF POSITIVE ATTITUDES AND VALUES ABOUT CULTURE

While the evidence for health disparities and rationale for understanding Social Determinants of Health in diverse populations is compelling, ultimately the relationship of the patient with each of their providers (e.g., primary care providers, pharmacists) is at the core of patient care. Do pharmacists have the values and attitudes to embrace diverse patients and their beliefs?

To aid in working across cultures, adopting an attitude of humility is valuable to a positive patient-provider relationship. With cultural humility, providers recognize that they will not be able to learn details of every culture. Rather they will approach working with patients and other providers from diverse cultures with the understanding that there are always new ways to learn to interact with persons from different backgrounds and perspectives.[42]

STEREOTYPES VS. GENERALIZATION

Pharmacist providers should recognize the **stereotypes** that they may have in working in diverse cultures. Stereotypes are "negative assumptions or biases about groups of people based on a common cultural characteristic (e.g., age, weight, sex, race, religion, country of origin)."[43] Providers and supportive staff should recognize that stereotypes are harmful and destructive in a patient care environment and can cloud provider and staff judgment. **Generalizations** are "common characteristics (positive or negative) that may be found within groups of cultures" and should be used cautiously. Generalizations can provide a framework for working in cultures to better understand potential behaviors or choices. For example, it is common to find a high plant-based and starch diet in the traditional foods among people from East Africa (e.g., Ethiopia, Somalia)[44,45] which could be problematic for blood sugar control in a patient with diabetes. However, when actually working with a patient who self-identifies with the Ethiopian culture, providers could offer a more individualized or family-centered approach to patient care.

> SN is a 45-year female who self-identifies with the Christian Ethiopian culture. She has two children and is at the pharmacy for diabetes management. The pharmacist, who is a 24-year-old African American male, sits down to review medications and diet. The following thoughts cross the pharmacist's mind:
>
> **Stereotype:** I won't be able to do much for this patient's diet—it's probably high starch and she won't change. I'll just focus on the meds.
>
> **Generalization:** This patient may eat a high starch diet that includes enjera (traditional Ethiopian flat bread). I will need to consider this possibility when exploring diet, medication, and exercise.
>
> **Individual/Family-oriented approach:** Mrs. N, please tell me about the type of foods you and your family eat throughout the day.

SELF-ASSESSMENT AND ORGANIZATIONAL ASSESSMENT

One way that pharmacists can better understand their own cultural perceptions, biases, and beliefs is to complete an individual self-assessment. If a pharmacy manager is committed to creating an environment that celebrates and serves diverse patients, the manager may find it helpful to have their staff (pharmacists, technicians, clerks, and students) also complete a self-assessment to provide opportunities for discussion about cultural practices in the community.

To provide more culturally competent care, pharmacists can be better supported if they work in a healthcare environment that values culture and diversity. A pharmacy manager could perform an organizational assessment to identify opportunities for the pharmacy to embrace and better serve patients from diverse cultures. In organizational assessments, leaders can evaluate domains such as the mission, recruitment, business and marketing strategies, and community involvement to address and support care for diverse communities and providers. The National Center for Cultural Competence based in Georgetown University provides some examples of individual assessments and guidance for organizational assessments.[46]

Through the process of self-assessment, pharmacists and organizational leadership can undertake a more objective process to benchmarking and improving care for diverse cultures. Pharmacists and leadership can then re-evaluate their assessments periodically to chart progress.

MODELS FOR UNDERSTANDING PATIENTS FROM DIVERSE CULTURES AND CULTURAL COMPETENCY

As the pharmacist continues to gain knowledge about cultures, it is important to recognize the roles of the patient's explanation of their health and acculturation. Further, various models for cultural competency exist that provide examples for understanding how to serve different cultures.

EXPLANATORY MODELS

While each individual has choices and perceptions about their health, their decisions are often influenced by their culture. At an individual level, pharmacist providers can elicit the patient's understanding of their illness using the Patient Explanatory Model.[47, 48] The explanatory model explores what a patient understands about their illness (e.g., diabetes, cough, fever) and its potential cause, therapy options, and perceived severity. This information can be helpful to providers to understand if the patient would accept or prefer pharmacologic and/or nonpharmacologic therapy. In general, the questions are:

1. What do you call the problem?
2. What do you think has caused the problem?
3. Why do you think it started when it did?
4. What do you think the sickness does to you? How does it work?
5. How severe is the sickness? Will it have a short or long course?
6. What kind of treatment do you think would be best? What are the most important results you hope to receive from this treatment?
7. What are the main problems the illness has caused you?
8. What do you fear most about your illness?[47]

ACCULTURATION

Another factor that can affect an individual's understanding and approach to healthcare is acculturation. On a simplistic level, acculturation may be described as how (well) a person adapts to and adopts a culture different from their own.[49,50] For example, a young child may be able to adapt to a learning a new language and living country more easily than a grandparent. Or, perhaps an adult who was raised with quick access to healthcare at a clinic with labs, x-rays, and medication may have a difficult time adjusting to going on a mission trip to a country where the closest healthcare option is a local healer who will use herbal products for most conditions. Each person has different abilities to adapt to new cultures and this comfort may affect their willingness to try or adopt ideas or customs that are different.

CULTURAL COMPETENCY MODELS

While assessing each individual is relevant to providing patient-centered care, the manner in which pharmacists approach care may take on different forms. While several examples exist, three models have been widely used in the literature to explore cultural competency: The Cultural Competency Continuum by Terry Cross, Campinha-Bacote Model, and the Purnell Model.[42,51,52] One commonality among all the models is that we are in a constant state of learning. We do not "arrive" at cultural competency. Rather, we continue to strive toward increased understanding and skills to navigate across cultures.

```
Cultural Proficiency

Cultural Competency

Cultural Pre-competency

**************

        Cultural Blindness

    Cultural Incapacity

Cultural Destructiveness
```

FIGURE 19-3: CROSS CULTURAL COMPETENCY CONTINUUM[52]

In the Cultural Competency Continuum by Cross, pharmacists may find themselves along a stair-step continuum that ranges from cultural destructiveness to cultural proficiency (Figure 19-3).[52] In the Cross model, those providers whose actions demonstrate blindness to destruction will likely have more challenges learning about new cultures and developing good cross-cultural skills. These providers may hold onto stereotypes about cultures. However, as pharmacists move from pre-competency towards proficiency, they are developing increased attitudes, knowledge, and skills to work more successfully across cultures.

When applying the Campinha-Bacote model, pharmacists may find their progression towards cultural competence involves an interplay among the number and types of cultural encounters with the acquired cultural knowledge, cultural skills, and cultural awareness by a provider.[42] In this model, one of the key factors that influences a person's more successful development is having a "positive desire" to learn about and engage with diverse cultures.

In the Purnell model, the competency framework can be visualized as concentric circles starting with the individual and their beliefs, practices and cultural influences in the middle.[51] The model continues to expand from the individual working outwards through the circular layers of family, the community, and finally society as a whole. The model can also be interpreted as looking from the society and inward toward the individual. As pharmacists or other providers learn the subtleties of how to interact with patients, family, and the community, they would move along a jagged line from being "unconsciously incompetent" towards becoming more "unconsciously competent" (Table 20-2).

TABLE 19:2 EXAMPLES OF PROVIDER RESPONSES USING THE PURNELL MODEL FOR CULTURAL COMPETENCY[51]

UNCONSCIOUSLY INCOMPETENT	CONSCIOUSLY INCOMPETENT	CONSCIOUSLY COMPETENT	UNCONSCIOUSLY COMPETENT
Providers are not aware that they cannot navigate across cultural issues	Providers are aware that they have challenges working through issues that arise with different cultures	Providers are aware that they are employing knowledge and skills to work across cultures and diverse problems	Providers are able to navigate more freely (almost without thinking) across cultures using their acquired attitudes, knowledge, and skills

Larry Purnell, Journal of Transcultural Nursing (13) pp. 193-196, copyright © 2002 SAGE Publications. Reprinted by permission of SAGE Publications.

While these three cultural competency models provide a framework for classifying oneself and improving cross-cultural care, it is important to recognize the atrocities that can happen in the health care system (organizational) and among providers (individuals) when they do not value cultures. This state of cultural destructiveness has often been described through the Tuskegee trials as one of the great injustices in US public health history.

During the infamous Tuskegee study, which began in 1932 in Alabama, 600 African-American men from modest economic and educational backgrounds were told that they had "bad blood" and were enrolled without informed consent into experimental and control "treatment" groups. In reality, these men had syphilis and were being studied to evaluate the sequelae of the disease. While therapy was not available when the study began, when penicillin became a standard treatment in the 1940s, it was withheld from both control and experimental groups. The study finally came to an end in 1972, nearly 40 years later, after the men and their families had been not been exposed to or provided treatment options.[53]

The Tuskegee study provides just one example of history and context (as highlighted under the "community competency" definition) and cultural destructiveness (Cross continuum) that are critical pieces to pharmacists developing skills to work across cultures. While providers should not necessarily dwell on the past, there are grave lessons to be learned to providing environments for caring for patients of the present and future.

BELIEFS, BEHAVIORS AND CULTURE-BOUND SYNDROMES

Imagine being the supervisor of a pharmacy with many patients of Slavic origin. An elderly man with limited English proficiency who identifies with this culture approaches the counter with a physician's prescription for an antibiotic. In a parental tone, one of the staff pharmacists reiterates the importance of using the medication, "no matter what," during the brief counseling session with the gentleman. With confidence bordering on smugness, your co-worker later mentions a cross-cultural colloquium she attended on "difficult" patients. This seminar included Eastern Europeans' attitudes toward prescription medications and how those people oppose antibiotics. Not surprisingly, the patient sensed the pharmacist's arrogance and took his business elsewhere from that point on.

This pharmacist possessed some facts, but sadly, little cultural humility or the abandonment of simplistic stereotyping for a continuous process of self-evaluation and analysis.[5] During his or her career, the pharmacist hoping to internalize this trait remains a lifetime learner. How can we use these models together to shape our understanding of becoming a more culturally competent pharmacist? What do we need to learn about the patient?

BELIEFS REGARDING HEALTH AND ILLNESS

Beliefs regarding the nature of health and causes of disease vary among cultures. The biomedical model of disease that permeates Western culture concentrates on the physical and biological processes (e.g., pathology, physiology) to explain the nature of disease and to guide diagnosis and development of treatment options.[54] As pharmacists practicing in the United States, the biomedical model is important to our understanding of disease and it influences how we approach care for our patients. Unfortunately, psychological, environmental and social influences on health are not necessarily components of the traditional biomedical model that many healthcare providers are trained to rely on. As a result, the inclusion of these key factors in our understanding of health, illness (vs. disease), and adherence to treatment modalities is something that must be incorporated into our training and development as culturally competent providers of care.

Outside the Western biomedical model of disease, we find that certain cultures have other explanations for the causes of or the descriptions of illness. Certain cultures describe illness as resulting from imbalances that may occur in the body.[43] In some Asian cultures, we find the belief that disease results from an imbalance between yin (cold) and yang (hot), with each of these terms referring to qualities not temperature. Other cultures including Hispanic, Middle Eastern, South Asian, and East Indian cultures may also incorporate the concepts of "hot" and "cold" properties as they relate to foods, illnesses, or treatments.[43] Within this cultural belief of a balance between hot and cold, a hot illness will require treatment with a cold remedy. Although the concept of hot and cold may be present among different cultures, what one culture considers to be "hot" may be considered to be "cold" in another culture. Therefore, it is difficult to generate a specific guide as it relates to this terminology that may be used across cultural groups.

Similar to the concept of "hot and cold," some cultures may also view balance within the body with terminology such as "high or low" or "wet and dry." In the African American culture, the concept of high/low blood has been described.[43] Certain foods may cause high blood (too much) or low blood (too little). Use of "high" and "low" terminology can lead to confusion between the healthcare provider and the patient when discussing concepts such as high blood pressure. This discrepancy can lead a patient to adopting practices such as eating certain foods aimed at restoring balance in their bodies while these practices may actually make the underlying condition worse. If patients use terms like "hot" or "cold" to describe properties of their illness, pharmacists should be aware that this terminology may mean something other than temperature based on the underlying beliefs of the patient.

Other cultures point to the existence of supernatural causes of disease such as spirits, demons, or "the will of God." **Fatalism**, the concept that life situations occur because they are willed or predetermined by a supreme being and that they are out of the control of the individual,[43,55] is a belief that has been documented in individuals from certain cultures, particularly Hispanic and Middle Eastern cultures. Research has shown that religious beliefs and practices lead to healthier behaviors and more positive health outcomes.[55] Practices such as prayer/relaxation/meditation, the availability of a social support network, and avoidance of risky behaviors (e.g., promiscuity, alcohol, drugs) are examples of practices that are associated with various religious beliefs that may contribute to positive health outcomes. In fact, every major world religion (i.e., Buddhism, Christianity, Islam, and Judaism) has teachings that promote care of the human body.[56] However, some researchers suggest that religious beliefs may reduce healthcare utilization and healthy behaviors leading to poorer health outcomes.[56,57]

There is data to suggest that religious beliefs may reduce detection of disease and adherence to treatment. For example, it has been documented that African American women who have fatalistic beliefs are less likely to be screened for cancer.[56] Research looking at treatment adherence and religious beliefs has shown a mixed association with some studies suggesting negative associations and others showing positive associations between religion and adherence. Thus, there is a concern amongst public health professionals including pharmacists that patients who believe that illness is something outside of their control may be less likely to adopt behaviors that may prevent the onset of disease (such as cancer screenings) or adhere to treatment regimens for the purposes of controlling existing illness or symptoms.

BEHAVIORS RELATED TO HEALTH AND ILLNESS

Behaviors and practices stemming from cultural beliefs about health and illness are as varied as the cultures that they represent. Dietary practices and preferences and the use of complementary and alternative methods of disease prevention and treatment are two examples of notable behaviors that should be highlighted for pharmacists seeking to expand their understanding of how these practices may influence care.

Cultural influences on dietary practices and preferences are important considerations for clinicians. Certain religions may require that patients fast during certain periods of time.[43] For example, Islamic patients observing religious practices during the month of Ramadan may fast from sunrise to sunset avoiding any food or drink during this period of time. Jewish patients observing holidays such as Yom Kippur and Catholics observing Lenten practices may also fast. These are just a few examples of fasting practices observed by members of major world religions.

Pharmacists should be concerned with whether or not fasting rituals observed by patients will be impacted by medication use or vice versa. For example, certain medications may need to be administered with meals. A common example includes diabetic patients who may be taking short- or rapid-acting insulins prior to meals. Patients who are fasting and continue to take their insulin may experience hypoglycemia and thus need to be counseled to refrain from injecting their insulin should they not eat a meal. On the other hand, there may be patients who avoid taking their medications altogether during a fasting period. In this situation, patients run the risk of losing the benefits of their medication during the fasting period and this can be life-threatening in certain situations depending on the medication and its indication.

There are several interventions that the pharmacist can recommend to accommodate fasting practices while maintaining appropriate medication use and administration. The pharmacist may be able to assist patients in deciding appropriate times for the medication to be administered so as not to break any fasting rules. For example, the Islamic patient who is observing a fast from sunrise to sunset during Ramadan may take their medications before sunrise or after sunset. Certain medications that are meant to be taken two or three times a day can be changed to extended release formulations, which may assist the patient in being adherent to medication use while still meeting the rules of the fast. The pharmacist working with patients who are skipping meals due to fasting and who take medications that require administration with food may be able to determine medication alternatives which do not require food for administration.

In addition to fasting, many religions may also promote certain dietary preferences which are required of individuals practicing the faith.[43] Jewish patients may observe strict *kosher* dietary laws which prohibit the consumption of pork and products as well as requiring kosher meat products. Islamic patients may also abstain from pork and pork products, which are considered *haram* (unlawful or prohibited). Medications may be derived from or contain pork or other animal products that may not be considered kosher or *halal* (lawful or permitted). For example, gelatin capsules, which are commonly used in the production of various pharmaceuticals are made from by-products of animals such as pigs and cows. Consumption of these pharmaceuticals may be objectionable to patients who adhere to strict dietary laws. Thus, pharmacists need to be aware that some patients may refuse to take medications that are not permitted based on their religious beliefs or dietary preferences (e.g., vegan). Fortunately, many pharmaceutical products are evaluated based on kosher and halal standards and list of acceptable medications are available to pharmacists and the general public on the Internet.[58-61]

Not all members of these religious cultures explored here will adhere to these specific examples of dietary practices and preferences. Additionally, many of these religious observances may allow exemptions for those who are ill or taking medications. Asking patients about their dietary habits and preferences can help the pharmacist determine the best way to optimize medication use and adherence without compromising the patient's personal beliefs and practices.

Complementary and alternative medicine (CAM) is a term that encompasses a variety of modalities and products used in prevention or treatment of illness which are considered to be outside the realm of traditional Western medicine. Examples of CAM include, but are not limited to, the use of herbs/herbal products, acupuncture, biofeedback, chiropractic care, massage, and yoga. The use of CAM is a practice that spans across cultures and goes back centuries. **Folk medicine** is a term that describes systems of healing "that have persisted since the beginning of human culture and flourished long before the development of conventional medicine."[62] An example of folk medicine is *curanderismo*, an approach to wellness and healing practiced in Mexican and other Latin American cultures. Traditional healers are known as *curanderos(as)* and may employ prayer, massage, spiritual cleansing rituals, use of herbs, and other CAM modalities.[63] Other examples of traditional medicine systems include *Ayurvedic* medicine, the traditional Hindu system of medicine, and Traditional Chinese Medicine (TCM).[43] Folk healers are found in various cultures although their names/titles and practices will depend on the culture of origin. In some cultures, religious leaders and communities of faith who pray for an individual who is not well could be considered a form of CAM.

Herbs have been used for centuries by individuals in almost every known culture. The types of products, indications and methods of use of herbs vary among cultures. In the United States, herbal product use is one of the most commonly used CAM modalities. According to a 2012 survey of households in the United States, approximately one-third of adults (33.2%) reported "any" use of CAM in the previous 12 months.[62] In this study, the most commonly used CAM modality was non-vitamin/non-mineral dietary supplements which included herbal products such as Echinacea, cranberry, garlic, and ginseng. The use of CAM may be more common in certain racial and groups across the United States including Hispanics and Asian-Americans.[64]

Despite the widespread use of herbal products, valid concerns regarding the use of these natural products exist among health professionals.[65] There is limited information evaluating the safety and efficacy of herbal products through conducting clinical trials. Additionally, concerns exist regarding the lack of regulations for quality standards in the manufacturing process of these products which may involve product contamination/adulteration. Use of herbal products in combination with pharmaceutical products is also another important consideration due to the potential for herb-drug interactions.

Pharmacists are well-positioned to promote the safe use of herbs and they should ask patients about the use of these products in a non-judgmental manner. Unfortunately, research shows that not all patients are comfortable disclosing the use of herbal products to their providers with estimates suggesting that only one-third or less of patients will tell their provider that they are taking herbal products.[66]

Rates of disclosure to providers are lower in ethnic minorities compared to whites.[64] It is also important to recognize that when asked about herbal product use, some patients may not consider the use of herbs in the form of teas, tinctures, or topical applications to be "herbal products" and they may be inclined to not report them as such if a provider does not ask questions that allow for patients to disclose products taken in a variety of formulations. Thus, pharmacists need to be proactive and specific in asking questions to elucidate the use of CAM modalities when taking a medication and treatment history.

It is important to recognize that a variety of modalities exist for administering traditional medicine remedies and healing practices. Some practices can leave unfamiliar markings on the body, which can be misinterpreted by health care professionals as signs of abuse or as symptoms that may lead to misdiagnosis of a medical condition. *Coining* is a traditional healing practice seen in Asian cultures in which coins are used to vigorously rub the body in order to promote healing.[43] There are variations in the practice that may involve heating the coins or dipping the coins in oil. This practice can leave red welts on the affected area, which can be concerning to those who are not familiar with the practice. Another practice that can lead to misunderstandings is the practice of *cupping*.[43] This is a practice that may be seen in various cultures including in which cups or drinking glasses are placed on the skin and heated, creating a vacuum in which the skin rises into the cup leaving bruises or red marks at the site. This process is intended to promote circulation in the area and is usually used to treat respiratory problems or sore muscles. Like coining, the presence of marks on the body after cupping can confuse health care providers who are not familiar with the practice.

Another example of differences that may be seen between traditional and Western medicine is the route of administration of medicines or remedies. Many cultures observe the administration of therapeutic remedies by applying them locally at the actual anatomical site where healing is needed. This practice may differ from Western medicine in which many medications are administered orally for effect at an anatomical site outside of the gastrointestinal tract. For example, case reports exist of patients opening antibiotic capsules in order to mix the powder with water to create a paste that is placed on an infected wound rather than taking the medication orally as indicated for the infection.[43] Differences among health beliefs stemming from cultural differences make counseling on the proper use of medications paramount for pharmacists working with diverse patient populations.

CULTURE-BOUND SYNDROMES

Illnesses that are only recognized as diseases within a specific culture are known as culture-bound syndromes. They are also sometimes referred to as folk illnesses. These syndromes usually include manifestations of behavior, affect and/or cognition with no signs that are able to be confirmed objectively.[43,67] Table 19-3 provides some examples of culture-bound syndromes that have been documented in various cultures. **Culture-bound syndromes** were formally recognized by the American Psychiatric Association in DSM IV as "locality-specific patterns of aberrant [deviant] behavior and troubling experience that may or may not be linked to a particular DSM-IV diagnostic criteria." It is important to recognize that there are also syndromes that are well-recognized in Western medicine and culture that are not recognized by other cultures in the world. Examples of conditions that have been previously considered to be Western culture-bound syndromes include anorexia nervosa and Type A personality/behavior pattern.[68,69]

TABLE 19-3: EXAMPLES OF CULTURE-BOUND SYNDROMES[43, 67, 70-73]

SYNDROME	CULTURE/REGIONA	DESCRIPTION	TREATMENT
Anorexia nervosa	Western culture (e.g., western/northern/central Europe, United States and the Americas)	Eating disorder characterized by extreme weight-loss caused by self-starvation; associated with a fear of weight gain or obsession with preventing weight gain	Cognitive behavioral therapy, pharmacotherapy may be used to treat associated psychiatric conditions, nutritional rehabilitation

Continued

TABLE 19-3: EXAMPLES OF CULTURE-BOUND SYNDROMES[43, 67, 70-73]

SYNDROME	CULTURE/REGION[a]	DESCRIPTION	TREATMENT
Dhat	Indian (Asian)	Weakness, fatigue, sexual dysfunction caused by loss of semen during urination, nocturnal emission or masturbation	Relaxation therapy, meditation, sex education, cognitive behavioral therapy
Empacho	Hispanic	Abdominal pain, indigestion thought to be caused by ball of food blocking the intestines	Massaging the abdomen or pinching the back to release the blockage; purgatives or teas may be given
Ghost sickness	Native American tribes	Weakness, bad dreams, fainting, dizziness, hallucinations and loss of consciousness thought to be associated with spirits or ghosts or preoccupation with death or the deceased	Religious/ceremonial rituals
Koro	South and East Asia	Extreme fear or anxiety of genitalia or nipples receding into the body	Prayer, traditional Chinese medicine remedies, psychotherapy, pharmacotherapy
Mal de ojo or "evil eye"	Hispanic	Poor health or illness (symptoms may include nausea caused by staring at an individual; may be caused by excessive admiration or jealousy	Prayer or cleansing rituals known as a *"limpia"* in which an egg is passed over the body to extract the heat or evil (seen in Hispanic cultures)
Susto or "fright-sickness"	Middle Eastern/Arabic South Asian	Symptoms of malaise, insomnia, fever, depression/anxiety caused by a traumatic experience	Prayer or cleansing rituals known as a *"limpia"*

[a]These syndromes are most commonly described in these cultures although they may not be restricted to only these cultures.

APPROACHES TO WORK WITH DIVERSE CULTURES

Pharmacists build frameworks for learning about cultures by recognizing personal and organizational values about culture that are positive as well as understanding the legal, educational, and accreditation expectations in healthcare. Knowledge of diverse cultures, models of cultural competency, health disparities, beliefs, and perceptions provide a context for care. However, what are some of the tools and skills that can help pharmacists to navigate across cultures?

EXPLORING COMMUNITIES

As highlighted in defining community competency, through recognizing Social Determinants of Health, and in reviewing The Joint Commission reports, it is important to understand the communities that are served by the pharmacy or health care organization. While this knowledge includes getting demographic data on cultures, religions, and languages found in the population served, it also includes reaching out to community leaders and learning about the culture and arts of the neighborhoods.[40,74-76]

CULTURAL BROKERING

Cultural brokers are liaisons, a "go-between" spanning the boundaries of two cultures; that of healthcare and that of the target community of which they are members. They can guide pharmacists and other clinicians to interact with the broker's own ethnic population. Cultural brokers understand the values of their own group and of the healthcare system that they have already navigated on their own behalf as well as of their relatives.[77] Cultural brokers are not language interpreters by training. However, they can have a sense respectful communication, taboos, and general health beliefs in a culture or community. If implemented properly, cultural brokering programs increase understanding and compliance and set the foundation for rewarding patient experiences. These endeavors substantially help establish the pharmacist as a respected clinician sincerely attempting to reduce disparities in a given community.[77] In some communities, cultural brokers might be called lay health workers, or community health liaisons, or health promoters.

Cultural brokering is "the act of bridging, linking, or mediating between groups or persons of different cultural backgrounds for the purpose of reducing conflict or producing change."[77] In the case of pharmacies, this process would involve the practitioner's increased use of cultural and clinical knowledge to negotiate an effective wellness plan with the patient and healthcare system.

COMMUNICATING RESPECT

One of the first ways pharmacists connect with a person from a different culture is through a simple greeting. Developing basic skills to greet patients in a manner that can cut across most cultures can help start the patient care encounter well. For example:

- Encounter each new patient with a "fresh" outlook. Do not pre-judge and do not let expectations from dealing with "similar" people lead you to act on stereotypes.[78]
- Refer to a patient as a "man" or "young man," "woman" or "young woman." Avoid using "girl" or "boy" except for very young children. Never say "honey," "dear," or refer to an elderly person as "Mom," "Grandma," "Pops," or "Grandpa."[78]
- Be cordial but not overly familiar. In many cultures, formality is a sign of respect, while informality is considered patronizing, as from a superior to an inferior.[78]

- While in Western culture, it is common to have direct eye contact and shake hands when meeting someone. However, these communication strategies may demonstrate lack of respect in some cultures.[79]

Across cultures, pharmacists can convey genuine concern can be communicated to patients by reflective responses that mirror the patients' worries and fears. Most people in any culture need to feel that the clinician is sufficiently experienced in his or her field. The "first impression" should convey this professionalism; otherwise, there is a loss of faith in the skill level of the provider.[78]

ELICITING PATIENT PERCEPTIONS OF THEIR HEALTH

The Kleinman Patient Explanatory Model has value for gaining a more comprehensive understanding of the patient's interpretation of their health. This model has been shortened and adapted by Galanti and called the 4C's of Culture 43. Pharmacists who find that they are having challenges helping a patient to understand their disease state or their medication can try eliciting the patient's understanding with the following abbreviated questions:

1. "What do you **CALL** the problem/condition?" Understanding the patient's own words used for the problem can help determine if the patient believes the condition is medical, spiritual, or of another cause.

2. "What do you think **CAUSED** your problem/condition?" The patient's perception of what has caused the health situation may be pathophysiologic, cultural, or spiritual. The perceived or real cause will help determine how the patient believes they should be treated.

3. "How do you **COPE** with the problem/condition?" A patient may have a variety of responses ranging from medicinal or procedural to physical or spiritual.

4. "What are your **CONCERNS** with the condition and/or recommended treatment?" The patient may have the perception that the condition is fatal, chronic, or temporary. They may also have concerns if the problem is infectious or if there is a cure.

The following fictional vignette provides an example of the value of the patient explanatory model.

Mrs. Khaya Movshevna, an elderly émigré, had gone through open heart surgery and had been given a series of tests to verify her current condition. The physician's office later telephoned Mrs. Movshevna and informed her through the interpreter (a family member) that she would need to add warfarin to her long list of medicines. Mrs. Movshevna and her relative went to the community pharmacy. There, the patient lamented having to ingest still another tablet. She feared a toxic reaction from this chemical overflow and asked the pharmacist clinician to recommend some sort of juice or nectar to "neutralize everything." Upon hearing the Mrs. Movshevna's request via her bilingual family interpreter, the pharmacist, Dr. Gladstone, smiled pleasantly, and told Mrs. Movshevna "Don't worry, Khaya," and handed the interpreter the medicine. Upon returning home, Mrs. Movshevna telephoned Regina, her friend and also an émigré, who agreed that "too much medicine is too much medicine." Regina promised to send a cleansing agent in the form of a liquid substance from "back home" that would prevent toxic reactions from the addition of warfarin to Mrs. Movshevna's other drugs. Mrs. Movshevna was relieved and commented to Regina that afterall, "I, not my clinician, understand my body best." The pharmacist clinician either failed to follow the line of questions or did not even reach this point while interacting with Mrs. Movshevna. Until further discussion with her physician, Mrs. Movshevna remained nonadherent with the warfarin regimen. Fortunately, no adverse event occurred.

INCORPORATING THE LEARN MODEL INTO OVERALL PATIENT CARE

The **LEARN** model provides a straightforward approach to interacting with patients across cultures.[80] Sadly, in the case above, the pharmacist, Dr. Gladstone did not do so in the preceding scenario. Several issues are relevant in this vignette and are outlined by incorporating the **LEARN** model into the case.

Listened to the patient. The initial communication barrier between Dr. Gladstone and Mrs. Movshevna was the lack of a common language, both spoken and written. This situation is not unique. It would be essential to use a trained and unbiased interpreter to explore the potential for nonadherence to the warfarin more carefully.

Dr. Gladstone's pleasant, non-condescending smile, and automatic phrase were positive but failed to compensate for his not "listening" to Mrs. Movshevna's nonverbal signs of distress and mistrust. Moreover, by speaking to her by her first name and giving the medicine to her family interpreter and not to her, he displayed disrespect for the patient and set a negative tone canceling out any later constructive interaction that should have taken place during this or future encounters.

If an appropriate interpreter could be acquired and the abbreviated 4C patient explanatory model had been used, the pharmacist, Dr. Gladstone might have discovered:

1. "Mrs. Movshevna, what do you **CALL** the problem that requires you take warfarin?" I am not really sure. I just know that I am taking a lot of medicine which is too many chemicals.
2. "And, what do you think **CAUSED** you to need to take this new medicine called warfarin?" Well, I had surgery on my heart. But I was taking too many medications... That is probably why I needed the surgery.
3. "How do you think you should **COPE** with the fact that you just had surgery?" I should stop taking the medicines and really don't want to take this new medicine. It seems toxic and the doctor said that I had to check my blood for an "eye and are" [INR] all the time. I would prefer to stop the medicines for a while and use the cleansing treatment that has worked for years in the family.
4. "What are your **CONCERNS** with this new medicine, warfarin?" It just doesn't seem safe. If I have to check my blood all the time, it is just not safe.

We cannot predict that if the pharmacist had used the "4C" approach, he could have actually convinced Mrs. Movshevna to take the warfarin. However, important information about the patient's concerns could be elicited.

Explained his perceptions of the problem and advice for treatment. With the information about fears of medication use and preference for family therapies, Dr. Gladstone may have been able to have a more candid conversation with the physician and with the patient about medication options. He could stress the particular importance of warfarin.

Acknowledged the patient's concerns. The relationship between Mrs. Movshevna and Dr. Gladstone should have been collaborative rather than purely prescriptive. Dr. Gladstone could provide a mirrored response with, "I understand that you are worried about the medication. I am also." Acknowledging the patient's understanding of her illness, her fears, and her ideas of treatment could help the pharmacist in building trust with the patient.

Recommended treatment while respecting the woman's individuality and cultural history. The pharmacist, Dr. Gladstone, initially failed to realize that Mrs. Movshevna would seek help elsewhere, most likely from a person in her own community. If he had set the mood for a constructive interchange and listened to her concerns and patient understanding, the pharmacist could have formulated a plan suitable to both parties.

Negotiated an agreement. One of Mrs. Movshevna's favorite phrases was "I, not my clinician, understand my body best." Dr. Gladstone's initial inability to acknowledge her views and include her as a team player contributed to her nonadherence.[81] After the above incident, this elderly patient probably spoke negatively about her experience to other émigrés. Her words, in turn, created reluctance among other potential patients to deal with the pharmacy, thus costing the establishment potential business. And in addition to reduced revenue from the surrounding community and to a tarnished reputation in the neighborhood, Dr. Gladstone missed the enjoyment he may have had from knowing Mrs. Movshevna for the years to come.[81]

SUMMARY

Working across cultures can be challenging and rewarding. Patients who seek medications at a pharmacy ARE seeking care from a pharmacist who will value their culture and identity and who will have the knowledge and skills to adapt and understand their genuine medication concerns. By taking time and gaining experience to understand the scope of diverse cultural beliefs and values influence medication use and recognizing the guiding legal and accrediting issues for culture and language competencies, pharmacists can develop the skills to successfully work across cultures.

REFERENCES

1. Gilbert, J., Goode, T.D., & Dunne, C. *Curricula enhancement module series.* http://www.nccccurricula.info/awareness/index.html. Accessed October 10, 2009.

2. Betancourt, J. in Diggs, A., & Berger, B. (2004). Cultural competence: Overcoming bias part 2: the pharmacist-patient relationship. *US Pharmacist* 29(06):94–97.

3. Robinson, R.G. (2005). Community development model for public health applications: Overview of a model to eliminate population disparities. *Health Promotion Practice* 6(3):338–346.

4. Banks, S. (October 20, 2014). Irrational Ebola fears make life difficult for Liberians in the U.S. *Los Angeles Times*.

5. Tervalon, M.G.J. (1998). "Cultural Humility Versus Cultural Competence" A critical distinction in defining physician training outcomes in multicultural education. *Journal of Health Care for the Poor and Underserved* 9:2:118.

6. Kaiser Family Foundation. (Dec 2012). Focus on health disparities: Five key questions and answers. #8396.

7. King, M.L. (2007). *Community health interventions prevention's role in reducing racial and ethnic disparities.* Washington, D.C.: Center for American Progress.

8. Institute of Medicine. (2012). *How far have we come in reducing health disparities?: Progress since 2000: Workshop summary.* Washington, D.C.: The National Academies Press.

9. Institute of Medicine. (2000). *Report brief: Examining the health disparities research plan of the National Institutes of Health: unfinished business.*

10. U.S. Department of Health and Human Services. (April 2011). *HHS action plan to reduce racial and ethnic disparities: a nation free of disparities in health and health care.*

11. U.S. Department of Health and Human Services, Office of Disease Prevention and Health Promotion. *Healthy People 2020: Disparities.* http://www.healthypeople.gov/2020/about/foundation-health-measures/Disparities. Accessed July 9, 2015.

12. Rastogi, S., Johnson, T.D., Hoeffel, E.M., & Drewery, Jr. M.P. (2011). *The Black population: 2010.* C2010BR-06.

13. Office of Minority Health, U.S. Department of Health and Human Services. *Minority population profiles: Black/African American.* http://minorityhealth.hhs.gov/omh/browse.aspx?lvl=3&lvlid=61. Accessed July 10, 2015.

14. Office of Minority Health, U.S. Department of Health and Human Services. *Minority populations: American Indian/Alaska Native.* http://minorityhealth.hhs.gov/omh/browse.aspx?lvl=3&lvlid=62. Accessed July 10, 2015.

15. Office of Minority Health, U.S. Department of Health and Human Services. *Minority population profiles: Asian American.* http://minorityhealth.hhs.gov/omh/browse.aspx?lvl=3&lvlid=63. Accessed July 10, 2015.

16. Office of Minority Health, U.S. Department of Health and Human Services. *Minority population profiles: Hispanic/Latino.* http://minorityhealth.hhs.gov/omh/browse.aspx?lvl=3&lvlid=64. Accessed July 10, 2015.

17. Office of Minority Health, U.S. Department of Health and Human Services. *Minority population profiles: Native Hawaiian/Other Pacific Islanders.* http://minorityhealth.hhs.gov/omh/browse.aspx?lvl=3&lvlID=65. Accessed July 10, 2015.

18. World Health Organization. (1946). *WHO definition of health.* From Preamble to the Constitution of the World Health Organization as adopted by the International Health Conference, New York, 19–22 June, 1946; signed on 22 July 1946 by the representatives of 61 States. http://www.who.int/about/definition/en/print.html. Accessed July 10, 2015.

19. US Department of Health and Human Services. *Healthy People 2020: Social determinants of health.* http://www.healthypeople.gov/2020/topics-objectives/topic/social-determinants-health. Accessed July 10, 2015.

20. ProLiteracy. *The crisis.* http://www.proliteracy.org/the-crisis. Accessed July 17, 2015.

21. Weiss, B. (2003). *Health literacy: A manual for clinicians: Part of an educational program about health literacy.* Chicago: American Medical Association.

22. National Commission on Adult Literacy. (2008). *Reach higher, America: Overcoming crisis in the U.S. workforce.*

23. U.S. Census Bureau. *State and county quickfacts.* http://quickfacts.census.gov/qfd/states/00000.html. Accessed July 17, 2015.

24. Weise, E. (July 20, 2006). Language Barriers Plague Hospitals. *USA Today.*

25. Agency for Healthcare Research and Quality. (May 2015). *2014 National Healthcare quality and disparities report.* AHRQ Pub. No. 15-0007.

26. US Health Resources and Services Administration. *About health literacy.* http://www.hrsa.gov/publichealth/healthliteracy/healthlitabout.html. Accessed July 15, 2015.

27. Vanderpool, H.K. (2005). Reportof the ASHP Ad Hoc Committee on Ethnic Diversity and Cultural Competence. *American Journal of Health System Pharmacists* 62:1929.

28. Taylor, D. & Taylor, J. (2014). The pharmacy student population: applications received 2012–13, degrees conferred 2012–13, Fall 2013 enrollments. *AJPE* 78(7):1–16.

29. Institute of Medicine of the National Academies. (2004). *In the Nation's Compelling Interest: Ensuring Diversity in the Health Care Workforce.* Washington DC: The National Academies Press.

30. Medina, M.S., Plaza, C.M., Stowe, C.D., et al. (2013). Center for the Advancement of Pharmacy Education 2013 educational outcomes. *Am J Pharm Educ.* 77(8):162–162. doi: 10.5688/ajpe778162.

31. Accreditation Council for Pharmacy Education. *Standards Revision 2016.* https://www.acpe-accredit.org/deans/StandardsRevision.asp. Accessed May 20, 2015.

32. Federal Interagency Working Group. *Limited English proficiency. Let everyone participate: meaningful access for people who are limited English proficient.* www.lep.gov. Accessed October 11, 2009.

33. U.S. Department of Health and Human Services, Office of Civil Rights. *Guidance to federal financial assistance recipients regarding title vi prohibition against national origin discrimination affecting limited English proficient persons.* http://www.hhs.gov/ocr/civilrights/resources/specialtopics/lep/lepguidance.pdf. Accessed July 20, 2015.

34. RxTran—*Pharmacy language solutions. regulatory environment for pharmacies serving customers with limited English proficiency.* http://www.rxtran.com/pharmacy-translation-regulations.html. Accessed July 20, 2015.

35. RxTran—Pharmacy Language Solutions. (2009). *Summary of regulations governing the provision of translation and interpreting services by pharmacies.* http://www.rxtran.com/pharmacy-translation-regulations.html. Accessed July 20, 2015.

36. RxTran—Pharmacy Language solutions. New York City LAW ON PROVISION OF TRANSLATION SERVICES IN PHARMACIES. http://www.rxtran.com/pharmacy-translation-regulations/pharmacy-translation-regulations-new-york-city.html. Accessed July 20, 2015.

37. The New York City Council. (2009). *Provision of language assistance services in pharmacies.* 2009/055.

38. Office of Minority Health, U.S. Department of Health and Human Services. *What are the National CLAS Standards?* https://www.thinkculturalhealth.hhs.gov/content/clas.asp. Accessed May 20, 2015.

39. Office of Minority Health, U.S. Department of Health & Human Services. *CLAS Legislation Map.* https://www.thinkculturalhealth.hhs.gov/Content/LegislatingCLAS.asp. Accessed July 20, 2015.

40. Kupka, N., Tschurtz, B., Wilson-Stronks, A., & Galvez, E. (2010.) The Joint Commission. *Cultural and linguistic care in area hospitals.* Oakbrook Terrace, IL: The Joint Commission.

41. The Joint Commission. (2010). *Advancing effective communication, cultural competence, and patient- and family-centered care: A Roadmap for hospitals.* 2010. Oakbrook Terrace, IL: The Joint Commission.

42. Campinha-Bacote, J. (2002).The process of cultural competence in the delivery of healthcare services: A model of care. *J Transcult Nurs* 13(3):181–184.

43. Galanti, G. (2008). *Caring for Patients from different cultures.* Fourth ed. Philadelphia, PA: University of Pennsylvania Press.

44. James, J. & Levine,Y. *How foods affect blood sugar: A guide for Somali patients with diabetes.* http://ethnomed.org/patient-education/diabetes/SomaliDMSlideshow.pdf/view?searchterm=ramadan. Accessed July 20, 2015.

45. Selinus, R. *The traditional foods of the central Ethiopian highlands* (research report no. 7). 1971; Accessed July 20, 2015.

46. National Center for Cultural Competence. *Self-Assessments.* http://nccc.georgetown.edu/resources/assessments.html. Accessed July 20, 2015.

47. Kleinman, A. (1980). *Patients and healers in the context of culture.* Berkeley, CA: University of California Press.

48. Johnson, T.M., Hardt ,E., & Kleinman, A. (1995). Cultural Factors in the Medical Interview In Lipkin, M., Putnam, S.M., & Lazare, A. (Eds.), *The medical interview: Clinical care, education, and research.* New York, NY: Springer.

49. Berry, J. (1980). Acculturation as varieties of adaptation. In Padilla, A.M. (Ed.), *Acculturation: Theory, models, and some new findings.* Boulder, CO: Westview Press.

50. Schwartz, S.J., Unger, J.B., Zamboanga, B.L., & Szapocznik, J. (2010). Rethinking the concept of acculturation: Implications for theory and research. *Am Psychol* 65(4):237–251. doi: 10.1037/a0019330

51. Purnell, L. (2002). The Purnell Model for cultural competence. *J Transcult Nurs.* 13(3):193–196.

52. Cross,T., Bazron, B., Dennis, K., & Isaacs, M. (1989). *Towards a culturally competent system of care: Volume I.* Washington, DC: CASSP Technical Assistance Center, Georgetown University Child Development Center.

53. Tuskegee University. *About the USPHS syphilis study.* http://www.tuskegee.edu/about_us/centers_of_excellence/bioethics_center/about_the_usphs_syphilis_study.aspx. Accessed July 13, 2015.

54. National Center for Cultural Competence. *Body/Mind/Spirit—Toward a biopsychosocial-spiritual model of health: definitions of health, illness and sickness.* http://nccc.georgetown.edu/body_mind_spirit/definitions_health_sickness.html. Accessed July 20, 2015.

55. Franklin, M.D., Schlundt, D.G., McClellan, L., et al. (2007). Religious fatalism and its association with health behaviors and outcomes. *Am J Health Behav.* 31(6):563–572.

56. Koenig, H.G., King ,D.E., & Carson, V.B. (2012). *Handbook of religion and health, 2nd ed.* New York, NY: Oxford University Press.

57. Johnson, K., Elbert-Avila, K., & Tulsky, J. (2005). The influence of spiritual beliefs and practices on the treatment preferences of African Americans: A review of the literature. *J Am Geriatr Soc.* 53:711–719.

58. Star-K Kosher Certifications. Approved over-the-counter medication list 2015. http://www.star-k.org/cons-appr-medicine.htm. Accessed July 20, 2015.

59. Islamic Food and Nutrition Council of America. *Halal.* http://www.ifanca.org/Pages/staticwebpages.aspx?page=whatisHalal. Accessed July 20, 2015.

60. Muslim Consumer Group. *Medicines.* http://www.muslimconsumergroup.com/medicine.html. Accessed July 20, 2015.

61. Halal Certified Medicine. *Introducing Halal medicine to your local pharmacy.* http://www.halalmedicines.com.au. Accessed June 1, 2015.

62. Clarke, T.C., Black, L.I., Stussman, B.J., et al. (2015). Trends in the use of complementary health approaches among adults: United States, 2002–2012. *National Health Statistics Reports* 79.

63. Padilla, R., Gomez, V., Biggerstaff, S.L., & Mehler, P.S. (2001). Use of curanderismo in a public health care system. *Arch Intern Med.* 161(10):1336–1340.

64. Gardiner, P., Whelan, J., White, L.F., Filippelli, A.C., Bharmal, N., & Kaptchuk, T.J. (2012). A systematic review of the prevalence of herb usage among racial/ethnic minorities in the United States. *J Immigr Minor Health* 1-12-doi:10.1007/s10903-012-9661-z.

65. Rivera, J.O., Loya, A.M., & Ceballos, R. (2013). Use of herbal medicines and implications for conventional drug therapy medical sciences. *Altern Integ Med.* 2:130.

66. Kennedy, J., Wang, C.C., Wu, C.H. (2008). Patient disclosure about herb and supplement use among adults in the US. *Evid Based Complement Alternat Med.* 5:451–456.

67. Balhara, Y.P.S. (2011). Culture-bound syndrome: Has it found its right niche?. *Indian J Psychol Med.* 33(2):210–215.

68. Helman, C.G. (1987). Heart disease and the cultural construction of time: The type A behavior pattern as a Western culture-bound syndrome. *Soc Sci Med.* 25(9):969–979.

69. Lee, S. (1996). Reconsidering the status of anorexia nervosa as Western culture-bound syndrome. *Soc Sci Med.* 42(1):22–34.

70. Prakash, O. (2007). Lessons for postgraduate trainees about Dhat syndrome. *Indian J Psychiatry.* 49(3):208–201.

71. Garlipp, P.(2008). Koro - a culture-bound phenomenon; Intercultural psychiatric implications. *German Journal of Psychiatry* 11:21–28.

72. Roufs, T.G. *Culture bound syndromes*. http://www.d.umn.edu/cla/faculty/troufs/anth4616/cpculture-bound_syndromes.html. Accessed May 22, 2015.

73. Putsch, III, R.W. (1988). Ghost illness: A cross-cultural expression of a non-western tradition in clinical practice. *American Indian and Alaska Native Mental Health Research* 2(2):6-26.

74. The Joint Commission. *The Joint Commission 2009 requirements that support effective communication, cultural competence, and patient-centered care Hospital Accreditation Program* (HAP). http://www.jointcommission.org/NR/rdonlyres/B48B39E3-107D-495A-9032-24C3EBD96176/0/PDF32009HAPSupportingStds.pdf. Accessed July 20, 2015.

75. The Joint Commission. *Office of Minority health national Culturally and Linguistically Appropriate Services (CLAS) Standards crosswalked to joint commission 2007 standards for hospitals, ambulatory, behavioral health, long term care, and home care.* http://www.jointcommission.org/NR/rdonlyres/5EABBEC8-F5E2-4810-A16F-E2F148AB5170/0/hlc_omh_xwalk.pdf. Accessed July 20, 2015.

76. Nichols-English ,G. (2000). Improving health literacy: A key to better patient outcomes. *J Am Pharm Assoc.* 40(6):835–836.

77. National Work Group Members. (2004). *Bridging the cultural divide in health care settings: The Essential role of cultural broker programs.*

78. Henry Ford Health System. (1999). General inter-cultural tips communicating respect. *Ethnic Resource Guide.* Detroit: Henry Ford Health System.

79. U.S. Department of Health and Human Services. *Indian health service pharmacists: Cultural considerations while serving the Indian health population.* https://www.ihs.gov/pharmacy/index.cfm?module=awareness. Accessed June 2, 2015.

80. Berlin, E.A., & Fowkes, W.C. (1983). A teaching framework for cross-cultural health care. *The Western Journal of Medicine* 139:934–8.

81. Desmond, J., & Copeland, L.R. (2000). *Communicating with today's patient essentials to save time, decrease risk, and increase patient compliance.* San Francisco, CA: Wiley, John & Sons.

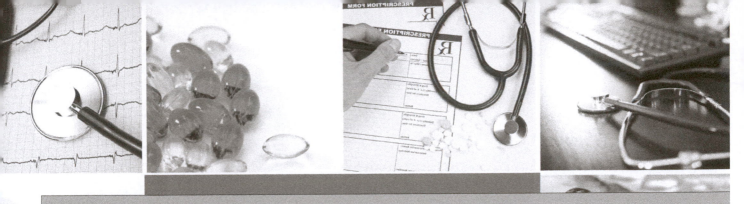

PART IV SYSTEM-LEVEL TOPICS INVOLVING PHARMACY PRACTICE

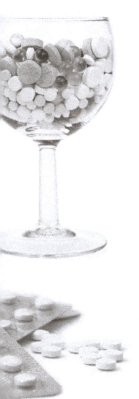
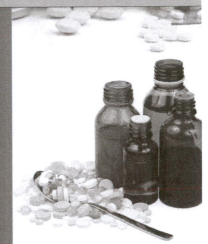
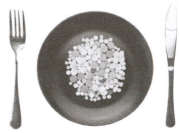
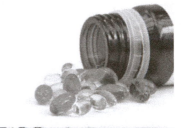
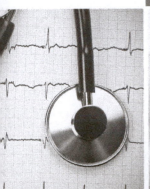
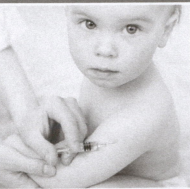
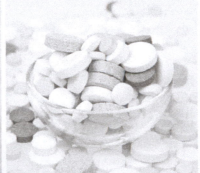
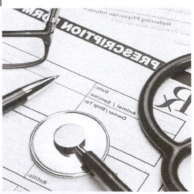

CHAPTER 20

A PSYCHOSOCIAL APPROACH TO MEDICATION ERRORS

Elizabeth Flynn, Kraig L. Schell, Jenny O. Rickles

LEARNING OBJECTIVES:

1. Evaluate medication errors from multiple perspectives, including psychosocial, system, patient, practitioner and societal.
2. Give examples of individual psychological attributes that have a role in the accuracy of performance.
3. Describe how often medication errors occur in different health care settings and at different stages of the medication distribution system.
4. Recommend interventions designed to prevent medication errors.
5. Explain different medication error detection techniques.

KEY TERMS

Adverse drug event

Error detection

Error prevention

Individual characteristics

Interpersonal perspectives

Medication errors

Medication safety

Psychosocial

Second victim

Situation-Background-Assessment-Recommendation (SBAR) technique

Work environment

INTRODUCTION

Alexander Pope said "To err is human, to forgive is divine."[1] Unfortunately, depending on the nature of a medication error (and the resilience of the victim), to err with medication can have life-changing consequences physically, psychologically, and socially for all involved and be difficult to forgive. Fatal medication errors often gain national media attention, and seem to occur at a frequency that keeps errors on the minds of health professionals. One example involved the death of three neonates after the administration of heparin overdoses where the staff did not recognize that the heparin retrieved from an automated medication dispensing device was 1,000 times greater than the normally-stocked concentration.[2] The death of Boston Globe health reporter Betsy Lehman at the Dana-Farber Cancer Institute due to administration of cyclophosphamide, 4,000 mg/ml[2] instead of 1,000 mg/ml[2] triggered widespread efforts to improve medication safety.[3] The goals of this chapter are to provide background on medication errors and describe the psychosocial aspects of errors.

The definition of a medication error has many components, and many definitions can be found in the literature. For example, one well-known definition suggests that a medication error must be preventable, directly or indirectly associated with some kind of patient harm, and can occur regardless of who controlled the medication at the critical point in time. The types of errors that have been identified in the literature are quite variable, including prescribing mismatches, dispensing irregularities, administration nonadherence, and incorrect compounding processes.[4] It is important to recognize that medication error is just one type of medical error; other types of medical errors include wrong medical procedures, non-adherence to treatment guidelines, etc. Also, the reader should note that adverse drug events (ADEs) are injuries related to medication use (e.g., allergic reactions) and errors; not all medication errors result in an ADE.[3]

It is important to recognize that medication error is just one type of medical error; other types of medical errors include wrong medical procedures, non-adherence to treatment guidelines, etc. Also, the reader should note that adverse drug events (ADEs) are injuries related to medication use (e.g., allergic reactions) and errors; not all medication errors result in an ADE.[3]

Medication safety (a recent term to recognize the goal of medication use) has received considerable attention and resources since the year 2000, when the Institute of Medicine (IOM) described the scope, severity, and impact of medical errors in the report "To Err is Human."[5] The impact of medication errors is astounding. Medication errors account for 20% of medical errors resulting in injury or death,[6] cause an estimated 7,000 deaths per year,[7] are associated with 3–7% of serious adverse events among those hospitalized[8], and increase hospital costs in the United States by about $2 billion annually.[9] The IOM report "Preventing Medication Errors" contains a comprehensive summary of the frequency of a wide variety of medication error types and adverse drug events in hospitals, nursing homes, pediatric, psychiatric and community settings.[3] The increasing number of organizations created to address medication errors and medication safety reflects a passionate desire to eliminate error—here is a list of selected groups and resources on medication errors:

1. U.S. Food and Drug Administration's Center for Drug Evaluation and Research (CDER) Division of Medication Error Prevention and Analysis (DMEPA)

2. Agency for Healthcare Research and Quality: Medical Errors and Patient Safety: http://www.ahrq.gov/qual/patientsafetyix.htm

3. Centers for Disease Control and Prevention: Medication Safety: http://www.cdc.gov/medicationsafety/

4. Department of Veterans Affairs National Center for Patient Safety: http://www.patientsafety.gov/

5. Institute for Safe Medication Practices: http://www.ismp.org/

6. To Err is Human: Building a Safer Health System (Institute of Medicine): http://www.iom.edu/Reports/1999/To-Err-is-Human-Building-A-Safer-Health-System.aspx

7. Preventing Medication Errors: Quality Chasm Series: http://www.iom.edu/Reports/2006/Preventing-Medication-Errors-Quality-Chasm-Series.aspx

8. National Patient Safety Foundation: http://www.npsf.org/

9. National Coordinating Council for Medication Error Reporting and Prevention: http://www.nccmerp.org/

MEDICATION ERROR LANDSCAPE FOR PRACTITIONERS

Physicians, nurses and pharmacists strive for 100% accuracy in the daily provision of pharmaceutical care. Demands for error-free work are placed on them by patients, families, employers, Boards of Medicine/Nursing/Pharmacy, peers, media, legal system, and liability insurance companies. Yet, medication administration errors have been shown to be common, occurring at a rate of two per patient day, based on the results of an observational study in 36 hospitals and skilled nursing facilities.[10] The medication administration errors occurred at a rate of 19% overall (605 errors detected on 3,216 doses), and 10% excluding wrong time errors. The most frequent types of errors were wrong time (43%), omission (30%), and wrong dose (17%). Seven percent of the errors were judged to have the potential for resulting in adverse drug events, or more than 40 per day in a 300-bed hospital.[10] Medication administration error rates in hospitals range from 0% to 18% measured by observational studies conducted since 1980 in several countries (excluding wrong time errors). Error rates as low as two to three per patient per week have been achieved by installing unit-dose systems. Comparison of error rates between studies should be made cautiously, considering differences in error category definitions and methodologies.[11] Observational studies of medication administration errors in hospitals before and after bar code verification technology have found accuracy rates ranging from 86% to 97%.[12-13] In the community pharmacy setting, a national observational study of prescription dispensing accuracy in 50 pharmacies found dispensing error rates ranging from 0% to 13%, with an overall error rate of 1.7% (77 errors on 4,481 prescriptions).[14] The ramifications are that a pharmacy dispensing 250 prescriptions per day would dispense four of them in error.

THE CONCEPTS OF FIRST AND SECOND VICTIMS

Adverse events ("errors") regarding medications have a unique characteristic that separates them from similar events in other industries. If an oilfield worker or a pilot triggers an adverse event, the negative effects of the event will probably include that individual as well as innocent others. However, the same cannot be said about errors triggered by healthcare professionals. The pharmacist that dispenses the wrong medication or the nurse that hangs the wrong bag suffers no ill effects from that event – the patient is the most obvious victim and historically has been described as the *only* victim. While there is a kernel of truth in this generalization (at least with respect to *physiological* effects), recent thinking in the field has raised awareness of the psychological and social effects of adverse events that are felt by all those connected in some way. The patient, the patient's family and friends, and the health care staff members all have stakes in proper and safe care. It is critical that we understand the ways in which adverse events affect healthcare professionals because it is the responsibility of healthcare organizations to support them.

In many available studies, the phrase "second victim" is used to identify the healthcare professional who triggered an adverse event that injured a patient.[15-16] Studies indicate that the effects felt by the second victim are strong and complex, and can affect the way in which this individual perceives themselves, their jobs, and their careers. Psychological literature helps to clarify why these effects occur. When an individual realizes that they have directly triggered an adverse event, he or she is motivated to find an explanation for it. Unfortunately, this process of explaining events (called *attribution* by psychologists) is not a rational, data-driven process. Instead, he or she is probably going to experience a variety of emotions and thoughts, including self-doubt, fear, anxiety and counterfactual thinking ("What if I had just...?"). These kinds of reactions tend to behave cybernetically, feeding back on themselves and becoming amplified in the process. She might begin to wonder if she will lose her job, if the patient's family will hate her, and if her colleagues will no longer trust her and view her favorably. Amidst all this chaos, she will ultimately decide whether the event was caused by factors inherent in her (an *internal* attribution) or factors outside of her control (an *external* attribution). Further, she may come to the conclusion about whether similar events can be controlled in the future, whether similar events are likely to occur with similar patients in the future, or whether she just doesn't want to decide anything at all. Regardless of how the organization chooses to support the employee (or not), this explanatory motive will be engaged in some way. For this reason, the scientific and institutional recognition of the "second victim" phenomenon is very important. In the past, adverse events were assumed to be caused by personal failings of the employee. Thus, the pharmacist who dispenses a medication improperly was labeled "at fault," subjected to organizational and regulatory punishments, and told to "be more careful" (if she kept her job at all). It is not hard to predict how the pharmacist in this situation will explain the event. She will see the error as an indictment of her abilities as a professional and feel that she is powerless to do anything to predict or prevent the next adverse event from occurring. She will begin to feel helpless, a debilitating psychological state that leads to a variety of negative and harmful psychological effects. Employees in this state will become more vulnerable to error, not less, because we cannot "punish the error out" of the healthcare system.

The case of Eric Cropp is an example of punishing a pharmacist responsible for a fatal error by revoking his Ohio pharmacist license, six months' imprisonment, six months of home confinement, three years of probation, and 400 hours of community service.[17] Julie Thao was a nurse in Wisconsin who faced felony charges after administering the anesthetic bupivacaine intravenously instead of an antibiotic—she served three years of probation.[18] Efforts to assist the second victim overcome survivor guilt are underway, including a Second Victim Committee at Johns Hopkins University.[19] The Institute for Safe Medication Practices has compiled a list of helpful resources on the ISMP web site for healthcare professionals who unintentionally commit errors.[20]

The acceptance and understanding of this "second victim" phenomenon will have a number of beneficial effects. First, the healthcare organization will be less likely to assume that adverse events are always caused by bad employees. Second, healthcare leaders will be more likely to create support systems for those who trigger adverse events that facilitate a healthier and more realistic explanation for the situation, rather than allowing employees to believe that it was their fault. Third, it will improve the quality and outcomes of error-oriented investigative processes, such as Root Cause Analysis, by incorporating employee feedback as neutral data rather than "the testimony of the accused." Fourth, it should contribute favorably to the creation and maintenance of "just culture" by demonstrating that the organization is willing to consider that adverse events may be caused by systemic and complex combinations of factors, rather than just incompetence or carelessness.[21] Fifth, and perhaps most importantly, it will force the industry to reconsider the prevailing definitions of "error" that can bias perceptions and reactions when adverse events occur.

UNDERSTANDING HOW ERROR EMERGES

This chapter presents errors from the individual, interpersonal and system/organizational perspective. As each perspective is described, we will discuss errors as they relate to the drug delivery process, including medication prescribing, dispensing, and administration. We will describe types of errors, psychosocial causes of errors, and possible interventions/solutions. Table 20-1 provides the reader with definitions of error types and points in the drug delivery system a particular error can occur. It is important to understand two characteristics of errors: first, "errors" are best thought of as emergent properties, events that "pop out" of the right combinations of factors such as the ones we will discuss. While we are categorizing errors as a convention for this chapter, it is not always scientifically useful to dogmatically cling to any error category scheme; instead, we can progress by understanding the characteristics of the environment that generate the error event. Second, it is important to understand that an error that occurs during administration could also have occurred at another stage in the drug delivery system (i.e. dispensing) but was not caught until the medication was administered.

TABLE 20-1

ERROR TYPE	DEFINITION	PRESCRIBING	DISPENSING	ADMINISTRATION
Wrong drug	Medication dispensed is different from medication prescribed	✓	✓	✓
Wrong strength	Dispensed dosage unit is different than prescribed dosage unit	✓	✓	✓
Wrong dose length	Number of doses dispensed per unit of time is different than number of doses prescribed per unit of time	✓	✓	✓
Wrong dosage form	Dispensed dosage formulation is different than prescribed dosage formulation	✓	✓	✓
Wrong quantity	Number of doses dispensed is different than number of doses prescribed	✓	✓	✓
Wrong label instructions	Directions dispensed to the patient are different than those prescribed by the provider; deviations must increase the probability of adverse events		✓	
Wrong label information (excluding instructions)	Information on label does not confirm to regulatory requirements		✓	
Deteriorated drug	Dispensed medication has surpassed its expiration date and/or has been stored inappropriately		✓	✓
Wrong patient	Medication is dispensed to incorrect patient	✓	✓	✓
Extra doses	Doses are administered after refills are expended or after "stop" orders have been charted		✓	✓
Missed doses	Doses are not administered at the appointed time		✓	✓
Wrong route	Doses are delivered using an incorrect route of administration	✓	✓	✓
Wrong time	Doses are administered later than intended (usually > 60 minutes)			✓
Wrong technique	Compounded medications are incorrectly manufactured, or the administration of a dose is not completed according to standard			✓

Figure 20-1 illustrates the three domains with respect to their proximity to a hypothetical error event (psychological, social, and organizational). It is adapted from a framework model proposed by Grasha and colleagues[22,23] and is based on the theories of error found in the literature.[24-26] The model suggests that some factors are proximal (near) to the error whereas others are typically distal (far). The "distance" from the error should not be interpreted to mean that distal factors are less important to error capture and prevention. The reader should understand that this is a "direct-influence" proximity; the factors closer to the error are usually more directly connected to its emergence, whereas distal factors may primarily affect the error by influencing the more proximal factors. Thus, our model should serve as an illustration of the typical relationship between the domains of influential factors as it relates to the individual, interpersonal, and system/organization perspective.

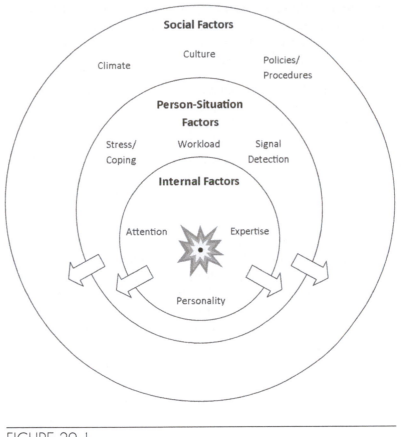

FIGURE 20-1

INDIVIDUAL PERSPECTIVES

Errors that can occur from the individual perspective can arise out of familiarity with procedures and materials. An individual has an innate tendency to perceive confirming evidence more readily than disconfirming evidence. Confirmation bias can occur when an individual interprets information in a way that confirms their preconceptions or beliefs. This also occurs when individuals become familiar with procedures.[27] Individuals can have unconscious "slips" that are errors that occur due to distractions or failure to pay attention at critical moments. Conditions that make slips more likely are fatigue, substance abuse, illness, emotions, and environmental factors.

As illustrated in the model in Figure 20-1, there are three internally-based factors that can contribute to the emergence of an error: attention, personality, and expertise. This is not an exhaustive list, but encompasses many factors that have been shown to influence error. Attention refers to one's focus on a particular stimulus;

attention can be singly-focused or focused across multiple tasks, and it can be sustained or varying amounts of time.[28] Attention allows the actor to detect "signals" in the environment and differentiate important information from distracting information.[29] With respect to medication error, individual differences in focused attention (i.e., resistance to attentional distraction) have been shown to be related to error rates in a stimulus checking task.[30] Attention is resource-dependent[28,31]—requiring "cognitive fuel" to maintain itself for extended periods. Finally, attention can be "captured" by stimulus characteristics.[32,33]

Personality includes traits and predispositions that inform and influence our behavioral choices.[34] With respect to specific traits, there is evidence that trait anxiety is related to error production in a simulated pharmacy task,[35] and that self-monitoring (a tendency to monitor and adjust behavior internally rather than relying on external information) has been connected to increased "false alarms", i.e., identifying an error that does not really exist.[23] Personality also influences attention by encouraging the actor to detect information more conservatively ("Everything is an error") or liberally ("Errors almost never happen").[36]

Expertise is defined as the degree to which a skilled behavior has become routine and, therefore, requires fewer cognitive resources to effectively complete.[37] Researchers usually describe expertise as a shift from effortful processing to automatic processing of tasks.[38,39] Most pharmacy staff with even just 6–12 months of experience are likely to be in "automatic mode" as they work. Expertise is important because it facilitates performance without sacrificing accuracy,[40,41] and does so with no discernable strain on short-term memory. It also facilitates adaptive error management through enhanced knowledge structures,[42] making memory more efficient. Errors may decline naturally as a function of expertise, but it is too extreme to say that experts do not make mistakes. Though expertise is seen as a benefit, individuals who are considered to have expertise may feel a false sense of security and the "automatic mode" in which they work could lead to errors.

PRESCRIBING ERROR RISKS

From the individual perspective the root of an error may begin when a provider sees a patient and handwrites a prescription or when the provider calls a prescription into a community pharmacy. This type of error may occur due to medications with sound-alike or look-alike names. For example, the prescriber writes for Taxol®, but the intent was to prescribe Paxil®.[43] An error may also occur when prescribing medications that have zeros or decimal points. As an example, a physician prescribes Vincristine 2.0 mg but later in the dispensing process is misread as Vincristine 20 mg. In the case of the Betsy Lehman overdose mentioned previously, an ambiguous or incomplete order for cyclophosphamide caused the fatal error as the order was written 4 g/ml days 1–4. This led to ambiguity as to whether the medication was to be given over 4 days or whether the total amount should be divided across 4 days. Errors can occur when mixing the metric and apothecary systems also. For example, 1/200 grain (0.3 mg) NTG tablets; gives 2 x 1/100 grain (0.6 mg each) = 1.2 mg total. Errors can also occur when using abbreviations. For example, U has been read as a 0, 4 or 6.[44]

DISPENSING ERROR RISKS

There are many different types of errors that can occur during dispensing (see Table 20-1 for specific definitions). For example, an error can occur when a prescriber calls a medication into a community pharmacy and a wrong drug is dispensed due to the nature of the oral communication. An example of a wrong dosage form error is giving a tablet when a suspension was ordered, or administering plain aspirin instead of enteric- coated aspirin. Instances in which tablets are crushed are not considered wrong dosage form errors because of inadequate knowledge of the effect of crushing the tablet.[11]

Dispensing errors can occur in different settings. In a community pharmacy setting there are many distractions during the dispensing of medication where an error may emerge. Many pharmacies experience high prescription volumes and thus have significant demands on their workload. Pharmacies have the additional burden of dealing with a multitude of insurance claims issues. These latter issues cause an enormous time strain on the pharmacy staff, which can stress individual cognitive resources to exhaustion. When this occurs, an error may more frequently emerge.

Past literature on error counts bears this out. The national study of prescription dispensing accuracy in 50 pharmacies measured an overall 1.7% dispensing error rate on 4,481 prescriptions.[14] Most deviations from the prescription were label errors, followed by wrong quantity, wrong strength, wrong drug, omission, and wrong dosage form.[14] Previous studies of error rates in prescription filling ranged from 1% to 24%.[45-48] Dispensing errors that could harm patients have been estimated to occur on 1.5% to 4% of erroneous prescriptions.[45,46,48] Ashcroft and colleagues studied the possible causes of near misses and dispensing errors in community pharmacies in the United Kingdom. The most common factors related to near misses and errors were misreading the prescription, similar drug names, selecting the wrong drug from the patient's profile, and similar drug packaging.[49]

Dispensing errors can occur in an inpatient hospital setting for similar reasons as community pharmacies: busy units, multi-tasking of staff, and strain of discharging patients by a certain time due to insurance or Medicare constraints. Pharmacy error rates involving doses dispensed during the cart filling process (picking errors) range from 0.04% to 2.9%.[50-55] In the most recent study, Cina and colleagues found a 3.6% pharmacy dispensing error rate (5,075 errors on 140,755 doses) on orders filled by pharmacy technicians.[56] Pharmacists inspecting these orders detected only 79% of the errors, for a final dispensing error rate of 0.75%. ADEs were judged to be possible on 23.5% of the undetected errors, with 28% of these deemed serious and 0.8% life threatening.

Some state boards of pharmacies have allowed technicians to check other technicians after filling patient medication drawers instead of requiring a pharmacist to perform this task.[57] A comparison of unit-dose medication drawer checking accuracy of technicians and pharmacists found that the error rates detected by each group did not differ significantly: both found a 1.2% cart fill error rate.[58] Pharmacists overlooked errors more often than technicians: 107 errors on 49,718 doses (0.21% error rate) versus 50 errors overlooked by technicians on 55,470 doses (0.09% error rate).

The authors noted that the percentage of missed errors that could have resulted in patient harm was not significantly different (25.2% for pharmacists versus 32.0% for technicians), but this means that 27 potentially serious errors were overlooked by pharmacists compared to 16 by technicians.

As illustrated in the model in Figure 20-1, we have identified three person-situation factors which can affect the dispensing process: stress and coping behaviors, signal detection factors, and workload. Stress and coping behaviors describe the interaction between stressful circumstances (stressors) and how we respond to them (coping).[59,60] The pharmacy literature includes a number of stress studies, most concluding that pharmacists must handle a considerable amount of stress at work.[61-63] But, we cannot assume that stress from work is the only relevant stress for work. Studies have shown consistently that stress from extra-work roles, such as family, can impact performance on the job.[64,65]

Signal detection factors refer to elements of the error detection environment that impact our ability to "find" errors amongst the "noise" of non-errors.[66] The theory suggests that we evaluate a stimulus on some criteria and then decide whether that stimulus is either a "target" or a "non-target." As it has typically been applied in pharmacy, the target would be an error (i.e., a mismatch between the expected and observed information), and the non-target would be a correct prescription (as far as we know). Our threshold for making that decision varies depending on a number of factors, which can encourage us to be more or less willing to interrupt the work process when we perceive the possibility of an error.[67] From this theory and studies of simulated pharmacy performance, we know that error probability,[68] costs and benefits of each decision possibility as well as signal strength[69] can "push" the person toward either a liberal decision threshold (greater willingness to identify suspicious targets) or a conservative one (lesser willingness to identify suspicious targets). Finally, workload can be composed of factors from a number of sources, including prescription volume, multiple tasks, interruptions and distractions, and poor environmental conditions for work. However, there is one pervasive assumption that persists about how workload affects errors in pharmacy. Workload is often thought by pharmacists to be a primary cause of error, but empirical investigations of this claim have shown that things are not quite that simple.[70] One study showed that the *lowest-volume* pharmacies produced the highest error rates, most likely through task disengagement and boredom.[71,72] Perceptions of workload are likely to be more important to errors in pharmacy[73] because they are indicative of how stressful the workload is to the person. This idea fits well with modern theories of stress as well.[74]

ADMINISTRATION ERROR RISKS

Medication administration errors are typically viewed as being related to drug administration in the hospital and are usually defined as any deviation from the prescriber's interpretable order.[11] There are many different types of errors that can occur during administration (see Table 20-1 for specific definitions). Administration errors can also occur at home when an older adult has multiple medications and confuses what should be taken, when to take their medication and takes too many, too few, at the wrong time, or forgets to take the medication altogether. Also, when a patient is discharged from a hospital with multiple medications and the patient has medications at home and confuses doses.

In a hospital setting, a wrong technique error can occur. For example, if the wrong rate of infusion is used but the patient receives the correct dose, a wrong technique error has occurred. If the prescriber ordered that the patient's heart rate or blood pressure meet a specific criterion prior to drug administration and the action was omitted, a wrong technique error has occurred. If the heart rate is measured, and the rate is too low for the dose to be given, but the nurse still administers the drug, an extra dose error has occurred.[11] One study defined intravenous drug errors as "any deviation in the preparation or administration of a drug from a doctor's prescription, the hospital's intravenous policy, or the manufacturer's instructions." However, it should be noted that this study only considered a dose to be in error if it had the potential to adversely affect the patient, which ignores error-related behavior that occurred without consequence.[75]

INTERVENTIONS

From the individual perspective, there are many interventions and solutions which could help to reduce errors. During prescribing, a double-check system can be put into place where a second person checks the written order. Read backs are also an important intervention. For example, if a prescriber were to call a medication into a community pharmacy or hospital pharmacy, the pharmacist on the phone would write down the verbal order, then repeat what he has written to receive confirmation of the correct prescription. This was incorporated into the Joint Commission National Patient Safety goals in 2003. The goal was to implement a process for taking verbal or telephone orders and requires a verification "read back" of the complete order by the person receiving the order.[76]

Another intervention/solution would be a model of patient empowerment. In 2007, the Joint Commission added a patient safety goal which encourages patients' active involvement in their own care.[30] There could be initiatives put into place which encourage patients and families to speak up and become an active participant in their care. For example, if a patient received a prescription and was not sure of the reason or dose, the patient would be encouraged to speak up and ask the prescriber or pharmacist. A great deal has been written on patient engagement/involvement in the past decade, and there are many examples in the literature of how it is being practiced.[77-79] It is important to recognize, however, that most of this work is centered on the care provider, with instructions on how to communicate, how to deal with patient literacy issues, and how to avoid paternalism and condescension. We must expand our viewpoint to include the patient as part of the dynamic, as well as to understand how a doctor-patient relationship should most beneficially unfold over time.

A sense of accountability is equally important from the individual staff perspective. Staff should have a sense of accountability for their responsibilities and how their actions can affect others that they work with and the patients that rely on them.

A sense of accountability will help staff feel empowered. Staff empowerment would include feeling comfortable and safe to tell another staff member, even a supervisor. that they question a particular dose or order that is written. Much of this is rooted in the culture and climate of the organization, and whether it is supportive of a collective "one for all, all for one" mentality. We will discuss culture more completely later in this chapter.

INTERPERSONAL PERSPECTIVES

Errors that can occur from the interpersonal perspective are complex. Interpersonal communications which occur between the pharmacist and patient, prescriber and patient, and prescriber and pharmacist all have their own particular challenges. For example, time and workloads limit the nature and extent of communication between different members of the healthcare team and between those members and the patient. Such communications are important for patient education, adequate provider assessment, and development of an optimal treatment plan. Inadequate patient education and patient assessment may lead to errors.

Communication and life stressors play a role in the interpersonal perspectives leading to errors. As described earlier, healthcare professionals continue to work in a fast-paced environment with increasing volume and acuity of patients. This is also compounded by the shortages of healthcare professionals in many disciplines. During these busy times teamwork is essential. Communication among team members was added as a Joint Commission National Patient Safety Goal in 2003 and then updated in 2006 to include the need to develop a standard approach for "hand-off" communication.[76] "Hand off" communication includes communication between health professionals, caregivers, and others during transitions in care and allowing enough time to ask questions and clarify issues. These and other interpersonal perspectives will be discussed further in the next paragraphs.

PRESCRIBING

The focus here is on inter-disciplinary communication as well the communication with the patient. Let us take an example of a provider not counseling the patient on the medication they are prescribing, or giving confusing information. The patient may not understand why they are taking it and be unclear of the risks or benefits. The patient may think they are taking a particular medication and not realize that the medication they were prescribed was not the intended one. Errors can occur through lack of proper assessment of the patient's background including medication history, adherence, illnesses, and/or barriers to taking medication.

DISPENSING

Poor exchange of patient information across shifts ("hand-off" communication) can lead to errors.[76] In a hospital setting, errors can be made due to miscommunication among team members regarding what medications are needed and doses needed. In a community pharmacy setting, there can be assumptions made about the medications being checked by someone else due to poor communication among staff members. An example of this is that a prescriber assumes that a pharmacist has checked for drug interactions and the pharmacist did not do so.

ADMINISTRATION

Errors can occur due to poor medication reconciliation between multiple healthcare providers. Medication reconciliation is a process where each patient's list of medications is cross-checked by a healthcare provider during each interaction or transition. For example, a patient being admitted to a hospital is asked to list all their current medications and then upon discharge the list is reconciled and decisions made about what medications to continue, new medications added, or other changes made. A complete list of medications is communicated to the next provider of service when they refer or transfer a patient to another setting. Medication reconciliation was added by the Joint Commission as a National Patient Safety Goal in 2006 and remains a goal as of 2015.[76,80]

Medication administration errors can occur when the pharmacist does not verify the patient's name and birthdate upon pick-up of medications. If the communication is poor between the patient and pharmacist and no counseling is performed during prescription pick-up, errors can occur during medication consumption by the patient at home.

INTERVENTIONS

Situation-Background-Assessment-Recommendation (SBAR) technique has long been used in the aviation industry and in recent years gained attention by healthcare organizations. SBAR provides a framework for communication between healthcare team members.[15] An example of way one could use SBAR in a community pharmacy setting would be: a pharmacist notices that the patient had recently refilled a prescription for a medication with similar mechanisms with the current prescription.

The pharmacist may call the prescriber and say:

S—Situation: "I am calling about Mr. Smith's prescription for fluoxetine."

B—Background: "The patient is already on a similar drug, paroxetine and refilled it two weeks ago."

A—Assessment: "If we give this medication then the patient may take both and have an interaction or excessive side effects."

R—Recommendation: "I suggest eliminating one of the medications"

In a community pharmacy setting, some ways to reduce dispensing errors are reviewing a patient's medication(s) during pick-up, creating distraction-free and interruption-free zones whenever possible, verifying each patient's name and birthdate (or another identifier) at pick up, and thorough patient counseling. The performance of show and tell counseling includes verifying the patient's identity (e.g., by viewing a driver's license), comparing the filled prescription to the original order, showing the medication to the patient, reviewing the label information, and counseling on key points. This technique detected 89% of dispensing errors.[81]

SYSTEM/ORGANIZATIONAL PERSPECTIVES

Errors that can occur from the system/organizational perspective are multi-faceted and quite complex. Many organizations have systems in place which may have worked decades ago but in today's environment are not feasible. The healthcare environment has become more complex and the regulations and policy implications, which we will discuss in the later part of the chapter, have increasingly become more prominent. For example, the nuclear power plant incident at Pennsylvania's Three Mile Island in 1979 was caused by a litany of factors, including some that were deliberately done by the maintenance workers. The design of the plant was actually quite good, but not everything can be designed out. No matter how well (or poorly) designed a system is, latent errors exist as emergent properties that can become observable in the right circumstances.[82]

We will discuss two main kinds of system failures: design failures and organizational/environmental failures. Design failures focus on process, task design, and environmental design. Organizational/environmental failures focus on psychological precursors, inadequate team building and training. Many obstacles exist such as system complexities and lack of ownership or accountability. Systems that are too complex may be open to failures because individuals do not find such complex systems intuitive or processes easy to remember. The lack of ownership can lead to system failures because individuals do not feel a sense of responsibility for a system they may not have had any input in developing. Individuals may also feel that they are not accountable for failures if the system was faulty to begin with and open to such failures. There is also a tolerance of faulty practices. For example, a new staff member may begin work in your pharmacy and ask "why do we take down the order in this particular area of the pharmacy but then need to walk across the pharmacy to input the order?" A person who has been working at the pharmacy a longer time may have adjusted well to this faulty practice and be surprised by the concern raised by the new staff member. We also may become less attune to potential error-causing situations due to the infrequent occurrence of events that lead to errors. There may be new technology in systems put into place and we may think that an error just could not occur and become too comfortable. Fear of punishment is also a growing concern from an organizational perspective. Many have adopted a blame-free and just culture environment. Everyone can learn from errors when the staff is comfortable analyzing and reporting errors.[83]

As illustrated in the model in Figure 20-1, organizational culture and climate sound quite similar, but they differ in that culture describes the often-embedded and unnoticed aspects of how employees are supposed to see the world and interpret it. Climate, by contrast, describes the general perceptions of the work environment by the workers with respect to their behavior. Climate can tap into culture, but it need not do so completely.[84] Many studies suggest that these two factors can impact employees' safety behaviors, particularly with respect to behaviors that might put themselves at risk, including one directly relevant to medication error.[85-87] Almost every organization must work within constraints outlined by the regulatory entities that govern them, and pharmacy is no exception. Professionally, pharmacists must behave according to guidance from a number of these entities, and on a smaller scale, the activities of a particular store in a chain pharmacy are determined in part by the decisions of the administration of the chain. This can impact perceptions of autonomy and self-determination, the lack of which many pharmacists consider to be a source of dissatisfaction with pharmacy practice.[88] In late 2014, the Joint Commission released its new chapter within its CAHP (Comprehensive Accreditation Manual for Hospitals) entitled, "Patient Safety Systems." Within this new chapter are a few key elements that would facilitate a culture of improving patient safety from leadership to those working on the floors. The new chapter includes additional resources for leaders and staff of hospitals to implement their safety goals. One key aspect is what is called the trust-report-improve cycle. The idea is that trust promotes reporting, which leads to improvement, which in turn fosters trust. This is clearly important with respect to medication safety as discussed within this chapter. One of the Joint Commission leadership standards already require leaders to have a code of conduct that all are required to abide by. This new patient safety system takes it a bit further by illustrating key elements of the code (i.e., accountability, identifying disruptive behavior, empowerment of staff and other leaders).[89]

PRESCRIBING

Errors that can occur during prescribing from a system/organizational perspective are multi-faceted. Errors can occur if a prescriber does not have access to the most current information, if the chart is not unavailable, not updated, or incomplete. A prescriber may feel rushed due to the nature of clinical practice and this type of environment does not allow for proper assessments. Allergies not properly incorporated into the chart can lead to errors as this information would be missing during drug selection. Awareness of national guidelines for prescribing of medications is crucial. Many prescribers may not be aware and prescribe a medication that is not the preferred therapy for a particular illness. Similarly, a prescriber may choose a drug that is on the hospital formulary or based on the patient's insurance coverage and it may not be the drug of choice.

DISPENSING

Errors can occur during dispensing at the system/organizational level depending on the equipment and products purchased and system of dispensing (e.g., when hospital floors use multiple-dose vials as floor stock). Errors may also occur when dispensing is based on computer-generated labels vs. original prescriptions. Organizations may also be vulnerable for dispensing errors for similar reasons as mentioned for prescribing errors. Busy hospital units or busy community pharmacies can create an environment prone to errors. Many community pharmacies rely on double checks of the pharmacist after a pharmacy technician has filled the prescription order. Safeguards may exist in some settings to avoid dispensing errors such as bar-coding and automated dispensing systems.

Bar code-based inspection systems have been studied in inpatient pharmacies to determine the effects on dispensing accuracy. Poon and colleagues evaluated pharmacy dispensing errors before and after implementation of a bar code verification system. Dispensing error rates before implementation were 0.25%–0.71% for four filling processes assessed, and 0.018%–0.026% after. A key recommendation of the study was to require bar code scanning of every dose dispensed, not just a single representative dose used to fill an order.[90]

Flynn and Barker conducted an observational study to assess the effect of an automated dispensing system (ADS) on dispensing error rates for all errors, and for target errors (those the ADS was designed to prevent) in one independent and one chain community pharmacies. The ADS had robotic controls for the top 200 most commonly dispensed tablets and capsules, as well as a bar code-based control system for all other medications dispensed. At the independent pharmacy, the authors noted a significant decrease ($p<0.10$) in percent dispensing error rate from 2.9% before ADS (99 errors on 3,427 prescriptions) to 2.1% *after* ADS (68 errors on 3,241 prescriptions). At the chain pharmacy, there was no significant difference between the error rate before and after ADS; 1.9% *before* ADS (64 errors on 3,424 prescriptions) and 2.4% *after* ADS (74 errors on 3,028 prescriptions). Target error rates decreased significantly at both pharmacies ($p = .002$ and $p = .07$, respectively). The most frequent source of errors that occurred after the intervention involved deliberate overriding of system controls by pharmacy staff. Most errors originated in the computer order entry process, which the ADS could not control.[91]

Teagarden and colleagues conducted an internal observational study of a high-volume, highly-automated mail order pharmacy operation.[92] Using the same definitions and methods as the national accuracy study by Flynn and colleagues,[14] the authors found 16 errors on 21,252 prescriptions for a 0.075% error rate. The errors found were believed to have originated during the initial tasks performed by the staff, such as order entry. No errors were associated with the automated parts of the prescription filling system.[92]

ADMINISTRATION

Medication administration errors that may occur from the system/organizational perspective will be briefly examined. Storing similar-looking medications next to each other may lead to errors. In a pharmacy, medications of different patients placed simultaneously on the counter may lead to errors if not separated from each other (e.g., with bins). In hospitals or nursing homes, errors may occur when discontinued medications are not removed from patient's medication boxes. Errors can occur due manufacturer and instrumentation problems such as near identical packaging (i.e., similar looking packaging for each manufacturer without highlighting the medication name). Errors can also occur due to inaccurate entry of rates and concentrations into infusion pumps and Patient Controlled Analgesia pumps (PCAs).

INTERVENTIONS/SOLUTIONS

There are several objectives in developing systems designed for safe medication practices. These objectives include making errors difficult to occur, creating redundancy (double-checks) in the system, and creating systems with automatically correct (buffers) errors. For example, Computerized Prescriber Order Entry (CPOE) systems have been gaining increasing use in hospital settings. CPOE is a valuable resource in providing patient medication history and other pertinent data. CPOE also provides clinical information such as drug interactions, adverse drug reactions, guidelines, and formulary/generic drug information. CPOE can reduce dispensing errors that occur from prescriber poor handwriting. CPOE can also reduce errors by taking into account the patient information and alerting the prescriber to potential errors. For example, if a prescriber ordered a medication dose based on the patient's weight and ordered an excessive dose, the system would prompt the prescriber to check the dosing. Some other key areas for systems/organizations to reduce medication errors are to create systems where process steps are simplified, standardization and simplification of communication, and creation of redundancies (such as double checks).[82]

In keeping with the framework displayed in Figure 20-1, interventions can be targeted at all three levels of analysis, but they will be most successful when they are supported by changes in the non-targeted levels simultaneously. At the most proximal level, error training has been used in other organizations to great effect.[93,94] The main idea of error training is to expose people to common errors in their tasks and allow for practice in handling those errors under controlled conditions. Frese and colleagues have reported not only better performance but deeper learning and development of expertise compared to controls.

A second intervention approach, this one at the interactive level, is stress inoculation, which is similar to error training in that it allows staff to practice responses in controlled conditions.[60] However, the intent of stress inoculation is to prepare the staff to cope with work-related stressors of all kinds, not just errors. Research in other domains has supported this approach as useful and beneficial.[95] At the organizational level, a stress audit can be useful to pinpoint areas of the work environment that may be contributed to perceived stress by employees. The stress audit can take a number of forms, but should include at minimum an assessment of the stress capacity of the employees (including stress tolerance and coping abilities), a detailed assessment of the work environment, and an historical survey of possible stress-related outcomes (errors, work injuries, absences, turnover, etc.).

Finally, culture and climate change can be instituted to support new approaches to error management.[96-98] Historically, reporting error events to administration has been a self-defeating exercise, leading to a number of reasons why front-line staff don't want to do it and why it often isn't feasible to expect them to do it.[99,100] Sidney Dekker argues that much of the just culture movement in health care has not been followed by real and systemic change at the organizational level, which contributes to a mistrust and suspicion among workers that self-reporting is actually a psychologically-safe behavior.[21]

One concrete idea that can be installed to facilitate these changes is error management meetings. The purpose of the meetings is to encourage organizational learning and reduce the stigma associated with errors; by doing this, the organization can develop expertise as a unit and should be better able to detect and intercept harmful errors before they reach the consumer.[101] However, use of these meetings should be relatively frequent (i.e., once a week), include actual errors and "near-errors" (captured before they exited the facility), and accompanied by clear changes in management priorities so as to emphasize their importance. Otherwise, they run the risk of being seen merely as superficial quality control devices. For example, in a hospital pharmacy setting it is important to consistently meet to discuss and evaluate sources of errors; develop interventions to reduce errors; assess impact of interventions on errors; and measure and track medication errors.

DETECTING AND REPORTING MEDICATION ERRORS

Detecting and reporting medication errors can be accomplished by many different methods. This section of the chapter will focus on the most common error detection mechanisms.

REPORTING MECHANISMS

ANONYMOUS SELF-REPORTS

Methods such as questionnaires can be used to provide the person who made or witnessed the error to report it but not be associated with it. Some advantages of this method are the low cost and avoiding fear of disciplinary action. A disadvantage is the person witnessing the error can report it only if he or she is aware that an error was made. In addition, anonymous reports do not allow for follow-up investigation and may end up contributing to a "file drawer" problem where many reports end up as just data points and nothing can be learned from them.

INCIDENT REPORTS

Incident reports are the most commonly used method for documenting medication errors. An incident report is the official written legal report of a medication error as documented by hospital staff. When staff detects an error, a standard form required by the hospital is completed to report the incident. Incident reports may or may not be anonymous. Voluntary reporting of medication errors in a culture of safety without fear of disciplinary action is promoted by The Joint Commission (TJC), Food & Drug Administration (FDA), United States Pharmacopeia (USP), and the Institute for Safe Medication Practices (ISMP). Medication use system processes that may have led to the error are analyzed in an attempt to prevent similar errors.[102]

The primary limitation of the incident report method is the under-detection of errors. The number of incident reports filed is not an accurate representation of the actual frequency of errors, and should not be used in research to evaluate the effects of interventions on errors. Flynn and colleagues compared observation methods to incident reports, and found one error detected by incident reports in the examination of 2,557 doses in a total of 36 hospitals and skilled-nursing facilities. Observation detected 456 errors among these doses.[103] Comparable results have been reported in other studies.[104-106] Cullen and colleagues studied the frequency of reporting adverse drug events (ADEs) and found under-reporting of ADEs as well.[107]

Several reasons may explain why a small percentage of medication errors are reported. For example, in a hospital setting, a nurse cannot report an error unless they are aware that an error has occurred. There is heavy reliance upon the nurse's motivation to report the error. Evidence suggests that the nurse is not likely to report the error if a physician advises against reporting the error, if the nurse believes that the drug involved will not lead to patient harm, or if the error involved is an omission or wrong time error.[108] An ethnomethodological study by Baker found some additional reasons that nurses do not report some errors, based on their own definition of what is and is not an error.[109] A recent survey of 1,105 staff nurses at 25 hospitals found three factors related to the frequency of error reporting: administrative response to reports, personal fears, and unit quality management.[110]

Incident reports have been used as a source of data in studies of clinical significance and possible causes of medication errors. Descriptions of the use of incident reports are available in a number of settings including anesthesia,[111-112] pediatrics,[113-115] tertiary care hospitals,[116] and community pharmacies.[117,118] An analysis of mortalities associated with medication errors from 1993–1998 in the FDA's Adverse Event Reporting System found that improper doses represented 41% of the fatal errors.[119]

CHART REVIEW

Chart review has been used to detect medication errors and adverse drug events. The chart review is focused on areas that are related to medication use such as medication orders, laboratory test results, physician progress notes, nurse notes, and the medication administration record (MAR). Trained nurses or pharmacists review information looking for clues that an error may have occurred. Clues include sudden acute changes in a patient's condition, clarification of an order, and lab results that exceed normal values to a degree that it was likely that an error occurred (e.g., blood glucose > 400 could indicate an omitted insulin dose).[120] Orders for red flag or trigger drugs such as naloxone and flumazenil may indicate that a medication error has occurred.[121] Chart review detected 24 medication administration errors compared to 456 detected using direct observation of the same 2,557 doses in one study.[103] Chart review is best used when patient harm resulting from medication errors is the focus of the research. Grasso and colleagues found that retrospective chart review identified 2,194 errors over 1,448 patient-days, compared to nine errors that were self-reported in a state psychiatric hospital.[122]

OBSERVATION

The observation technique was developed for the detection of medication administration errors by Barker and McConnell.[123] A nurse or pharmacist trained in the observation technique accompanies the person administering medications and witnesses the preparation and administration of each dose. The observer writes down exactly what the subject does, including all details of the medication and noting consumption of the medication by the patient.[33] The observer's notes are then compared to the original prescriber orders to identify discrepancies. An error is counted if there are any differences between what was ordered and what was administered. The accuracy rate is calculated as the percent doses administered correctly.[124]

The observation method overcomes many of the limitations of the incident report method because it does not require the nurse to be aware of the error, be willing to report it, and memory of the error. As noted earlier, observation detects many more errors and types per unit time than other methods—it can detect 24 times more errors than chart review, and 456 times more than incident reports.[103] The potential disadvantages of the observation method include:

- Fatigue: Observation is a physically and mentally demanding activity if performed for more than a few hours each day;
- Staff: A trained nurse or pharmacist is required, and may be difficult to arrange during staff shortages;
- Influence of observer: the effects of close observation upon the subjects can be minimized by striving to remain unobtrusive and nonjudgmental; and
- Observer inference: Careful training of observers and proper category definitions can minimize this problem.[123]

Dean and Barber confirmed that if the observer is unobtrusive and nonjudgmental, the subject will resume normal work patterns within a brief period.[125]

How accurately do pharmacists fill prescriptions? Methods for answering this question include having a pharmacist double-check the filled orders,[14] self-report by pharmacists,[126] and analyzing patient reports of errors on prescriptions. Observation has also been used to identify system problems and technology workarounds that may contribute to medication errors.[127]

COMPUTERIZED ERROR MONITORING

Computerized error monitoring detects medication errors and ADEs by screening for trigger drug orders, and evaluating lab test results for outliers that may have resulted from an error. Hospital personnel are alerted that follow-up is needed to confirm the error and treat the patient if necessary.[128,129] Jha and colleagues compared computerized monitoring of ADEs to chart review and voluntary reporting. Chart review identified the most ADEs (398), followed by computerized monitoring (275), and voluntary reporting (n=?) for a total of 21,964 patient-days.[130] Chart review and computerized monitoring identified 67 of the same ADEs, while two ADEs were detected by both voluntary reporting and computerized monitoring.[116] Retrospective computerized analysis of outpatient medication records for ADEs found a rate of 5.5 per 100 patients.[131]

SYSTEMS APPROACH TO ERROR DETECTION AND REDUCTION

Root Cause Analysis (RCA) can be used to identify critical underlying reasons for the occurrence of the adverse event or near miss. The major steps of an RCA are convening a team, documenting and researching the incident, and identifying its possible root causes. The RCA is an analytical approach used in organizations to find out what happened, why it happened, and what will prevent it from happening again. Key learning can occur from a RCA and a system/organization can use the findings to improve their processes. The RCA should include all the key staff that is associated with the incident. The RCA also provides managers an opportunity to implement more reliable and cost-effective processes. In order for an RCA to be effective, an organization needs to be open to realizing that there may be system flaws discovered by performing this analysis.[132]

The purpose of failure mode effects analysis (FMEA) is to discover potential risks in a product or system by identifying ways in which a failure could occur. FMEA is a risk assessment method that identifies where a potential error could occur at each step in a process. In a FMEA, one may ask what happens if a prescriber mistakes one medication for another because of similar packaging; administers a dose by the wrong route; or gives a drug at the wrong time. Once these potential failures are identified potential stop gaps can be put into place to assist in preventing an error.[82]

Several promising interventions could lead to reductions in medication error through enhancements in detecting and learning from the errors that occur. It is important to clarify that a successful intervention need not reduce the overall number of self-reporting errors; in fact, it may increase them. Thus, the most appropriate outcome measure is the ratio of errors that reach the patient to overall prescriptions produced; this is a "batting average" of sorts and considers the probability of error in its correct form. Also, data regarding the number of recurrences of the same error over time is also useful to chart the learning ability of the organization.

PUBLIC POLICY IMPLICATIONS

Data about patient safety indicators and medical errors has been publically available due in part to Centers for Medicare and Medicaid Services (CMS) regulations. The move to publically report data is a move towards transparency in hospital outcomes. In August of 2008, CMS began displaying hospital mortality rates from certain disease groups and procedures. Many hospitals will now also receive a reduced payment from CMS for what is seen as hospital-acquired conditions including preventable injuries (i.e., injuries from falls/fractures, hospital acquired infections). Could publically reporting medication errors and adverse events be next?[133]

Continuous Quality Improvement Programs (CQI) is a system of standards and procedures to identify and evaluate quality-related events (QRE)—(247 CMR 15.00). An example of a QRE is an incorrect dispensing of a prescribed medication that is received by a patient. The CQI requirements were to be implemented for each pharmacy in the State of Massachusetts by December 2005. The implementation required each pharmacy to identify individual(s) to monitor CQI program compliance, identify and document QREs, minimize impact of QREs on patients, analyze QRE data to determine causes and identify interventions to prevent QREs, and an annual CQI education for pharmacy staff.[134]

SUMMARY

Why is it important for pharmacists to understand the importance and implications of psychosocial aspects of medication errors? Could we have an error-free environment? Errors can occur at any time and to anyone. If we can understand why they occur, when they can occur, as well as how to detect and report an error, we can learn how these errors could potentially be prevented. In a fast-paced community pharmacy or hospital unit we can all become familiar with processes and make critical judgments that can affect patients. The judgments are based on the best available resources and information. One of the reasons why we all need to understand the importance of this chapter is that each of us is vulnerable to an error. We are all going to be in a situation where we rely on others to work together to provide the safest care possible in any number of the care settings mentioned. Medication errors as discussed in this chapter are a vast topic that has received much attention over recent years. Hopefully, this chapter will guide the reader to learn more about individual, interpersonal and organizational perspectives of medication errors that occur throughout the drug delivery system and discover innovative ways to reduce medication errors.

REFERENCES

1. Pope, A. (1711). *An essay on criticism, Part II.* Accessed February 2015, http://www.ourcivilisation.com/smartboard/shop/popea/critic.htm

2. Davies, T. (2006). Deaths of 3 babies in Indiana spotlight medication mix-ups. (2006). [cited 2007 May 23]; web site]. *Boston.com.* Available from: http://www.boston.com/news/nation/articles/2006/09/23/ deaths_of_3_babies_in_indiana_spotlight_medication_mix_ups/

3. Aspden, P., Wolcott, J., Bootman, J.L., & Cronenwett, L.R. (Eds.). (2007). *Preventing medication errors.* Washington, D.C.: National Academies Press.

4. National Coordinating Council for Medication Error Reporting and Prevention (NCCMERP). © 1998–2008. Accessed August 2008, www.nccmerp.org.

5. Kohn, L.T., Corrigan, J.M., & Donaldson, M.S. (Eds.). (2000). To err is human: Building a safer health system. Washington, DC: National Academies Press.

6. Leape, L.L., Brennon, T.A., & Laird, N., et al. (1991). The nature of adverse events in hospitalized patients. Results of the Harvard Medical Practice Study II. *N Engl J Med* 324:370–76.

7. Agency for Healthcare Research and Quality. (2000). *Medical errors: the scope of the problem.* Available at: http:www.ahrq.gov/qual/errback/htm. Accessed October 15, 2005.

8. Bond, C.A., Raehl, C.L., & Franke, T. (2002). Clinical pharmacy services, hospital pharmacy staffing, and medication errors in United States hospitals. *Pharmacotherapy* Feb;22(2):134–47.

9. Quality Interagency Coordination Task Force. (February 2000). *Report of the Quality Interagency Coordination Task Force* (QuIC) to the President. Available at http://www.quic.gov/report/errors6.pdf. Accessed October 15, 2005.

10. Barker, K.N., Flynn, E.A., Pepper, G.A., Bates, D.W., & Mikeal, R.L. (2002). Medication errors observed in 36 healthcare facilities. *Archives of Internal Medicine* 162(16):1897–1903.

11. Flynn, E.A. & Barker, K.N. (2006). Medication error research. In Cohen, M.R. (Ed.), *Medication errors* 2nd ed. Washington, DC: American Pharmaceutical Association.

12. Seibert, H.H., Maddox, R.R., Flynn, E.A., & Williams, C.K. (2014). Effect of bar code technology with electronic medication administration record on medication accuracy rates. *Am J Health-Syst Pharm* 71:209–18.

13. Paoletti, R.D., Suess, T.M., Lesko, M.G., et al. (2007). *Am J Health-Syst Pharm* 64:536–43.

14. Flynn, E.A., Barker, K.N., & Carnahan, B.J. (2003). National observational study of prescription dispensing accuracy and safety in 50 pharmacies. *J Am Pharm Assoc* 43(2):191–200.

15. Dekker, S. (2013). *Second victim: Error, guilt, trauma, and resilience.* Boca Raton, FL: CRC Press.

16. Scott, S.D., Hirschinger, L.E., Cox, K.R., McCoig, M., Brandt, J., & Hall, L.W. (2009). The natural history of recovery for the healthcare provider "second victim" after adverse patient events. *Quality and Safety in Health Care*, 18, 325–330.

17. Acute Care ISMP Medication Safety Alert, Eric Cropp weighs in on the error that sent him to prison. December 3, 2009. http://ismp.org/Newsletters/acutecare/ articles/20091203.asp, accessed 12/20/14.

18. Nurse charged with felony in fatal medical error. Medical Ethics Advisor, February 2, 2007; http://asq.org/qualitynews/qnt/execute/displaySetup?newsID=1056 accessed 12/20/14.

19. Manfuso, J. The second victims. *The Dome.* http://www.hopkinsmedicine.org/news/ publications/dome/files/bin/c/c/A20EA21617EAAF4FAA40C310CAF37F1A.pdf. Accessed February 17, 2015.

20. Acute Care ISMP Medication Safety Alert. Too many abandon the "second victims" of medical errors. July 14, 2011. http://www.ismp.org/Newsletters/acutecare/ articles/20110714.asp. Accessed February 17, 2015.

21. Dekker, S. (2012). *Just culture: Balancing safety and accountability.* Burlington, VT: Ashgate.

22. Grasha, A.F., & O'Neill, M. (1996). Cognitive processes in medication errors. *US Pharmacist*, 21, 96–109.

23. Schell, K.L., Grasha, A.F., Reilley, S., & Tranum, D. (2001). *Improving accuracy in simulated product assembly tasks using workspace interventions to enhance the cognitive environment.* (Technical report 06-1201: 1–13). Cincinnati, OH: Cognitive Systems Performance Laboratory, University of Cincinnati.

24. Reason, J. (1990). *Human error.* New York: Cambridge.

25. Reason, J. (1997). *Managing the risks of organizational accidents.* Aldershot, England: Ashgate.

26. Moray, N. (1994). Error reduction as a systems problem. In M.S. Bogner (Ed.), *Human error in medicine*, pp. 67–92. Hillsdale, NJ: Erlbaum.

27. Nickerson, R.S. (1998). Confirmation bias: A ubiquitous phenomenon in many guises. *Review of General Psychology*, 2, 175–220.

28. Johnson, A., & Proctor, R.W. (2004). *Attention: Theory and practice.* Thousand Oaks, CA: Sage.

29. Johnston, W.A. & Dark, V.J. (1986). Selection attention. *Annual Review of Psychology*, 37, 43–75.

30. Schell, K.L., Kelley, K., & Hunsaker, C. (2005). Focused attention and error detection in a prescription checking task. *Poster presented to the Society for Industrial-Organizational Psychology annual conference*, Los Angeles, CA.

31. Norman, D.A. & Bobrow, D.B. (1975). On data-limited and resource-limited processes. *Cognitive Psychology*, 7, 44–64.

32. Franconeri, S.L., Hollingworth, A., & Simons, D.J. (2005). Do new objects capture attention? *Psychological Science*, 16, 275–281.

33. Franconeri, S.L. & Simons, D.J. (2003). Moving and looming stimuli capture attention. *Perception & Psychophysics*, 65, 999–1010.

34. Ozer, D.J, & Benet-Martinez, V. (2006). Personality and the prediction of consequential outcomes. *Annual Review of Psychology*, 57, 401–421.

35. Schell, K.L. & Grasha, A.F. (2000). State anxiety, performance accuracy and work pace in a simulated pharmacy dispensing task. *Perceptual and Motor Skills*, 90, 547–561.

36. Parasuraman, R., Warm, J.S., & Dember, W.N. (1987). Vigilance: Taxonomy and utility. In L.S. Mark, J.S. Warm, & R.L. Huston (Eds.), *Ergonomics and human factors* (pp. 11–31). New York: Springer-Verlag.

37. Ericsson, K.A., & Charness, N. (1994). Expert performance: Its structure and acquisition. *American Psychologist*, 49, 725–747.

38. Shiffrin, R.M. & Schneider, W. (1977). Controlled and automatic human information processing: II. Perceptual learning, automatic attending and a general theory. *Psychological Review*, 84, 127–190.

39. Logan, G.D. (1992). Attention and preattention in theories of automaticity. *American Journal of Psychology*, 105, 317–339.

40. Anderson, J.R. (1983). *The architecture of cognition.* Hillsdale, NJ: Lawrence Erlbaum.

41. Anderson, J.R. (1993). *Rules of the mind.* Hillsdale, NJ: Lawrence Erlbaum.

42. Shallice, T. (1988). *From neuropsychology to mental structure.* Cambridge: Cambridge University Press.

43. Institute for Safe Medication Practices. (February 2015). *List of confused drug names...* http://www.ismp.org/Tools/confuseddrugnames.pdf

44. National Patient Safety Goals Official "Do Not Use" List. The Joint Commission. 2015 (Accessed September 4, 2015, http://www.jointcommission.org/standards_information/npsgs.aspx).

45. Guernsey, B.G., Ingrim, N.B., Hokanson, J.A., Doutre, W.H., Bryant, S.G., Blair, C.W., et al. (1983). Pharmacists' dispensing accuracy in a high-volume outpatient pharmacy service: focus on risk management. *Drug Intelligence & Clinical Pharmacy* 17(10):742–6.

46. Kistner, U.A., Keith, M.R., Sergeant, K.A., & Hokanson, J.A. (1994). Accuracy of dispensing in a high-volume, hospital-based outpatient pharmacy. *American Journal of Hospital Pharmacy* 51(Nov 15):2793–2797.

47. Buchanan, T.L., Barker, K.N., Gibson, J.T., Jiang, B.C., & Pearson, R.E. (1991). Illumination and errors in dispensing. *American Journal of Hospital Pharmacy* 48(10):2137–45.

48. Allan, E.L., Barker, K.N., Malloy, M.J., & Heller, W.M. (1995). Dispensing errors and counseling in community practice. *American Pharmacy* NS35(Dec):25–33.

49. Ashcroft, D.M., Quinlan, P., & Blenkinsopp, A.(2005). Prospective study of the incidence, nature and causes of dispensing errors in community pharmacies. *Pharmacoepidemiology & Drug Safety* 14(5):327–332.

50. Woller, T.W., Stuart, J., Vrabel, R., & Senst, B. (1991). Checking of unit dose cassettes by pharmacy technicians at three Minnesota hospitals: pilot project. *American Journal of Hospital Pharmacy* 48(Sep):1952–1956.

51. Becker, M.D., Johnson, M.H., & Longe, R.L. (1978). Errors remaining in unit-dose carts after checking by pharmacists versus pharmacy technicians. *American Journal of Hospital Pharmacy* 35(Apr):432–434.

52. Mayo, C.E., Kitchens, R.G., Reese, L., Spruill, W.J., Taylor, A.T., et al. (1975). Distribution accuracy of a decentralized unit-dose system. *American Journal of Hospital Pharmacy* 32(Nov):1124–1126.

53. Taylor, J. & Gaucher, M. (1986). Medication selection errors made by pharmacy technicians in filling unit dose orders. *Canadian Journal of Hospital Pharmacy* 39(Feb):9–12.

54. Hassall, T.H. & Daniels, C.E. (1983). Evaluation of three types of control chart methods in unit dose error monitoring. *American Journal of Hospital Pharmacy* 40(Jun):970–975.

55. Hoffmann, R.P., Bartt, K.H., Berlin, L., & Frank, B.M. (1984). Multidisciplinary quality assessment of a unit dose drug distribution system. *Hospital Pharmacy* 19(Mar):167–169, 173–174.

56. Cina, J.L., Gandhi, T.K., Churchill, W., Fanikos, J., McCrea, M., Mitton, P., et al. (2006). How many hospital pharmacy medication dispensing errors go undetected? *Joint Commission Journal on Quality & Patient Safety* 32(2):73–80.

57. Chi, J. (1994). Tech-check-tech, as sanctioned practice, gaining in states. *Hosp Pharm Rep* 8:14,17.

58. Ness, J.E., Sullivan, S.D., & Stergachis, A. (1994). Accuracy of technicians and pharmacists in identifying dispensing errors. *American Journal of Hospital Pharmacy* 51(Feb 1):354–357.

59. Lazarus, R.S. & Folkman, S. (1984). *Stress, appraisal and coping.* New York: Springer.

60. Quick, J.C., Quick, J.D., Nelson, D.L., & Hurrell, J.J., Jr. (1997). Preventive stress management in organizations. Washington, DC: American Psychological Association.

61. Wolfgang, A.P. (1987). Is pharmacist turnover a function of job stress? *American Pharmacy*, NS27, 33–37.

62. Lapane, K.L. & Hughes, C.M. (2004). Baseline job satisfaction and stress among pharmacists and pharmacy technicians participating in the Fleetwood Phase III study. *The Consultant Pharmacist*, 19, 1029–1037.

63. Lapane, K.L. & Hughes, C.M. (2006). Job satisfaction and stress among pharmacists in the long-term care sector. *The Consultant Pharmacist*, 21, 287–292.

64. Judge, T.A., Ilies, R., & Scott, B.A. (2006). Work-family conflict and emotions: Effects at work and at home. *Personnel Psychology*, 59, 779–814.

65. Somech, A. & Drach-Zahavy, A. (2007). Strategies for coping with work-family conflict: The distinctive relationships of gender role ideology. *Journal of Occupational Health Psychology*, 12, 1–19.

66. Davies, D.R. & Parasuraman, R. (1982). *The psychology of vigilance.* London: Academic Press.

67. Wickens, C.D. & Hollands, J.G. (2000). Engineering psychology and human performance (3rd Ed). Upper Saddle River, NJ: Prentice Hall.

68. Bilsing-Palacio, L., & Schell, K.L. (2003). Signal probability effects on error detection performance in a quality control task. *Psychological Reports*, 93, 343–352.

69. Schell, K.L., Hunsaker, C., & Kelley, K. (2006). Extending effects of salience and payoffs on stimulus discrimination: An experimental simulation of prescription checking. *Perceptual & Motor Skills*, 103, 375–386.

70. Marken, R.S. (2003). Errors in skilled performance: A control model of prescribing. *Ergonomics*, 46, 1200–1214.

71. Prinzel, L.J. III, Freeman, F.G., & Prinzel, H.D. (2005). Individual differences in complacency and monitoring for automation failures. Individual Differences *Research*, 3, 27–49.

72. Young, P.T. (1967). Affective arousal: Some implications. *American Psychologist*, 22, 32–40.

73. Hart, S.G. & Staveland, L.E. (1988). Development of NASA-TLX (Task Load Index): Results of empirical and theoretical research. In P.A. Hancock & N. Meshkati (Eds.), *Human mental workload* (pp. 139–183). Amsterdam: North-Holland.

74. Svenson, O. & Maule, A.J. (Eds.). *Time pressure and stress in human judgment and decision making.* New York: Plenum.

75. Taxis, K., & Barber, N. (2003). Ethnographic study of incidence and severity of intravenous drug errors. *British Medical Journal* 26(7391):684–687.

76. National Patient Safety Goals. The Joint Commission. 2008 (Accessed September 8, 2008 http://www.jointcommission.org/AccreditationPrograms/Hospitals/NPSG/).

77. Guglielmi, C.L., Stratton, M., Healy, G.B., Shapiro, D., Duffy, W.J., Dean, B.L., & Groah, L.K. (2014). The growing role of patient engagement: Relationship-based care in a changing health care system. *AORN Journal*, 99, 517–528.

78. Burns, K.K., Bellows, M., Eigenseher, C., & Gallivan, J. (2014). 'Practical' resources to support patient and family engagement in healthcare decisions: a scoping review. *BMC Health Services Research*, 14, 1–25.

79. Pelletier, L.R. & Stichler, J.F. (2014). Patient-centered care and engagement. *Journal of Nursing Administration*, 44, 473–480.

80. National Patient Safety Goals. The Joint Commission. 2015 (Accessed September 7, 2015 http://www.jointcommission.org/assets/1/6/2015_NPSG_HAP.pdf).

81. Kuyper, A.R. (1993). Patient counseling detects prescription errors. *Hospital Pharmacy* 28(Dec): 1180–1181, 1184–1189.

82. Leape, L. L. (2007). Systems analysis and redesign: The foundation of medical error prevention. In Cohen, M.R., *Medication errors,* 2nd Edition. American Pharmacists Association, 3–14.

83. Smetzer, J. L. (2007). Managing medication risks through a culture of safety. In Cohen, M.R., *Medication errors*, 2nd Edition. American Pharmacists Association, 613–614.

84. Schneider, B., Brief, A.P., & Guzzo, R.A. (1996). Creating a climate and culture for sustainable organizational change. *Organizational Dynamics*, 24, 7–19.

85. Parker, D., Lawrie, M., & Hudson, P. (2006). A framework for understanding the development of organisational safety culture. *Safety Science*, 44, 551–562.

86. Wiegmann, D.A., Zhang, H., von Thaden, T.L., Sharma, G., & Gibbons, A.M. (2004). Safety culture: An integrative review. *International Journal of Aviation Psychology*, 14, 117–134.

87. Hofmann, D.A., & Mark, B. (2006). An investigation of the relationship between safety climate and medication errors as well as other nurse and patient outcomes. *Personnel Psychology*, 59, 847–869.

88. Mott, D.A. (2000). Pharmacist job turnover, length of service, and reasons for leaving. *American Journal of Health-System Pharmacy*, 57, 975–984.

89. Patient safety systems chapter for the hospital program. Joint Commission. 2015. (http://www.jointcommission.org/assets/1/6/PSC_for_Web.pdf accessed September 8, 2015).

90. Poon, E.G., Cina, J.L., Churchill,W., Patel, N., Featherstone, E., Rothschild, J.M., et al. (2006). Medication dispensing errors and potential adverse drug events before and after implementing bar code technology in the pharmacy. *Annals of Internal Medicine* 145(6):426–434.

91. Flynn, E.A. & Barker, K.N. (2006). Effect of an automated dispensing system on errors in two pharmacies. *Journal of the American Pharmacists Association* 46(5):613015.

92. Teagarden, J.R., Naglem B,, Aubert, R.E., Wasdyke, C., Courtney, P., & Epstein, R.S. (2005). Dispensing error rate in a highly automated mail-service pharmacy practice. *Pharmacotherapy* 25(11):1629–1635.

93. Heimbeck, D., Frese, M., Sonnentag, S., & Keith, N. (2003). Integrating errors into the training process: The function of error management instructions and the role of goal orientation. *Personnel Psychology*, 56, 333–361.

94. Keith, N. & Frese, M. (2005). Self-regulation in error management training: Emotion control and metacognition as mediators of performance effects. *Journal of Applied Psychology*, 90, 677–691.

95. Southwick, S.M., Vythilingham, M., & Charney, D.S. (2005). The psychobiology of depression and resilience to stress: Implications for prevention and treatment. *Annual Review of Clinical Psychology*, 1, 255–291.

96. Kaissi, A. (2006). An organizational approach to understanding patient safety and medical errors. *The Healthcare Manager*, 25, 292–305.

97. Milligan, F.J. (2007). Establishing a culture for patient safety - the role of education. *Nurse Education Today* Feb; 27(2): 95–102

98. Vogus, T.J., & Sutcliffe, K.M. (2007). The Safety Organizing Scale: Development and validation of a behavioral measure of safety culture in hospital nursing units. *Medical Care*, 45, 46–54.

99. Kaldjian, L.C., Jones, E.W., Rosenthal, G.E., Tripp-Reimer, T., & Hillis, S.L. (2006). An empirically-derived taxonomy of factors affecting physicians' willingness to disclose medical errors. *Journal of General Internal Medicine* 21, 942–948.

100. Karsh, B-T., Escoto, K.H., Beasley, J.W., & Holden, R.J. (2006). Toward a theoretical approach to medical error reporting system research and design. *Applied Ergonomics* 37, 283–295.

101. Argyris, C. & Schon, D.A. (1996). *Organizational learning II: Theory, method and practice.* Reading, MA: Addison-Wesley.

102. Phillips, M.A. (2002). Voluntary reporting of medication errors. *American Journal of Health-System Pharmacy* 59(23):2326–2328.

103. Flynn, E.A., Barker, K.N., Pepper, G.A., Bates, D.W., & Mikeal, R.L. (2002). Comparison of methods for detecting medication errors in 36 hospitals and skilled-nursing facilities. *American Journal of Health-System Pharmacy* 59(5):436–446.

104. Barker, K.N., Kimbrough, W.W., & Heller, W.M. (1966). *A study of medication errors in a hospital.* Fayetville, AR: University of Arkansas.

105. Barker, K.N., Harris, J.A., Webster, D.B., Stringer, J.F., Miller, G.J., et al. (1984). Consultant evaluation of a hospital medication system: analysis of the existing system. *American Journal of Hospital Pharmacy* 41(Oct):2009–2016.

106. Borel, J.M. & Rascati, K.L. (1995). Effect of an automated, nursing unit-based drug-dispensing device on medication errors. *American Journal of Health-System Pharmacy* 52(17):1875–1879.

107. Cullen, D.J., Bates, D.W., Small, S.D., Cooper, J.B., Nemeskal, A.R., & Leape, L.L. (1995). The incident reporting system does not detect adverse drug events: a problem for quality improvement.[see comment]. *Joint Commission Journal on Quality Improvement* 21(10):541–8.

108. Barker, K.N. & McConnell, W.E. (1962). The problems of detecting medication errors in hospitals. *Am J Hosp Pharm* 19:360–69.

109. Baker, H.M. (1997). Rules outside the rules for administration of medication: A study in New South Wales, Australia. *Image—the Journal of Nursing Scholarship* 29(2):155–8.

110. Blegen, M.A., Vaughn, T., Pepper, G., Vojir, C., Stratton, K., Boyd, M., et al. (2004). Patient and staff safety: Voluntary reporting. *American Journal of Medical Quality* 19(2):67–74.

111. Chopra, V., Bovill, J.G., Spierdijk, J., & Koornneef, F. (1992). Reported significant observations during anaesthesia: A prospective analysis over an 18-month period. *British Journal of Anaesthesia* 68(1):13–7.

112. Currie, M., Mackay, P., Morgan, C., Runciman, W.B., Russell, W.J., Sellen, A., et al. (1993). The Australian Incident Monitoring Study. The "wrong drug" problem in anaesthesia: An analysis of 2000 incident reports. *Anaesthesia & Intensive Care* 21(5):596–601.

113. Wong, I.C., Ghaleb, M.A., Franklin, B.D., & Barber, N. (2004). Incidence and nature of dosing errors in paediatric medications—A systematic review. *Drug Safety* 27(9):661–670.

114. Ross, .LM., Wallace, J., & Paton, J.Y. (2000). Medication errors in a paediatric teaching hospital in the UK: Five years operational experience.[see comment]. *Archives of Disease in Childhood* 83(6):492–7.

115. Wilson, D.G., McArtney, R.G., Newcombe, R.G., McArtne,y R.J., Gracie, J., Kirk, C.R., et al. (1998). Medication errors in paediatric practice: Insights from a continuous quality improvement approach. *European Journal of Pediatrics* 157(9):769–774.

116. Winterstein, A.G., Johns, T.E., Rosenberg, E.I., Hatton, R.C., Kanjanarat, P., et al. (2004). Nature and causes of clinically significant medication errors in a tertiary care hospital. *American Journal of Health-System Pharmacy* 61(18):1908–1916.

117. Kennedy, A.G. & Littenberg, B. (2004). Medication error reporting by community pharmacists in Vermont. *Journal of the American Pharmaceutical Association* 44(4):434–438.

118. Quinlan, P,. Ashcroft, D .M., & Blenkinsopp, A. (2002). Medication errors: A baseline survey of dispensing errors reported in community pharmacy. *Int J Pharm Pract* 10(supplement):R68.

119. Phillips, J., Beam, S., Brinker, A., Holquist, C., Pame,r C., et al. (2001). Retrospective analysis of mortalities associated with medication errors. *American Journal of Health-System Pharmacy* 58(Oct 1):1835–1841.

120. Kausha,l R. (2002). Using chart review to screen for medication errors and adverse drug events. *American Journal of Health-System Pharmacy* 59(23):2323–5.

121. Dalton-Bunnow, M.F. & Halvachs, F.J. (1993). Computer-assisted use of tracer antidote drugs to increase detection of adverse drug reactions: retrospective and concurrent trial. *Hospital Pharmacy* 28(Aug):746–749, 752–755.

122. Grasso, B.C., Genest, R., Jordan, C.W., & Bates, D.W. (2003). Use of chart and record reviews to detect medication errors in a state psychiatric hospital. [see comment]. *Psychiatric Services* 54(5):677–81.

123. Barker, K.N. (1980). Data collection techniques: observation. *American Journal of Hospital Pharmacy* 37(Feb):1235–1243.

124. Barker, K.N., Flynn, E.A., & Pepper, G.A. (2002). Observation method of detecting medication errors. *American Journal of Health-System Pharmacy* 59(23):2314–2316.

125. Dean, B. & Barber, N. (2001). Validity and reliability of observational methods for studying medication administration errors. *American Journal of Health-System Pharmacy* 58(1):54–59.

126. Chua, S.S., Wong, I.C., Edmondson, H., Allen, C., Grantham, J., et al. (2003). A feasibility study for recording of dispensing errors and "near misses" in four UK primary care pharmacies. *Drug Safety* 26(11):803–813.

127. Patterson, E.S., Rogers, M.L., Chapman, R.J., & Render, M.L. (2006). Compliance with intended use of Bar Code Medication Administration in acute and long-term care: An observational study. *Human Factors* 48(1):15–22.

128. Classen, D.C., Pestotnik, S.L., Evans, R.S., & Burke, J.P. (1991). Computerized surveillance of adverse drug events in hospital patients. *JAMA* 266(Nov 27):2847–2851.

129. Bates, D.W. (2002). Using information technology to screen for adverse drug events. *American Journal of Health-System Pharmacy* 59(23):2317–9.

130. Jha, A.K., Kuperman, G.J., Teich, J.M., Leape, L., Shea, B., Rittenberg, E,. et al. (1998). Identifying adverse drug events: development of a computer-based monitor and comparison with chart review and stimulated voluntary report. *Journal of the American Medical Informatics Association* 5(3):305–14.

131. Honigman, B., Lee, J, Rothschild, J., Light, P., Pulling, R.M., Yu, T, et al. (2001). Using computerized data to identify adverse drug events in outpatients. *Journal of the American Medical Informatics Association* 8(3):254–66.

132. Burkhardt, M., Lee, C., Taylor, L., Williams, R., & Bagian, J. (2007). Root cause analysis of medication errors. In Cohen, M.R., Medication errors, 2nd Edition. *American Pharmacists Association*, 67–86.

133. FY 2008 Inpatient prospective payment system proposed rule improving the quality of hospital care. Centers for Medicare and Medicaid Services (Accessed September 8, 2008 http://www.cms.hhs.gov/apps/media/press/factsheet.asp? Counter=2119)

134. 247 CMR 15: Board of Registration in pharmacy: Continuous quality improvement program (Accessed September 8, 2008; http://www.mass.gov/Eeohhs2/docs/dph/regs/247cmr011.pdf)

CHAPTER 21

ETHICAL ISSUES AND THE PROVISION OF PHARMACEUTICAL CARE

Amy M. Haddad, PhD and Amy F. Wilson, PharmD

LEARNING OBJECTIVES:

1. Determine when a clinical situation involves ethics.
2. Apply a normative decision-making model to an ethical issue in pharmacy practice.
3. Distinguish the contributions to ethical deliberation among principles, virtues and care-based ethics.
4. Identify differences in moral obligations on individual, institutional and societal levels.
5. Justify a resolution to moral conflicts between duties or obligations.

KEY TERMS

Beneficence

Ethics

Fidelity

Justice

Moral intuition

Nonmaleficence

Respect for autonomy

Values

INTRODUCTION

As health care continues to grow and evolve, so too do the types and numbers of ethical problems that health care professionals, patients, and families encounter. There are many factors that contribute to the incidence and complexity of ethical issues in health care including marketplace and governmental regulations, changes in financing and places where care is delivered, health disparities, sophisticated technology, and the emphasis on "rescue" treatment in acute care, to name a few. Within the larger health care system, pharmacy practice continues to grow and evolve particularly regarding responsibilities within the pharmacist/patient relationship.

This chapter examines ethics in the provision of pharmaceutical care and reviews cases that represent the most common types of ethical issues in pharmacy practice in a variety of clinical settings—community pharmacy, hospital and outpatient care. The major concerns of ethics are addressed in light of common clinical experiences. The first case explores how to determine when a situation involves ethics; expectations of the moral conduct of pharmacists on an individual, institutional, and societal level; and the impact of values on ethical decisions. The second case focuses on the process of ethical decision making and provides a framework to resolve ethical issues with a five-step model. The final case explores the potential conflict between two moral obligations, that is, duties that benefit individual patients versus duties that benefit society as a whole.

ETHICS AND HEALTH CARE

Ethics is a branch of philosophy that examines the rightness of human behavior. Normative or applied ethics is that level of ethical analysis that asks "whether there are any general principles or norms describing the characteristics that make actions right or wrong."[1] A complete view of normative ethics encompasses not only principles or action guides to moral behavior but also virtue, which explores moral character and care-based reasoning that encompasses our obligations to care for others and to acknowledge our connectedness as human beings.

The application of ethics to the practical problems engendered by technological developments began in the United States in the late 1960s. As modern health professions began to differentiate from each other and define their respective scopes of practice, so too did specific standards of professional conduct. Codes of ethics for pharmacists in the United States date back to 1848 at the Philadelphia College of Pharmacy. The present version of the code is the Code of Ethics for Pharmacists that was approved by the American Pharmaceutical Association in 1995.[2] All professional codes affirm high ideals of a profession and commit members of the profession to honor them. Codes indicate in general terms the ethical considerations a professional should take into account in deciding on conduct. Although codes of ethics are helpful, they are not without their flaws. There can be conflicts between personal values and the values embedded in the code. When there are value conflicts, which code takes priority—the personal or professional? Also, codes are general not specific, leaving gaps between actual practice and what is included in the code. Codes of ethics are another source of guidance for ethical decisions and a public pronouncement of professional values.

ETHICS AND PHARMACY PRACTICE

Applied ethics, in this case pharmacy ethics, focuses on principles and norms for right action, virtue, and care-based reasoning for the pharmacy profession. Ethics provides insights into "right-making" characteristics of professional standards in pharmacy practice. The types of ethical issues encountered in the provision of pharmaceutical care in the contemporary health care system reflect the more patient-centered care the public has come to expect whenever they encounter a pharmacist. Additionally, new responsibilities such as counselling about health and wellness or activities that focus on public health broaden the scope of possible ethical issues that pharmacists may encounter. Pharmacists continue to deal with abiding ethical issues such as how to fairly allocate scarce and expensive resources, informed consent, conscientious refusal regarding dispensing certain drug products, and concerns about the competency of colleagues. New ethical questions arise as scientific advances move from the laboratory to the clinical setting. New drugs and delivery systems lead to questions such as whether to support "right-to-try" statutes allowing providers and patients to bypass the FDA and obtain untested drugs from manufacturers or how to balance respect for personal decisions about health care with potential negative consequences for the public as a whole.

The following case shows how pharmacists and pharmacy interns encounter situations in a community pharmacy setting that may not at first glance raise questions about ethics. However, there are certainly a number of evaluations in every patient interaction, many of which are evaluations of values an important component of ethical judgments. Consider the values and expectations of moral conduct of the individuals involved in the case.

CASE ONE—INFORMING A PATIENT ABOUT A POTENTIAL DRUG INTERACTION

Maddison is a second-year pharmacy student who works as an intern on the weekends at a national pharmacy chain store. She spends much of her time stocking shelves and working at the counter, but as she is learning more through her coursework, she is trying to become involved in the patient interactions that occur in the pharmacy. She frequently hears patients ask questions about drug interactions, and she listens in to learn as much as she can. She is currently taking her pharmacotherapeutics course, and is excited because she is learning about things she hears patients talking about at work.

She asks a lot of questions of the pharmacist related to drug interactions, because she is trying to learn how the pharmacist clinically judges a situation when an interaction occurs. Maddison has noticed that sometimes an immediate contact to the physician office is necessary, at other times a chat with the patient is needed, and sometimes there is nothing significant that actually needs to be addressed. Multiple pharmacists have relayed to Maddison that learning to discern how to address drug interactions takes experience and clinical judgment, which will come with time.

Today, Maddison is helping up front when a technician is checking out a patient. The patient is starting itraconazole therapy for toenail onychomycosis and has replied that he had no questions for the pharmacist, as he had taken this medication once in the past. As an afterthought he states, "Oh wait, I do have a question. I have heard that there are a lot of interactions with my Lipitor. Does this toenail drug cause any interaction?" The technician says there should be no concerns as she hands the bag to the patient. Maddison recalls recently learning about drug interactions with atorvastatin that can be serious.[3]

DETERMINING WHEN A SITUATION INVOLVES ETHICS

Although all of human behavior and interactions could be said to involve ethics, it is helpful in clinical practice to be able to sort through the facts of a situation to identify the significant ethical elements. Maddison is involved in a situation that starts with the patient's question, "Does this toenail drug cause any interaction?" and ends when she recalls what she knows about a possible drug interaction leaving the reader at a decision point. What should Maddison do next is a question that comes to mind, but does this question involve ethics? Three simple questions can serve as a guide as to whether a situation involves ethics.[4] Each question will be answered in reference to Case One. First, is there more than one morally plausible resolution? The question qualifies the type of resolution to be considered, i.e., that is it "morally plausible" meaning that the resolution must be judged good based on some basic value. When we make a judgment about a person's conduct, we are actually judging the act itself, the values attached to the action, and accountability for the action. One action that has already occurred in the case is the technician's response to the patient's question about a possible drug interaction between an existing prescription for Lipitor and a new one for itraconazole. It is hard to tell from the information in the case about the underlying values of the pharmacy technician regarding counseling patients. However, one could judge the response of the pharmacy technician by examining what technicians are accountable for in their interactions with patients. Are pharmacy technicians qualified to independently offer counseling on drug interactions especially those that are potentially serious? Perhaps the pharmacy technician has no idea about the potential seriousness of this drug interaction. If that is the case, then the morally appropriate response should have been for the technician to say that she didn't know and ask one of the pharmacists to counsel the patient. Certainly, one has to know when something is wrong in order to be accountable for an action. The key point is that what the technician needed to know was not the specific drug interactions in the case, but the limits or boundaries of her obligations to counsel patients and when to seek assistance or "hand-off" a particular question from a patient.

Since the pharmacy technician sent the patient on his way, Maddison is left to consider what is required of her. What steps should she take based on her recollection about potential serious drug interactions for this patient? She has several options. For example, Maddison could intervene and ask the patient to wait while she finds a pharmacist to handle the patient's question, she could talk to the patient directly about what she recalls about the potential drug interaction, she could let the patient leave and look up information on the two drugs and call the patient later, or she could do nothing. Of these options, at first glance it would appear that involving the pharmacist in some way before the patient leaves the pharmacy is a morally justifiable option if the aim is to provide reliable information and protect the patient from unnecessary harm. Each option contains underlying principles that would need to be explored to determine the best option. At a minimum, there could be more than one morally plausible resolution to the issue so the answer to the question is at least "maybe" which would warrant exploring the additional two questions.

The second question asks, is there no clear-cut resolution? In this case, there doesn't seem to be very many morally plausible options. Perhaps what is difficult in this case is not a moral issue, but a contextual one involving the hierarchy of a community pharmacy. Maddison knows that there is the risk of potential harm to the patient so she should do something to protect that patient from that harm. However, she is only a pharmacy student and arguably the lowest ranked staff member in the pharmacy at this time in her career. She has been advised by more experienced pharmacists that it will take time for her to learn how to handle drug interactions. Perhaps she is mistaken about the potential drug interaction. What Maddison is weighing is the possible embarrassment she might suffer if there is no serious drug interaction involved against protecting the patient. She also has to consider how this might reflect on the performance of the pharmacy technician who would be responsible for performing a task for which she is not prepared. All of these evaluations are likely occurring in mere moments as Maddison considers them while the patient is walking away. At this point, Maddison may think that she is the only one who knows about the potential drug interaction so she has, at a minimum, the obligation to share what she knows with a pharmacist. However, Maddison isn't the only one involved in this case. A pharmacist filled the prescription and should have made a judgment (although possibly an inappropriate one) about this interaction as part of the dispensing process. Given the fact that this is a documented interaction, the system should have flagged a concern to alert the pharmacist. Knowing about a possible harm to another person includes bearing the responsibility of preventing or protecting the other person from harm unless you can safely transfer the burden to someone who is more qualified. Thus, the answer to the second question appears to be "yes" as well.

The third question asks, is there a direct reference to the welfare or dignity of others? The pharmacy intern, Maddison, recalls that drug interactions could be serious between itraconazale and atorvastatin, so the patient's welfare could be at risk. Maddison may not be sure about the details of this particular drug interaction but the fact that she remembers that they can be serious is enough to answer the third question about ethics in the case with a "yes." The second, subtler harm is to the pharmacy technician and perhaps to the pharmacy as a whole. If Maddison stops the patient from leaving the pharmacy so as to ensure that he gets the correct drug counseling he needs, it might result in embarrassment for the technician in front of the patient and perhaps the rest of the pharmacy staff. Harm might also come to the reputation of the pharmacy if Maddison decides not to intervene and the patient was harmed because of inappropriate drug therapy counseling. Again, all of these possible consequences hinge on whether the pharmacist who filled the prescription verified the seriousness of the drug interaction for this particular patient. Therefore, because the answer was "yes," to more than one of the questions, Case One involves ethics.

MORAL CONDUCT ON AN INDIVIDUAL, ORGANIZATIONAL AND SOCIETAL LEVEL

Glaser proposes a conceptual model of ethics that is beneficence-based.[5] By beneficence-based, he is invoking a basic ethical principle that requires us to act for the good of others in all of our human interactions. He recognizes that we not only come into contact with the individuals closest to us, literally and figuratively, but also in larger groups that eventually comprise society. As one moves from the individual to the organizational level of ethics, the conflicts become more complicated as to the resolutions. The tools, principles and rules we use on these different levels change to accommodate the increasing complexity of the issues and number of individuals involved.

At the individual level, we are concerned with the well-being of individuals and their relationships.[5] Case One generally deals with ethics on the individual level in that in that it deals with "weighing and balancing the values/good/loyalties that stand in tension between two or more individuals."[5] However, individuals are also part of institutions, organizations, groups, etc. At an organizational level, there are commitments, responsibilities, values that are shared by the group whether it is a family or employees at a community pharmacy. The aim of benefitting others at this level of ethics requires us to recognize the individuals within the organization, such as the community pharmacy where Maddison works, and to work to achieve net good to the organization within and without. That means attending to the responsibilities that people have to each other within the organization like providing accurate drug therapy consultation and complying with rules and regulations external to the organization where it interacts with society at large. Community pharmacies that live up to the responsibilities that society requires of them have a great deal of impact on the health and well-being of the people they serve. Finally, beneficence on a societal level deals with the common good. The good of all differs from individual good and may at times conflict with it. In other words, in order to achieve the well-being of society as a whole, individuals have to sacrifice at least some of their own good for others, many of whom they will never know.

The balancing act of attending to all of the goods that a society must have to thrive is a complicated one and health care is but one of the many social goods that call for our attention and resources. The important points here are two-fold. First, as human beings we are called to accomplish more good than we are capable of within and between the individual, organizational, and societal levels of ethics. Therefore, our moral lives are comprised of almost constant choices as to where we put our efforts to achieve good. Most of the time people are unaware that they make choices that prioritize goods and where they direct their energy and attention. Second, many ethical issues clearly reside in a specific level of ethics, yet most of the work in contemporary health care ethics has focused on the individual level. Therefore, health professionals often attempt to use tools, guiding principles, or methods that work well on an individual level but are ill-equipped for the higher levels of organizational and societal levels of ethics. It is important therefore that we discern what level of ethics is of primary concern in a specific case before embarking on ethical analysis. Case One generally involves individual level ethical issues with its focus on specific benefits and harms for a small number of identified people. In other words, the question revolves around what it means to do good for a particular patient.

VALUES AND VALUE CONFLICTS

The final major concern of all ethical analysis, regardless of the level in which the issue or problem resides, is the identification of values. "Values are concepts we use to explain how and why various realities matter. Values are not to be confused with concrete goods. They are ideas, images, notions. Values attract us. We aspire after the good they articulate."[6] Simply put, values are internal motivators for our actions. Because basic values are instilled in us from childhood on, we may not be conscious of some of the values that we hold most dear until they are challenged. Strong emotions are tied to important values. Therefore, an emotional reaction in a situation, whether negative or positive, can be a sign that there are important values in conflict, which is often the genesis of an ethical problem. In addition to personal values, individuals can also hold professional values that are shared by other members of the profession. These professional values can have a profound effect on how a pharmacist views his or her obligations to patients, peers and society. Many core values in pharmacy are reflected in the Code of Ethics for Pharmacists and standards for professional responsibility such as the primacy of patient safety and benefit, respect for privacy and confidentiality, honesty, and fairness.[2] Regardless if a value has a personal or professional origin, it can have an impact on how an ethical situation is viewed and resolved. The following underlying values in the case help explain why the issue of accurate drug counseling is so important in ethical pharmacy practice. One reason providing drug counseling holds so much value to the pharmacy profession is that without it serious harm could result to patients. Maddison seems to understand how important drug counseling and clinical judgment are and the central role these tasks will play when she becomes a pharmacist. Her thoughts immediately turned to potential problems when the patient asked, "Does this toenail drug cause any interaction?" indicating that the patient wasn't counseled on the drug interaction or didn't comprehend what he had been told. She also understands that her role will involve preventing harm to patients and working with other members of the team to benefit patients. Additionally, there is a corollary value to obtain adequate information before making a judgment whether the information is from the patient, the prescriber or a pharmacy peer. Another value is that of respect for the knowledge that experience and education bring. Maddison may be uncertain about what she knows at this time in her educational program and doesn't want to step out of line within the hierarchy of the community pharmacy. She is an intern after all. But her sense of responsibility, her value system, is already developed enough for her to immediately stop and recall what she knows about the possible drug interaction because she was attuned to the type of knowledge that could be of benefit to the patient.

A MODEL TO RESOLVE ETHICAL PROBLEMS

Many ethical problems are full of tension, anxiety, and other emotions that make it difficult to see matters in an objective and clear manner. Given the emotional nature of ethical problems in health care and the general lack of time to reflect on what would be the best course of action in a busy practice setting, it is helpful to have a decision making model that prescribes steps to reach a morally justifiable decision. A five-step decision-making model is proposed but there are similar models in the literature to assist in this process.[7-9] The five steps provide the structure for a decision making process but also acknowledges that thinking about complicated issues like ethical problems don't always move in a linear fashion. Therefore, although the steps will be applied in the order listed to Case Two to illustrate the process and components of decision-making, it is likely in reality, people could work through ethical issues in a more random fashion. For example, one might jump to a familiar and safe decision then go back and collect additional information to see if the facts support the initial choice. Some individuals might decide to seek input from trusted colleagues about the issue in general and then seek a resolution. The order of the steps is not as important as the content of each step. The steps are listed below:[10]

- Respond to the sense or feeling that something is wrong.
- Gather clinical and contextual information.
- Identify the ethical problem.
- Seek a resolution.
- Work with others to determine a course of action.

The five-step model will be applied to Case Two to illustrate the process of decision making when a situation involves ethics.

CASE TWO—PRIORITIZING DECISIONS IN AN EMERGENCY SITUATION

Thomas is a pharmacist working in the central pharmacy of an academic medical center. Tonight has been especially busy, with a trauma arriving at the facility earlier in the evening. As is the usual on Saturday evenings, the pharmacy has a limited staff scheduled and things have been very hectic. It has been a struggle just to keep up with all the medication orders that are coming in.

Normally, nurses in the emergency department (ED) are required to enter medication orders into the system before pharmacy will dispense the medications. This evening, however, an ED nurse called down with two verbal orders that were needed stat: a cefazolin 2 gm IV piggyback for a patient who was being sent to surgery for a hip open reduction and internal fixation (ORIF) and a pantoprazole 80 mg IV infusion for a bleeding ulcer. John, a fellow pharmacist, had answered the phone and written the orders down on a piece of paper, along with patient name and allergy information. Thomas offered to get those orders started as John headed back to check IV preparations in the hood.

As Thomas was entering the two orders, he noted one of the two patients was allergic to penicillin. The words "pcn allergy" were scrawled on the paper, at the bottom of the page. Although it wasn't clear to Thomas, the penicillin allergy information appeared to be associated with the pantoprazole order. He made a quick call to the ED for clarification, but no one picked up at the nurses' station. To keep things moving, he decided to go ahead with the assumption that the penicillin allergy was related to the pantoprazole patient. In addition, he realized that the crossover sensitivity between penicillin-allergic and cephalosporin-allergic reactions was low.[11]

Approximately 30 minutes later, things were still hectic in the pharmacy when a Code Blue was called from the ED. John headed up to respond to the code. A few minutes later, a technician returned from restocking the Pyxis in the ED. When Thomas asked how things were going upstairs, the technician replied that things were a little chaotic, as the patient with a hip fracture had "anaphylaxed" after receiving his cefazolin, just before heading to the orthopedic surgical suite.

RESPOND TO THE SENSE OR FEELING THAT SOMETHING IS WRONG

The first step in the ethical decision-making process encourages those involved to respond to their moral intuition, i.e., those "gut instincts" about what is potentially harmful, fair, loyal, subversive, or degrading that precede any type of moral reasoning.[12] Unlike clinical, factual data such as a laboratory value or heart rate, there are no set objective signs that an ethical problem has occurred or is likely to occur. However, there are other clues that indicate well before the end of the case that something is wrong and could lead to a significant problem. The first sign that something is amiss in the case is that the nursing staff didn't follow standard procedures for entering medication orders from the ED to the pharmacy. This departure from standard procedure was explained because the ED was "especially busy." The pharmacy had limited staff which made things "hectic." The pharmacy staff struggled to keep up. When the environment is emotionally charged and there is stress and interpersonal tension, these are often indicators that a potential ethical issue is brewing. The second sign in the case is when Thomas noted that one of the two patients was allergic to penicillin. He is concerned enough about getting clarity about the allergy that he calls to confirm the information with someone in the ED, but he cannot reach anyone. So, he decides to proceed on the assumption that the penicillin allergy belongs to the patient who is to receive the pantoprazole. If that isn't the case, Thomas is willing to risk the small chance of crossover sensitivity between penicillin and cephalosporin-allergic reactions. Of course the news that the patient with the hip fracture "anaphylaxed" would seem to indicate that there was crossover sensitivity and a serious allergic reaction when he received the cefazolin. Thomas's initial intuition that something could go wrong was correct.

What prevented Thomas from following his moral intuition? He correctly determined that it was important to know which patient had the penicillin allergy. Why did he stop trying to find out this information when he did? Perhaps the urgent nature of the clinical setting, the drive to keep things moving, trumped his sense that something could go wrong.

GATHER CLINICAL AND CONTEXTUAL INFORMATION

Case Two is an excellent example of an organizational level ethical problem for several reasons. First, there are several people and departments involved in the case. Second, the organization has obligations to the people within the hospital including personnel and patients as well as obligations to the broader community to follow best practices and standards to deliver safe, appropriate care. The case isn't the usual "pro-active" case in clinical ethics in which the health professional stands at the point of making a decision. Rather it is a retrospective case in which decisions were made and actions were taken that lead to a bad outcome for the patient with the hip fracture. In a case like this, when the harm has already happened, it is helpful to analyze such "sentinel events" which includes the various actions of the players involved. A sentinel event is defined by the Joint Commission as a patient safety event that reaches a patient and results in any of the following: death, permanent harm, or severe temporary harm and intervention to sustain life.[13] Such events signal the need for investigation and response. One such tool for investigating sentinel events is Root Cause Analysis (RCA) that helps identify what, how and why something happened, thus preventing its recurrence.[14] The information gathered through the RCA process fits well with the information gathering step in the model for ethical decision making because it is important to have accurate information about what and how an event occurred but also why it happened. Regarding the information we have in Case Two, it is too simple to say that Thomas is the one responsible for the severe harm to the patient because he didn't confirm which patient had the penicillin allergy. Thus, the RCA process would contribute to the ethical analysis but is not a substitute for it as the RCA process has different aims.

Prospectively, in order to make an informed decision, one needs facts. In health care, one needs clinical facts that include pertinent data related to patient care. In the case of pharmacy practice, clinical data would include diagnosis, drug therapy, allergies, present clinical status, relevant laboratory values, etc. Situational or contextual information includes background data on the individuals involved and the environment in which they interact including communication tools such as electronic medical records or other means of transferring data between departments and individuals. The relationships between those involved also can have an impact on an ethical problem.

Since the case is being reviewed retrospectively, the clinical information that was used to make the decision to dispense the medications is relatively clear. In other words, we know the information that Thomas had when he made the decision to prepare and dispense the medications that were ordered over the phone from the nurse in the ED. One patient had a hip fracture and was to receive a pre-operative dose of cefazolin IV piggyback. There is no more information about this specific patient. The other verbal order was for pantoprazole IV infusion for a patient with a bleeding ulcer. Again, there is no additional information about this specific patient. Both patients urgently need their medications so they share that clinical fact in common. There is no information about age, other medications the patients might be on, clinical status beyond what brought them to the ED, etc. Finally, the most important clinical fact that is absent in the case is which patient has the penicillin allergy.

The situational information includes data regarding the values, perspectives, and relationships of the principals involved. There are several individuals in the case who had a clear role in the actions and decisions that took place, but not all of them are identified by name. There is Thomas one of the pharmacists who worked in this short-staffed, busy, inpatient pharmacy. Next, there is John, a fellow pharmacist, who took the phone order, wrote down the drugs, dosage, and patients' names, but didn't specifically identify which patient had the penicillin allergy. John seems to disappear after this critical action until he leaves the pharmacy to assist with the code team in the ED. We are given to understand that John is unavailable to clarify what he wrote. There is also the nameless nurse from the ED who called the pharmacy with the medication orders rather than following procedure that required the orders to be entered in the clinical record. There is no information about the prescriber or prescribers in the ED so it is hard to tell what type of working relationship the pharmacy has with the

ED personnel. Thomas learned that the patient with the hip fracture "anaphylaxed" because a technician relayed the news on his return from the ED. In fact, we do not know if this is because of the penicillin allergy or some other problem. This is an important point and supports the root cause analysis process mentioned earlier. Based on the low risk of cross-reactivity, one shouldn't automatically assume that there are no other possible contributing factors to the outcome. There are likely others who have a stake in the outcome of the decisions and actions taken in this case such as the patient's family, surgical team members, and other staff in the ED who might have been taking care of the patient who had the anaphylactic reaction.

The other situational information that is important in retrospective reviews is the conflict of values of those involved. It is at this point that it makes sense to view values at an institutional level rather than the individual level because many people are involved in the actions that led to a bad outcome for the patient. The institutional values that are in conflict are the demands of urgency, in this case the need to move a patient with a broken hip into the operating room as soon as possible, versus the need for safe, accurate care, in this case medication therapy that takes into account potentially life-threatening consequences from a penicillin allergy. In the heat of the moment, when personnel are working beyond their capacity, the institution may unconsciously value speed over accuracy. Beyond the exploration of values such as these, there are other values at stake such as the trust and respect members of the health care team have for each other. Trust and respect among all members of the health care team is important so that when someone stops the action, as it were, to ask a question or verify important information this is seen as appropriate and necessary step to protect patients from harm and not as a sign of disrespect or perhaps insubordination.

IDENTIFY THE ETHICAL PROBLEM

- Gathering information can be an end in itself and in proactive cases, there is usually very little time for doing so given all of the other responsibilities of busy clinicians. Even in retrospective case review, there is a point when the most important facts have been outlined and key people have had a chance to share their views and concerns. At that time, the information can be examined to see whether there is an ethical issue involved and what type of ethical issue it is. As was noted previously, the case involves ethics because there is a direct reference to the welfare of someone, in this case a patient in the ED who is in serious condition. Ethics deals with a wide-range of obligations and duties. Ethical principles can serve as action guides as to right-making characteristics of actions, which duties should take priority in a given situation, or help determine what ethical values are at stake. The ethical principles most often encountered in clinical practice are those described by Beauchamp and Childress in the four principles approach to ethics.[15] The principles include respect for autonomy, nonmaleficence, beneficence, and justice.

Respect for autonomy requires that we respect the right of competent adults to make decisions about their life and well-being without undue interference from others. Pharmacists need to be aware of the autonomy of their patients. For example, patients have the right to weigh the benefits risks that commonly occur with a drug to determine if they are willing to take it. Some patients may judge a side effect as too bothersome to continue on a medication. In Case Two, there is little evidence that the principle of respect for autonomy is at work in any significant way. Some of the individuals involved in the situation appear to have acted autonomously in that the nurse decided to call the order to the pharmacy rather than enter the order in the medical record. Thomas decided to fill the prescriptions and assumed which patient had the penicillin allergy and what risk he was willing to bear.

The principle of nonmaleficence is often referred to as the most basic of ethical principles in our interactions with others in that we are always bound to avoid harming others. In health care settings, this prohibition against harm is often balanced against the good that might be achieved with certain types of therapies and treatment. In Case Two, Thomas didn't put the principle of nonmaleficence as his first priority unless he hypothesized that greater harm would come to both patients if he took the time to confirm the penicillin allergy with the prescriber. It is unlikely that a prescriber would knowingly write a prescription that would harm a patient. If there are there no alternatives to a drug with known risks, prescribers should work with pharmacists to choose an option that has the least amount of risk. It should always be the aim of pharmacotherapy to prescribe a drug with the greatest benefit and the least amount of side effects. If informed about the potential drug reaction in this case, it is likely that a different drug could have been prescribed.

Beneficence is the duty to do good or prevent harms from occurring to others. All of the pharmacist's efforts should be to advance the good of the patient in the sense that drug therapy should improve overall well-being. The very act of providing drug therapy is a beneficent act because it is for the patient's welfare whether in the long or short term. Even if we put the welfare of the patient as being of the highest priority, there could be disagreement about what is the appropriate action to achieve such a goal. For example, some might argue that it is worth the risk of a possible crossover sensitivity to get the cefazolin started and the patient on his way into surgery to repair the hip as quickly as possible. Others might argue that the extra time that it takes to confirm just who has the penicillin allergy is worth it in the long run to prevent anaphylaxis that could have fatal consequences, as is the situation in Case Two, or they weaken the patient and further delay the surgery. What is important here is insight into how those involved calculate the benefit to the patient.

The fourth principle is justice which mediates claims between individuals and other groups or even the community as a whole. Justice encompasses the idea of fairness in our interactions with others. Nonmaleficence and beneficence are focused, respectively, on minimizing harms and maximizing good as much as possible. Justice is concerned about the way these goods and harms are distributed. Case Two does not seem to include a direct conflict between the interests of different patients. It appears that Thomas treated both patients the same way in that he filled the prescriptions as quickly as possible and accurately in that it was the right dose for the right patient. The principle of justice will be discussed in greater detail in regard to Case Three.

An additional ethical principle that may not be as obvious as those already mentioned in the case is the principle of fidelity or promise keeping. Other things being equal, it is important to keep promises to others. One of the implicit promises in the workplace is to be loyal to co-workers so that they can work to the best of their abilities. In a work setting, particularly in health care since the stakes are so high, "Loyalty is important from an ethical point of view because it creates a framework of trust. In an ambience of trust, individuals presume each other's good will, make allowances for personal and professional short-comings, and generally support each other's highest level of achievement."[16] An atmosphere of trust is necessary for members of a health care team to work through an error of this type because it requires probing into the actions of others. Misplaced loyalty in these sorts of organizational level cases may work against honesty. In order to arrive at recommendations that are ethically justifiable to prevent a recurrence, conflicts in loyalties need to be critically examined. At this point, it is appropriate to analyze different courses of actions that could have prevented the problem and that would be ethically justifiable for future such incidences.

SEEK A RESOLUTION

The next step is to seek a justifiable resolution. Proposing more than one course of action and examining the ethical justification of various actions is the working phase of ethical decision making. Since this is a retrospective case review, the recommendations for changes to process or systems will not have an impact on Case Two and its outcomes but could have an impact on future cases. We know, for example, that the pharmacy is routinely short-staffed on weekend nights. What are the patterns for admissions to the ED at that time? Is there a mismatch between the staffing in the pharmacy and the needs of the ED at those times? We know that the order was given verbally over the phone by the nurse in the ED and not written into the medical record. Was this purely to save time? Are there other variables at play? If so, why does it take longer to enter orders in the medical record? Answers to these questions and others will inform the formulation of corrective actions to help prevent recurrence.

WORK WITH OTHERS TO DETERMINE A COURSE OF ACTION

No one works alone in health care and Case Two is a perfect example of how the actions of many people have to align for an error to occur. Thus, it takes the input and actions of many people to craft a workable and justifiable course of action. Ethical decision making is often richer when it encompasses a range of views of the people who have a legitimate stake in the outcome. Although many of the ethical problems encountered in an institution such as a hospital involve the principles of respecting autonomy, balancing harms and goods, telling the truth, and keeping promises, there are cases that require pharmacists to consider broader goods that affect the health and well-being of society versus individual welfare. In the next section, we will examine how moral principles are factored into decisions confronting pharmacists at the societal level of ethics.

DOING GOOD FOR INDIVIDUALS VERSUS THE COMMON GOOD

Pharmacists are often involved in situations where there are conflicts between patients and others. In fact, the Code of Ethics for Pharmacists anticipates this sort of situation in Principle VII that states,

> **A pharmacist** serves individual, community, and societal needs. The primary obligation of a pharmacist is to individual patients. However, the obligations of a pharmacist may at times extend beyond the individual to the community and society. In these situations, a pharmacist recognizes the responsibilities that accompany these obligations and acts accordingly.[2]

Although the Code of Ethics for Pharmacists anticipates these conflicts, the means to resolve such conflicts is absent in the Code except for the general advice to recognize responsibilities and act accordingly. What are the responsibilities of a pharmacist when the perceived good of an individual conflicts with those of society? The following case poses such a dilemma for a pharmacist.

CASE THREE—THE PROBLEM OF CONFLICTING ETHICAL OBLIGATIONS

Lori is a pharmacist who works in a pharmacy located within a family medicine clinic. The pharmacy has gotten more involved with vaccinations over the past year, and all pharmacists at the clinic are certified to administer immunizations. In an effort to make the clinic more efficient, pharmacists are often called upon to help with the vaccination process. This can involve actually administering the vaccination, but often the pharmacists are also used as an information resource for patients and caregivers to answer questions. Today Lori is being asked to speak with a mother who is uncomfortable with the routine vaccinations associated with a two-month old infant's checkup.

Mrs. Eicher, the mother in question, is visiting the clinic with her 9-week old daughter, Lillian, for a routine infant follow-up appointment. This is the visit where the first series of vaccinations are generally initiated. As Lori speaks with Mrs. Eicher about her concerns, she indicates that although she has vaccinated her 7-year old son, she no longer believes in the safety of immunizations. Upon questioning, Mrs. Eicher tells Lori that her 2-year old nephew was recently diagnosed with autism and she has been doing a great deal of Internet research on the safety of immunization. "I am not uninformed—there is a lot of information out there, and most of it is pretty scary. I know researchers are saying that vaccinations are not linked to autism, but how do we really know? Plus, what about all the other potential hazards associated with putting these chemicals into our children?" Mrs. Eicher also relays that when Tommy, her son, received his kindergarten vaccinations, he had a high fever afterward and his leg swelled up for a week. "How can you say they are safe? Does that sound normal? I don't want to risk anything happening to Lillian!"

As a parent, Lori empathizes with Mrs. Eicher. She realizes that she is trying to protect her child. At the same time, as a pharmacist Lori recognizes that the true protection comes from the vaccinations themselves. She is also aware that there is always a risk of an adverse reaction. However, most reactions, such as the one experienced by Tommy, are generally not associated with any lasting harm. As a healthcare professional, Lori feels the responsibility to not only her patients, but also the public at large. There have been many recent examples of disease outbreaks being tracked to a lack of immunization and the effect on herd immunity. In addition, Lori is particularly concerned for the infant as one of the recommended vaccinations at the two-month visit is pertussis.[17]

Lori must wrestle with an ethical problem that is a head-on conflict between the principles of respect for individual autonomy, or in this case the autonomy of a parent to make decisions about her infant, and the good of the public at large which in this case is the prevention of potentially life-threatening communicable diseases by vaccinations. The underlying question is: where does the pharmacist's duty lie? Is Lori's primary duty to serve the welfare of the patient exclusively or do other parties have a claim on the pharmacist's attention? Even a cursory review of Case Three would uncover the following conflicting responsibilities that Lori faces: 1) provide the best possible care to the child, 2) maintain the relationship that has been established with the parent/family, 3) respect parent's/parents' preferences and beliefs, and 4) protect the public's health. There is obvious tension in the case of vaccine hesitancy or refusal because it pits individual goods or perceived goods against the common good. In other words, Lori cannot meet all of these responsibilities because they are conflicting.

She could, for example, provide clear and understandable information about the safety and benefit of compliance with full vaccination and still not convince Mrs. Eicher. If Mrs. Eicher wants to continue to bring Lillian to the clinic, Lori and the medical staff have a decision to make of their own. Should they dismiss unvaccinated children from their practice? They might decide to do this as a matter of course because they believe that the risk to other children they interact with in the clinic setting. They might decide to not let unvaccinated children stay in the practice because it sends a message that immunizations are optional.[19] Some clinicians have gone so far as to consider the involvement of legal authorities to intervene on the child's behalf if parents continue to refuse immunization to protect the child. Conversely, they might decide to let unvaccinated children stay in the clinic but provide a different waiting area, appointment times, etc. This final option is the course that the American Academy of Pediatrics has affirmed in a policy statement on vaccine refusal arguing that keeping children under the care of pediatricians allows for continuing dialogue and opportunities to change the parents' minds on vaccination.

All of these options must take into account not only the well-being of the child and the parents' satisfaction but the harms and risks to unknown others. Vaccination is a community intervention. It is especially hard for people in the United States to comply with public health mandates because of the emphasis on individualism and self-determination. On the societal level, it is a given that individuals have to accept serious and often burdensome limits on individual freedoms. However, health is not only limited to individuals. From a public health perspective, health is best understood in a collective sense because the majority of people are embedded in communities.

A remedy to the focus on individualism in our society is to engage and involve the community, as much as is practical and possible, in discussion over these difficult health questions that pit individual choice against public good. Societal level ethical questions deserve this kind of energy and effort because of their serious consequences for future generations, the complexity of the interdependence of the various systems involved in their resolution and the complicated coordination and integration of different systems to effect a resolution to name a few.[5] Regarding vaccine hesitancy or refusal, pharmacists like Lori should work with others to achieve high acceptance of vaccines by proposing and testing interventions that lead to full compliance and parent satisfaction built on trust.[20] Pharmacists are strategically placed in a variety of accessible community settings to assist in empowering people with accurate information and guidance about vaccinations and other types of health information.

RESOURCES TO ASSIST IN ETHICAL DECISION MAKING

Ethical decision making is never easy, but it is especially challenging as one moves from the kind of issues encountered at an individual level to organizational problems and those that occur at the societal level. This chapter is an overview of some of the ethical issues that pharmacists encounter in their daily practice in a variety of settings and provides sources of support for working through questions of ethics. The Code of Ethics for Pharmacists and other professional codes and position statements or "white papers," can provide practice standards and professional values to serve as a guide for clinicians and administrators. Other resources that could be helpful for individuals or groups faced with ethical choices could look to the standards promoted by the Joint Commission or for Catholic institutions the Ethical and Religious Directives for Catholic Health Care Services.[21] Tools such as decision making models and literature on basic ethical principles or theories of ethics such as virtue that focuses on the character of moral agents or care-based reasoning that takes into account relationships and the context of the moral life can assist in ethical reflection and the soundness of decisions. Pharmacists who work within hospitals could also turn to the institutional ethics committee, if one exists, for assistance and consultation on ethical issues or questions. The arrangement and range of approaches to ethical analysis presented in this chapter can improve the quality of ethical decisions by pharmacists as they strive to fulfill professional standards in pharmacy practice.

REFERENCES

1. Veatch, R., Haddad, A., & English, D. (2010). Case studies in biomedical ethics: *Decision-making, principles and cases.* New York, NY: Oxford University Press, 10.

2. American Pharmaceutical Association. (1995). *Code of ethics for pharmacists.* Washington, DC: American Pharmaceutical Association.

3. Mazzu, A.L., Lasseter, K.C., Shamblen, E.C., Agarwal, V., Lettieri, J., & Sundaresen, P. (2000). Itraconazole alters the pharmacokinetics of atorvastatin to a greater extent than either cerivastatin or pravastatin. *Clin Pharmacol Ther.* 68(4);391–400.

4. Chater, R., Dockter, D., Haddad, A., et al. (1991). Ethical decision making in pharmacy. *American Pharmacy* NS33(9):48–50.

5. Glaser, J. (1998). *Three realms of ethics.* Kansas City, MO: Sheed and Ward, 12, 23.

6. Ogletree, T.W. (1995). Value and valuation. In: Reich, W.T. (Ed.), *Encyclopedia of bioethics.* New York, NY: Macmillan Library Reference, 2151–2520.

7. Fletcher, J.C. (Ed.). (2005). *Fletcher's introduction to clinical ethics.* 2nd ed. Frederick, MD: University Publishing Group.

8. Jonsen, A., Siegler, M., & Winslade, W. (2015). *Clinical ethics: A practical approach to ethical decisions in clinical medicine* 8th ed. New York, NY: McGraw Hill Medical.

9. Lo, B. (2005). *Resolving ethical dilemmas: A guide for clinicians* 3rd ed. Philadephia, PA: Lippincott, Williams, and Wilkins.

10. Haddad, A. & Kapp, M. (1991). *Ethical and legal problems in home health care.* Norwalk, CT: Appleton and Lange.

11. Terico, A.T. & Gallagher, J.C. (2014). Beta-lactam hypersensitivity and cross-reactivity. *J Pharm Pract* 27(6):530–544.

12. Haidt, J. (2007). The new synthesis in moral psychology. *Science* 316;998–1002.

13. The Joint Commission. (2014). *Sentinel event policy and procedures.* www.jointcommission.org/Sentinel_Event_Policy_and_Procedures. Updated November 19, 2014. Accessed July 10, 2015.

14. Rooney, J.J. & Vanden Heuvel, L.N. (July 2004). Root cause analysis for beginners. *Quality Progress* 45–53.

15. Beauchamp, T. & Childress, J. (2012). *Principles of biomedical ethics* 7th ed. New York, NY: Oxford University Press.

16. Haddad, A. & Dougherty, C. (1991). Whistleblowing in the OR: the ethical implications. *Todays OR Nurse* 13(3)30–3.

17. Centers for Disease Control and Prevention. *Recommended immunization schedule for persons aged 0 through 18 years.* http://www.cdc.gov/vaccines/schedules/downloads/child/0-18yrs-child-combined-schedule.pdf. Effective January 1, 2015. Accessed July 17, 2015.

18. Jakinovich, A. & Sood, S.K. (2014). Pertussis: Still a cause of death, seven decades into vaccination. *Curr Opin Pediatr* 26(5):597–604.

19. Opel, D.J., Feemster, K.A., Omer, S.B., Orenstein, W.A., Richter, M., & Lantos, J.D. (2014). Ethics rounds: A 6-month-old with vaccine-hesitant parents. *Pediatrics* 133: 526–530.

20. Leask, J. & Kinnersley, P. (2015). Physician communication with vaccine-hesitant parents: The start, not the end, of the story. *Pediatrics* 136:180–182.

21. United States Conference of Catholic Bishops. (2009). *Ethical and religious directives for Catholic health care services.* Washington, DC: United States Catholic Conference.

CHAPTER 22

NETWORKS OF CARE: SOCIAL NETWORKS IN HEALTH AND CARE DELIVERY

Andrea L. Kjos and Daniel G. Ricci

LEARNING OBJECTIVES:

1. Describe what is meant by the use of a network perspective.
2. Define key terms in understanding empirical assessment of social networks.
3. Synthesize how social networks impact health by way of the structure and function to provide information and resources.
4. Summarize how socio-behavioral concepts such as social support and social capital are related to a network perspective.
5. Describe how health care can use social network applications and interventions to promote health.

KEY TERMS

Social capital

Social integration

Social network

Social network analysis

Social network function

Social network structure

Social support

INTRODUCTION

Patient-centered practice occurs when those involved in providing care consider a patient's medical needs within the context of the patient's overall life and wellbeing. In order to achieve this model of practice, those involved in providing care must consider the complex social environment, within which each patient is uniquely situated. Failure to acknowledge a patient's social environment when considering individual risk factors, specific symptoms, and treatment options reduces the quality of care provided. These often-overlooked social and environmental factors reside in what is known as a social network. In the broadest sense, a social network is a set of connections or relationships among people. Our day-to-day understanding and experience of the world is filtered through our connections with others, our social networks. This is also true for the experience of health and illness. For example, when a patient receives a diagnosis of diabetes, their outlook and understanding of the disease will be heavily influenced by societal beliefs, the beliefs of their immediate social contacts, and family. The link between the "social environment" and mental and physical health is supported with a large and continuously growing body of evidence. Further, it is the existence of human relationships that impacts an individual's health and the well-being of entire communities. Considering these relationships and the networks that surround patients are essential for designing optimal patient-centered care. These networks may include relationships with family, friends, co-workers, acquaintances, or healthcare providers. Thinking more broadly, these may also include organizational networks that connect patients to providers, providers to each other, or even inter-organizational connections (such as insurance coverage networks); or even community or neighborhood networks that link patients to others within a common geographic context. It is within these social structures that communication and information processes operate to impact patient outcomes.

The purpose of this chapter is to provide an introduction to the sociological concept of social networks and how this concept can be applied in the context of pharmacy practice. The chapter will define key terms in understanding empirical assessment of social networks using a network perspective. Additionally, this chapter will review how the social networks impact health by way of the structure and function of the social networks that operate to provide information and resources. Finally, this chapter will describe how health care interventions may be able to use social network applications and interventions to promote health.

BACKGROUND

Health science researchers in disciplines such as medical sociology, epidemiology, public health, medicine, and policy have been intrigued by the ways that relationships and social support impact patient behavior. This intrigue has led to a proliferation of growth in the last decade, lending to a wealth of theoretical and empirical work. This growing body of literature is helpful in advancing our understanding of the factors that impact health. However, in part due to the abundance of interest, in combination with the distinct disciplines involved in its use, there has been little dissemination across the various fields of study resulting in limited integration of findings. This has led to a diverse theoretical landscape of terminology and paradigms that make the practical application of empirical findings difficult to implement from a provider standpoint.

To assist in one's understanding of the social environmental impact on health, an orientation to the major terminology encountered in this area of inquiry is warranted.

Social integration is a broad concept that is used to indicate something about a person's number of social ties. Level of social integration could be related to any social situation that creates relationships with others. Social integration can also be measured as number of ties in one's family structure as well as religious, occupational volunteering, recreational activities, or within other relational basis for interacting with others.

Social capital is conceptualized as either an individual or group-level attribute to conceptualize the collective benefits that come from being part of a larger community of other people.[1] The term is often related to the nature of the norms within the relationships and interactions of the group as well as a level of cohesiveness. A common presumption is that having more social capital is a good thing; these interactions are positive in nature and include characteristics of being cooperative, trusting and helpful. In contrast, social capital can also be related to the accessibility to resources available to a person or a group by way of simply being part of that community or group. Resources derived from social capital can be information, skills, financial, or assistance with various functions.

A *social network* is a defined group of individuals who are connected to each other in some way.[2] The theories of social networks operate under the assumption that the social network *structure*, or presence or absence of connections between the people within the network, as well as the *function* (i.e. results, or product) of the connections can be taken together to explain and possibility even predict behavior.

A much more individually measured attribute is that of *social support*. Social support is a way to conceptualize the outcomes of assistance that originates from interpersonal relationships. The kinds of aid that come from having relationships with others has been categorized in different ways such as provision of information or resources, as well as emotional or decision-making support.[3] Table 22-1 summarizes these related social environmental terms, yet distinct constructs. There are dozens of ways these constructs have been measured in empirical research across these disciplines previously mentioned. Providing the extensive listing of operational measurement scales for each of these constructs is beyond the scope of this chapter. However, excellent summaries of measurements for social ties can be located in the monographs, "Social Epidemiology" by editors Berkman and Kawachi in addition to "Social Capital and Health" by editors Kawachi, Subramaniea and Kim.[1,4]

TABLE 22-1: SUMMARY OF FOUNDATIONAL SOCIAL ENVIRONMENT CONSTRUCTS

CONSTRUCT	DESCRIPTION
Social Network	A defined group of people who are connected.
Social Capital	Quality of social trust and accessibility of resources as a result of being part of a group.
Social Support	Specific types of assistance as a result of social interactions.
Social Integration	Presence or absence of social ties in any setting (family, religious, occupation)

A social network framework uses the focus on relationships that are defined by families, communities, or organizations to build directly on the key concept of social network structure. It is believed that these social structures can be measured and assessed to determine the structural features that help explain behavioral patterns, especially when these behavioral patterns have been unexplained or only partly explained using traditional individual psychological approaches.

In recent decades, scientists in the area of social epidemiology have developed conceptual models for describing how social networks link to health. One such model can first be described in terms of the **structure** of the social environment that shape the existence and nature of specific social networks within communities and organizations. These structural features have been called "upstream" factors that can be contributory features impacting health. For example, the level of social integration and the qualities of the *social network* itself would be considered structural factors. What results from these social structures are resultant aspects, or "downstream" factors. These downstream factors describe the **function** of the relationships and characterize the individual-level impact of the social structure in terms of *social support* or the *social capital* related outcomes. (Berkman & Glass, 2000, Ch 7)[4] Some of the downstream factors can be further expanded into psychological pathways that are commonly reviewed in the literature as health promoting and adherence behaviors, as well as self-esteem and self-efficacy. This conceptual model is depicted in Figure 22-1.

THEORY

There is no single theory of social networks. Rather, the consideration of social networks is a paradigm or perspective that uses consistent ideas and concepts from various frameworks and models. To organize theoretical perspectives some have used a separation between what may *cause* certain types of networks to exist in contrast to what network properties may explain the *effects* of specific networks.[5,6] For example, the cause-focused "theories of networks" was described by Borgotti and Halgin as it related to understanding why networks obtain certain structures. For example, theories of networks can be used when network properties may explain other network properties (i.e. network variables are both the independent and dependent variables). In contrast, the frameworks that have been called "network theories" are concerned with the outcomes of either the individuals or groups.[5] Network theories can use network variables as either the independent or dependent variable in comparison to some other non-network property, such as individual demographics.

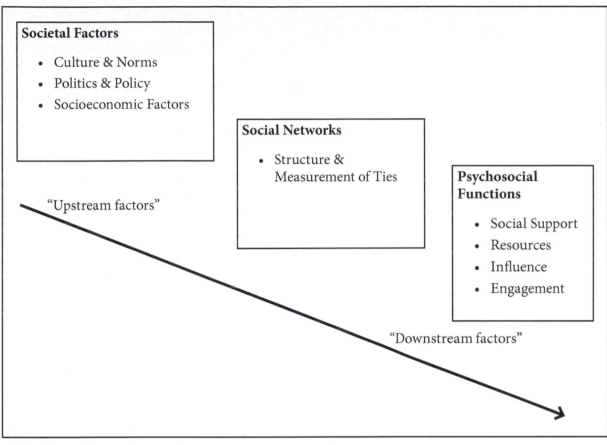

Societal Factors

- Culture & Norms
- Politics & Policy
- Socioeconomic Factors

Social Networks

- Structure & Measurement of Ties

Psychosocial Functions

- Social Support
- Resources
- Influence
- Engagement

"Upstream factors"

"Downstream factors"

(Adapted from Berkman Fig 7-1, pp. 143)[4]

FIGURE 22-1: CONCEPTUAL MODEL FOR LEVELS OF SOCIAL ENVIRONMENT IMPACTING HEALTH*

In an attempt to address the need for further theoretical development, Kildruff and Brass published a review and outlined the dominant ideas that supply a framework for further theory development in the field.[7]

There are numerous social network models that are progressing the theoretical foundations of the paradigm (i.e., the reviews by Borgatti et al. 2011 and Brass et al. 2011). The most commonly cited and used application of social networks models in the context of health care include the Structural Holes (SH) framework[8] and the Strength of Weak Ties (SWT).[9] Both the Structural Holes theory and the Strength of Weak Ties theory focus on how the structure of the network will be positioned in a such a way as to allow novel, non-redundant information to pass within the network. The SH theory focuses on the number of non-redundant ties in the network, where as the SWT theory focuses on how bridging ties between more dense networks may also yield opportunities for new information.[10] As application, the theories imply that by having less new information available as a resource, individual actors' behaviors may be more constrained that they otherwise would be if they had the full and complete information. However, the Network Episode Model (NEM) was created as a way to bring together both structural and functional ideas and how both types of network features may interact to effect health.[11] For a more comprehensive review of specific social network models in application to existing social behavior theory and pharmacy administration research, see the article by Kjos, Worley, and Schommer, 2013.[12]

STRUCTURAL ASSESSMENT OF SOCIAL NETWORKS

A social network can be defined as a structure comprised of a set of people (actors) who are connected to each other by one or more relationships (i.e. a "tie").[2] A basic concept in models of social networks is that individual attributes matter in the context of how they predict interaction with others. Social networks can be visualized as a web of social ties.

Social networks can be thought to take one of two perspectives; an **egocentric** or **a whole network** perspective. An egocentric network considers the perspective of a social network with one person at the center. Networks can also be considered from a whole network perspective. In a whole network perspective, all ties within specified boundaries can be assessed to characterize a broader network of a community or an organization.

Although social researchers can agree with near certainty to the contribution of social networks to predict health outcomes, there is considerable debate about measurement of social networks. For those researchers focused on the structural aspect of social ties; it has been the "upstream" features that help us to understand larger networks, communities, and organizations. The specific set of measurement techniques is known as **social network analysis**. Social network analysis is characterized by measurement of the relationships that exist within a specified group of people. The analysis will be different depending on variables of interest. For example, measure can be at the individual level, the dyadic level or the whole network level.[13]

Social network analysis and its quantitative methods have disseminated into health care research. Application in areas such as public health (e.g. health awareness/media campaigns), social support and patient outcomes, and HIV/AIDS programs have been topics using the approaches of social network analysis to understand how relationships with others impact health.[14]

Social network structural analysis can be measured based on characteristics about **complexity and dynamics of relationships** that are within the network. Characteristics are described by variables and measures that are unique to network analysis. A summary of definitions for important measures are summarized in Table 22-2.

TABLE 22-2: SOCIAL NETWORK ANALYSIS MEASURES

CONCEPT	DEFINITIONS
Whole Network Characteristics	All of these concepts are considered to be network structural properties of a network as defined by specified boundaries. These are useful to compare a network with other networks.
Network size	The number of people, or "actors" in a social network.
Density	The extent to which people in the network are connected to each other.
Closeness	The proximity of persons within a network.
Homogeneity	The extent to which people in the work are similar to each other.
Dyadic/Relationship Characteristics	Additional assessments of social network structure relate to the characteristics of the relationships or ties within the specified network.
Frequency	The extent of contact made between people.
Reciprocity	The extent to which interactions between people are reciprocal, i.e. the degree to which information or exchange is bi-directional.

FUNCTIONAL ASSESSMENTS OF SOCIAL NETWORKS

Measuring social networks provide a structural or architectural representation of our social environment. The complexity of this approach quickly amplifies in acknowledgement that these structural elements only reveal part of our complex social stories. Measuring the frequency of contact as well as the duration of relationships give us useful information related to a patient's social environment. However, it is also important to measure **content** or what flows between people. Another way to think about this would be measurement of the **function** to individuals as a direct result of personal relationships. Most often, content as derived from relationships is conceptualized as something positive, or protective to health.

Social interactions may tell something about a person's behavior in collective settings (drinking, smoking, exercise). But also knowing with whom patients discuss important matters reveals something about their sources of social support and information. What happens as a result of ties in the social environment may have clear implications for health behavior interventions as well as help-seeking and provision of health services.

Individuals' experiences of illness are not static, and often patient's illness trajectories change over time. Likewise, relationships of patients are just as complex in the context of illness. For example, chronic illness can introduce tension and lead to a destabilization of norms within relationships. Understanding the effects of social networks on health means studying social relationships that contain elements of both conflict and support. Most often, scientists have been interested in the positive functions provided by social relationships. However, more recently there has been interest on the negative impact of relationships to health. As one major example, consider the highly cited Christakis et al. study on the spread of obesity.[15] Other applications on the network effects of networks have been in illicit drug use, and HIV/AIDS. Networks can have the potential for positive as well as negative functions on patient's behavior.

SOCIAL SUPPORT

It has been explained that **social support** is something that enhances health and reduces mortality by way of its ability to buffer stress.[1] Similarly, **social isolation** has been shown to be linked to worse health outcomes.[16] It is not yet well understood what aspects of social relationships are most protective in terms of health outcomes (e.g. advice, information, financial). While researchers readily acknowledge that social relationships are impacting the health of people, it is difficult to isolate the specific effects emanating from those relationships. Some believe that social support is the most important construct in explaining the link between social relationships and health. However, similar to other work in ideas about the social environment the development of the construct of social support has occurred across multiple disciplines spanning several decades of theory development.

The first development of the concept of social support was in the 1970s, resulting today in a body of work that has been proliferated with attempts to conceptualize and describe the aspects that might be causing health effects. Are beneficial effects derived from the use of *information* provided by others? Is social support *help* that family members provide to a patient when they fall ill? Is social support a perception of *emotional affirmation* or validation that comes from just being part of broader community?

The question of primary focus remains as what *is it about social support that causes* health to improve. Clues to this answer can be found in the ways that social support has been defined. Although definitions vary, most come together to describe the concept as a *relationship-based resource* that is *beneficial*.[10] Further, operational definitions remain diverse within the literature, but commonly social support conceptualizations can be described by subtypes.[17] The **subtypes of social support** explain the nature of *resources* that flow within social relationships. Distinguishing these resources can help determine the causal mechanism underlying the beneficial effects of social support. Common subtypes of social support are **emotional support** or **instrumental support**. Emotional support has been defined as "love and caring, sympathy and understanding and/or esteem or value available from others."[18] Instrumental support implies assistance with day to day needs and may be given as time, money, or labor. Another type of support has been described as **appraisal support**, that is, assisting with decision-making. Finally, **informational support** is that by which someone give information or advice. These types have been conceptualized in order to more precisely measure social support.[3] Conflicting evidence exists on which particular component of social support is more strongly linked to health related outcomes. Because of this, researchers continue to look for both direct and indirect effects that may explain the link between social support and health.[10]

Closely related to social support are additional concepts that describe the function of social networks on health. As mentioned earlier as foundational concepts, **social cohesion, social integration**, and **social capital** are all discrete but interrelated concepts.[10] **Social cohesion** has been described as the degree of connection and equality within a network. **Social integration** has been described as active participation in a network. Social integration has also been called social engagement, which describes someone's ability to have an obligation of participation within a community.[4] Finally, **social capital** is a collection of resources within the network. **Social capital** is a more commonly understood idea, especially in public health. This is a construct to imply the level of social cohesion that exists in a group or community. Ideas about social capital have been derived from a social networks perspective to measure properties of groups to allow for exchange of resources and information[10] (Song, Son and Lin, pg 119 Ch 9).

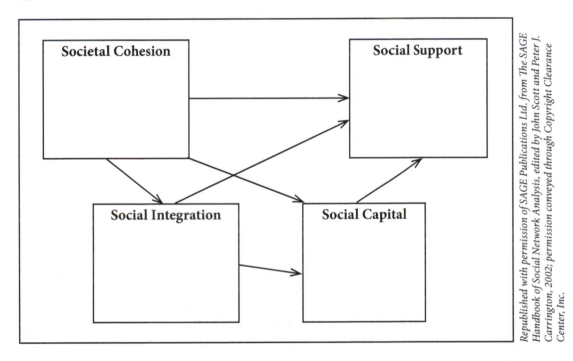

Republished with permission of SAGE Publications Ltd. from The SAGE Handbook of Social Network Analysis, edited by John Scott and Peter J. Carrington, 2002; permission conveyed through Copyright Clearance Center, Inc.

FIGURE 22-2: CONCEPTUAL MODEL OF SOCIAL CONNECTEDNESS

Song, Son and Lin have conceptualized these constructs to come together in a way that social support is a "downstream" result of the preceding constructs (Figure 22-2), and that they are generally related in a positive direction. For example, as social cohesion or social integration increases, so does social capital and social support. Song et al. discussed how social support is reciprocal, such that feedback mechanisms exist so that social support (or lack thereof) can reinforce or change group properties that are "upstream" related to social cohesion, social integration and social capital. The work by Song and Lin in 2009 was foundational to theorizing the differences between social capital and social support, and have advocated for differentiation in measurement.[19] However, because of the interrelated nature of all of these constructs, social cohesion, social integration, and social capital have sometimes been used as approximating measures of social support. (For a comprehensive listing of social relationship measurement scales, see Kawachi I, Berkman LF. *Social epidemiology*.[4] This will be an important area of work as social scientist work to tease apart more valid and reliable measurement for each of these fundamental constructs in the field.

No matter the specific measurement of resources that flow as a byproduct of the relational environment, there is a high degree of empirical evidence that suggests receipt of social resources serve as a *buffer to stressors*. Reduction of stressors has been linked to more positive health outcomes. It is this connection that many theorists believe to be the explanation for why social support resources act in a way to promote health.[3] In additional, some postulate that the impact of the social environment can be more readily understood as the cumulative impact over the life course as opposed to a cross-sectional view of one point in time.[20] Therefore, in addition to more internally valid measurement, scientists will be challenged by a call for a more longitudinal understanding of social environments in health care.

SOCIAL NETWORK APPLICATIONS IN PROVISION OF PHARMACEUTICAL CARE

Previous work has clearly reiterated the beneficial effects of social networks on health,[11] and there have been published reviews on the use of social network applications in health.[21-26]

Findings have additional application and direct implications for pharmacy practitioners. Although these reviews are helpful to researchers, the current approach will be to review application from both outside and within the pharmacy literature and demonstrate how social environmental questions and issues can be also be shaped using a social network approach. Most of these studies have been descriptive and observational; however, it is still known that both structural and functional features can be related to health status. For example, research that provides **structural** descriptions reporting network size, density, and frequency of interaction between people can advance our understanding of how these structural features are related to health delivery and health behavior.

Further, **functional** assessments of types of support such as emotional and instrumental support can provide opportunities to strengthen patients' unmet resource-related or psychosocial needs. Applications exist in both **clinical assessments of individual patients** as well as **community level** characteristics.

Social network principles in practice start with an assessment of a particular network, and who within given network is involved. Once network information has been obtained and described, subsequent intervention could occur.

WHO: Beneficial functions derived from social networks can come from informal networks including, family, friends, and co-workers. In contrast, inside formal medical care settings providers may act as important sources of appraisal and informational support. As such, pharmacy providers may often find themselves as a key bridge in a patient's social network bringing together aspects of both informal and formal networks.

WHAT: Social ties in these applications can influence patient behaviors at the psychosocial level through things such as 1) patient perceptions of illness severity, or perceived risk; 2) adherence to medical advice in a context of symptom severity; 3) help-seeking behaviors, especially for stigmatized conditions; and 4) financial resource barriers to care or treatment.[27]

HOW: One area that has been discussed is that providers already act as people who can influence network ties at the individual patient level. For instance, in a study by Lau in 2010, it was found that providers could act as important resource for caregivers in medication management.[28] When a provider identifies that a chronically ill patient does not have informal supports, an intervention could be created to connect the patient to more formal support and available professional services.[29]

Communication with other providers may be thought by pharmaists to be somewhat of a hassle, as pharmacists can be organizationally and geographically isolated from many other providers in the health care team. However, one way that pharmacists can influence a patient's formal care network is to foster collaboration and trust with patients' other providers. It is important that pharmacists develop expectations that enhancing the formal medical care network for a patient will improve the quality of patient care.[30]

Pharmacists can also be involved in helping patients develop new linkages in their social networks. For example, some research has suggested that health professionals do not typically provide information to patients about support groups, and that this can be an important emotional and informational support.[31] In the future, community pharmacists could play a more central role in being an active referral center for patients, especially those who may have complex illnesses and require added guidance in navigating the health care system. Being proactive to intervene on patient's formal network for things such as consumer health organizations and support groups may raise the level of trust and rapport that the pharmacist maintains within the community of patients they serve.[32]

In addition, health system pharmacists may serve a similar role as *transitions-of-care* experts as hospitalized patients make their way back into the community and ambulatory care settings. A *transitions-of-care* pharmacist can serve to connect the patient with their primary care provider, reinforce information, as well as communicate with caregivers or other informal network members in order to help the patient successfully integrate their care into their normal environment.[33]

WHEN: As a natural consequence of communicating with patients on a regular basis, pharmacists learn about the challenges patients may face in the health care system and especially as it related to medication use. As a part of their regular accessibility to patients in the community, pharmacists have an opportunity to intervene in the context of the patient's social environment. There is no formal insurance billing, there are no protocols to follow, but individually focused social network interventions in practice become possible when providers operate using their assessments to overcome barriers to care and with being a reliable and trusted source of support and information.

SYSTEM-LEVEL APPLICATIONS

WHO: A number of social network studies in health care have focused on provider interactions. These studies have evaluated how relationships between and among various types of professionals which can characterize the type and level of collaboration and support. Studies have investigated intent to implement "evidence-based" medicine as well as prescribing behavior. In alignment with other studies, most of these investigations have been cross-sectional and focused on description. For example, physician studies in this area have shown that similarities in geographic proximity, health care specialty, demographics, and attitudes are all common in provider networks.[25,34]

Further, studies have investigated specific professionals. For example, nursing staff studies have found prevalence in social support and trust relationships to be more important than hierarchical ones. Similar to physicians, nursing-focused network studies have found that nursing relationships occur more frequently with other nurses of similar backgrounds. Of note, some of these studies have also shown how professionally-supportive intra-professional nurse networks promoted increased patient satisfaction and reduction of adverse drug events.[25]

The recent drive in interest for integration and collaboration within health care multidisciplinary teams has created much attention to the problem of a fragmented US health care system. This is an area with a large potential for application with the social network paradigm. For example, one study of teams found network differences existed in teams who had more external influence compare to those with more internal communication and coordination of information.[35]

At the broader level, public health systems have been evaluated using social network methods. This application is useful to demonstrate that networks can represent various levels of relationships at the individual level as well as at the organizational level. In these cases, researchers have found that characteristics for how connections surround key public agencies subsequently impact collaboration in data collection in assessment initiatives and building advocacy, similar to social capital.[21] Outside of public organizations, private health organization such as managed care companies, have evaluated coordinated service networks to specifically determine what influential characteristics may be most important for addressing change in the area of reducing racial and ethnic disparities in large populations of covered patients. Important application of this work allows for leaders and administrators to assess group processes in a formal way, to help document change and provide feedback.

One interesting finding in this area has been that a fully-integrated and collaborative model may be counterproductive to organizations that may find themselves in competition with other organizations in the private health care market. Therefore, network studies can bring to light important decision-making thresholds for organizational collaborations that are more likely to exist in these competitive markets, and when organizations will shy away from sharing information or resources when this sharing presents a threat to proprietary information.[36] Applications such as these will be important to examine new models in the area of health care reform such as structure and functions of specific accountable care organizations, when government incentives are linking financial incentives to coordination, collaboration, and improving patient outcomes.

Social networks can also be considered in the bringing together of informal and formal groups in the delivery of health care. In additional to health care provider networks and health care organizations working together amongst themselves, health care providers and organizations can also be purposefully linked to informal patient's community networks. Examples of for this type of collaboration has been described as purposeful community-based participatory inventions using "community helpers" that create infusion of health promotion knowledge, support, and behaviors that come to a community from key community members within the informal network itself. More importantly, health care organizations that use informants directly from the communities they serve, can have a more enriched understanding of issues and barriers faced within communities allowing for more specific health promotion program design and intervention.[17,24,37]

WHAT: Interprofessional studies that have utilized social network analysis have focused on a mixture of **structural** and **functional** aspects. The structural features of focus have related to knowledge sharing, professional connections within and between different professional designations, reciprocity of communication, and clinical exchanges. Functionally, these applications have aimed to point to specific strategies to illuminate what social environment creates a supportive, collaborative professional environment to maximize patient care coordination.[38]

Some of these applications have been used to explore more than just than just a cross-sectional snapshot of provider-provider care networks. For example, a longitudinal study found that networks can change over time from initial creation with a collaboration and relationship building phase, into a longer term communicative and cooperative phase. This change in health care teams over time will be useful as interprofessional practice becomes a normative occurrence in health care, and be a useful benchmark to guide professional development in this area.[39]

Network strategies can be applied to community health education initiatives. As mentioned earlier, "community helpers" can be mobilized.[24,37] The function of directly acting in coordination with community-based helpers could be to increase access to locally held skills and resources, as well as a way to provide training to key individuals who could bring new knowledge to infuse within the community. Usually the goals of this type of intervention are to strengthen the community networks by building social support, cohesion, engagement, and overall level of social capital.

Not as much literature is related to how the **structure** and **function** of patient's social networks impact their **utilization** of health care services. Some research has suggested that increased family availability and support or other informal sources of connection may lead to a **decrease** in the use of health promotion and preventative services, especially as these services related to a patient's need for information.[40] It is unknown as to whether this decreased use means that services are being used more prudently or whether needed care is being substituted for self-care.

Networks involve a variety of actors within the entire health care system. Networks considered will be dependent on the issue or problem of interest, as well as the structural and functional characteristics of the networks that are hypothesized to matter the most. Most attention to system-level networks will be from administrators, managers, policy makers, and others who have an interest in optimizing outcomes in provision and receipt of health care for entire populations of patients.

WHEN: It has been discussed that to improve care delivery, coordination, and efficiency among providers, that network research could be applied.[41] Time spent in describing the whole network factors, such as structural relationships and functions such as knowledge sharing may be a good investment by administrators who would like to prioritize higher-level team functioning and improving the quality and outcomes that result from these interactions. However, more research is still needed to understanding the precise causal mechanisms from which structural and functional network changes can improve specific care delivery outcomes. At present, although intervening on certain aspects of an interprofessional network may improve collaboration and professional relationships, there is not a strong amount of evidence that these positive outcomes would systematically occur in all cases.[42] Additionally, some have discussed that because of the nature of the assumptions of the social network paradigm that are context dependent, there is not a way to easily allow for generalizability of research findings from network studies.

Nonetheless, there is still much that can be acquired from reading of reports, assessments, and interventions that have used a social network framework in their approach to improve health and the delivery of health care. The social network paradigm has been applied when objectives were to 1) improve safety, efficiency and quality of care;[41,43] 2) increase social support, social capital and partnerships within specific communities;[44] 3) optimize collaboration and research sharing 6; and 4) intensify cost-effectiveness.[45,46]

Beyond just the organizational level, social network analysis can be applied to international health care system benchmarking as a way to help policy makers understand how the relational **structure** of the entire health care system may change over time. Likewise, **functional** assessment of any inefficiencies in current operations, duplication or underperformance can allow for a finer level of policy planning regarding capacity to innovate service provision to the people served. This usefulness may be especially prevalent for low- and middle- income countries where resource allocation is a high priority.[47]

The ways in which the social connectedness impact a population's utilization of services is of particular interest to those who wish to maximize the most efficient use of resources; matching patient need with optimization of services. There has been a growing body of evidence in this area especially with respect to mental health and aging service **utilization**. In these domains, there have been an increasing number of investigations on the integration of formal and informal support and how these differences impact utilization of services.[48] More specifically, support networks may change over time during stressful illness disruption such as inpatient treatment and initial diagnosis compared to illness maintenance phases.[49] Stability of a patient's social network can impact their experience of their illness over time as well as how this stability or lack therefore may in turn, impact outcomes and quality of life. Among older adults, a lack of social connectedness, measured as chronic loneliness, was associated with greater use of provider services.[50] Utilization assessment across countries and global regions have concluded that social connections and social resources have a large amount of contextual and cultural variation. Therefore, on a global health scale, it is unlikely that a common model can exist for how social network structure and function impacts health care service utilization at the population level across different counties.[51]

PERSONAL COMMUNITIES/ PEER-PEER LEVEL APPLICATION

WHO: Informal networks that comprise people friends and acquaintances have experienced a perceptional shift, such that relationships within these networks may not only be comprised of face-to-face contact and communication, but electronic as well. How people are defining their "communities" are changing, and venues such as the Internet and subsequent use of social media make geographic proximity less important to those who may be considered part of your personal community. For a review on the growing application of new communication technologies including the uses of the Internet and mobile phones communication on our understanding for the change in reach and influence of social networks, see the chapter by Chau et al. in Scott & Carrington (2011)[10]

With regard to particular application to health care, some have begun to discuss the impact of online communication and information sharing among patients surrounding certain diseases and illnesses. Online communities and virtual networks have developed to provide additional avenues of patient participation and empowerment in the face of diagnoses that may be accompanied with uncertainty and stigma. One such online community is known as "patientslikeme.com."

WHAT: The research that has been generated from this type of community has been focused primarily on collation of individually-based reported outcomes such as quality of life issues, and adverse events. The utility of information from these communities from a clinical perspective is that providers may have a more generalizable understanding of patients' experiences of illnesses in a practical way. Data provided from these sites may complement post-marketing trial information about specific treatments. Further, data reported by patients within these online environments may be an additional way to validate patient-reported outcomes.[52]

WHEN: The degree of **social support** that may be a byproduct of these social networking sites continue to be of interest to the clinical community. There has been some evidence that patients' participation in online support systems may lead to behavior change; however more research is needed.[53] A review of online, peer-to-peer support communities found that most commonly assessed patient outcomes measured were depressive symptoms and levels of social support. This review found that the communities had little to no effect on these outcomes; however, the research also found little support for any negative or harmful effects on patients.[54] The real implications appear to be surrounding creating a platform for advocacy within segments of patients or to influence health policies indirectly by raising awareness, education, and sharing experiences.[55]

Social theory developing out of this area may be applicable to examining how social influence and social support may differ in a virtual compared to a face-to-face environment. Confounding these variables may also be to determine which circumstances and in which clinical conditions would patients benefit the most. These applications would be of interest to health practitioners who may be involved with virtual care delivery, telehealth initiatives, or with other populations that encounter issues in health care access.[56]

SUMMARY

The social environment and the imperceptible powers of the people within it work continuously to impact health at the patient level, as well as the delivery of health care at a population level. In the current area of reform, the specific social environment of patients' receipt of care and provision of services are changing. The fragmentation and silo approaches of the past are being replaced with more integration, collaboration, and coordination. Concurrently, social scientists that study health have found the social network paradigm to be a useful framework to study the way people behave in the context of the broader communities where we live and work. Social network analysis is not a specific theory or method, rather it is a way of collecting data about the **structure** and **functions** of groups to understand and predict behavior. Using a social network paradigm allows scientists to draw on decades of work across numerous disciplines to synthesis theories and methodology and contribute to an ever-growing body of empirical research. In an environment where patient-centered care is prioritized, our understanding of how the social environment impacts patient outcomes and utilization of care service are becoming important areas of growth and development.

Health care systems have focused more on integration across medical specialties in the effort to reduce the problems associated with fragmented and disorganized service delivery. As such, a social network perspective would be a way to use a common language to describe, assess, and intervene when planning quality improvement initiations in the delivery of health care.

Additionally, either at the patient level or system level, experimental and intervention research will be important to determine exactly what social network variables can be influenced to optimize structural aspects of the network. Additionally, intervention research will also help identify what network modifications are best matched to impact functions of the network. In either case, work in the context of health should conscientiously consider the growing number of peer-reviewed published reviews in scientific journals as well books and monographs in the area of social network research. New application and research should draw upon growing consensus to progress the application of theory and methods, and be cognizant against further dividing the field. Work is needed to validate the conceptual linkages between the **structural** and **functional** characteristics of social networks and how these match to specific outcomes of interest. Findings about how these characters impact outcomes have important implications for health providers at any level, who want to make a difference in their communities.

REFERENCES

1. Kawachi, I, Subramanian, S.V., & Kim D (2008). p. 16 Social capital and health. New York: Springer.

2. Knoke, D. & Young, S. (2008). *Social network analysis.* 2nd ed. SAGE Publications, Inc.

3. Berkman, L.F., Glass, T., Brissette, I., & Seeman, T.E. (2000). From social integration to health: Durkheim in the new millennium. *Soc Sci Med.* 51(6):843–857.

4. Kawachi, I. & Berkman L.F. (2000). *Social epidemiology.* New York: Oxford University Press, USA.

5. Borgatti, S.P. & Halgin, D.S. (2011). On network theory. *Organization Science* 22(5):1168–1181.

6. Brass, D.J. (2011). A social network perspective on organizational psychology. In: Kozlowski, S.W.J. (Eds.), *The oxford handbook of organizational psychology.* New York: Oxford University Press.

7. Kilduff, M. & Brass, D.J. (2010). Organizational social network research: Core ideas and key debates. *Academy of Management Annals* 4:317–357.

8. Burt, R.S. (1992). *Structural holes: The social structure of competition.* Cambridge, MA: Harvard University Press.

9. Granovetter, M.S. (1973). The strength of weak ties. *American Journal of Sociology* 78(6):1360–1380.

10. Scott, J., Carrington, P J. (2011). The SAGE handbook of social network analysis. Los Angeles: SAGE Publications.

11. Pescosolido, B.A. (2006). Of pride and prejudice: The role of sociology and social networks in integrating the health sciences. *J Health Soc Behav* 47(3):189–208.

12. Kjos, A.L., Worley, M., & Schommer, J.C. (2013). The social network paradigm and applications in pharmacy. *Research in Social & Administrative Pharmacy* 9(4):353–369.

13. Borgatti, S.P., Everett, M.G., & Johnson, J.C. (2013). *Analyzing social networks.* Los Angeles i.e. Thousand Oaks, Calif. London: SAGE Publications.

14. Valente, T. (2010). *Social networks and health*. Oxford: Oxford University Press, Inc.

15. Christakis, N.A. & Fowler, J.H. (2007). The spread of obesity in a large social network over 32 years. *N Engl J Med.* 357(4):370–379.

16. Link, B.G. & Phelan, J. (1995). Social conditions as fundamental causes of disease. *J Health Soc Behav* 35 (Extra issue: Forty years of medical sociology: The state of the art and directions for the future):80–94.

17. Glanz, K., Rimer, B.K., & Viswanath, K. (2011). Health behavior and health education: *Theory, research, and practice*. 4th ed. Hoboken: Jossey-Bass.

18. Thoits, P.A. (1995). Stress, coping, and social support processes: Where are we? What next? *J Health Soc Behav* 53.

19. Song, L. & Lin, N. (2009). Social capital and health inequality: Evidence from Taiwan. *J Health Soc Behav* (2):149.

20. Bird, C.E. (2010). *Handbook of medical sociology*. Nashville: Vanderbilt University Press; 2010.

21. Wholey, D.R., Gregg, W., & Moscovice, I. (2009). Public health systems: A social networks perspective. *Health Serv Res* 44(5):1842–1862.

22. Chambers, D., Wilson, P., Thompson, C., & Harden, M. (2012). Social network analysis in healthcare settings: A systematic scoping review. *PLoS One.* 7(8) :e41911–e41911.

23. Levy, J.A. & Pescosolido, B.A. (Eds.). *Social networks and health*. Oxford, UK: Elsevier Science Ltd. No. 8.

24. Israel, B.A. (1982). Social networks and health status: Linking theory, research, and practice. *Patient Couns Health Educ.* 4:65–79.

25. Bae, S., Nikolaev, A., Seo, J.Y., & Castner, J. (2015). Article: Health care provider social network analysis: A systematic review. *Nurs Outlook* 63:566–584.

26. Benton, D.C., Pérez-Raya, F., Fernández-Fernández, M.P., & González-Jurado, M.A. (2015). A systematic review of nurse-related social network analysis studies. *Int Nurs Rev.* 62(3):321–339.

27. Pescosolido, B. A. (2006). Of pride and prejudice: The role of sociology and social networks in integrating the health sciences. *Journal of Health & Social Behavior* 47(3):189–208.

28. Lau, D.T., Berman, R., Halpern, L., Pickard, A.S., Schrauf, R., & Witt, W. (2010). Exploring factors that influence informal caregiving in medication management for home hospice patients. *J Palliat Med* 13(9):1085–1090.

29. Crotty, M.M., Henderson, J., Ward, P.R., et al. (2015). Analysis of social networks supporting the self-management of type 2 diabetes for people with mental illness. *BMC Health Services Research* 15(1):1–12.

30. Bardet, J., Vo, T., Bedouch, P., & Allenet. B. (2015). Review article: Physicians and community pharmacists collaboration in primary care: A review of specific models. *Research in Social and Administrative Pharmacy* 11:602–622.

31. Guidry, J. J., Aday, L.A., Zhang, D., Winn, R.J. (1997). The role of informal and formal social support networks for patients with cancer. *Cancer Pract.* 5(4):241–246.

32. McMillan, S.S., Wheeler, A.J., Sav, A., et al. (2013). Original research: Community pharmacy in australia: A health hub destination of the future. *Research in Social and Administrative Pharmacy* 9:863–875.

33. Fera, T., Anderson, C., Kanel, K. T., Ramusivich, D.l. (2014). Role of a care transition pharmacist in a primary care resource center. *American Journal of Health-System Pharmacy* 71(18):1585–1590.

34. Landon, B.E., Keating, N.L., Barnett, M.L., et al. (2012). Variation in patient-sharing networks of physicians across the United States. *JAMA* 308(3):265–273.

35. Meltzer, D., Chung, J., Khalili, P., et al. (2010). Exploring the use of social network methods in designing healthcare quality improvement teams. *Soc Sci Med* 71(6):1119–1130.

36. Gold, M., Doreian, P., Taylor, E.F. (2008). Understanding a collaborative effort to reduce racial and ethnic disparities in health care: Contributions from social network analysis. *Soc Sci Med.* 67(6):1018–1027.

37. Israel, B.A. (1985). Social networks and social support: Implications for natural helper and community level interventions. *Health Education & Behavior* 12(1):65.

38. Uddin, S., Hossain, L., Hamra, J., & Alam, A. (2013). A study of physician collaborations through social network and exponential random graph. *BMC Health Serv Res* 13:234–234.

39. Ryan, D., Emond, M., & Lamontagne, M. (2014). Social network analysis as a metric for the development of an interdisciplinary, inter-organizational research team. *J Interprof Care* 28(1):28–33.

40. Birkel, R.C. & Reppucci, N.D. (1983). Social networks, information-seeking, and the utilization of services. *Am J Community Psychol* 11(2):185–205.

41. Lewis, V.A. & Fisher, E.S. (2012). Social networks in health care: So much to learn. *JAMA* 308(3):294–296.

42. Cunningham, F.C., Ranmuthugala, G., Plumb, J., et al. (2013). Health professional networks as a vector for improving healthcare quality and safety: A systematic review. *BMC Health Services Research* 21; 13(3):239–249.

43. Siriwardena, A.N. (2014). Understanding quality improvement through social network analysis. *Qual Prim Care* 22(3):121–123.

44. Provan, K.G., Veazie, M.A., Staten, L.K., & Teufel-Shone, N. (2005). The use of network analysis to strengthen community partnerships. *Public Adm Rev* 65(5):603–613.

45. Goehl, L., Nunes, E., Quitkin, F., & Hilton, I. (1993). Social networks and methadone treatment outcome: The costs and benefits of social ties. *Am J Drug Alcohol Abuse* 19(3):251–262.

46. Blanchet, K. & James, P. (2012). How to do (or not to do)...a social network analysis in health systems research. *Health Policy Plan* 27(5):438–446.

47. Cummings, S.M. & Kropf, N.P. (2009). Formal and informal support for older adults with severe mental illness. *Aging Ment Health* 13(4):619–627.

48. Perry, B.L. & Pescosolido, B.A. (2012). Social network dynamics and biographical disruption: The case of 'first-timers' with mental illness. *American Journal of Sociology* (1):134.

49. Gerst-Emerson, K. & Jayawardhana, J. (2015.) Loneliness as a public health issue: The impact of loneliness on health care utilization among older adults. *Am J Public Health* 105(5):1013–1019.

50. Burholt, V., Windle, G., Ferring, D., et al. (2007). Reliability and validity of the older americans resources and services (OARS) social resources scale in six european countries. *J Gerontol B Psychol Sci Soc Sci* 62(6):S371–S379.

51. Frost, J., Okun, S., Vaughan, T., Heywood, J., & Wicks, P. (2011). Patient-reported outcomes as a source of evidence in off-label prescribing: Analysis of data from PatientsLikeMe. *J Med Internet Res* 13(1):e6–e6.

52. Staccini, P. & Fernandez-Luque L.(2015). Health social media and patient-centered care: Buzz or evidence? findings from the section "education and consumer health informatics" of the 2015 edition of the IMIA yearbook. *Yearb Med Inform* 10(1):160–163.

53. Eysenbach, G., Powell, J., Englesakis, M., Rizo, C., & Stern, A. (2004). Health related virtual communities and electronic support groups: Systematic review of the effects of online peer to peer interactions. *BMJ: British Medical Journal* (7449):1166.

54. Griffiths, F., Dobermann, T., Cave, J.A.K., et al. (2015). The impact of online social networks on health and health systems: A scoping review and case studies. *Policy & Internet* n/a-n/a. doi: 10.1002/poi3.97

55. Rock, M.J. (2010). Harnessing social networks along with consumer-driven electronic communication technologies to identify and engage members of 'hard-to-reach' populations: A methodological case report. *BMC Med Res Methodol* 10:8–8.

INDEX

CPSIA information can be obtained
at www.ICGtesting.com
Printed in the USA
BVHW061920100922
646698BV00004B/20

9 781465 252579